HISTOLOGY
A TEXT AND ATLAS

SECOND EDITION

HISTOLOGY
A TEXT AND ATLAS

SECOND EDITION

MICHAEL H. ROSS, Ph.D.

Professor and Chairman
Department of Anatomy and Cell Biology
University of Florida School of Medicine
Gainesville, Florida

EDWARD J. REITH, Ph.D. †

Professor and Chairman
Department of Anatomical Sciences
Temple University School of Dentistry
Philadelphia, Pennsylvania
† *Deceased*

LYNN J. ROMRELL, Ph.D.

Professor
Department of Anatomy and Cell Biology
University of Florida School of Medicine
Gainesville, Florida

With Illustrations by Lydia V. Kibiuk

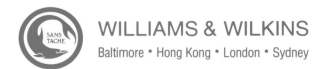

WILLIAMS & WILKINS
Baltimore • Hong Kong • London • Sydney

Editor: Kimberly Kist
Associate Editor: Victoria M. Vaughn
Copy Editor: Shelley Potler
Design: JoAnne Janowiak
Illustration Planning: Wayne Hubbel
Production: Barbara Felton

Copyright © 1989
Williams & Wilkins
428 East Preston Street
Baltimore, Maryland 21202, USA

Printed in the United States of America

First Edition 1985

Library of Congress Cataloging in Publication Data

Ross, Michael H.
    Histology : a text and atlas / Michael H. Ross, Edward J. Reith, and Lynn J. Romrell;
        with illustrations by Lydia V. Kibiuk. — 2nd ed.
        p. cm.
    Includes index.
    ISBN 0-683-07368-0
        1. Histology. 2. Histology—Atlases.   I. Reith, Edward J. II. Romrell, Lynn J.
        III. Title.
        [DNLM: 1. Histology—Atlases. QS 516 R825h]
    QM551.R67 1989
    611'.018—dc19
    DNLM/DLC   88-20811
    for Library of Congress   CIP

89 90 91 92 93
1 2 3 4 5 6 7 8 9 10

Dedicated to Edward J. Reith (1925–1985)—and his wife, Addie, and his children, John, Christopher, Mary Ann, and Paul—all of whom contributed to Ed's qualities as a gifted teacher, scientist, and concerned individual.

Preface to the Second Edition

The first edition of *Histology: A Text and Atlas* was conceived at a time when advances in cell and tissue biology were being made in a rapidly moving stream, as continues to be the case today. The question faced was how does one incorporate this burgeoning new knowledge into a text in a manner that enables the student of histology to absorb the "pertinent" new information along with basic information on the microstructure of cells, tissues, and organs. Clearly numerous compromises needed to be made to attain a text of manageable scope for professionals as well as undergraduate students. Moreover, the concept of incorporating a free-standing atlas as an addendum to the text also presented some uncertainty. While an atlas has its place largely in the lab (as well as for review), it was felt that the appending of the atlas to the text, or vice versa, depending on how one wishes to view it, would have considerable value. This enables students to have the text at hand when in the laboratory and, thus, to resolve many questions relating to didactic information.

With respect to the use of color in the Atlas section of the book, other uncertainties emerged, particularly related to the possibility that we were doing a disservice to our students by suggesting to them that color itself is important. We clearly do not feel that students should rely on color as they study and interpret the structure of the cells and tissues of the body. However, we judge the book a success in meeting students' needs on the basis of selling out three substantial printings in less than 3 years. The success of the book and its increasing popularity resulted in its being unavailable for a short period before this new edition published by Williams & Wilkins.

This brings us to two important questions: How does this second edition differ from the first edition, and why a new publisher? The major change that is evident as one peruses this second edition of the book is the addition of text in two chapters where previously only the Atlas section was included. These are the chapters on the Eye and the Ear. Other chapters have been revised to varying degrees; many of the changes were the outcome of suggestions of our colleagues. New figures have been added, other figures were deleted or modified, and, of course, identified errors have been corrected. Pertinent new information has been included. To help make the text manageable, items that can be regarded as significant, but to some extent outside of the direct scope of histology, have been boxed to identify their ancillary significance to the basic information. The least changed area in this new edition is the Atlas section. Here major emphasis has been directed toward simplifying the text while maintaining a concise descriptive account of cell and tissue structure and organization. Because histological structure is not a changing entity, the basic pictorial material in the Atlas section did not require dramatic revision at this time.

With considerable regret we made the decision to leave Harper & Row Publishers. We have had an extremely long and enjoyable association with them. Our departure was based on uncertainties where buy-outs and takeovers in the corporate world can create changes that are not always in the best interest of each of the internal parts. Facing the possibility that the College and Medical Divisions could be divested we felt that problems might arise in the preparation of the second edition of the book. Therefore, we made the decision to go with our new publisher, Williams & Wilkins. The strong interest on the part of Williams & Wilkins led us to believe that an equally good relationship would exist for the production of the second and future editions of *Histology: A Text and Atlas*.

Michael H. Ross
Lynn J. Romrell

January 1989

Preface to the First Edition

In recent years a variety of new histology textbooks have been published. In many ways these books are in contrast with the more traditional texts that had been the mainstay for teaching the subject matter of histology over the decades. The impetus for this new generation of books—though they are varied in approach, content, and design—appears to have one common denominator, which is to provide for the student the kind of basic information that can be assimilated in a reasonable but shortened time frame. In a sense we are faced with a paradox, for, on the one hand, there has been a major growth of information in all areas of histology and, at the same time, these newer books are reduced in length; and, unfortunately, explanations of important background material are often omitted.

In writing this book an attempt has been made to present the student with the pertinent subject matter of histology and, at the same time, to focus on many of the newer salient findings of cell biology as they relate to the understanding of cell, tissue, and organ structure and function. In effect, we too have presented a condensation of what is found in many of the larger textbooks, but every attempt has been made to create a condensation of information that will fulfill the student's needs in histology. In addition, we have made an attempt to present the information so that it will serve as an effective building block for understanding the cellular basis of pathology, physiology, endocrinology, and other basic sciences.

An attempt has also been made to maximize the number of photographs and other illustrations to complement the general text material. To this end, color has also been used lavishly. This has been done with the realization that color has become an increasingly stronger element in the way that we learn. Indeed, we are firmly entrenched in media color. In effect, the color that is used here is simply an extension of another mode of color in communication.

The present book departs from previous histology texts in that it has been combined with an atlas. To this end, we have attempted to incorporate the positive aspects of our previous book, *Atlas of Descriptive Histology*. The one major change relating to the atlas material that is included in this book is, as we have mentioned, the utilization of color. The authors preach just as vehemently as before that it is structure that is important in the understanding of histology, and consequently there is no need to excuse black and white as a basis for learning. However, it is clearly evident that color captures a reality, perceived or otherwise, that is more consistent with the mode of learning of most of today's students. With the patience of the instructor, the student can still be taught the value of basic structure in the learning of histology and at the same time benefit from the new dimension of color which is so much a part of learning in other fields.

The reader will also note that there is a certain repetition between the text and the atlas sections that follow most chapters of the book. It is hoped that this repetition will create a reinforcement in learning. However, it should also be recognized that the text portion of the book restricts itself in large part to theoretical aspects of cells, tissues, and organs, whereas the atlas section restricts itself to the identification of structure and the reasoning that should go into learning how to identify structures.

In summary, it is hoped that this book will satisfy the student's need in learning and, despite its brevity, create sufficient stimulation so that the learning process is enhanced, not diminished.

Acknowledgments

As we publish this second edition of *Histology: A Text and Atlas,* we again express our appreciation to those individuals who have made this work possible through their help, advice, and inspiration. We are particularly grateful for the opportunity to have known and worked with Dr. Edward J. Reith. His excellence in teaching, passion for discovering the essence of things around him, and enthusiasm for science and life, in general, continue to be an inspiration to us and to all those who had the opportunity to know him.

The impetus to write the first edition grew from our positive experiences with students and colleagues with whom we have worked in teaching and in a variety of other roles. We wish to acknowledge the many kind and supportive words of former students who used the *Atlas of Descriptive Histology* in their study of histology and also of colleagues who recommended the *Atlas of Descriptive Histology* to their students. We are also grateful to those who have responded positively to the first edition of *Histology: A Text and Atlas* and especially to those who have offered suggestions for improving the book. These suggestions have been extremely helpful in the preparation of this second edition.

We again thank Carl Zeiss Inc. for providing a grant, which defrayed much of the cost of producing the photomicrographs, Ernst Keller of Carl Zeiss Inc., U.S.A., and Heinz Gundlack of Carl Zeiss, Oberkochen, West Germany, provided technical assistance and invaluable information. The section on the proper use of the microscope written by Mr. Keller is also acknowledged. Finally, with respect to color photomicrographs, the quality of these reproductions is due to the efforts, patience, and technical skill of Denny Player. His contribution in preparing the enlarged positive transparencies from which the color separations were made is evident throughout the book.

A major contribution was made by Dr. Kyle Rarey of the Department of Anatomy and Cell Biology, University of Florida College of Medicine. He contributed the text and many of the illustrations and micrographs in Chapter 24. His expertise on the anatomy and physiology of the ear will be appreciated by all who read this chapter. We also appreciate the efforts of Dr. Christopher West whose critical reading and suggestions on the first seven chapters of the text have been extremely helpful in updating this section of the text which covers various aspects of cell and molecular biology.

Special thanks also go to a number of our colleagues. We appreciate the suggestions and other contributions of Drs. Johannes Rhodin, George Pappas, Gordon Kaye, Bernard Tandler, Tom Hollinger, Kelly Selman, John Terzakis, Ernest Kallenbach, Bryce Munger, Dorothy Zucker-Franklin, Carl Feldherr, Albert Farbman, Toichero Kuwabara, Craig Tischer, and Wilhelm Kriz. We thank them and other unnamed colleagues for their positive impact on this book.

We are also indebted to Lisa Booher and Christi Hughes who played an important role in the preparation and review of the manuscript. Their careful attention to detail has made possible the efficient preparation of the manuscript for this edition. Finally, we acknowledge the advice and assistance provided by the staff of Williams & Wilkins; special thanks are due to Vicki Vaughn, Bob Och, Wayne Hubbel, and Barbara Felton.

Michael H. Ross
Lynn J. Romrell

Contents

5 Connective Tissue 85

6 Adipose Tissue......................... 117

7 Cartilage 123

8 Bone 141

14 The Integumentary System **347**

15 Digestive System I: Oral Cavity and Pharynx **379**

16 Digestive System II: Esophagus and Gastrointestinal Tract **421**

20 Endocrine Organs 563

21 Male Reproductive System 603

22 Female Reproductive System 649

23 The Eye **711**

24 The Ear **739**

Methods

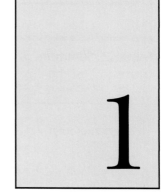

Most of the materials examined on a firsthand basis by students taking a histology course are routine paraffin sections stained with hematoxylin and eosin (H&E). These specimens are on the "slides" handed out during laboratory sessions; they are examined with the light microscope and they represent a major part of the histology course. The subject matter of histology, however, goes far beyond what can be learned by the examination of routine H&E paraffin sections. Indeed, it is the objective of histology to understand not only the microanatomy of cells, tissues, and organs, but also to learn as much as possible about their function in structural terms. The methods employed by histologists are extremely diversified and, while much of the histology course content can be framed in terms of light microscopy, the more detailed interpretation of microanatomy rests with the electron microscope, both transmission and scanning, because of its greater useful magnification, that is, its greater resolving power.

Histologists also utilize specialized procedures such as histochemistry and autoradiography, specialized methods for examining tissues such as cell, tissue, and organ culture, and specialized microscopic techniques to visualize the specimen. The student might feel removed from such procedures because direct experience with them may not be available in a busy curriculum. Nevertheless, it is important to know something about specialized procedures and the data that they yield. This chapter provides a survey of methods and offers an explanation of how the data provided by these methods can help the student acquire a sound appreciation of histology.

TISSUE PREPARATION FOR HEMATOXYLIN AND EOSIN STAINED PARAFFIN SECTIONS

The preparation of a stained tissue section on a slide is described in greater detail than other topics presented in this chapter, because this is the type of specimen examined most often by the student and because the methods involve certain basic principles that also apply to other methods.

The first step in preparing a tissue sample for examination with the light microscope is fixation. This step preserves the structure of the tissue and prepares it for future treatments. Numerous chemicals and mixtures of chemicals are used as fixatives; one of the most widely used is formaldehyde. This fixative, a solution of which is called *formalin,* may be used simply with buffers or it may be used in combination with other fixatives. Formaldehyde reacts with amino groups of proteins and, thus, is a good fixative for preserving the general structure of the cytoplasm and the nucleus because of their protein content.

After the tissue has been fixed, the fixative is washed out of the sample and the tissue is dehydrated so it can be embedded in a hard substance, such as paraffin, for slicing it into thin sections. Dehydration is typically accomplished by passing the tissue through a graded series of alcohol solutions up to 100 percent. This step removes the water from the tissue and permits it then to be placed in a nonaqueous liquid, such as xylene, which is miscible with melted paraffin. Next, the tissue is infiltrated with melted paraffin and allowed to cool and harden. The hardened paraffin, containing

TABLE 1.1. Summary of H&E Staining

CELL AND EXTRACELLULAR COMPONENT	STAIN REACTION
Nucleus	
Heterochromatin	Blue
Euchromatin	Negative
Nucleolus	Blue
Cytoplasm	
Ergastoplasm	Blue
General cytoplasm	Pink
Cytoplasmic filaments	Pink
Extracellular material	
Collagen fibers	Pink
Elastic fibers*	Pink, but not usually distinguishable from collagen fibers
Reticular fibers†	Pink, but not usually distinguishable from collagen fibers
Ground substance	Blue, but only if present in large amounts as in cartilage matrix
Bone matrix (decalcified)	Pink
Basement membrane†	Pink

* Special staining procedure used for their demonstration, such as one containing resorcin fuchsin or orcein.
† Special staining procedure used for their demonstration, such as silver impregnation or PAS.

the tissue, is trimmed, usually into some block form; it is mounted on a cutting machine called a **microtome;** and tissue sections (slices) are cut. The sections are placed on a slide with a small amount of albumin serving as an adhesive.

The sections are not yet suitable for examination with a microscope, since the tissue is infiltrated with paraffin and the section is colorless. The paraffin is removed by dissolving it with xylene and the tissue is then rehydrated by being passed through a graded series of alcohol solutions back to water. The tissue is then stained with H&E.

At this point, the slide is still unsuitable for microscopic examination and storage. In order to obtain a permanent preparation, the stained tissue section must be dehydrated again with alcohols and, using a nonaqueous mounting medium, covered with a coverslip. When the mounting medium dries, the specimen is ready for microscopic examination and storage. A summary of H&E staining reactions is presented in Table 1.1.

OTHER STAINING PROCEDURES

Generally speaking, H&E are used in histology because they display structural features and not because they provide information on the chemical characteristics of tissue sections. Despite the merits of H&E staining, the procedure does not adequately reveal certain structural components of histological sections, including elastic ma-

terial, reticular fibers, basement membranes, and lipids. When it is desirable to display these components, other staining procedures, most of them selective, can be used. These procedures include the use of orcein and resorcin fuchsin for elastic material and silver impregnation for reticular fibers and basement membrane material. The chemical basis for these methods is not well understood, but they work. For the student of histology, knowing what the procedure reveals is often more important than knowing why the procedure works.

Lipids can also be displayed by selective procedures, but the utility of these methods is limited. It needs to be emphasized that in preparing a histological display of lipids, it is necessary to avoid any step, such as the use of fat solvents, which will cause the loss of the lipid by dissolution. Therefore, frozen sections of formalin-fixed tissues are typically employed to display neutral lipids. Essentially the method calls for the use of dyes that are fat soluble, such as one of the Sudans. The dye is prepared in a solvent in which it is not very soluble, such as 70 percent alcohol, and it is applied to the frozen section. The dye then "stains" the lipid because it is more soluble in the lipid than in the carrying solvent. Glycerol can be used as a mounting medium. The procedure outlined is useful for the display of neutral lipids, such as triglycerides, a storage form of energy. Neutral lipids are found in the fat droplets of fat cells. Complex lipids such as the phospholipids of membranes require more elaborate procedures for their display.

CYTOCHEMISTRY AND HISTOCHEMISTRY

In addition to routine H&E and special staining of paraffin sections, histologists regularly apply specific chemical procedures to tissues. These procedures provide more detailed information about a tissue and often provide information on the function of the cells and extracellular components of the tissues. These chemical procedures, which include the use of enzymes, antibodies, and radioactive isotopes, are grouped under the heading of cytochemistry and histochemistry. Often special optical methods are used in conjunction with the cytohistochemical method as in immunocytochemistry. Some of the cytohistochemical procedures can be used not only with the light microscope, but also with the electron microscope. Before some of the cytohistochemical methods are outlined, it will be useful to examine briefly what is contained, in chemical terms, in a routine tissue section.

Chemical Composition of Histological Tissue Samples

The chemical composition of a tissue sample ready for routine staining differs greatly from the tissue in the living state. Many tissue components are lost during the preparation of the H&E-stained section. To a large extent the components that remain consist of large molecules that are not readily dissolved, especially after treatment with the fixative. The large molecules, particularly those that are complexed with other large molecules to form macromolecular complexes, are most consistently preserved in a tissue section. Examples of such large macromolecular complexes are nucleic acids complexed with protein to form nucleoproteins; intracellular cytoskeletal proteins complexed with other proteins; extracellular proteins in large, insoluble aggregates complexed with similar molecules due to crosslinking of neighboring molecules, as in collagen fiber formation; and phospholipids of membranes, some of which are also complexed with proteins or carbohydrates. For the most part, these molecules constitute the structure of cells and tissues in the sense that they make up the formed elements of the tissue. They are the basis for the organization that is seen in the tissue with the light microscope. It should be noted that in many cases a structural element is at the same time a functional unit. For example, in the case of proteins that make up the contractile filaments of muscle cells, the filaments are the visible structural components and they are the actual participants in the contractile process; the RNA of the cytoplasm is visualized as part of a structural component (ergastoplasm of gland cells, Nissl bodies of nerve cells) and at the same time it is the actual participant in the synthesis of protein.

Despite the fact that nucleic acids, proteins, and phospholipids are for the most part retained in tissue sections, many are also lost. Small proteins and small nucleic acids, such as transfer RNAs, are generally lost during the preparation of the tissue. In addition, large molecules may be lost. For example, they may be hydrolyzed by an unfavorable pH of the fixative solutions. Examples of large molecules lost during routine fixation in aqueous fixatives are glycogen (an intracellular storage carbohydrate) and proteoglycans and glycosaminoglycans (two components of the extracellular ground substance). They can, however, be preserved by the use of nonaqueous fixatives for glycogen or by the addition to the fixative solution of specific binding agents that preserve the extracellular carbohydrate-containing molecules of the ground substance. Also usually lost during routine tissue preparation are neutral lipids, such as those within the fat droplets of fat cells. They are lost when the tissue is treated with a fat solvent prior to paraffin imbedding. As with the carbohydrates, lipids can be retained in tissue if appropriate steps are taken to prevent their loss as outlined above.

Small soluble ions and molecules are also lost from the tissue samples during the preparation of paraffin sections. Thus, water, intermediary metabolites, glucose, sodium, chloride, and similar substances are no longer present in the tissue. Although these small substances are lost during the preparation of routine H&E paraffin sections, many of these substances can be studied in special preparations, usually with considerable loss of structural integrity. These small soluble ions and molecules do not make up the formed elements of a tissue; they constitute substances being processed or participating in cellular reactions. Water, a highly versatile molecule, participates in these reactions and contributes to the stabilization of structure.

Chemical Basis of Staining

As already mentioned, H&E are the most commonly used dyes in histology. Eosin is an acid dye and its staining properties can be explained on the basis of what is understood about the action of acid dyes. Hematoxylin, while not a basic dye, has staining properties that closely resemble those of a basic dye, and the term *basophilia*, a tissue property displayed with basic dyes, is used in conjunction with hematoxylin staining. Accordingly, it is advisable to define a basic and acid dye and examine their method of action. A basic dye is a dye molecule that carries a positive charge (or charges) on the colored part of the molecule; it is represented by the general formula Dye^+Cl^-. An acid dye molecule carries a negative charge on the colored portion; it is represented by the general formula Na^+Dye^-. The color of the dye is not related to whether it is basic or acid, as can be noted by the list of some basic and acid dyes in Table 1.2.

Basic Dyes. Basic dyes react with anionic groups of tissue components. These include phosphate groups of nucleic acids (DNA and RNA), sulfate groups of glycosaminoglycans, and carboxyl groups of proteins. The reaction of the anionic groups varies with pH. At a high pH (about 10), all three groups are ionized and available for reaction by electrostatic linkages with the basic dye; at a slightly acid to neutral pH (5 to 7), sulfate and phosphate groups are ionized and available for reaction with the basic dye by electrostatic linkages; and at the lowest pH (below 4), only sulfate groups remain ionized and react with basic dyes. Thus, staining with basic dyes at controlled pH can be used to focus on specific anionic groups, and because the specific anionic groups are found predominantly on certain macromolecules, the staining serves as an indicator of these macromolecules.

An additional procedure used in conjunction with staining at controlled pH is the use of enzymes to remove selectively substrates from the tissue section prior to staining (Fig. 1.1).

As already mentioned, hematoxylin is, strictly speaking, not a basic dye. It is used with a mordant, that is, an intermediate link between the tissue component and the dye, and it is due to the mordant that hematoxylin staining resembles the staining of a basic dye. The linkage in the tissue-mordant-hematoxylin complex is not a simple electrostatic linkage, and when placed in water, hematoxylin does not dissociate from the tissue, but remains firmly adherent. Because of this, hematoxylin lends itself to those staining sequences in which hematoxylin is followed by eosin or other acid dyes. True basic dyes are not generally used in sequences wherein a basic dye is followed by an acid dye because the basic dye tends to dissociate from the tissue during the subsequent washes in aqueous solutions.

Acidic Dyes. Acid dyes bind primarily to tissue components by electrostatic linkages in a manner similar to but opposite that of basic dyes. Acid dyes react with cationic groups, namely the ionized amino groups of proteins. While the electrostatic linkage is the major factor in the primary binding of the dye to the tissue, it is not the only one, and because of this, acid dyes are sometimes used in combinations to color different tissue constituents selectively. For example, three acid dyes are used in the Mallory staining technique: aniline blue, acid fuchsin, and orange G. These selectively stain collagen, ordinary cytoplasm, and red blood cells, respectively. The acid fuchsin also stains the nuclei. In other multiple acid dye techniques, hematoxylin is used to stain nuclei first, then the acid dyes are used to stain cytoplasm and extracellular fibers selectively. The selective staining of tissue components by acid dyes is not due to specific properties of the dye or tissue, but rather to relative factors. They include such factors as size and degree of aggregation on the part of the dye and permeability and degree of "compactness" on the part of the tissue. Basic dyes can also be employed in combinations, but these combinations are not as widely used as acid dye combinations.

Acidophilia and Basophilia. Any tissue component that reacts with a basic dye (or with hematoxylin) is said to be *basophilic* and to display *basophilia*. Tissue components that are stained with basic dyes are heterochromatin and nucleoli of the nucleus (both due chiefly to ionized phosphate groups), some cytoplasmic components such as the ergastoplasm (also due to ionized phosphate groups), and some extracellular materials such as the matrix of cartilage (due to ionized sulfate groups). Tissue components that stain with acid dyes are said to be *acidophilic* and to display *acidophilia*. Such tissue components include most cytoplasmic filaments, much of the otherwise unspecialized cytoplasm, and extracellular fibers (all due primarily to ionized amino groups).

Metachromasia. A phenomenon whereby a dye (such as toluidine blue) changes color after reacting with a tissue component is referred to as

TABLE 1.2. Some Basic and Acid Dyes

	COLOR
Basic Dyes	
Methyl green	Green
Methylene blue	Blue
Pyronine G	Red
Toluidine blue	Blue
Acid dyes	
Acid fuchsin	Red
Aniline blue	Blue
Eosin	Red
Orange G	Orange

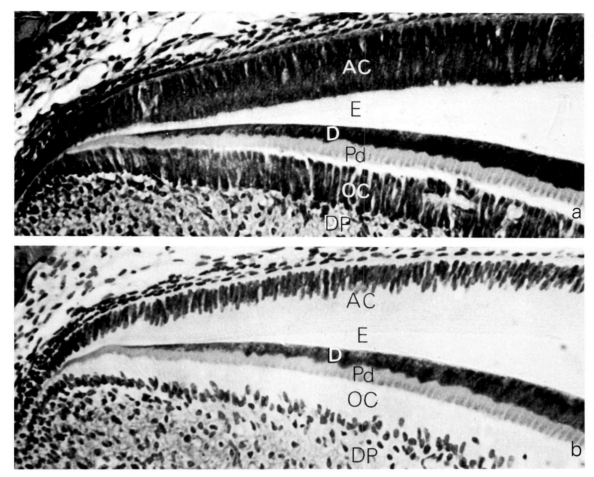

Figure 1.1(a). Developing tooth germ stained with toluidine blue at pH 6.5. Note the staining of ameloblast cytoplasm (AC), dentin (D), predentin (Pd), odontoblast cytoplasm (OC), and components of the dental papilla (DP). The developing enamel (E) is unstained. The toluidine blue stains anionic groups, for example, COO^-, PO_4^{3-}, SO_4^{2-}; consequently little specificity is displayed by the dye. **(b)** This specimen [a serial section to the specimen shown in Figure 1.1(a)] was treated with the enzyme RNAse to remove RNA from the tissue prior to staining with toluidine blue, again at pH 6.5. Note that the ameloblast cytoplasm (AC) and the odontoblast cytoplasm (OC) have lost their intense staining due to digestion of the RNA. Since the nuclei contain chiefly DNA, which is unaffected by the RNAse, they retain their intense staining and resemble the same structures seen in Figure 1.1(a). In like manner, the matrix of dentin (D), predentin (Pd), and dental papilla (DP) retain their staining, probably due to presence of sulfated compounds within the matrix. In this example, the enzyme RNAse was employed as a reagent prior to staining in order to aid in the identification of RNA when used in combination as in Figures 1.1(a) and (b). A variety of other enzymes, for example DNAse, and enzymes used to focus on the presence of polysaccharides can be employed accordingly to the same principles.

metachromasia. The underlying mechanism for the phenomenon is the presence of polyanions within the tissue. When stained with a more concentrated basic dye solution, the dye molecules are sufficiently close to form aggregates whose absorption properties are different from those of the individual nonaggregated dye molecules. Metachromasia is interpreted to reflect the presence of numerous closely positioned anionic charges in the tissue, a condition which prevails in the ground substance of cartilage and in mast cell granules.

Reactions of Schiff Reagent with Aldehyde Groups

There are two well-known applications of the Schiff reagent in histochemistry. One is the *Feulgen reaction* for DNA, and the second is the *periodic acid-Schiff (PAS)* reaction for carbohydrates and for carbohydrate-rich macromolecules.

In the Feulgen reaction mild acid hydrolysis with hydrogen chloride (HCl) cleaves the purine groups from deoxyribose. The deoxyribose then opens and forms aldehyde groups. These, in turn, react with Schiff reagent to produce a magenta-colored reaction product. The reaction is specific for DNA because the HCl hydrolysis causes only the deoxyribose to form aldehyde groups. RNA, which in chemical composition closely resembles DNA, fails to react in this procedure because it lacks the deoxyribose sugar. A type of control commonly employed by histochemists is to predigest a tissue with a specific enzyme to remove a specific substrate in question and then apply the staining reaction. Thus, after treatment of tissue with deoxyribonuclease, the enzyme that specifically digests DNA, the Feulgen reaction will be negative. The Feulgen reaction displays DNA of chromatin within the nucleus and DNA that might be present in the phagosomes of macrophages; DNA of mitochondria is not present in sufficient concentration to yield a positive Feulgen reaction.

The PAS reaction is useful in the detection of glycogen and carbohydrate-containing molecules. It is based on the fact that hexose rings of carbohydrates contain adjacent carbons each of which bears a hydroxyl (—OH) group, and hexosamines of glycosaminoglycans contain adjacent carbons one of which bears an —OH group, while the other bears an amino (—NH$_2$) group. Periodic acid cleaves the bond between these adjacent carbon atoms and forms aldehyde groups, which in turn react with the Schiff reagent. Since many tissue components give a positive PAS reaction, other factors must be considered and further procedures followed for the specific identification of PAS-positive material. In the case of glycogen, which is known to be an intracellular carbohydrate, it is customary to employ amylase, an enzyme that specifically digests glycogen. Thus, intracellular PAS-positive material, which is unreactive after pretreatment with amylase is interpreted to be glycogen. Enzymes are also used to aid in the identification of complex polysaccharides of ground substance. However, the issue is not as straightforward as the identification of glycogen, and several different enzymes may be necessary. The PAS reaction also serves the histologist in the identification of basement membrane material and reticular fibers (Fig. 1.2). Each of these extracellular formed tissue constituents contains PAS-positive sugar groups and each has a characteristic location. Both the positive reaction and the location contribute to their identification. Thus, the PAS-positive band at the interface of epithelium and connective tissue is the basement membrane. The PAS reaction serves as an alternate method to silver impregnation methods for the display of basement membranes and reticular fibers.

Enzymes

Enzymes can be used as control reagents in histochemical procedures as outlined in the above examples relating to predigestion of RNA, DNA, and glycogen. In addition, an entire section of histochemistry deals with the localization of enzyme activity in cells and tissues. In these procedures the reaction product of the enzyme activity, rather than the enzyme itself, is visualized. In a typical reaction to display a hydrolytic enzyme, the tissue section is placed in a solution containing a substrate (AB) and a trapping agent (T) which will precipitate one of the products as follows:

$$AT + T \xrightarrow{\text{Enzyme}} AT\downarrow + B$$

Figure 1.2. A photomicrograph of kidney tissue stained by the PAS method to demonstrate and localize histochemically carbohydrate. The basement membranes are PAS positive as evidenced by the deep pink staining of these sites. The kidney tubules (T) are sharply delineated by the stained surrounding basement membrane. The glomerular capillaries (C) and the epithelium of Bowman's capsule (BC) also show PAS-positive basement membranes.

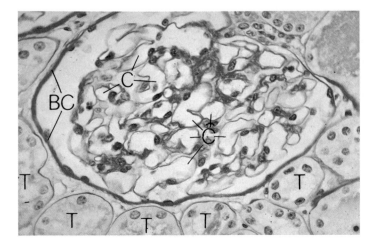

In performing enzyme histochemistry, it is important to avoid inactivation of the enzyme by the action of the fixative and to avoid conditions that will lead to false localization. One of the most useful enzyme methods is that for acid phosphatase because the enzyme is located within lysosomes. Thus, the procedure for acid phosphatase serves to identify lysosomes both at the level of the light and electron microscope. Methods are also well established for ATPase, alkaline phosphatase, respiratory enzymes, and several other enzymes (Fig. 1.3).

Immunocytochemistry

If one injects a foreign substance into an animal, **antibodies** are produced in response to the injected substance. The antibody reacts specifically with the foreign substance (called the *antigen* because of its ability to stimulate antibody formation). The reaction between antigen and antibody is the underlying basis of immunocytochemistry. In one procedure, a specific protein under investigation (for example, actin) is isolated from some source (for example, rat muscle) and injected into another

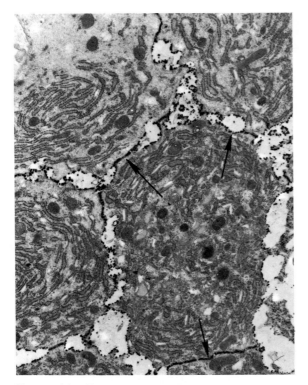

Figure 1.3. The localization of enzyme activity, namely ATPase, is displayed at the ultrastructural level in this electron micrograph. The activity of the enzyme is localized on the plasma membrane. It appears as the black reaction product (arrows) at the perimeter of the cells.

species of animal (for example, rabbit). The actin (the antigen) stimulates the formation of antiactin antibodies that circulate in the blood of the rabbit. The antibodies are removed from the blood of the rabbit, conjugated with a fluorescent dye, and used to stain tissues or cells suspected of containing actin (such as fibroblasts in connective tissue). If actin is present, the antibodies bind to it, and the reaction is visualized by virtue of the fluorescent dye bound to the antibodies (Fig. 1.4). A fluorescence microscope is used to display the fluorescein now attached indirectly to the antigen. It is also possible to conjugate substances such as gold or ferritin (an iron-containing molecule) to the antibody molecule. These markers can be directly visualized with the electron microscope.

Another approach is to bind enzymes (such as peroxidase) to antibody molecules. The labeled tissue is then reacted with the appropriate enzyme substrate to produce a reaction product that may be visualized with a light or an electron microscope to determine the location of the labeled antibodies that are bound to the antigen of interest. The marker used to visualize the location of an antigen can be bound to a second antibody, which is specific to the antibody that was raised in the rabbit (for example, goat antirabbit antibodies). Using a second antibody in the labeling procedure is called *indirect* labeling. When using this method, the tissue is first treated with the primary antibody (produced in the rabbit) and then treated with the second antibody (produced in the goat and tagged with marker used to visualize the location of the bound antibody). A major advantage of the indirect labeling method is that an investigator can produce a number of specific *primary* antibodies (for example, in rabbits). A single tagged *secondary* antibody (goat antirabbit antibody) can be used to identify the location of the various bound *primary* antibodies.

Autoradiography

Autoradiography makes use of a photographic emulsion, placed over a tissue section, in order to localize radioactive material within the tissue. The procedure has been used effectively by injecting precursor molecules needed by cells in the synthesis of large molecules such as DNA and collagen. For example, thymidine is used by the cell in DNA synthesis. The thymidine is incorporated into the DNA by cells about to divide and, therefore, need to double their DNA content. Once incorporated into the DNA, the thymidine stays. In practice, radioactive (tritiated) thymidine is injected into an animal. Cells in the process of

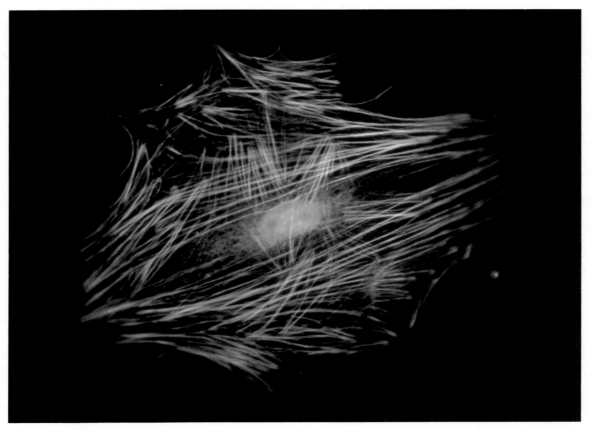

Figure 1.4. A human skin fibroblast in culture photographed in the fluorescence microscope. The cell was "stained" with an actin specific antibody conjugated with the dye fluorescein. The antigen-antibody reaction, performed directly in the culture, results in localization of the actin. The actin filaments organized in linear bundles fluoresce and thus show their distribution in this nonmigrating cell. (Courtesy of Dr. E. S. Lazarides, 1984.)

synthesizing DNA use the tritiated thymidine and these cells become radioactive. The tissue is processed in the usual manner up to the point where the tissue section is on the slide. At this point, in a dark room, the slide with adherent tissue is dipped into a photographic emulsion and stored for an appropriate period of time during which radiation from the isotope reacts with the photographic emulsion. The photographic emulsion is developed and black silver grains indicate the location of the radioactive tissue component. The tissue may then be stained if this has not already been done, covered with a coverslip (using alcohols to remove water, etc., as outlined above) and examined with the light microscope (Fig. 1.5). Autoradiography can also be performed using thin plastic sections for examination with the transmission electron microscope (TEM).

Historadiography

Historadiography is actually the production of an x-ray photograph, that is, a microradiograph, of a specimen on a slide. It displays mass just as a regular x-ray does. While x-rays can be used to examine soft tissues, their greatest utility is in the examination of ground sections of bone or other mineralized tissue. In practice, the ground section of bone is placed in contact with a photographic emulsion on a glass slide and exposed to a beam of x-rays. The photographic emulsion is then developed and viewed with a microscope (Fig. 1.6). Standards of known mass can be added to the slide or to a companion slide treated in the same manner in order to provide semiquantitative information on the amount of bone mineral in different parts of the ground section.

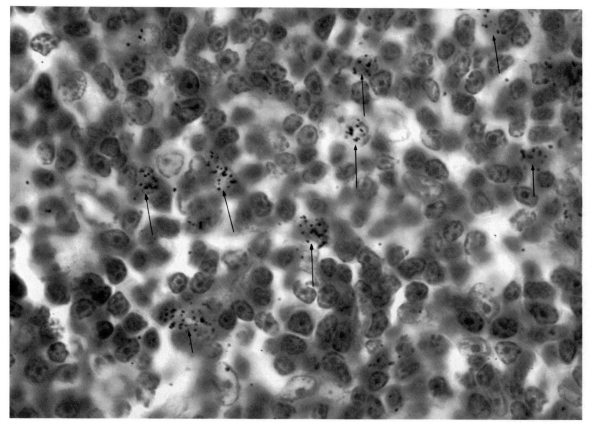

Figure 1.5. Photomicrograph of a lymph node section from an animal treated with tritiated thymidine. Some of the cells exhibit aggregates of metallic silver grains, which appear as small black particles **(arrows)**. These cells are preparing for division and have incorporated the thymidine into their nuclei. The low energy radioactive β particles emitted from the tritiated thymidine, upon striking silver halide crystals in a photographic emulsion covering the specimen over a period of time (exposure), create a latent image (much like light striking photographic film in a camera). Upon photographic development of the slide with its covering emulsion, the latent image, actually the activated silver halide in the emulsion, is reduced to the metallic silver which then appears as the black grains in the microscope. (Original slide specimen courtesy of E. Kallenbach.)

MICROSCOPY

Light Microscopy

Bright-field Microscope. The microscope used by the student in the histology laboratory is referred to as the light microscope, the compound microscope, or perhaps more appropriately, the bright-field microscope. It is the direct descendent of the microscopes that became widely available in the 1800s and opened the first major era of research in histology. Essentially, the bright-field microscope consists of a light source, a condenser that focuses rays of light on the specimen, a stage on which the specimen is placed, an objective lens, and an ocular lens through which the specimen

may be directly viewed (Fig. 1.7). A specimen to be viewed with the light microscope needs to be sufficiently thin so that the light can pass through it. Some light is absorbed while passing through the specimen and differences in light absorption by different parts of the specimen produce contrasts that reveal structural detail. Because the optical system of the light microscope does not reveal much contrast in the unstained specimen, contrast is enhanced by staining the tissue specimen.

The usefulness of the light microscope is its ability to magnify and, more importantly, its ability to resolve structural detail. Resolving power is the ability of a lens or optical system to produce separate images of closely positioned objects. The degree of resolution depends not only on the optical

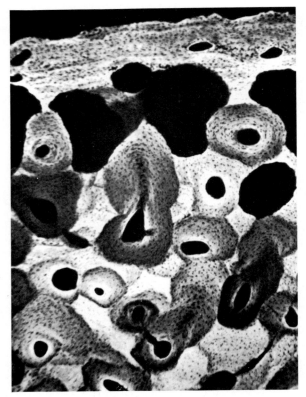

Figure 1.6. A microradiograph of a 200-μm-thick section of bone. Black areas are sites of soft tissue. The white areas contain high concentrations of calcium salts; the light gray to dark gray areas reflect decreasing amounts of calcium salts. (Courtesy of Dr. J. Jowsey, 1984.)

system, but also on the wavelength of the light source and on other factors such as specimen thickness. With light whose wavelength is 540 nm (see Table 1.3 for linear equivalents), a green filtered light to which the eye is extremely sensitive, and with appropriate objective and condenser lenses, the greatest attainable resolving power would be about 0.2 μm (see page 14 for method of calculation). This is the theoretical resolution and, as already mentioned, it depends on all conditions, including tissue sample, being optimal. The ocular lens magnifies the image produced by the objective, but it does not increase resolution.

TABLE 1.3. Linear Equivalents

1 Angstrom (Å)	= 0.1 nanometer (nm)
10 Angstroms	= 1.0 nanometer [formerly millimicron (mμ)]
1000 nanometers	= 1.0 micrometer (μm) [formerly micron (μ)]
1000 micrometers	= 1.0 millimeter (mm)

Phase Contrast Microscope. The phase contrast microscope enables the viewer to examine unstained cells and tissues and, thus, it is especially useful for the examination of living cells. There are small differences in the index of refraction in different parts of a cell and in different parts of a tissue sample. Light passing through regions of greater refractive index is deflected and becomes out of phase with the main stream of light waves. Such differences in refraction are not evident with the light microscope, but with the phase contrast microscope the out-of-phase wavelengths are matched with other induced out-of-phase wavelengths, which cancels their amplitude. In essence, the light waves initially retarded by the specific tissue component have been further diminished by a set of rings in the optical system and the object can be visualized with a useful amount of contrast. The phase contrast microscope is commonly used not only for examining living cells and tissues, but also for examining unstained, plastic thick sections.

Two further modifications of the phase contrast microscope are the *interference microscope,* which also allows for quantitation of tissue mass, and the *differential interference microscope* (using Nomarski optics), which is especially useful for assessing surface properties of cells and other biological objects.

Fluorescence Microscope. The fluorescence microscope detects molecules with fluoresce, that is, emit light of wavelengths in the visible range when exposed to an ultraviolet light source. The fluorescence microscope is used to display naturally occurring fluorescent (autofluorescent) molecules, such as vitamin A, but since autofluorescent molecules are not numerous, its most widespread application is the display of introduced fluorescence, as in the detection of antigens or antibodies in immunocytochemical staining procedures (see Fig. 1.4). Specific fluorescent molecules can also be injected into an animal or directly into cells and used as tracers. Such methods have been useful in studying intercellular (gap) junctions, in tracing the pathway of nerve fibers in neurobiology, and in detecting fluorescent growth markers of mineralized tissues.

Confocal Scanning Microscope. This is a relatively new microscope system being used to study the structure of biological materials. The confocal scanning microscope combines components of a light optical microscope, fitted with fluorescence equipment, with a scanning system that employs a laser beam. The illuminating laser light is very strongly convergent and, therefore, produces a very shallow scanning spot. The light emerging from the spot is directed to a photomulti-

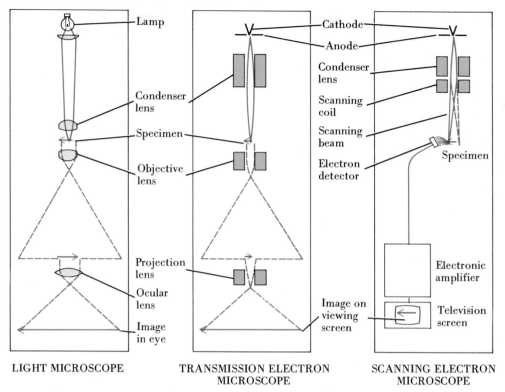

Figure 1.7. Diagram comparing the optical paths of the light microscope, **left** (shown as if it were turned upside down); the transmission electron microscope, **middle**; and the scanning electron microscope, **right**. The specimen and the projected magnified image are depicted by the **arrows**. (Based on Ham AW, Cormack DH: *Histology*, 8th ed. Philadelphia, JB Lippincott, 1979.)

plier tube where it is analyzed. A mirror system is used to move the laser beam across the specimen illuminating a single spot at a time (Fig. 1.8). The data from each point of the specimen scanned by this moving spot is recorded and stored in a computer. The information can then be displayed on a high resolution monitor to create a visual image. The major advantage of this system is its ability to image the specimen in very thin optical sections (approximately 1 μm thick). The out-of-focus regions are subtracted from the image by the computer program, thus creating extreme sharpness of the image. Ordinary, or nonconfocal, light imaging contains superimposed in-focus and out-of-focus specimen parts, therefore the image quality is not as sharp. In addition to utilizing only the narrow depth of the in-focus image, it is possible to create multiple images at varying depths within the specimen. Thus, one can literally dissect layer by layer through the thickness of the specimen. It is also possible to use the computer to make three-dimensional (3-D) reconstructions of a series of these images. Since each individual image located at specific depths within the specimen is extremely

sharp, the resulting assembled 3-D image is equally sharp. Moreover, once the computer has assembled each of the sectioned images, one can rotate the reconstructed 3-D image and view from any orientation desired.

Ultraviolet Microscope. The ultraviolet (UV) microscope uses an ultraviolet light source and depends on the absorption of UV light by molecules in the specimen. UV microscopy is not unlike the workings of a spectrophotometer in principle, but the results are recorded photographically. The specimen cannot be inspected directly through an ocular since the UV is not visible and it is injurious to the eye. The method is useful in detecting nucleic acids, specifically the purine and pyrimidine bases of the nucleotide. It is also useful for detecting proteins that contain certain amino acids.

Polarizing Microscope. The polarizing microscope is a simple modification of the light microscope in which polarized light is passed through the specimen and another polarizer is used as a rotator to detect molecular orientation within a tissue sample. Crystalline substances and well-ordered fibrous molecules alter the plane of the en-

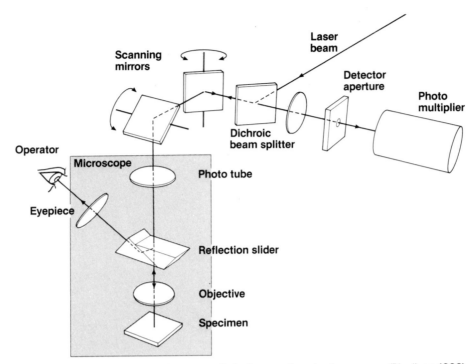

Figure 1.8. Diagram of the beam path in the confocal microscope (Phoibos 1000) by Sarastro. (Courtesy Sarastro, Inc., USA.)

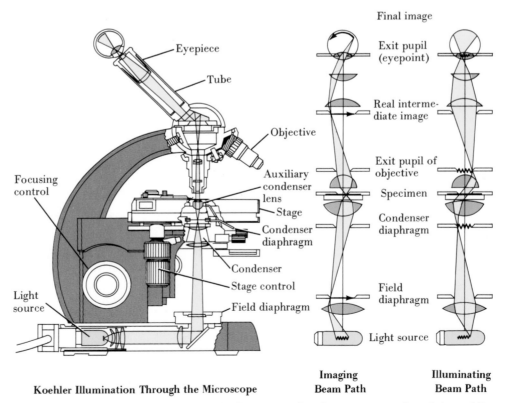

Koehler Illumination Through the Microscope

Imaging Beam Path

Illuminating Beam Path

Figure 1.9. Diagram of a modern light microscope showing a cross-sectional view of its operating components and light path. (Courtesy of Carl Zeiss, Inc., Thornwood, NY, 1984.)

tering polarized light and the altered plane of light is noted with the detector lens. The rotation of polarized light due to the molecular orientation of tissue components is referred to as **birefringence**.

Electron Microscopy

Two kinds of electron microscopes provide essentially morphological data: the transmission electron microscope (TEM) and the scanning electron microscope (SEM).

Transmission Electron Microscope. The TEM utilizes a beam of electrons instead of light in producing an image. The essential components of an electron microscope are (Fig. 1.7): (1) the cathode, a heated tungsten filament (this is the electron source); (2) an anode, which imparts a difference of potential between the cathode and anode ranging from 60,000 to 100,000 volts (this drives the electron through the column); (3) a system of electromagnets that serve as the condenser lens, objective lens, and projection lens (the magnets create electromagnetic fields that bend and thereby focus the beam of electrons); (4) a specimen holder (this accepts a very thin plastic section on a grid through which the electrons pass); (5) a viewing screen; and (6) provision for the image to fall on a photographic film.

Thin sections for transmission electron microscopy are prepared using essentially the same principle as for light microscopy. There are, however, certain differences related to the use of electrons as the "light source." The electrons are made to pass through the specimen and then impinge on photographic film (or on a screen for direct visualization). Image formation in the electron microscope is dependent upon the fact that some electrons do not pass through the specimen to fall on the photographic film; rather, they are deflected by substances of high mass normally within the specimen or added to the specimen during fixation and staining.

Because of the higher resolution of the electron microscope, it is necessary to use fixatives that maximally preserve structure. These fixatives retain many of the substances ordinarily lost during the preparation of tissue for the light microscope. Current fixation procedures use glutaraldehyde to retain protein constituents of the cell and osmium tetroxide to retain the lipid components, especially phospholipid. Because it contains a heavy metal, osmium tetroxide also plays a major role in electron deflection and consequent image formation. Instead of paraffin, the tissues are embedded in plastic, which is harder than paraffin, thereby permitting extremely thin sections to be cut. Special

microtomes, usually equipped with diamond knives, are used. The sections are placed on a copper-mesh grid and then stained. The stains employed contain heavy metals, for example, uranyl acetate and lead citrate. In contrast to the procedure for light microscopy, where paraffin must be removed before staining, the plastic preparation does not require removal of the embedding medium. The grid containing the stained section is then placed in the electron microscope, and the portion of the specimen which spans the openings in the grid may be visualized and photographed.

Freeze Fracture. A special method of sample preparation for TEM, especially important in the ultrastructural study of membranes, is the procedure of **freeze fracture**. The tissue to be examined may be fixed or unfixed; if it has been fixed, the fixative is washed out of the tissue before proceeding. A cryoprotectant, such as glycerol, is allowed to infiltrate the tissue. The tissue is then rapidly frozen to about −160°F. Ice crystal formation is prevented by the use of cryoprotectants, rapid freezing, and extremely small tissue samples. The frozen tissue is placed into the freeze fracture apparatus. The apparatus contains a chamber in which the frozen tissue can be maintained under vacuum. The tissue is then fractured, usually with a cutting device on a swing arm. The tissue is not actually cut, but rather it is fractured along a plane approximately that of the plane of the cutting device. Preferential rifts occur along the hydrophobic plane within the membrane that are parallel or close to the fracture plane, thereby exposing the inner faces of the membrane. The fractured tissue may be allowed to remain for a variable, but short, period of time in the apparatus during which frozen water evaporates causing certain structural details to stand out in greater relief. The specimen is then coated, typically with platinum, to create a shadow cast. In essence, the platinum becomes a replica of the fracture surface. The tissue is removed and the surface replica, not the tissue itself, is picked up on grids to be examined with the TEM. Such a replica displays details at the macromolecular level.

Scanning Electron Microscope. Scanning electron microscopy differs from transmission electron microscopy in that the electrons do not pass through the specimen as part of the image-making process. Instead, a beam of electrons is made to scan the sample surface. Electrons reflected from the surface are collected by a detector and processed so that they can be displayed as a 3-D image on a television screen. The SEM, with a resolution of about 10 nm, allows for a great range of magnifications. In addition, a great variety of methods can be employed in preparing samples for SEM. In the case of mineralized tissues, it is possible to remove all the soft tissues with a bleach and then examine the structural features of the mineral. For the examination of soft tissue, the sample is fixed, dehydrated either by critical point drying or by freeze drying, coated with a film (such as gold or carbon), mounted on a stub, and then examined with the SEM.

Electron Microprobe X-ray Analysis. When the electron beam of the TEM or SEM bombards the tissue sample, x-rays are produced that are characteristic of the specific elements hit by the electron beam. Both the SEM and TEM can be fitted with detectors to collect these x-rays and, with appropriate analyzers, the identity of the element can be ascertained. In effect, with the appropriate accessories both the TEM and SEM can be converted into analytical tools that can detect the presence of elements whose atomic number is greater than about 12.

PROPER USE OF THE LIGHT MICROSCOPE

This brief introduction to the proper use of the light microscope is directed to those students who will be utilizing the microscope for the routine examination of tissues. If the following comments appear elementary, it is only because so frequently many users of the microscope fail to use it to its fullest advantage. Despite the availability of today's fine equipment and its widespread use, there is relatively little formal instruction on the use of the light microscope.

Expensive and highly corrected optics can perform optimally only when the illumination and observation beam paths are centered and correctly adjusted. The use of proper settings and proper alignment of the optic pathway will contribute substantially to the recognition of minute details in the specimen and to the faithful display of color for the visual image and for photomicrography.

Kohler illumination. *Kohler illumination* is one key to good microscopy and is incorporated in the design of practically all modern laboratory and research microscopes. Figure 1.9 shows the two light paths and all the controls for alignment on a modern laboratory microscope and should be referred to in following the instructions given below to provide appropriate illumination in your microscope.

The alignment steps necessary to achieve good Kohler illumination are few and simple. They are:

1. Focus the specimen.
2. Close the field diaphragm.
3. Focus the condenser by moving it up or down until the outline of its field diaphragm appears in sharp focus.
4. Center the field diaphragm with the centering controls on the (condenser) substage. Then open the field diaphragm until it covers the full field observed.
5. Remove the eyepiece (or use a centering telescope or a phase telescope accessory if available) and observe the exit pupil of the objective. You will see an illuminated circular field, the radius of which is directly proportional to the numerical aperture of the objective. As you close the condenser diaphragm, its outline will appear in this circular field. For most stained materials, set the condenser diaphragm to cover approximately two-thirds of the objective aperture. This setting results in the best compromise between resolution and contrast.

By using only these five simple steps, the image obtained will be as good as the optics allow. Now let us find out why.

Principles of bright-field microscopy. First, why do we adjust the field diaphragm to cover only the field observed? Illuminating a larger field than the optics can "see" only leads to internal reflections or stray light, resulting in more "noise" or a decrease in image contrast.

Second, why is there emphasis on the setting of the condenser diaphragm or, in other words, the illuminating aperture? This diaphragm greatly influences the resolution and the contrast with which specimen detail can be observed.

For most practical applications the resolution is determined by

$$d = \frac{\lambda}{NA_{objective} + NA_{condenser}}$$

where d = point-to-point distance of resolved detail (in nm)

λ = wavelength of light used (green = 540 nm)

NA = numerical aperture or sine of half angle picked up by the objective (condenser) of a central specimen point multiplied by the refractive index of the medium between objective (condenser) and specimen

How do wavelength and numerical aperture directly influence resolution? Specimen structures diffract light. The diffraction angle is directly proportional to the wavelength and inversely proportional to the spacing of the structures. According to Ernst Abbe, a given structural spacing can be resolved only when the observing optical system (objective) can see some of the diffracted light produced by the spacing. The larger the objective's aperture, the more diffracted light participates in the image formation, resulting in resolution of smaller detail and sharper images.

Our simple formula, however, shows that the condenser aperture is just as important as the objective's aperture. This is only logical when you consider the diffraction angle for an oblique beam or one of higher aperture. This angle remains essentially constant, but is represented to the objective in such a fashion that it can be picked up easily.

How does the aperture setting affect the contrast (contrast simply being the intensity difference between dark and light areas in the specimen)? The closest to the real contrast transfer from object to image theoretically would be obtained by the interaction (interference) between nondiffracted and all the diffracted wavefronts.

For the transfer of contrast between full transmission and complete absorption in a specimen, the intensity relationship between diffracted and nondiffracted light would have to be 1:1 in order to get full destructive interference (black) or full constructive interference (bright). When the condenser aperture matches the objective aperture, the nondiffracted light enters the objective with full intensity, but only part of the diffracted light can enter, resulting in decreased contrast. In other words, closing the aperture of the condenser to two-thirds of the objective aperture brings the intensity relationship between diffracted and nondiffracted light close to 1:1 and thereby optimizes the contrast. Closing the condenser aperture (or lowering the condenser) beyond this equilibrium will produce interference phenomena or image artifacts such as diffraction rings or lines around specimen structures. Most microscope techniques used for the enhancement of contrast, such as dark field, oblique illumination, phase contrast, or modulation contrast, are based on the same principle, that is, they suppress or reduce the intensity of the nondiffracted light to improve an inherently low specimen contrast.

By observing the steps outlined above and maintaining clean lenses, the quality and fidelity of visual images will vary only with the performance capability of the optical system.

The Cell

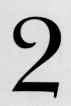

All cells engage in a number of activities that classical cytologists designate as vital or basic functions, that is, activities that serve to maintain the life of the cell. To a very large extent, similar mechanisms are used by cells of different types to perform such activities. Thus, cells use similar mechanisms to synthesize protein, to transform energy, to move essential substances into the cell; they utilize the same kinds of molecules to engage in contraction; they duplicate their genetic material in the same manner. Many of these specific activities have been identified as being the work of distinctive structural components within the cell. For example, certain kinds of filaments are involved in contraction, and, as one might expect, muscle cells (which are specialized to contract) contain large numbers of these contractile filaments. While the muscle cell is an obvious example of a specialized cell, it turns out that most cells of the body are specialized (differentiated) in that they are able to perform one or more specific activities with great efficiency. Not only does the muscle cell have large numbers of filaments, but it is also elongated and organized in parallel with its neighbors. These structural features at different levels of organization are manifestations of the muscle cell's specialized activity of contraction. The specialized activity may be reflected not only by the presence of a larger amount of the specific structural component performing the activity, but also by the shape of the cell, by its organization with respect to other similar cells, and by its products (Fig. 2.1).

The purpose of this chapter is to examine those structural components common to virtually all cells. Cells can be divided into two major compartments, the **cytoplasm** and the **nucleus.** [The term **protoplasm** applies to both compartments.] The cytoplasm and the nucleus not only manifest distinct functional roles, but they work in concert to maintain the cell's viability as well as contributing to the viability of the organism as a whole.

CYTOPLASM

Organelles, Inclusions, and Cytosol

The structural components of the cytoplasm have been traditionally classified as being either organelles or inclusions. This classification, while not as useful as when it was originally introduced, is nevertheless still retained. Organelles, the "little organs" of the cell, possess a distinctive structure and perform specific energy-requiring activities within the cell. Inclusions, on the other hand, are storage components of the cell such as pigment granules, secretory granules, glycogen, and lipid. The portion of the cytoplasm that surrounds the organelles and inclusions is referred to as the **cytosol,** the **cytoplasmic ground substance,** or the **cytoplasmic matrix.**

Many of the organelles and inclusions are membrane-limited structures, that is, they are surrounded by a membrane. The membranes form vesicular, tubular, and other structural patterns that may be convoluted (as in the case of the smooth-surfaced endoplasmic reticulum) or plicated (as in the case of the inner mitochondrial membrane). These convoluted and plicated membrane configurations provide an immense augmentation of surface within the cell on which physiological reactions occur. Moreover, the spaces enclosed by the membranes constitute intracellular microcompartments in which substrates, products, or other substances can be segregated or concentrated. For example, the enzymes of lysosomes are

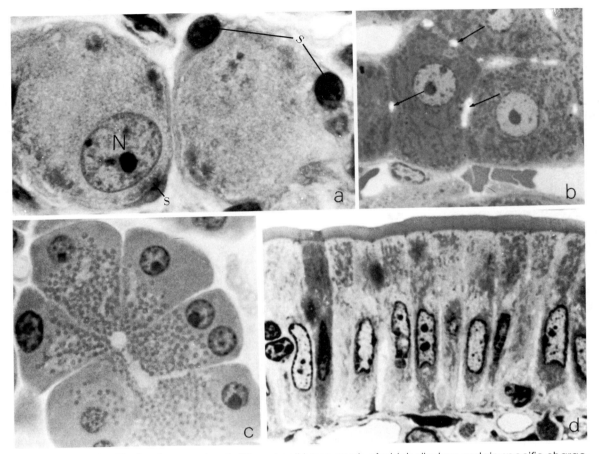

Figure 2.1 (a–d). Photomicrographs of different cell types, each of which displays certain specific characteristics, such as size, shape, orientation, and cytoplasmic contents, that can be related to its specialized activity or function. All figures are from plastic-embedded specimens and are of the same magnification. **(a)** Two ganglion cells. Note the large size of these cells and the large nucleus (N) compared to the surrounding satellite cells (S) and the cells seen in the other figures. The size of the ganglion cell reflects the extensive synthetic activity required in providing for the exceedingly long processes (axons) that these cells possess. **(b)** Several liver cells. They are generally cuboidal in shape and exhibit small spaces or canaliculi **(arrows)** between neighboring cells into which they secrete bile. The small and very numerous dark bodies within the cell are mitochondria, a reflection of the liver cells' high metabolic activity. **(c)** An acinus or secretory unit comprised of pancreatic cells. Note how the cells here tend to have a pyramidal shape. The narrow apical end of the cell faces a lumen, created by the organization of the cells, into which the enzyme precursor, the small granules within the cell, are emptied. The basal part of the cell (the part away from the lumen) is highly basophilic, reflecting the abundant RNA localized in this region of the cytoplasm, which is related to enzyme production. **(d)** The tall (columnar) epithelial cells of the small intestine. The apical surface of these cells has minute cytoplasmic processes known as microvilli, which when seen at the light microscope level appear as a dark band across the top of the cells. The processes greatly expand the apical surface area of the cell to facilitate absorption. (Fig. 2.2 provides a TEM of the apical part of one of these cells and shows to advantage the microvilli.)

separated by a membrane from the cytosol since their hydrolytic activity might be detrimental to the cell.

In addition to the membrane-limited organelles, the cell contains organelles that are not surrounded by membranes. To emphasize this point, organelles belonging to these two categories are listed below.

1. The membranous organelles are:

Plasma (cell) membrane
Rough-surfaced endoplasmic reticulum (rER)
Smooth-surfaced endoplasmic reticulum (sER)
Golgi apparatus
Mitochondria
Lysosomes

Endosomes
Peroxisomes

2. The nonmembranous organelles

Microtubules
Filaments
Centrioles
Ribosomes

Plasma Membrane

The plasma membrane (cell membrane) is not visible with the light microscope. However, even when the light microscope was the only optical tool of the cytologist, it was known that some boundary structure enclosed the cell and that the integrity of this boundary structure was essential to the integrity of the cell. It is now known that the plasma membrane is more than a simple boundary structure and that it participates in numerous functions of the cell. In diagrams, the plasma membrane is usually drawn as a single line. However, when stained with osmium, sectioned, and viewed on edge with the electron microscope, the plasma membrane displays a characteristic trilaminar appearance which has been designated as the *unit membrane.* The components referred to by the designation trilaminar are an outer electron dense layer, an inner electron dense layer, and the intermediate, electron lucid, or nonstaining layer (Fig. 2.2). The total thickness of the plasma membrane is about 8 to 10 nm. On its outer surface, the plasma membrane has a coat consisting of a high density carbohydrate, which is covalently attached to proteins and lipids in the membrane.

The current interpretation of how the plasma membrane is organized at the molecular level, referred to as the *modified fluid-mosaic model,* is shown in Figure 2.3. The membrane consists primarily of phospholipid, cholesterol, and protein molecules. The lipid molecules form a bilayer; they are arranged with the fatty acid chains facing each

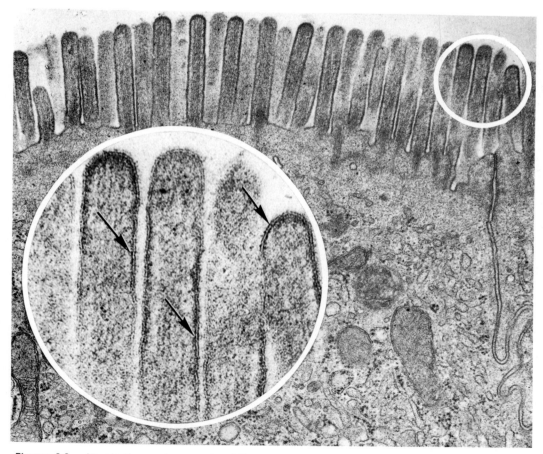

microvilli

Figure 2.2. An electron micrograph of the apical portion of an absorptive cell of the small intestine. The inset is a higher magnification (× 95,000) of the area within the circle. Note that at this magnification the plasma membrane appears as a trilaminar structure **(arrows),** that is, there are two electron dense lines separated by a clear or electron lucid intermediate layer.

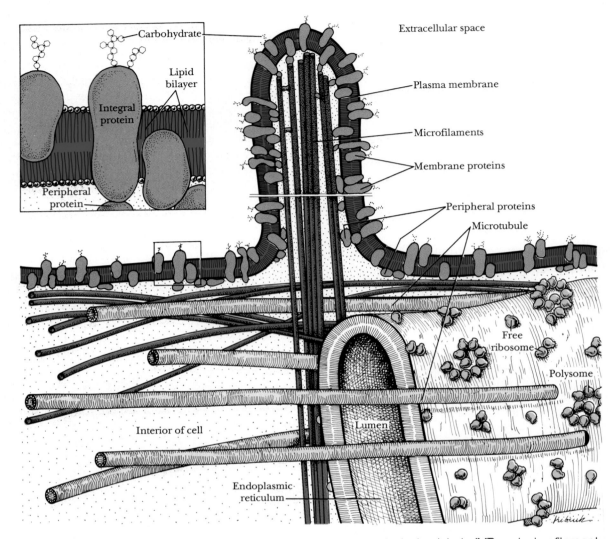

Figure 2.3. Hypothetical interactions between membrane-associated microtubule (MT) and microfilament (MF) systems involved in transmembrane control over cell surface receptor mobility and distribution. This model envisages opposite, but coordinated, roles for microfilaments (contractile) and microtubules (skeletal) and suggests that they are linked to one another or to the same plasma membrane (PM) inner surface components. This linkage may occur through myosin molecules (either in small bundles or the larger filaments [*my*]) or through cross-bridging molecules such as α-actinin. In addition, peripheral membrane components linked at the inner or outer plasma membrane surface may extend this control over specific membrane domains (Modified from Nicolson et al., 1977).

other, thereby making the inner portion of the membrane hydrophobic. The cytoplasmic and extracellular surfaces of the membrane are formed by the polar head groups of the lipid molecules. Hydrophobic regions of proteins extend through or partially through the lipid bilayer as integral proteins of the membrane. On the extracellular surface of the plasma membrane, carbohydrate is attached to protein forming a glycoprotein or to lipid, thereby forming a glycoplipid. These surface molecules constitute a layer at the surface of the

cell, referred to as the *cell coat,* and contribute to the establishment of specific extracellular microenvironments.

Confirmation for the existence of protein within the substance of the plasma membrane came from studies by the method of freeze fracture. When tissue is prepared for electron microscopy by the process of freeze fracture, membranes typically split or cleave along the hydrophobic plane to expose two interior faces of the membrane, an E face and a P face (Figs. 2.4, b and c).

The E-face is backed by *E*xtracellular space, whereas the P-face is backed by *P*rotoplasm. The numerous particles seen on the E- and P-faces are protein. Usually, the P-face displays more particles, thus more protein, than the E-face.

Categories of Membrane Proteins

Six categories of membrane proteins have been identified in functional terms: pumps, channels, receptors, enzymes, transducers, and structural proteins. These categories are not mutually exclusive in that a structural protein might simultaneously serve as a receptor, enzyme, pump, or combination of these.

Pumps serve to transport certain ions actively, for example, Na^+ pumps or metabolic precursors of macromolecules.

Channels allow for the passage of small ions and molecules between cells (down concentration or voltage gradients). Gap junctions (see below) formed by the membrane components of adjacent cells are an example of channels.

Receptor proteins allow for the recognition and localized binding of substances to the outer surface of the plasma membrane in such processes as hormone response, coated vesicle pinocytosis, and antibody reactions.

Transducers are involved in the coupling of receptors to enzymes following the binding of a *ligand,* such as a hormone, to the receptor. (The term ligand refers to any molecule that binds to a receptor on the surface of a cell). Through the action of a transducer, an enzyme may activate the formation of a second messenger such as cyclic adenosine monophosphate AMP.

Several *enzymes* (for example, certain adenosine triphosphatases ATPases) have been shown histochemically to be membrane bound.

Structural proteins have been specifically visualized by the freeze fracture method where they form tight junctions with neighboring cells. Often specific proteins and lipids are concentrated in regions of the plasma membrane that carry out specific functions. An example of such regions can be recognized in the polarized cells shown in Figure 2.1**(b–d)**.

The fluidity of the plasma membrane is not revealed in static electron micrographs of cells. However, experiments reveal that the membrane behaves as though it were a two-dimensional lipid fluid. Proteins that bathe their hydrophobic regions in the interior of the lipid bilayer are free to diffuse laterally. Such movement may occur in order for the membrane molecules to mediate a hormone response (as receptors are coupled with transducers) or to sort (or move) to a different membrane component of the cell. It is important to recognize that the lateral diffusion of proteins is often limited by physical connections between membrane proteins and intracellular or extracellular structures. Such connections may exist between proteins associated with cytoskeletal filaments of the cell and the portion of the membrane proteins that extend into the adjacent cytoplasm, the cytoplasmic domains of membrane proteins, or between proteins associated with the extracellular matrix and the portion of the membrane proteins that extend from the surface of the cell, the extracellular domain. By these mechanisms proteins can be localized, or restricted, to specific "specialized" regions of the plasma membrane or act as transmembrane linkers between intracellular and extracellular filaments (see below). Because these contacts restrict the mobility of proteins, our understanding of the lipid membrane is often referred to as the modified fluid-mosaic model, as stated earlier.

Endocytosis and Exocytosis. As already noted, certain substances enter or leave the cell by passing through the plasma membrane by means of diffusion, pumps, or channels. In addition, substances can enter or leave the cell by processes that are designated as *endocytosis* and *exocytosis,* respectively. These processes involve changes in the configuration of the plasma membrane at localized sites. Moreover, they can be visualized with the electron microscope.

Two forms of endocytosis are recognized: *phagocytosis,* the ingestion of particulate matter; and *pinocytosis,* sometimes referred to as micropinocytosis, the ingestion of substances initially in molecular dispersion (Fig. 2.5). There are two forms of pinocytosis, one involving the formation of smooth *pinocytotic vesicles* and the other involving the formation of *coated vesicles.*

In the formation of pinocytotic vesicles, the plasma membrane invaginates to form small pits, or *caveolae,* which project into the cell. The opening of the pit constricts into a narrow neck, and further constriction results in a pinching off of a vesicle. Such pinocytotic vesicles are especially numerous in the endothelium of blood vessels, but are present in nearly every cell type. The second type of pinocytosis is similar except that where the pinocytosis is to occur, the plasma membrane acquires a localized concentration of short bristles on its inner surface. In the formation of vesicles by this method, the coated membrane first forms a

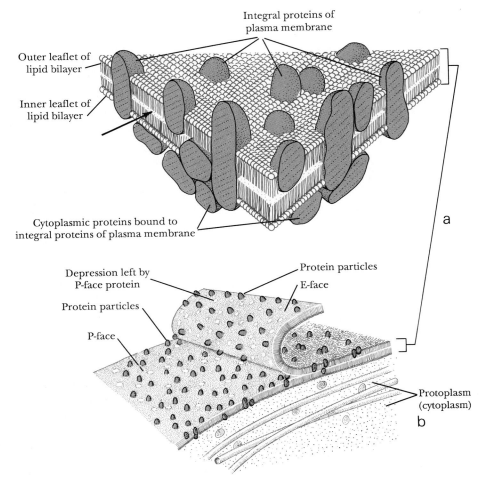

Integral proteins of
plasma membrane

Outer leaflet of
lipid bilayer

Inner leaflet of
lipid bilayer

Cytoplasmic proteins bound to
integral proteins of plasma membrane

a

Depression left by
P-face protein

Protein particles

E-face

Protein particles

P-face

b

Protoplasm
(cytoplasm)

Figure 2.4(a,b). Diagram showing where cleavage occurs in *freeze fracture* of a plasma membrane. **(a)** View of plasma membrane seen on edge with **arrow** indicating preferential split of lipid bilayer along the hydrophobic plane of the membrane. Some proteins are carried with the outer leaflet; most proteins are retained within the inner leaflet. **(b)** Inner leaflet after fracture. Before examination with the TEM, the surface is coated, forming a replica; the replica is separated from the tissue and it is the replica that is examined microscopically. Proteins appear as bumps. The replica of the inner leaflet is called the P-face, it is backed by protoplasm; a view of the outer leaflet is called the E-face, it is backed by extracellular space.

depression, then a small pit, and finally, the coated pit pinches off to become a ***coated vesicle.***

Experimental studies of the pinocytotic process involving coated vesicles indicate that it is a selective process of absorption (also referred to as ***receptor-mediated endocytosis***) whereby certain molecules within the plasma membrane recognize and bind specific substances coming in contact with the plasma membrane. In contrast, nonselective uptake, or absorption, of fluid components occurs in smooth-surfaced pinocytotic vesicles.

Exocytosis is the reverse process of endocytosis. It involves the movement of a membrane-limited structure, such as a secretory granule or a synaptic vesicle, to the plasma membrane, fusion of the membrane of the vesicle (or granule) with the plasma membrane, and then opening and discharge of the vesicular or granular contents.

There are two general pathways of exocytosis, the ***constitutive pathway*** and the ***regulated secretory pathway.*** The ***constitutive pathway*** identifies a process that is continual (rather than induced). Proteins that leave the cell by this process are secreted immediately after their synthesis and exit from the Golgi apparatus (for example, in the secretion of immunoglobulins by plasma cells and tropocolla-

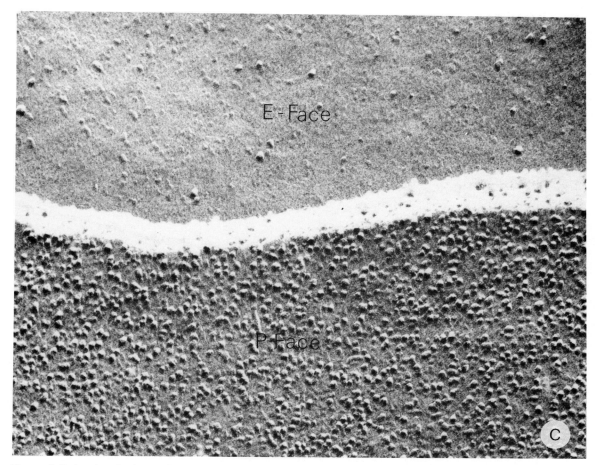

Figure 2.4(c). An electron micrograph of a freeze-fracture replica showing the E-face of the membrane of one epithelial cell and the P-face of the membrane of the adjoining cell. Note the paucity of particles in the E-face as compared to those present in the P-face from which the majority of the globular proteins project. (Courtesy of Dr. G. Raviola.)

gen by fibroblasts). Proteins that are transiently stored in secretory granules pass along the *regulated secretory pathway,* which is named in reference to the regulatory event that must be activated for secretion to occur (for example, in the release of zymogen granules by chief cells and pancreatic acinar cells).

Gap Junctions. Another significant feature of the plasma membrane is its ability to create special channels that bridge the space or gap between adjacent cells. These junctions are called *gap junctions.* Various experiments have been used to study these junctions including, for example, the injection of fluorescent dyes into cells and electrical conductance studies. In the dye studies, a fluorescent dye is injected with a micropipette into one cell of an epithelial sheet. The readily visualized dye can be seen to pass to the immediately adjacent cells. Experiments of this sort have led to the con-

clusion that adjacent cells share communicating channels that allow small molecules and ions to pass between cells without entering the extracellular space.

The electrical conductance studies involve the introduction of microelectrodes into neighboring cells of a cell aggregation and measuring the current flow between the cells as a voltage difference is applied to the electrodes. If there are no gap junctions between the neighboring cells, the current flow is low due primarily to the high electrical resistance of the plasma membranes. In contrast, when electrodes are placed into neighboring cells joined together by gap junctions, there is little electrical resistance between them. The low resistance is a reflection of the direct cytoplasmic continuity between the two cells due to the presence of the gap junctions, which are also called *low resistance junctions.*

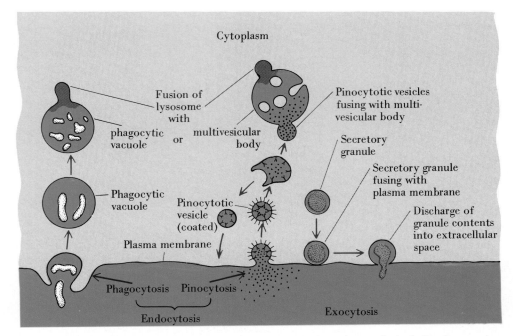

Figure 2.5. Endocytosis (phagocytosis and pinocytosis) and exocytosis. Both phagocytosis and pinocytosis are mechanisms whereby substances are brought into the cell. Phagocytosis involves the ingestion of particulate substances. The particles make contact with the outer surface of the membrane; the plasma membrane may partially enclose or envelope the particles, then the membrane and particles are internalized by the cell; finally, the invaginated membrane becomes pinched off from the plasma membrane; it is then a phagocytic vacuole. Pinocytosis involves the ingestion of nonparticulate substances (e.g., molecules in solution). Again, contact is made with the outer surface of the plasma membrane, it becomes indented, and finally pinches off from the membrane to become a pinocytotic vesicle within the cell. Exocytosis is the discharge of a substance from the cell. The illustration shows a secretory granule, surrounded by a membrane. This membrane makes contact and fuses with the inner surface of the plasma membrane. The fused region then opens, allowing the contents of the secretory granule to escape from the cell.

The existence of gap junctions has been verified by ultrastructural studies. When viewed with the electron microscope, the gap junction has a characteristic appearance. With conventional staining, the gap junction appears as an area where the plasma membranes of adjacent cells have come into contact. With the application of uranyl acetate as a "stain" before embedding the tissue (*en bloc staining*), the gap junction appears as two parallel, closely apposed plasma membranes separated by a gap of 2 nm (Fig. 2.6). Other studies, including freeze fracture procedures, have demonstrated the channels that pass from the cytoplasm of one cell to that of the other.

All of the above aspects of the plasma membrane indicate that it is both a dynamic structure and a boundary structure. It participates in the functional activities of the cell; it serves as a barrier between the inside and the outside of the cell, allowing the cell to maintain a distinctive intracellular environment different from the extracellular environment; and, as will be explained in the chapter on epithelium, it participates in the formation of several other types of intercellular junctions including, for example, adhering junctions and tight junctions.

Ergastoplasm, Rough-surfaced Endoplasmic Reticulum, and Ribosomes

The cytoplasm in the basal portion of pancreatic acinar cells and certain salivary gland cells stains with basic dyes. The basophilic staining is due to the presence of RNA, and the cytoplasmic compartment that stains with the basic dye is called the *ergastoplasm.* Comparable areas of basophilia due to RNA are also present in other cells, and in all cases the staining is indicative of protein synthesis.

The ergastoplasm in the base of pancreatic acinar cells is the light microscopic image of the organelle that cell biologists call the *rough-surfaced reticulum* or *rER.* With the TEM, sections through

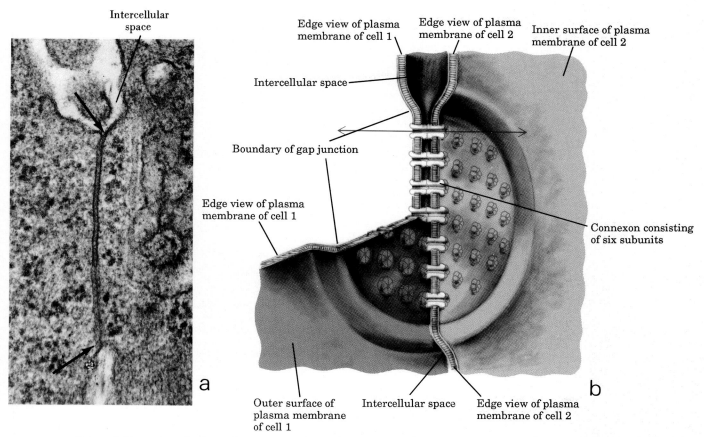

Figure 2.6(a). An electron micrograph showing the plasma membranes of two adjoining cells forming a gap junction. The unit membranes **(arrows)** approach one another (note **top** and **bottom** of micrograph) narrowing the intercellular space to produce a 2-nm wide gap. **(b)** A model representation of a gap junction showing the membranes of adjoining cells creating the 2 nm gap and the structural components of the membrane that form channels or passageways between the two cells (see **double-headed arrow**). Each passageway is formed by a circular array of six subunits, dumbbell-shaped particles, that span the membrane of each cell. These complexes, called connexons, have a central opening of about 2 nm in diameter. The channels formed by the registering of the adjacent complementary pairs of connexons permit the flow of small molecules through the channels but not into the intercellular space. Conversely, substances in the intercellular space can permeate the area of a gap junction by flowing around the connexon complexes but cannot enter into the channels. (From Junqueira LC, Carneiro J: *Basic Histology,* 3rd ed. Los Altos, CA, Lange, 1980.)

the rER appear as membrane-limited flattened sacs referred to as *cisternae.* In the pancreatic cells and other secretory cells active in protein synthesis, the cisternae appear as parallel membranous profiles delineating the cavity of the rER from the cytoplasmic matrix (Fig. 2.7). The cisternae are interconnected, forming a continuous system of membrane-limited cavities.

An essential feature of the rER is the presence of small particles, 15 to 20 nm in diameter, called *ribosomes,* which are transiently attached to the outer, or cytoplasmic, surface of the membrane by proteinaceous receptors called *ribophorins.* When these particles are seen in a face view of the membrane, it becomes evident that groups of ribosomes

are arranged in a short spiral, or rosette, pattern. Such groups are called *polysomes,* or *polyribosomes* (Fig. 2.8). Although not evident in conventional transmission microscopy, the ribosomes in a polysome are joined by a thread of messenger RNA. In addition to ribosomes which are attached to membranes, ribosomes also occur scattered throughout the cytoplasmic matrix, either singly or as polysomes. Such unattached ribosomes are called *free ribosomes* or *free polysomes.* All ribosomes contain RNA; it is the RNA of the ribosomes, and not the membranous component of the endoplasmic reticulum, that accounts for the basophilic staining of the rER.

The rER, as already noted, is well developed

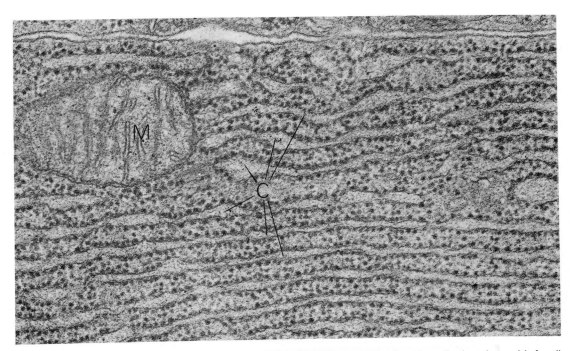

Figure 2.7. Electron micrograph showing the rough-surfaced endoplasmic reticulum in a chief cell of the stomach. Note the cisternae (C) are closely packed in parallel arrays. Each is bounded by a ribosome-studded membrane. M, mitochondrion. × 50,000.

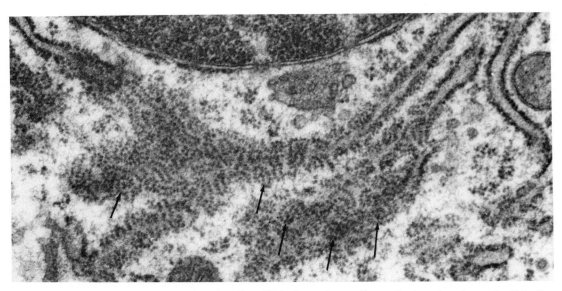

Figure 2.8. A fortuitous section showing the rER in two planes. The reticulum has turned within the section. Thus, in the **upper right** and **left** of the electron micrograph, the membranes of the reticulum have been cut at a right angle to their surface. In the **center** area the reticulum has twisted and it is seen as though one were looking down on the surface of the membrane. Viewed in this aspect, it becomes evident that most of the ribosomes are arranged in a spiral configuration on the membrane **(arrows)**. × 38,000.

in cells that synthesize protein for export. Included among these are glandular secretory cells, fibroblasts, plasma cells, odontoblasts, ameloblasts, and osteoblasts. The rER is not limited to synthetic-secretory cells. Virtually every cell of the body contains profiles of rER but these are usually small in amount and dispersed so that they are not evident with the light microscope as areas of basophilia.

In agreement with the observation that the rER is most highly developed in active secretory cells, secretory proteins are exclusively synthesized on the ribosomes of the rER. Proteins that are to become permanent residents of the lysosome, Golgi, rER, or nuclear envelope (these structures are discussed below), or integral components of the plasma membrane, are also synthesized on the ribosomes of the rER. These proteins are unique in that they have a hydrophobic signal domain, or region of the molecule, at their initial forming end. The signal domain of the forming protein induces its receptor-mediated attachment to the membrane of the rER and then its cotranslational insertion into and through the membrane. If the forming protein is not to be threaded in its entirety through the membrane, a new hydrophobic domain will stop the threading process and cause the protein to be anchored permanently in the membrane at this site. Upon completion of the protein synthesis, the ribosome detaches from the rER membrane and is then free in the cytoplasm. The region of the newly formed protein that extends into the lumen of the rER is exposed to modification by enzymes present there. For example, most proteins receive an oligosaccharide transferred from a lipid donor to the amide N of certain asparagine residues (thus referred to as N-linked oligosaccharide). The initial hydrophobic domain is usually cleaved by a protease. Disulfide bonds are established to achieve the correct conformation of the molecule. Except for those few proteins that are to remain permanent residents of the rER, the newly synthesized proteins are delivered to the Golgi apparatus (see below) within several minutes.

Cells that produce large amounts of protein for internal use also display cytoplasmic basophilia. This basophilia is also designated as ergastoplasm, but it is due to the presence of numerous free ribosomes and free polysomes and not to ribosomes which are attached to membranes as rER. Examples of such cells are keratinocytes of skin, which produce large amounts of keratin (an intercellular protein); developing muscle cells, which produce large amounts of the contractile proteins actin and myosin; and developing red blood cells, which produce large amounts of hemoglobin. Nerve cells display areas of basophilia called Nissl bodies. This

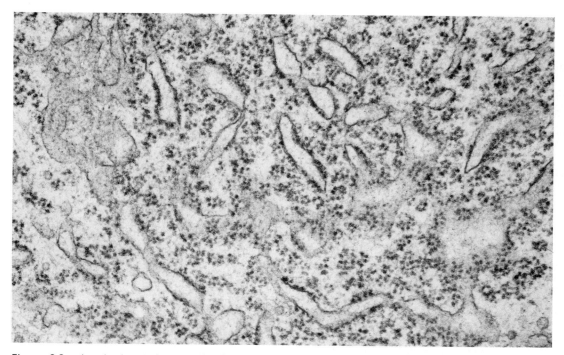

Figure 2.9. An electron micrograph of a nerve cell body showing profiles of endoplasmic reticulum with attached ribosomes. The cytoplasm between the reticulum contains numerous free ribosomes. Collectively, the free ribosomes and membrane attached ribosomes are responsible for the cytoplasmic basophilia observed in the light microscope. × 45,000.

basophilia is due to the presence of large numbers of ribosomes which occur both as free ribosomes and in the form of rER (Fig. 2.9).

Smooth-surfaced Endoplasmic Reticulum

The *smooth-surfaced* or *smooth endoplasmic reticulum* (*sER*) typically consists of short anastomosing tubules (Fig. 2.10). These membranous formations do not contain attached ribosomes. Without the attached ribosomes, regions of cells containing large amounts of sER fail to display basophilia. On the contrary, such cells display pronounced cytoplasmic acidophilia (i.e., staining with eosin). The sER has been implicated in a multitude of seemingly unrelated functions. It is found in large amounts in cells that secrete steroids, such as the cells of the adrenal cortex and the interstitial cells of the testes. Large amounts of sER are found in liver cells exposed to certain drugs; enzymes involved in detoxification of the drugs are attached to the sER. It is present in a specialized pattern in skeletal muscle cells (in this location it is named the sarcoplasmic reticulum), where it functions to seg-

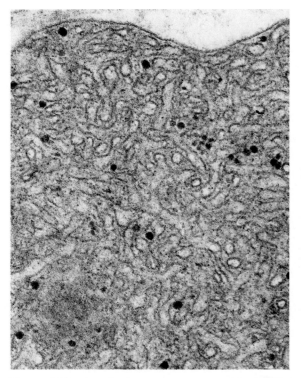

Figure 2.10. An electron micrograph of the sER in an interstitial cell of the testis. The reticulum seen here is a complex system of anastomosing tubules. The small dense objects are glycogen particles. × 60,000.

regate calcium. The sER has also been shown to be involved in lipid absorption, glycogen metabolism, and membrane formation.

Golgi Apparatus

The Golgi apparatus was known to early cytologists because it can be displayed with osmium and viewed with the light microscope. It was discovered originally in nerve cells, where it forms networks around the nucleus. In this cell type, the Golgi apparatus serves to process the relatively large amount of membrane protein that enters into neuronal processes to mediate electrical conductance and synaptic signalling. The Golgi apparatus is also well developed in active secretory cells. In these cells the Golgi apparatus carries out the finishing steps of secretory protein synthesis, referred to as post-translational modifications, and helps to sort these proteins to the proper plasma membrane domain across which they will be exocytosed.

The Golgi apparatus does not stain with hematoxylin or eosin (H&E). In secretory cells that have a large Golgi apparatus (for example, plasma cells, osteoblasts, or cells of the epididymis), it typically appears as a clear area, often referred to as a negative image partially surrounded by the basophilic ergastoplasm (Fig. 2.11). In electron micrographs, the Golgi appears as stacks of flattened membrane-bound sacs, or cisternae, closely associated with vesicles (Fig. 2.12). Often, the Golgi is polarized so that an outer (convex) or inner (concave) part can be identified. These are referred to as the *forming face* and *maturing face*, respectively.

The role of Golgi has been studied most intensively as it relates to protein secretion. The nature of the process makes it necessary to include the role of the rER and secretory granules in interpreting the role of the Golgi. In gland cells secreting protein, these structures are typically juxtaposed with the forming face of the Golgi adjacent to the rER, and the mature face of the Golgi directed toward the secretory granules (Fig. 2.12). Small vesicles, called *transport vesicles,* are interposed between the rER and the forming face of the Golgi. These vesicles convey secretory product from the rER to the Golgi.[1] Secretory proteins to be stored before secretion are found first in precursor struc-

---

[1] Movement from the forming to the maturing face of the Golgi is associated with successive changes in the N-linked oligosaccharides from the high-mannose type, delivered from the rER, to complex forms. On some proteins, a distinct class of oligosaccharides becomes attached to the hydroxyl moieties of selected serine and threonine amino acid residues (O-linked oligosaccharides) and with sulfate and/or phosphate residues on selected oligosaccharides and amino acids.

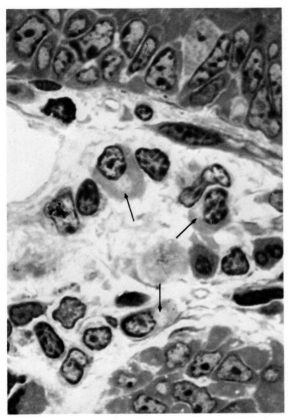

Figure 2.11. A light micrograph of a plastic embedded specimen from the intestine stained with toluidine blue. The plasma cells, where appropriately oriented, exhibit a clear area in the cytoplasm (i.e., negatively stained), which represents the Golgi area. The surrounding cytoplasm is deeply stained due to the presence of the ribosomes associated with the extensive rER. × 1200.

tures called ***condensing vacuoles*** (Fig. 2.13). The condensing vacuoles form as dilatations of the inner (mature) Golgi membranes that pinch off and become relatively large free vacuoles. There is, however, no complete agreement on how the secretory product in the transport vesicle is moved through or around the flattened Golgi cisternae to the condensing vacuoles.

The Golgi is also involved with the rER in lysosome production. The lysosomes contain hydrolytic enzymes that are proteins. These proteins carry a signal that triggers an enzyme to attach phosphate residues to their N-linked oligosaccharides. This post-translational modification occurs in the forming face of the Golgi before the N-linked oligosaccharides are processed from high-mannose to complex forms at more distal levels of the Golgi stack. The lysosomal proteins exit from the maturing face of the Golgi by a receptor-

mediated process, which ensures that they are segregated from secretory proteins entering condensing vacuoles at the same level of the Golgi. The maturing face of the Golgi and the associated tubolovesicular array, referred to as the ***trans-Golgi network***, thus serves as the sorting station for shuttling vesicles that deliver protein to various locations, such as the basolateral membrane of an epithelial cell, its luminal surface, or the lysosomes.

The Golgi also processes proteins that are to remain membrane-associated throughout their lifetime. The principles involved in modifying and sorting these proteins is similar to those described for proteins that pass through the Golgi lumen. This type of protein is subject to an additional class of modifications that involves the addition and/or alterations of fatty acids or glycolipids, which may influence the subsequent association of these proteins with the membrane.

Mitochondria

Mitochondria were known to early cytologists who speculated that they were "elementary" cell structures. The idea was forwarded that they evolved from an ancestral procaryote that established a symbiotic existence with the host eucaryotic cell by way of an aborted endocytotic event. While this idea is speculative, it should be noted that mitochondria do possess DNA and a variety of RNAs, which enable them to produce some of their constituents proteins. However, the genetic system of the nucleus is needed for the production of the remaining mitochondrial proteins, indicating that the mitochondria are no longer entirely autonomous. These cytoplasmically derived proteins are synthesized on cytoplasmic (not rER-associated) ribosomes and are post-translationally transported into mitochondria by a receptor-mediated mechanism at sites of contact between the inner and outer mitochondrial membranes. Mitochondria divide to produce new mitochondria.

Mitochondria are present in all cells except red blood cells and terminal keratinocytes from which they have been lost by autophagy. The mitochondrial number and arrangement for a specific cell type, while not fixed, are usually characteristic of that cell type. While they display no specific staining properties in routine histological sections, mitochondria, especially when present in large numbers, contribute to the eosinophilic staining of the cytoplasm.

Mitochondria contain the enzyme system that generates ATP by means of the Krebs cycle and oxidative phosphorylation. Cells that expend large amounts of energy, such as striated muscle cells or

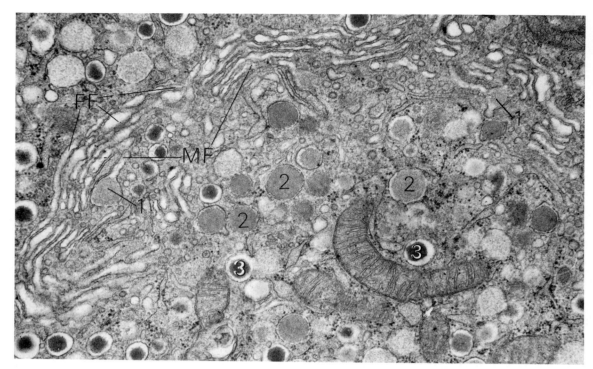

Figure 2.12. Electron micrograph of the Golgi apparatus in an islet cell of the pancreas. The flattened membrane sacs of the Golgi are arranged in layers. The forming face (FF) of the Golgi is represented by the flattened vesicles on the outer convex surface, whereas the flattened vesicles of the inner convex region constitute the maturing face (MF) of the Golgi. Budding off the maturing face are several condensing vacuoles (**1**). These are released (**2**) and eventually become the mature secretory granules (**3**).

kidney tubule cells, have large numbers of mitochondria. Typically, they are localized in those regions of the cell where energy is needed, for example, adjacent to the membrane infoldings of the proximal convoluted tubules of the kidney. Mitochondria also contain granules in their matrix that are divalent cation binding sites. The matrix granules are known to increase in size and number when cation levels in the cytosol are increased above a certain apparently critical level. Thus, in addition to ATP production, mitochondria also function to regulate the concentration of certain ions of the cytosol; a role they share with the endoplasmic reticulum.

The mitochondrion presents a distinctive appearance when examined with the electron microscope (Fig. 2.14). It is comprised of two parallel unit membranes, each of which has a specific arrangement. The outer membrane is smooth and about 6 to 7 nm in thickness. The inner membrane is slightly thinner and forms a variable number of sheet-like folds, called *cristae,* which project into the inner portion of the organelle. In certain cell types, the inner mitochondrial membrane forms tubular or vesicular invagination rather than the flat, shelf-like cristae. With high-resolution elec-

tron microscopy and negative-staining, spherical bodies with a stalk, called ***elementary particles,*** can be seen attached to the inner surface of the inner membrane. The elementary particles contain the enzymes of the electron transfer system (for oxidative phosphorylation); they also contain ATPase activity (Fig. 2.15). The inner chamber of the mitochondrion contains a more or less dense-appearing material known as the ***mitochondrial matrix.*** The mitochondrial (matrix) granules, DNA, RNA, and ribosomes are contained within the mitochondrial matrix.

Lysosomes

The lysosome was not known before the era of electron microscopy. In order to identify lysosomes with light microscopy, special histochemical procedures (such as the acid phosphatase reaction, immunolabeling, or staining with a vital dye) must be employed. Biochemical techniques (cell fractionation) combined with electron microscopy has revealed that the lysosome contains hydrolytic or "digestive" enzymes separated from the cytosol by a surrounding membrane.

Lysosomes are involved in digesting sub-

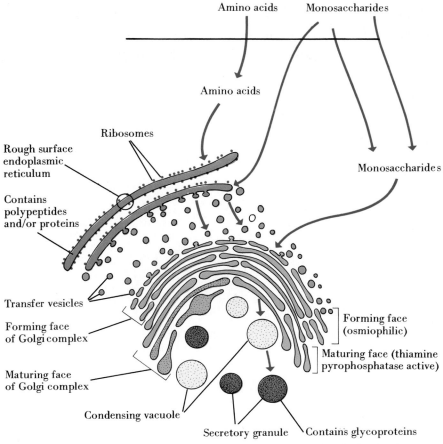

Amino acids   Monosaccharides

Amino acids

Ribosomes

Rough surface
endoplasmic
reticulum

Monosaccharides

Contains
polypeptides
and/or proteins

Transfer vesicles

Forming face
of Golgi complex

Forming face
(osmiophilic)

Maturing face (thiamine
pyrophosphatase active)

Maturing face
of Golgi complex

Condensing vacuole

Secretory granule   Contains glycoproteins

Figure 2.13.   Diagram of relationship between rER, Golgi apparatus, and secretory granules. The rER synthesizes polypeptides and protein from amino acids; these are conveyed to the Golgi apparatus by transfer vesicles; carbohydrates are added to the protein in the rER and in the Golgi to form glycoproteins. The product is condensed in vacuoles to form secretory granules, which are discharged from the cell by exocytosis. (Based on Bloom W, Fawcett DW: *A Textbook of Histology,* 10th ed. Philadelphia, WB Saunders, 1975.)

stances brought into the cell by means of *endocytosis* (see above) or the autophagy pathway; they also participate in the hydrolysis of cellular constituents. A list of enzymes demonstrated to be present in lysosomes is given in Figure 2.16. These digestive enzymes are adapted to function in the low pH environment created within of the lysosome by proton pumps located in the lysosomal membrane. As already mentioned, lysosomes are diverted from the secretory pathway at level of the trans-Golgi network. The newly produced lysosome is referred to as a *primary lysosome.* When a primary lysosome contacts and fuses with the structure that contains the substance to be digested, the contents of the two are mixed, the newly formed structure is referred to a *secondary lysosome.* A secondary lysosome may be given an additional name (for example, phagosome, digestive vacuole, autophagic vac-

uole) depending on the origin of the material that is being digested (see also Fig. 2.17).

In certain cells with a long life-span (such as nerve cells or cardiac muscle cells), pigment granules can be detected with the light microscope. These granules are large *residual bodies,* which contain accumulated material not digested by lysosomal enzymes. In the classical histological literature, the pigment was referred to as "wear and tear" pigment and as lipofuscin. The presence of residual bodies is not considered pathological. On the other hand, failure of lysosomes to function in their normal capacities can result in several disorders known collectively as *lysosomal storage disease.* One such disorder, Tay-Sachs disease, affects nerve cells. It is caused by the absence of a lysosomal enzyme that ordinarily digests a galactoside in nerve cells. The substrate accumulates as concen-

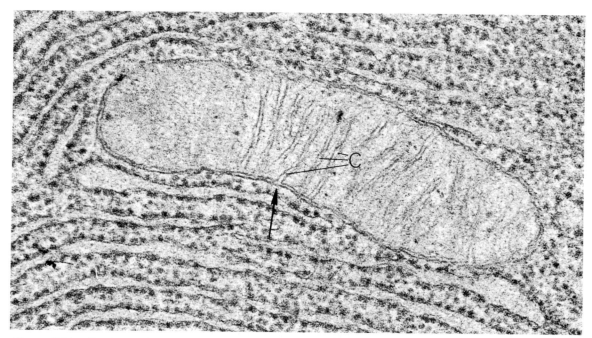

Figure 2.14. Electron micrograph of a mitochondrion in a pancreatic acinar cell. Note the inner mitochondrial membrane forms the cristae (C) through a series of infoldings. This is evident in the region of the **arrow**. The outer membrane is a smooth continuous envelope, which is separate and distinct from the inner membrane.

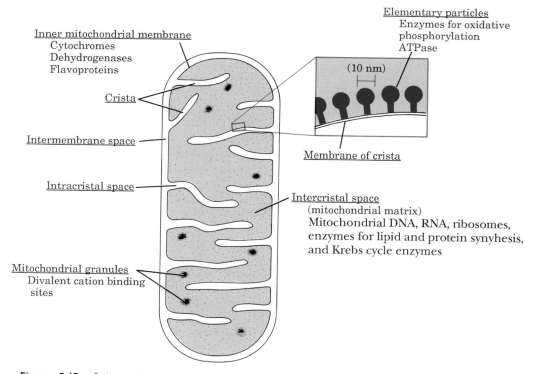

Figure 2.15. Schematic diagram of a mitochondrion and some activities of mitochondrial components. (Based on Bloom W, Fawcett DW: *A Textbook of Histology,* 10th ed. Philadelphia, WB Saunders, 1975.)

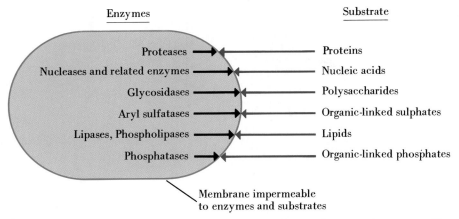

Figure 2.16. Diagram of a lysosome and a list of some lysosomal enzymes. The respective substrates are listed outside of the lysosome. In order to act, the lysosome typically discharges the enzyme into the cellular microcompartment containing the substrate. More than 40 lysosomal enzymes have been identified. (From Novikoff AB, Holtzman, E: *Cells and Organelles,* 2nd ed. New York, Holt, Rinehart and Winston, 1976. Copyright © 1970, 1976 by Holt, Rinehart and Winston, Inc. Reprinted by permission of CBS College Publishing).

tric lamellae in residual bodies that fill up the nerve cell and interfere with its function.

Examples of cell types with large numbers of lysosomes as a regular component of their cytoplasm are the polymorphonuclear leukocytes and macrophages.

Endosome-associated Vesicles

As was previously explained, vesicles formed as the result of phagocytosis typically fuse with lysosomes leading to the degradation of the phagocytosed material. The vesicle formed by pinocytosis is generally referred to as an **endosome**. The fate of pinocytosed material depends on the nature of the material and may follow one of three pathways once it is within the cell.

1. The endosomes may fuse with another domain, or region, of the plasma membrane to release its product from the cell; this process is referred to as **transcytosis**. This pathway allows substances altered and transported across the cells of an epithelium, such as the secretion of immunoglobulins into the saliva or milk.

2. The endosomes may fuse with a lysosome, forming a **phagosome**. As explained above, this pathway allows substances taken into the cell to be digested or hydrolyzed.

3. The endosomes may fuse with a vesicular structure, sometimes referred to as the **compartment for uncoupling of receptor and ligand** (**CURL**) (Fig. 2.17). This pathway allows a **ligand** (as stated previously, a general name for any molecule that is recognized by a receptor) to be segregated from its

receptor.[2] This pathway is important because it allows surface receptors to be recycled. As explained above, the receptors allow the cell to bring substances selectively into the cell through the process of endocytosis. Tracer-ligands can be used as markers which are taken up by the cell to identify the vesicles of the three pathways described above.

Peroxisomes (Microbodies)

Peroxisomes are spherical, membrane-limited structures, about 0.5 μm in diameter. They are found in most cell types, but are especially numerous in the cells of the liver and kidney. The number of peroxisome present in a cell increases in response to diet, drugs, and hormonal stimulation. In some species, the peroxisome exhibits a characteristic dense core referred to as a **nucleoid**. Peroxisomes have been shown to contain catalase, an enzyme that hydrolyzes hydrogen peroxide (H_2O_2); this is the basis for their designation as peroxi-

---

[2] In the CURL pathway, the phase of the process involving the dissociation of the ligand and receptor is usually mediated by the acidic pH of this compartment. After dissociation, the ligand leaves the CURL en route to the lysosome by way of the vesicle-mediated pathway and the receptor typically returns to the plasma membrane along another vesicle-mediated pathway. Ligand-receptor dissociation does not always accompany receptor recycling. For example, the low pH of the endosome and CURL dissociates iron from the iron-carrier protein-transferrin, but transferrin remains associated with its receptor. However, once the transferrin-transferrin receptor pair returns to the cell surface, transferrin is released because at the neutral extracellular pH transferrin requires bound iron to be recognized by its receptor.

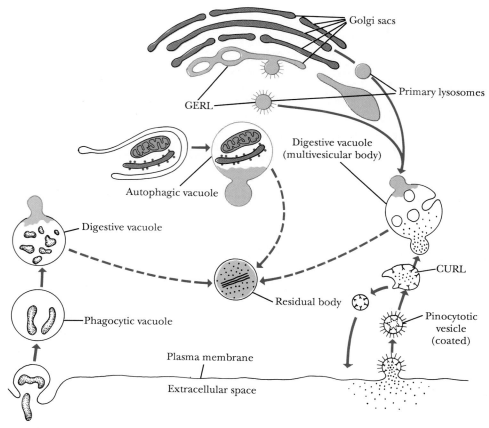

Figure 2.17. Origins of primarily lysosomes from the Golgi and trans-Golgi network. Primary lysomes fuse with and discharge hydrolytic enzymes into autophagic, pinocytotic (or endosome), and phagocytic vacuoles to form secondary lysosomes (digestive vacuoles). Residual bodies contain undigested residue. Endosomes fuse to form a compartment where uncoupling of the ligands and surface receptors occurs (CURL, see text for explanation). The compartment containing the free ligands subsequently fuses with the lysosome; the receptors remain bound to the membrane of vesicles which is partitioned off from the CURL and recycle to the plasma membrane. (Modified from Novikoff AB, Holtzman E: *Cells and Organelles,* 2nd ed. New York, Holt, Rinehart and Winston, 1976.)

somes. Since catalase hydrolyzes hydrogen peroxide, it has been postulated that peroxisomes serve to protect the cell against this substance. They have also been implicated as being involved in the degradation of purines (found in nucleic acids), D-amino acids, and fatty acids, and in lipid absorption and metabolism. The proteins contained in the peroxisome lumen and membrane are synthesized on cytoplasmic ribosomes and appear to gain entry into the peroxisome by a receptor-mediated mechanism.

NONMEMBRANOUS ORGANELLES

Microtubules

Microtubules are hollow, nonbranching cylinders about 22 nm in diameter and many microme-

ters in length (Fig. 2.18). They are distributed throughout the cytoplasm in patterns, not always obvious, BUT which reflect their special functions. In addition to their general distribution through the cytoplasm, short microtubules arranged as triplets are present in centrioles (see Fig. 2.21) and basal bodies. They are also present in cilia and flagella, and they are the spindle filaments of the mitotic spindle. Microtubules are involved in the elongation of cells, movement of cilia and flagella, maintenance of asymmetry in cells, intracellular transport of secretory granules, and movement of chromosomes during mitosis.

Microtubules are made up of a protein called *tubulin,* which occurs in two forms, α-*tubulin* and β-*tubulin*. Two tubulin proteins, which differ slightly in composition and are arranged as dimers, are the basic subunit of the microtubule (Fig. 2.19).

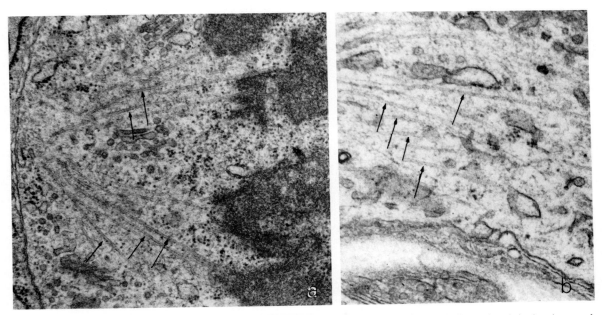

Figure 2.18. Electron micrograph of cytoplasmic microtubules. Figure **(a)** reveals the microtubules **(arrows)** associated with the chromosomes in a dividing (metaphase) cell. Figure **(b)** shows the microtubules **(arrows)** in the axon of a nerve cell. In both examples the microtubules are seen in longitudinal profile. × 30,000.

Microtubule formation is easily inhibited, or arrested, by dimer-binding drugs (such as vinblastine and colchicine). Microtubules are easily dissociated into their dimeric subunits by decreased temperature, and by increased hydrostatic pressure. When microtubules are disrupted by these means, mitosis is arrested because spindle filaments are dissociated and the chromosomes fail to move apart; secretory granules fail to reach the cell surface due to the absence of microtubules involved in their movement; and axon formation is halted due to the absence of microtubules (neurotubules) involved in cell elongation. In these processes, microtubules are understood to serve as guides for molecular motors, which are attached to the moving structures and are fueled by ATP hydrolysis.

Filaments

Two basic types of filaments occur within cells—*microfilaments* and *intermediate filaments*.

Histologists first recognized the abundant and orderly array of cytoplasmic filaments in muscle cells. With the advent of electron microscopy, two types of filaments, one thick and one thin, were noted and were collectively referred to as *myofilaments* (myo-muscle). The thin filaments are composed of a protein called *actin;* the thick filaments are composed of a protein called *myosin.* The mechanism by which these filaments interact is described in the chapter on muscle. In those cells not specialized for contraction, nonmuscle cells, the actin filaments are designated as *microfilaments.* Mi-

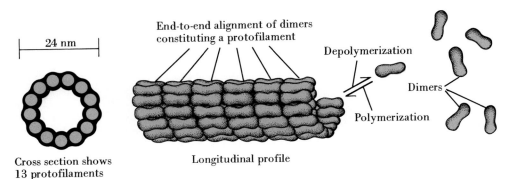

Figure 2.19. A microtubule in cross-section and in longitudinal profile showing depolymerization of the microtubule into dimers. (From Junqueira, Carneiro J: *Basic Histology,* 3rd ed. Los Altos, CA, Lange, 1980.)

crofilaments are found in all cell types. Myosin is also present in most cell types where it interacts with the actin, but the myosin is often not found in a filamentous state. The actin and myosin are responsible for the contractile and viscoelastic properties of the cytoplasm.

Microfilaments. Microfilaments, approximately 5 to 7 nm in diameter, are composed of actin. They are often grouped as bundles close to the plasma membrane. These membrane-associated microfilaments function in the anchorage and movements of membrane proteins, movement of the plasma membrane (such as movement of the plasma membrane during endocytosis, exocytosis, and cytokinesis), extension of cell processes, and locomotion of the cell. Other microfilaments are distributed in three-dimensional networks throughout the cell (Fig. 2.20**a**; see also Fig. 1.4). These microfilaments are considered to be active in cytoplasmic streaming, that is, the stream-like movement of cytoplasm that can be observed within cells in culture. In muscle cells, contraction involves the interaction of actin-containing filaments, myosin-containing filaments, and the accessory proteins including tropomyosin. This is also the case in nonmuscle cells, but the myosin and tropomyosin molecules in nonmuscle cells are not usually aggregated or evident as filaments. They can, however, be demonstrated with immunocytochemical techniques. It is now apparent that some movements relative to microfilaments are due to "molecular motors" as described above for microtubules. Nonfilamentous myosin may function in this manner. Other possible mechanisms of movement involving microfilaments include the force exerted by polymerization at the growing end of

the filaments and syneresis (the contraction of a gel, such as a blood clot, by squeezing out some of the dispersion medium). Crosslinked microfilament networks are also suspected to be important for maintenance of static structures within the cell.

Unlike most organelles, microfilaments and microtubules are transient structures which, unless organized into specialized arrays (as in myofilaments, of muscle cells or microtubules of cilia), persist for periods of time ranging from only minutes to hours. The cell, thus, can regulate the activity of microfilaments and microtubule activity by their selective placement during polymerization. This placement is achieved, in part, by local fluctuations in the concentration of divalent calcium ions, the concentration of specific actin-binding proteins (both monomer-binding and filament-end-binding proteins), and the pH. It is because of the dynamic nature of microtubules and microfilament networks that antipolymerization agents (such as colchicine for microtubules) can result in their disappearance.

Intermediate Filaments. Intermediate filaments are a heterogeneous group of filaments. Five major classes of intermediate filaments have been identified on the basis of protein composition and their cellular distribution: *cytokeratin (or prekeratin)*, *vimentin, desmin, neurofilament,* and *glial fibrillary acidic protein.* These chemically distinct types of intermediate filaments are composed of subunits that differ in molecular weight. Immunolabeling techniques have been used to determine the distribution of these five types of intermediate filaments (see Table 2.1). The use of antibodies, which are specific to the various filament types, has also been useful in clinical medicine to aid in the

---

TABLE 2.1. Distribution of the Primary Types of Intermediate Filaments

TYPE OF FILAMENT (m.w.)*	CELL(S) WHERE FOUND
Cytokeratin (Prekeratin) (40,000–65,000)	Epithelial cells
Vimentin (55,000)	Cells of mesenchymal origin—including endothelial cells and some smooth muscle and myofibroblasts; and some cells of neuroectoderm origin
Desmin (51,000)	Muscle cells
Neurofilament (70,000, 140,000, and 210,000)	Neuronal cells
Glial fibrillary acidic protein (50,000)	Neuroglial cells—including oligodendroglia, astrocytes, microglia, Schwann cells, and ependymal cells and pituicytes

* The approximate molecular weight values of the polypeptide subunits are listed in the table. The neurofilament consists of three different filament polypeptides, which are sometimes referred to as a neurofilament triplet. Cytokeratin is a family of polypeptides that have a range of molecular weights.

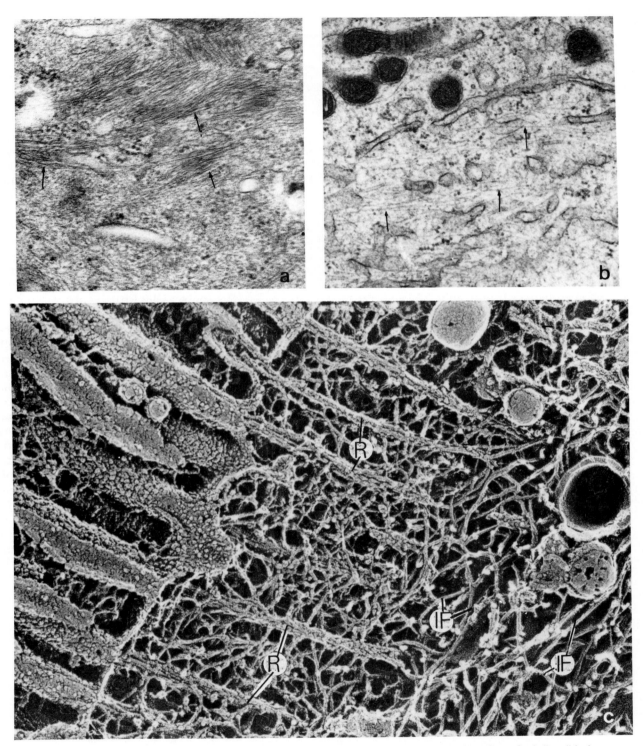

Figure 2.20(a). Electron micrograph showing the very thin microfilaments **(arrows)** within a Sertoli cell in human testis. × 45,000. **(b)** Electron micrograph showing aggregates of intermediate filaments **(arrows)** in the cytoplasm of a urinary bladder epithelial cell. The filament bundles are passing through the thickness of the section at oblique angles. Thus, their length within the cell cannot be appreciated. × 45,000. **(c)** Electron micrograph showing terminal web portion of an epithelial cell and underlying intermediate filaments. The epithelial cells were treated with glycerin after incubation in a medium containing no ATP. The long straight rootlets extending from the bases of the microvilli are cross-linked by a dense and complicated network of cross-linkers. Intermediate filaments can be seen at the base of the rootlets forming a foundation for these processes. (From Hirokawa et al: *J Cell Biol* 96:1325, 1983.)

diagnosis of tumors. For example, in the diagnosis of gliomas, a pathologist can utilize immunolabeling techniques and look for cells that are reactive with antiglial fibrillary acidic protein antibody.

The intermediate filaments appear to have a supporting or general structural function. The various classes of filaments differ in their amino acid sequence and show large variation in their molecular weight. They all share a homologous region, which is important in filament self-assembly and contain a region of variable length which is available for molecular contact with other intracellular structures and other functions within the cell. Intermediate filaments are approximately 8 to 11 nm in diameter (Fig. 2.20**b**). The intermediate filaments found in neurons and neuroglial cells are called **neurofilaments** and **glial filaments,** respectively. In epidermal cells, intermediate filaments include the filaments referred to as **tonofibrils** and are composed of proteins of the cytokeratin family. Some of the intermediate filaments of muscle and epidermis connect internal structures or organelles to transmembrane proteins that are bound to similar transmembrane proteins of neighboring cells or to extracellular matrix filaments (see Chapters 4 and 5). Intermediate filaments also do not typically disappear and reform in the continuous manner characteristic of most microtubules and microfilaments. It is for these reasons that intermediate filaments are believed to play a primarily structural role within the cell and to comprise the cytoplasmic link of a tissue-wide continuum of cytoplasmic, nuclear and extracellular filaments (Fig. 20**c**).

Centrioles

Classical cytologists identified a part of the cell near the nucleus as being important in the early stages of cell division. This part of the cell is called the **cell center centrosome,** or **centrosphere.** The special structural components of the cell center that are involved in mitosis are the centrioles. Each is comprised of nine sets of microtubule triplets arranged to form a short cylinder-like structure. The centrioles occur in pairs with one oriented at right angles to the other, that is, they have a T-shaped configuration (Fig. 2.21). Two of the microtubules in each triplet share a wall with an adjacent microtubule. Thus, in a cross-sectional profile the two microtubules appear to be C-shaped, while the third is O-shaped (CCO). Before cell division, each centriole duplicates itself. Duplication begins with the formation of a procentriole at a right angle to the surface of each of the original centrioles. The procentriole initially consists of nine single tubules arranged as a cylinder. An additional pair of tubules forms in association with each, thus giving rise to the nine triplet microtubules characteristic of the mature centriole. After duplication, the two centriolar pairs move to opposite poles in the cell and serve as the organizing centers for the formation of the mitotic spindles.

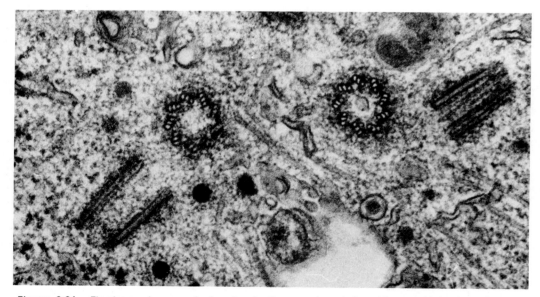

Figure 2.21. Electron micrograph showing both parent and daughter centrioles in a Chinese Hamster fibroblast. Note the transverse-sectioned centriole in each of the pairs reveals the triplet configuration of microtubules. The centriole in the **lower left** represents a midlongitudinal section, whereas the **upper right** centriole has also been longitudinally sectioned, but along the plane of its wall. × 90,000. (Courtesy of M. McGill, D. P. Highfield, T. M. Monahan, and B. Brinkley.)

Centrioles are known to be equally important in organizing the new microtubule system that forms in daughter cells from the tubulin dimers resulting from dismantling of mitotic spindle. The centriole and adjacent paracentriolar material thus constitute a general microtubule organizing center (MTOC) in both interphase and mitosis. The presence of a single MTOC in interphase cells, together with the inherent polarity of microtubules derived from the polarity of tubulin dimers (see above), provides a radial coordinate system by which the cell can distinguish center from periphery for the localization of its organelles and enzymes.

During the formation of cilia (and the flagellum that is often considered to be a modified cilium), centrioles replicate and migrate to the surface of cells on which cilia will develop. Each centriole serves as the organizer for assembly of the microtubules in the cilium. The core structure of a cilium is a complexly organized set of microtubules, consisting of two central microtubules surrounded by microtubule doublets (see Fig. 4.23). The organizing role is different from that in the MTOC for in this case axonemal microtubules are continuous with the microtubules of the centriole. The centriole then remains as the **basal body** of the cilium.

Inclusions

Inclusions are construed to be "nonliving" components of the cell; they do not participate in energy-requiring reactions. Included in the category of inclusion bodies are secretory granules and pigment granules, which are bounded by a membrane, and lipid and glycogen, which are not. The density of secretory granules in secretory cells is sensitive to the presence or absence of signalling agents, or "secretagogues," which trigger granule exocytosis by a receptor-activated second messenger cascade. Some highly active secretory cells lack secretory granules altogether because they exocytose their secretory proteins constitutively rather than in a secretagogue-dependent regulated manner. The hepatocyte, which continuously synthesizes and releases serum proteins, provides an example of constitutive exocytosis. In electron micrographs, glycogen appears as large granules about 25 to 30 nm in diameter or as clusters of such granules (see Fig. 2.10). Unless special steps are taken to preserve the glycogen, it is lost during the routine preparation of sections for light microscopy. Liver cells, which may contain large amounts of glycogen, display empty regions where the glycogen was formerly located.

Certain cells contain crystalline inclusions that are recognized with the light microscope. In the human, such inclusions are found in Sertoli and interstitial (Leydig) cells of the testis. With the electron microscope, crystalline inclusions have been found in many cell types and in virtually all parts of the cell including the nucleus and organelles. While some of these inclusions are storage material, the significance of others is not known.

Cytoplasmic Matrix

Morphologic techniques have provided relatively little information about the composition and organization of the cytoplasmic matrix (cytoplasmic ground substance or cytosol). It has an amorphous, structureless appearance with the light microscope (and with conventional thin-section TEM). It is considered to contain soluble electrolytes and molecules, including proteins and metabolites, that play a role in metabolism of the cell. More recent work, using the high voltage electron microscope and thicker specimens than conventionally used, or embedment-free sections, has shown that the ground substance contains a fine 3-dimensional network, or **cytoskeleton,** composed in part of the filaments and tubules which have been identified above (Fig. 2.3). Biophysical studies indicate that the distances between the components of the network approach but do not agree with the molecular dimensions of proteins dissolved in the cytosol. There is controversy, however, over whether conventional "soluble" proteins spend more time immobilized transiently onto this network or more time solvated in the aqueous fluid. This answer to this question surely will shed important light on the suspected microcompartmentalization of proteins in the cytoplasm of cells.

THE NUCLEUS

The nucleus plays a central role in gene expression, heredity, and cell division. It contains DNA (the macromolecule that contains the genetic information). Two activities of DNA, transcription and replication, provide for the expression of genetic information and for cell division, respectively. DNA, along with associated protein, is organized as chromosomes. However, the chromosomes themselves are not evident as discrete bodies except during cell division (mitosis or meiosis). During cell division the chromosomal material is coiled and gathered into the compact configurations described as **chromosomes.** In the nondividing cell, also referred to as the **interphase cell,** the chromosomal material is less tightly packed and it is designated as *chromatin.*

The nucleus of the interphase cell includes the following components: *chromatin,* the *nucleolus,* the *nuclear envelope,* the *nuclear cytoskeleton,* and the *nucleoplasm.*

Chromatin

Two arrangements of chromatin occur in the nucleus: *heterochromatin* (condensed chromatin) and *euchromatin* (extended chromatin). Heterochromatin is disposed in three locations (Fig. 2.22): (1) the *marginal chromatin,* at the perimeter of the nucleus (the structure light microscopist formerly referred to as the *nuclear membrane* actually consists largely of marginal chromatin); (2) the *karyosomes,* discrete bodies of irregular size and shape throughout the nucleus; and (3) the *nucleolar associated chromatin,* in association with the nucleolus. Heterochromatin stains with basic dyes and hematoxylin (because of the phosphate groups of the DNA); it is also readily displayed with the Feulgen procedures (a specific histochemical reaction for the deoxyribose of DNA) and fluorescent vital dyes such as Hoechst dyes and propidium iodide. It is the heterochromatin that accounts for the conspicuous staining of the nucleus in hematoxylin and eosin preparations.

Euchromatin is not evident with the light microscope. It is present with the nucleoplasm in the "clear" areas between the heterochromatin. In routine electron micrographs, there is no sharp delineation between euchromatin and heterochromatin; both have a granular-filamentous appearance, but the euchromatin is less tightly packed. Euchromatin is indicative of active chromatin; heterochromatin is regarded to be inactive chromatin. Generally, metabolically active cells, such as large neurons and liver cells, possess large amounts of euchromatin. An example of inactive chromatin is to be found in the head of the sperm, a very condensed package indeed.

The correlation between the chemical composition of chromatin and its structure as seen in sections with the electron microscope has not been entirely clarified. Special preparations of chromatin viewed with the electron microscope display long chains of particles joined by a thin thread. Each particle with its connecting thread is called a *nucleosome.* The thin thread consists of the portion of the DNA molecule in its double helical configuration which has unwound from the particle, whereas the particles consist of the DNA coiled about a core of histones.

Chromosomes

Human cells (except the gamete cells, the egg, and the sperm) contain 46 chromosomes organized as 23 homologous pairs (Fig. 2.23). In 22 of these homologous pairs, the partners are morphologically similar; these are called *autosomes.* One pair of chromosomes, the twenty-third pair, is comprised of the *sex chromosomes,* designated X and Y. In the female there is a homologous pair consisting of two X chromosomes; in the male the pair consists of an X and a Y chromosome. The chromosomal number 46, found in most *somatic cells* (cells of the body other than the *gametes,* or sex cells), is designated as *diploid* (*2n*). Each gamete, as a result of meiosis, have only 23 chromo-

---

CHROMOSOMAL PREPARATION

Because of its clinical importance, the student should know how chromosomes are examined by the cytologist. As already stated, the chromosomes are evident as individual bodies only during cell division. A brief account of how a chromosomal preparation is made follows:

Since all the somatic cells of the body contain similar chromosomes, it is convenient to use blood as a source of cells in making a chromosome preparation. Having obtained a sample of blood, the white blood cells are separated by standard procedures. The cells are placed in a special medium containing phytohemagglutinin, which stimulates the lymphocytes to undergo mitosis. The mitosis is interrupted in metaphase by the addition of colchicine, a drug that disrupts the microtubules of the mitotic spindle. The cells are then placed on a glass slide, fixed, stained, and viewed as a spread preparation. They are not sectioned in the usual manner of preparing a specimen for viewing with the microscope, but rather they are made to flatten and spread out on the glass slide by appropriate techniques. Figure 2.23 shows the chromosomes of a male and a female prepared in this manner. By cutting a photomicrograph of the specimen so that each segment contains one chromosome, it becomes possible to match chromosome pairs and arrange them in a sequence similar to that seen in the illustration. Such an arrangement is referred to as a *karyotype.* It allows the cytologist to study the chromosomal makeup of the individual. Special stains (banding techniques) allow the study of localized regions of specific chromosomes.

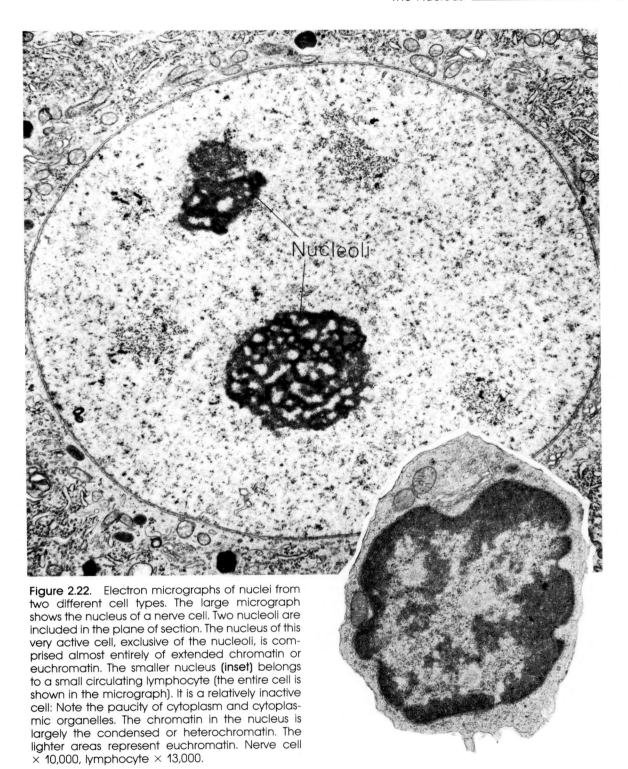

Nucleoli

Figure 2.22. Electron micrographs of nuclei from two different cell types. The large micrograph shows the nucleus of a nerve cell. Two nucleoli are included in the plane of section. The nucleus of this very active cell, exclusive of the nucleoli, is comprised almost entirely of extended chromatin or euchromatin. The smaller nucleus **(inset)** belongs to a small circulating lymphocyte (the entire cell is shown in the micrograph). It is a relatively inactive cell: Note the paucity of cytoplasm and cytoplasmic organelles. The chromatin in the nucleus is largely the condensed or heterochromatin. The lighter areas represent euchromatin. Nerve cell × 10,000, lymphocyte × 13,000.

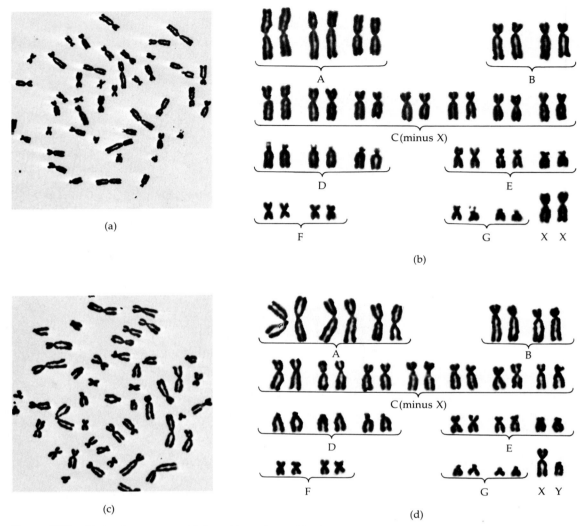

Figure 2.23. Metaphase spread **(a)** and karyotype **(b)** of a normal female; metaphase spread **(c)** and karyotype **(d)** of a normal male. Note that the only difference in the karyotypes is the sex chromosomes: Females have two X chromosomes, and males have one X chromosome and one Y chromosome. (Identification of the X chromosome among the C-group chromosomes is somewhat arbitrary without special staining procedures.) (Courtesy of Dr. M. W. Shaw. From Hartl DL: *Human Genetics.* New York, Harper & Row, 1983.)

somes, one member of each homologous pair. This number is designated as **haploid** (***n***). At the time of fertilization, the chromosomal number is again reestablished at 46; 23 from the egg and 23 from the sperm.

Barr Body

Some chromosomes are repressed in the interphase nucleus and exist in the tightly packed heterochromatic form. One X chromosome of the female is an example of such a chromosome. This chromosome was discovered in 1949 by Barr and Bertram in nerve cells of female cats where it ap-

pears as a well-stained round body, now called the **Barr body,** adjacent to the nucleolus. Although it was originally found in sectioned tissue, it was subsequently learned that any relatively large number of cells prepared as a smear (for example, scrapings of the oral mucous membrane from the inside of the cheeks) might be used in a search for the Barr body. In cells of the oral mucous membrane, the Barr body is located adjacent to the nuclear envelope (Fig. 2.24). Obviously, both in sections and in smears, many cells need to be examined in order to find those whose orientation is suitable for the display of the Barr body.

Figure 2.24. Photomicrograph of nuclei of oral mucosal cells showing Barr bodies in female (**arrows**). (K. I. Moore and M. L. Barr, 1955).

Sex chromatin

of infant female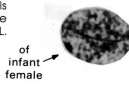

of adult female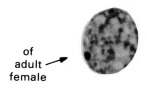

Not seen in male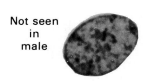

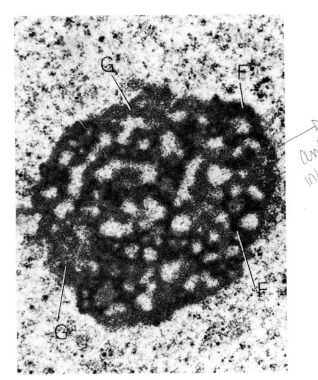

Figure 2.25. Electron micrograph of the nucleolus from a nerve cell showing the DNA-containing interstices (the light areas), the pars granulosa (G)-containing accumulated ribonucleoprotein particles, and the pars fibrosa (F), which has a more electron dense appearance.

Nucleolus

The nucleolus is a spherical body within the nucleus. It varies in size, being especially well developed in cells active in protein synthesis. It is the site of ribosomal RNA production and initial ribosomal assembly. In some cells, there may be more than one nucleolus.

The nucleolus consists largely of RNA and protein. Some DNA is present (nucleolar organizer regions), but the amount is so small that Feulgen-stained specimens viewed with the light microscope react negatively for DNA. The nucleolus is, however, often rimmed by DNA-positive reaction product that is identified as the nucleolus associated chromatin. The nucleolus stains well with hematoxylin; it also stains well with basic dyes. Predigestion of the specimen with the enzyme RNase can be used to demonstrate that the basophilia of the nucleolus is due to RNA.

With the electron microscope the nucleolus is seen to consist of a network of granular and fibrillar material (Fig. 2.25). The *pars granulosa* is that portion of the nucleolus that consists of granular material (RNA). The *pars fibrosa* consists of extremely fine filaments (also RNA) packed very tightly and seen as the "darkest" component of the nucleolus. The network formed by the pars granulosa and pars fibrosa is referred to as the nucleolonema. The interstices of the network (that is,

the "clear" areas) contain DNA in small amounts, and they are the regions where ribosomal RNA is synthesized.

Nuclear Envelope

The nuclear envelope is comprised of two parallel membrane with an intervening perinuclear space (Fig. 2.26). At numerous points over the surface of the nucleus there are small "openings," approximately 70 nm in diameter, in the nuclear envelope, which have been designated *nuclear pores*. The pores are not true unrestricted channels since a selective transport mechanism operates to transport proteins and RNAs that are too large to diffuse through the channels. Although the nuclear pores appear to be more or less circular in face view, they are, in fact, octagonal at their circumference. The nuclear pores have been shown to be channels through which substances pass from the nucleus to the cytoplasm and vice versa.

The outer membrane of the nuclear envelopes may be studded with ribosomes, and in places the

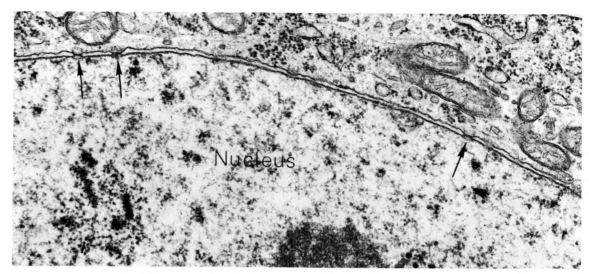

Figure 2.26. Electron micrograph of the nuclear envelope showing the nuclear pores **(arrows)** and the two membranes that constitute the "envelope." At the periphery of each pore the outer and inner membranes of the nuclear envelope are continuous. × 30,000.

outer membrane is continuous with the rER. In these places the perinuclear space and the cisternae of the rER are continuous.

The inner membrane of the envelope is lined at its nucleoplasmic surface by a filamentous mat referred to as the *nuclear lamina*. Evidence is accumulating that some of the protein lamins that comprise the lamina are related to intermediate filament subunits. The lamina has been suggested to serve as a scaffolding for chromatin, chromatin-associated proteins, nuclear pores, and the nuclear membranes themselves.

Nucleoplasm

All of the material enclosed by the nuclear envelope excluding the chromatin and the nucleolus is referred to as the *nucleoplasm*. It is amorphous. Not much is presently known about its composition, although it seems that it must contain proteins and metabolites diffusing throughout the nucleus.

CELL DIVISION

Cells divide by two processes, *mitosis* and *meiosis,* which are fundamentally different and serve two distinctly different purposes. Mitosis is the process of cell division by which somatic cells divide. It assures that each daughter cell receives a diploid set of (2n) chromosomes (46 in the human) just as the parent cell. In mitosis, the continuity of the chromosome number and genetic complement is preserved through successive cell divisions. In

contrast, meiosis, the process that gives rise to the gametes, brings about a reduction in the number of chromosomes from 46 (2n) to 23 (n), and it allows for the interchange of hereditary material between chromosomes. Thus, whereas mitosis ensures a continuation of identical hereditary material, meiosis provides for the diversification of the hereditary material (see also Chapter 21).

CELL CYCLE

Cells of the adult body can be classified into three populations, static, stable, and renewing, according to the amount of mitotic activity displayed by the tissue. (Mitotic activity may be judged by autoradiographic studies of the incorporation of tritiated thymidine, indicative of DNA doubling before mitosis; see Fig. 1.5). *Static cell populations* include cells that no longer divide (nerve and skeletal muscle cells) or rarely divide (smooth and cardiac muscle cells). *Stable cell populations* engage in relatively little mitotic activity, but are able to divide more vigorously under certain conditions, such as in the repair of a tissue after an injury. Included in this category are fibroblasts, osteoblasts, and the epithelium of many organs. *Renewing cell populations* display regular mitotic activity. The cell divisions typically result in the production of one cell that is similar to the parent cell and another cell that becomes differentiated. Moreover, the differentiated cell may be dispensable. Examples of renewing cell populations are blood cells, epithelial cells of the skin, and epithelial cells of the lining of the alimentary canal.

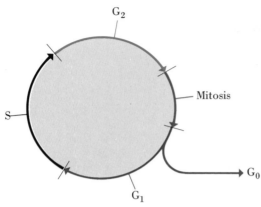

Figure 2.27. Scheme of cell cycle of rapidly dividing cells in relation to DNA synthesis. After *mitosis*, the cell is in interphase. G_1 represents the period in which there is a lull or gap in DNA synthesis. S represents the period during which DNA synthesis occurs. This is the period during which (tritiated) thymidine is incorporated into the DNA to serve as an experimental tracer. G_2 represents a second lull, or gap, in DNA synthesis. G_0 represents the path of a cell that no longer stays in the compartment of rapidly dividing cells. Such a cell is said to be outside of the cycle.

For renewing cell and stable cell populations and cells that constitute a growing population (embryonic cells, cells in culture, cells in tumors), it is possible to outline a cell cycle in terms of the changes in DNA synthesis during repeating cell divisions (Fig. 2.27). The cycle is divided into two principal stages, mitosis and interphase. Interphase is further divided into G_1, S, and G_2 phases. The G_1, or gap 1, phase is a period of time after a mitotic division during which cell growth occurs. G_1 is also the stage at which exogenous factors regulate when the next cell cycle will be activated. It is followed by a period of DNA synthesis, the S phase, during which the amount of DNA is doubled. The S phase is followed by a period of time during which no DNA synthesis occurs. This is the G_2, or gap 2, phase.

Cells that no longer divide, such as those belonging to the static or stable populations, are best thought of having left the cycle. These cells are "outside" the cycle and they may be designated as G_0. Typically, G_0 cells leave the cycle from the G_1 phase. Occasionally some cells leave the cycle in G_2 after DNA synthesis (i.e., after the S phase); they possess twice the amount of DNA as G_1 cells, although the chromosome number has not changed. Cells identified as *reserve stem cells* may be thought of as G_0 cells that may be induced to reenter the cell cycle in response to injury of the cell populations within the tissues of the body. Such activation of the reserve stem cells may occur in the repopulation of the seminiferous epithelium after intense acute exposure of the testis to X-irradiation or during regeneration of an organ, such as the liver, after removal of a major portion of it. If the damage to the tissues is too severe, even the reserve stem are killed and there is no potential for regeneration.

Tissues: Concept and Classification

3

In examining the structure of the body at the light microscopic level, it soon becomes apparent that the cells and extracellular substances comprising the various organs and parts of the body exhibit a variety of recognizable, often distinctive, organizational patterns. Indeed, it is usually the orderly arrangement and distinctive patterns of the cells that tend to catch the eye. This organized arrangement is a reflection of the cooperative efforts that like cells perform in carrying out a particular function. When we speak of an organized aggregation of cells that function in a collective manner, we are, by definition, referring to a tissue. Although it is frequently said that the cell is the functional unit of the body, it is really the tissues through the collaborative efforts of their individual cells that are responsible for maintaining body functions. Furthermore, it is now well known that cells within a tissue can communicate through specialized intercellular junctions, thus facilitating collaborative effort. Such junctions (gap junctions) represent sites that not only mediate electric coupling between cells, but also permit the preferential passage of small molecules from one cell to the next.

The concept of tissues provides a basis for understanding and recognizing the many cell types within the body and how they interrelate. Despite variations in general appearance, structural organization, and physiological properties of the various body organs, the cell aggregations that make them up are reduced to and classified under four tissue types. These *basic* or *fundamental tissues* are: (1) *epithelial tissue (epithelium)*; (2) *connective tissue;* (3) *muscular tissue;* and (4) *nervous tissue.* Each of these basic tissues is defined by a set of general morphological characteristics or by functional properties. Each type may be further subdivided

on the basis of more specific characteristics of the various cell populations (as well as intercellular substances in those cases where they present special characteristics). In considering the basic tissues, it should be recognized that two different definitional parameters are employed. The basis for the definition of epithelium and connective tissue is primarily morphological, the basis for the definition of muscular and nervous tissue is functional.

Epithelium is characterized by the close apposition of its constituent cells and their presence at a free surface. A free surface is one to which no cellular or extracellular formed elements adhere, such as the surface that forms the outer covering of the exterior of the body, the outer covering of some internal organs, or the lining of body cavities, tubes, or ducts, both those that ultimately communicate with the exterior of the body and those that are enclosed. The various types of epithelia are subclassified on the basis of location as well as the shape and arrangement of the cells.

Connective tissue, unlike epithelium, contains cells that noticeably are separated from one another. The intervening spaces are occupied by intercellular material formed by the connective tissue cells. The cells and intercellular material vary according to the particular type of connective tissue. Consequently, the subclassification of connective tissue considers not only the cells, but also the composition and organization of the intercellular material. Figure 3.1 shows the essential differences between a typical epithelium and its subjacent connective tissue. Note the relative position of the cells within each tissue.

In contrast to epithelium and connective tissue, nerve and muscle are classified on the basis of their functional roles. Strictly speaking, *nervous tis-*

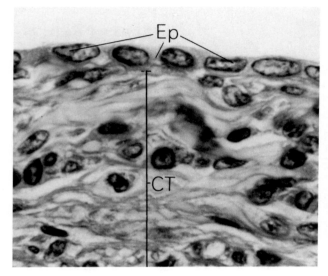

Figure 3.1. Comparison of an epithelium (Ep) and connective tissue (CT). Note that the epithelial cells possess one surface that is not adherent to other cells. This is the free surface. Furthermore, the epithelial cells have established themselves in a single layer to form a continuous surface cover. Their nuclei have a uniform appearance and orientation. The cells of the connective tissue are of several types and appear randomly disposed. The nuclei exhibit varied sizes and shapes. The cytoplasm is difficult to discern and tends to blend with the connective tissue fibers.

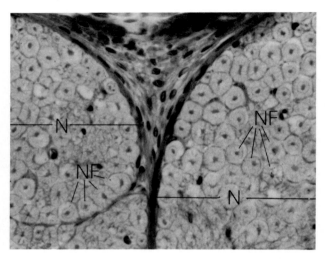

Figure 3.2. A section through a nerve showing part of two smaller nerve bundles (N). The bulk of the nerve is comprised of long thread-like nerve fibers (NF). The fibers are tightly packed together, and because they have been cut in cross-section, they give a circular profile pattern. The dot-like units represent the thin cytoplasmic processes or axons of the nerve fibers. The surrounding material is myelin, which forms a highly specialized "insulating" cover.

sue consists of nerve cells, called **neurons,** and associated supporting cells of various types. In the central nervous system, the supporting cells are referred to as **neuroglia** and in the peripheral nervous system they are referred to as **Schwann** and **satellite cells.** While all cells exhibit electrical properties, neurons are highly specialized to transmit electrical impulses from one site in the body to another and to integrate such impulses. This functional capacity is reflected in the morphology of the neuron, particularly the cytoplasmic processes that emanate from the cell body and the interconnections between these cell processes. In an ordinary tissue section, nervous tissue may be observed in the form of a nerve, consisting of varying numbers of neuronal processes along with their supporting cells (Fig. 3.2), or in the form of a ganglion, where the nerve cell bodies are present (Fig. 3.3).

Muscle tissue is also categorized as a fundamental tissue on the basis of a functional property, namely, the ability of the cells to contract. The appearance of the several types of muscle tissue is such that, with few exceptions, they are easily recognized. In order to form an effective contractile unit, the muscle cells, or fibers as they are usually called, tend to be aggregated in bundles that have a

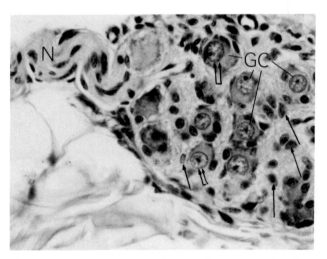

Figure 3.3. A section through a small ganglion. Here the principal feature is the relatively large ganglion cells or nerve cell bodies that possess large nuclei **(double arrows)**. Many other smaller cells are present, as evidenced by the small nuclei **(arrows)**. Most of these are supporting or satellite cells, which are intimately associated with the nerve cell bodies. A longitudinal section of a nerve (N) leaving (or entering) the ganglion is also evident. The nerve fibers are longitudinally disposed in this section. Furthermore, they are unmyelinated, and without a myelin cover the small nerve process is difficult to define.

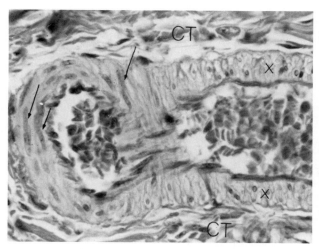

Figure 3.4. A section of a small artery making a right angle turn within the section. The right portion of the micrograph shows the vessel longitudinally cut, whereas on the left it has been cross-sectioned. The wall of the vessel is comprised largely of smooth muscle cells, which have an elongate shape. They are packed together, parallel to one another, and tend to circumscribe the lumen of the vessel. Thus, where the vessel is longitudinally sectioned the smooth muscle cells are seen in cross-section (X) and the elongate nuclei appear as small circular profiles. Where the vessel has turned and is cross-sectioned, the nuclei of the smooth muscle cells are seen as elongate profiles (arrows). The pattern of the nuclei is distinctive in both instances.

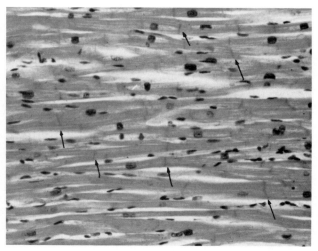

Figure 3.5. A section of cardiac muscle, which consists of elongate cells, larger in size than the smooth muscle cells just examined. As in the case of smooth muscle, the muscle cells seen here are arranged in parallel arrays, and when longitudinally sectioned, a linear pattern is readily discernible. The cells are attached end-to-end, forming a "fiber" structure. The muscle fibers anastomose with one another as evidenced by branching of the fibers. The faint vertical lines (arrows) seen at this magnification are specialized sites, which maintain adhesion between adjoining cells.

distinctive appearance, usually quite different from the surrounding tissues. Figures 3.4 and 3.5 show two types of muscle, *smooth* and *striated.* Note that the cells are oriented in the same direction, as evidenced by the arrangement of their nuclei. While the cells that comprise each of these muscle types appear distinctly different, they share one property, namely, the bulk of their cytoplasm is occupied by the contractile proteins *actin* and *myosin.* It is the interaction of these two proteins that effects shortening of the cells. Actin and myosin are not limited to those cells that are traditionally categorized as muscle tissue; they are also found in a wide variety of cells belonging to the other types of tissues. In these cases, however, the contractile components usually do not constitute a substantial portion of the cytoplasm and they usually are encoded by duplicate genes with subtly different sequences. They may be present in a cell whose principal role has nothing to do with organ movement, but rather the contractile components may serve only in providing localized shape changes within the cell.

By keeping in mind the few basic facts and concepts concerning the fundamental tissues, the task of examining and interpreting histological slide material can be greatly facilitated. The first goal is that of recognizing aggregates of cells as tissues and determining what special characteristics they present. Are the cells present at a surface? Are they in contact with their neighbors or are they separated by a definable intervening material? Do they belong to a group having special properties such as muscle or nerve?

The elements that characterize each of the fundamental tissues and relate to its functional aspects will be examined in the following chapters. It is important to realize that in focusing on a single specific tissue we are, in a sense, artificially separating the constituent tissues of organs. However, only after having dealt with each of the basic tissues and its subtypes in this way is it possible to understand and appreciate the histology of the various organs of the body and the means by which they operate as functional units.

Epithelium

4

CHARACTERISTICS AND FUNCTION

Epithelium is comprised of cells that cover the exterior surfaces of the body and line both the internal closed cavities of the body and those body tubes that communicate with the exterior (the alimentary, respiratory, and genitourinary tracts). Epithelium also forms the secretory portion (parenchyma) of glands and their ducts and the receptors of certain sensory organs.

The cells forming epithelium are in close apposition with one another. They may be arranged in multiple layers, as in the covering of the exterior surfaces of the body where protection and impermeability are primary requirements, or in a single layer, as in the lining of most of the internal surfaces of the body. By virtue of their location and organization, epithelia also exhibit a free surface, one at which there are no adherent cellular or extracellular formed elements other than coating substances. The opposite surface, that part which adjoins the underlying connective tissue, adheres to the **basement membrane** (Fig. 4.1). This is a noncellular, protein-polysaccharide-rich layer demonstrable at the light microscopic level by histochemical methods.

In some locations, cells are found aggregated in close apposition with one another, but lack a free surface. While the close relationship of these cells would lead to their classification as an epithelium, the absence of a free surface is sufficient to justify terming such cell aggregates as epithelial-like or **epithelioid tissues.** Examples of epithelioid tissues include the interstitial cells of Leydig in the testis, the luteal cells of the ovary, the parenchyma of the adrenal gland, and the epithelioreticular cells of the thymus.

A given epithelium may serve one or more functions, depending upon the cell types present.

It may be an almost impervious barrier, as in the epidermis of skin and urinary bladder; it may be secretory, as in the stomach; or it may be both secretory and absorptive, as in the intestines. Covering and lining epithelia form a continuous, sheet-like cellular investment that separates the underlying connective tissue from the external environment and from the environment of internal cavities. This investment serves as a selective barrier capable of facilitating or inhibiting the passage of specific substances between the exterior (as well as the body cavities) and the underlying connective tissue compartment. In the study of the various organs it will be seen that any substance that enters the body or is discharged from the body as a waste product must literally pass through the epithelial cells, not between them (Fig. 4.2).

CLASSIFICATION OF EPITHELIA

Classification of the various epithelia of the body is based on the arrangement and shape of the cells. Thus, the terminology used is unrelated to function but is related to structure. Epithelium may be described as **simple,** consisting of one cell layer, or **stratified,** consisting of two or more cell layers. The individual cells may be described as **squamous,** where the width and depth of the cell is greater than its height; **cuboidal,** where the width, depth, and height are approximately the same; or **columnar,** where the height of the cell appreciably exceeds the width and depth. The term **low columnar** is often used where a cell's height only slightly exceeds its other dimensions. The cells in a number of exocrine glands have a more or less pyramidal shape with their apices directed toward the lumen of the glands. These cells are classified either as cuboidal or columnar depending on their height. In a stratified epithelium, the shape and

51

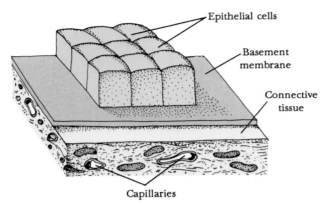

Epithelial cells

Basement membrane

Connective tissue

Capillaries

Figure 4.1. Diagram showing location of basement membrane interposed between the epithelium and the underlying connective tissue. Note the epithelial cells are in close apposition and their basal surface rests on the basement membrane.

height of the cells usually vary from layer to layer, but only the shape of the cells forming the surface layer is utilized in categorizing the epithelium. Thus, in designating an epithelium as stratified squamous, we are stating that it consists of more than one layer of cells and that the surface layer is comprised of flat or squamous cells.

Two special categories of epithelium are typically included in classification, namely, ***pseudostratified*** and ***transitional epithelium.*** A pseudostratified epithelium has the appearance of being stratified. Some of the cells do not reach the free surface, but all rest on the basement membrane. Thus, it is actually a simple epithelium. Because pseudostratified epithelium has a rather limited distribution in the body, its identification usually

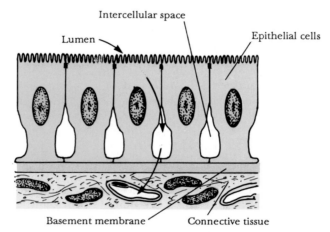

Intercellular space

Lumen

Epithelial cells

Basement membrane

Connective tissue

Figure 4.2. Diagram of absorptive cells, like those of the intestine. The pathway of fluid movement, indicated by the **arrows**, is from the intestinal lumen into the cell, then to the lateral intercellular space, and across the basement membrane to the connective tissue.

depends on the knowledge of where it exists rather than on the ability to discern that all of the cells contact the basement membrane. ***Transitional epithelium*** is a special name applied to the epithelium lining the pelvis of the kidney, ureters, urinary bladder, and part of the urethra. It is a stratified epithelium that has rather specific morphological characteristics and functionally accommodates well to the distension these organs undergo. This epithelium will be dealt with in more detail in the urinary system.

It should also be pointed out that specific names are applied to epithelium in certain locations. ***Endothelium*** is the name given to the epithelial lining of the vascular system. ***Mesothelium*** is the epithelium that lines the walls and covers the contents of the thoracic, pericardial, and abdominal cavities of the body. Both endothelium and mesothelium are almost always classified as simple squamous epithelia.

The morphology of the epithelium and its resident cells can often be correlated with functional activity. For example, epithelia involved in secretion or absorption are typically simple or pseudostratified. The height of the cells often reflects the level of secretory or absorptive activity. Simple squamous epithelia are compatible with a high rate of transepithelial transport if no intracellular processing of the transported substance occurs. Stratification of the epithelium usually correlates with transepithelial impermeability. Finally, the pseudostratified arrangement of some epithelia reflects the role of stem cells in maintaining a stable population of cells to balance cell turnover. The basal cells in epithelia of this type are often members of a renewing cell population.

The cellular configurations of the various types of epithelia and their appropriate nomenclature are illustrated in Figure 4.3.

BASEMENT MEMBRANE

Structure of the Basement Membrane

Basement membrane is the term originally given to a layer of variable thickness and distinction found at the basal surfaces of epithelia. It was believed that this layer consisted of a condensed, gel-like substance and delicate reticular fibers, which together served to attach the epithelium to the underlying connective tissue. In a few instances, the basement membrane is seen as a prominent structure in hematoxylin and eosin (H&E) preparations, a typical example being the trachea (Fig. 4.4). In most organs, the basement membrane

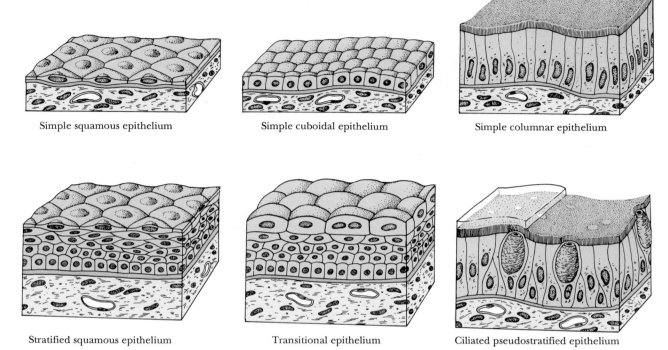

Simple squamous epithelium

Simple cuboidal epithelium

Simple columnar epithelium

Stratified squamous epithelium

Transitional epithelium

Ciliated pseudostratified epithelium

Figure 4.3. Diagrams illustrating the three-dimensional arrangements of cells in different types of epithelia and their descriptive nomenclature.

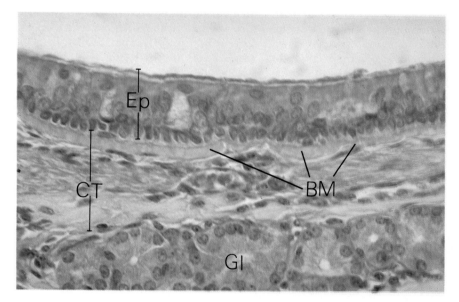

Figure 4.4. Photomicrograph of an H&E preparation showing the basement membrane of the trachea. It appears as a thick homogeneous structure lying immediately below the epithelium (EP). It is actually a part of the connective tissue (CT) and is comprised largely of densely packed connective tissue fibrils (collagen). Note that the epithelia forming the glands (GI) in the tracheal wall do not exhibit a similar structure. In order to demonstrate the basement membrane associated with the epithelium of the glands, as is the case with most other epithelia, special staining techniques, such as the PAS technique, are required. × 450.

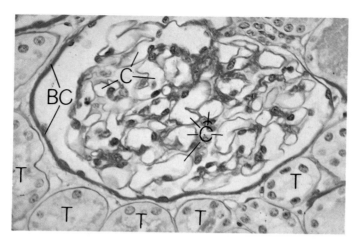

Figure 4.5. Photomicrograph of a PAS kidney preparation. The deep pink staining sites represent basement membrane. The kidney tubules (T) are sharply delineated by the stained surrounding basement membrane. The glomerular capillaries (C) and the parietal epithelium of Bowman's capsule (BC) also show PAS-positive basement membrane.

appears much thinner and is usually indistinct. With the development of the periodic acid–Schiff (PAS) technique, it was shown that the site of the basement membrane gives a positive reaction, appearing as a well-defined pink layer (Fig. 4.5). A technique involving the reduction of silver, wherein the basement membrane is blackened, also has been utilized to demonstrate this structure. While the basement membrane was classically described as being exclusively associated with epithelia, PAS-positive and silver reactive sites can

also be demonstrated in relation to nerve supporting cells, adipocytes, and muscle cells (Fig. 4.6). In these tissues, the PAS reaction product sharply delineates the cells from the surrounding connective tissue. The cells of the connective tissue (other than adipocytes), in contrast, do not show a similar PAS-positive reaction.

Examination of the site of epithelial basement membrane with the electron microscope reveals a continuous layer of electron-dense material, 50 to 100 nm thick (Fig. 4.7), which can often be further

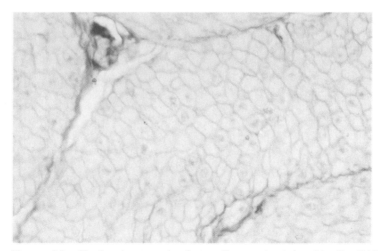

Figure 4.6. Photomicrograph of smooth muscle stained by the PAS method and counterstained with hematoxylin. The muscle cells have been cut in cross-section and appear as polygonal profiles due to the presence of PAS reactive material surrounding each cell. As the plane of section passes through each smooth muscle cell it may or may not pass through the portion of the cell that includes the nucleus. Therefore, in some of the polygonal profiles, pale staining nuclei can be seen; in other profiles, no nuclei are seen. The cytoplasm is not stained by the method used. × 850.

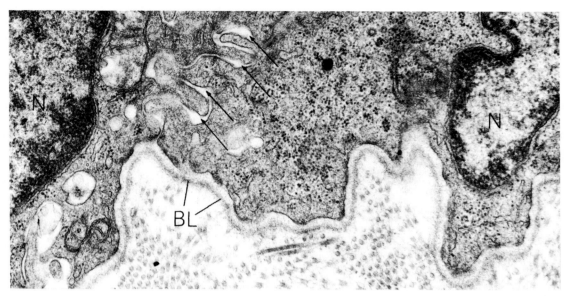

Figure 4.7. An electron micrograph showing only the very basal portion of two adjoining epithelial cells and part of their nuclei (N). The intercellular space is partially obscured by lateral interdigitations between the two cells (**arrows**). The basal lamina (BL) appears as a thin band, which follows the contours of the basal aspect of the overlying cell. Below the basal lamina are numerous cross-sectioned connective tissue fibrils (collagen). × 30,000.

resolved to contain a network of extremely fine (3 to 4 nm) filaments embedded in an amorphous matrix. This thin layer intervening between the epithelium and the adjacent connective tissue is referred to as the **basal lamina.** Between the basal lamina and the overlying epithelial cell plasma membrane is a narrow electron-lucid region, which is referred to as the lamina lucida (or lamina rara). Examination of muscle and nerve fibers reveals a surrounding extracellular electron-dense material having the same appearance as the basal lamina of epithelium. It is, thus, not surprising that the immediate extracellular environs of the cells belonging to these tissues are also PAS reactive. While the term basement membrane has not been applied to the extracellular stainable material of nonepithelial cells in light microscopy, the term basal lamina is typically used at the electron microscope level.[1]

Chemical analysis of the basal lamina derived from the epithelia in several locations (kidney glomeruli, lung, cornea, lens of the eye) indicates that it consists principally of collagen, proteoglycans rich in heparan sulfate, laminin, and other glycoproteins. Immunolocalization studies have generalized these findings to all basal laminae. The collagen is designated type IV collagen and represents one of approximately ten types of collagen in the body. Type IV collagen does not form fibrils as do the other types. Moreover, it has a much higher content of hydroxyproline, hydroxylysine, and carbohydrate side chains. Collagen of basal laminae has been shown to be a product of the epithelial cells, whereas the connective tissue collagens are produced by fibroblasts and related cell types. It is generally thought that the collagen provides a property of structural integrity to the basal lamina. It is also likely (see below) that the basal lamina collagen is responsible for the silver reaction observed in the light microscope. The PAS-positive reaction is (of course) due to its carbohydrate moiety.

Much of the bulk volume of the basal lamina is probably contributed by the heparin sulfate proteoglycan molecules that, owing to their highly anionic character, are extensively hydrated (see Chapter 5). Laminin is believed to bridge the lamina lucida to link the basal lamina with the basal plasma membrane surface of the overlying epithelial cells. Collagen fibrils of a different type may anchor the basal lamina to the underlying connec-

---

[1] At the present time there is some confusion in the usage of the terms **basement membrane** and **basal lamina.** Some authors use basement membrane interchangeably for light and electron microscopy. Others dispense with the term basement membrane and use basal lamina for light and electron microscopy. Since the term basement membrane originated with light microscopy, it will be used in this book only in the context of light microscopic descriptions and then only in relation to epithelia. The term basal lamina will be reserved for the ultrastructural level to denote the thin extracellular layer present at the interface of connective tissue with epithelial cells, Schwann cells, and smooth, cardiac, and skeletal muscle cells. The term **external lamina** may be a more appropriate term to use to identify this layer when it forms a circumferential cellular investment as opposed to basal lamina when dealing with epithelium.

tive tissue or reticular lamina (see below). These molecular associations are reinforced by additional glycoproteins, which interconnect or cross-link the molecules to achieve even greater stability between the basal lamina and the structures that interface with it.

There is currently lack of agreement as to what extent the basal lamina corresponds to the basement membrane of light microscopy. Some investigators contend that the basement membrane includes not only the basal lamina, but also a secondary layer, the *reticular lamina,* which is comprised of small unit fibrils of collagen (reticular fibers of light microscopy) that immediately underlies the basal lamina. The reticular lamina, as such, belongs to the connective tissue and is not a product of the epithelium. These investigators regard the reticular lamina as the component that is reactive with silver, while the PAS reaction is thought to stain principally the polysaccharides of the basal lamina and perhaps also the adjacent ground sub-

stance associated with the reticular fibers. However, convincing arguments can be made for the basal lamina alone to be responsible for both the PAS and silver reactions. For example, in normal kidney glomeruli there are no collagen (reticular) fibrils in relation to the basal lamina of the epithelial cells (Fig. 4.8), yet a positive reaction occurs with PAS and the silver impregnation. Also, in the case of the venous sinuses of the spleen, where the basal lamina forms a unique pattern consisting of ring-like bands around the vessel rather than a thin sheath-like layer, a complementary picture can be seen in the light microscope with both the silver and PAS techniques. Thus, the pattern of the reactive sites corresponds to the unusual configuration of the basal lamina as seen with the electron microscope (Fig. 4.9).

Function of the Basement Membrane

The role of basement membrane (basal lamina) is not well understood. It is generally

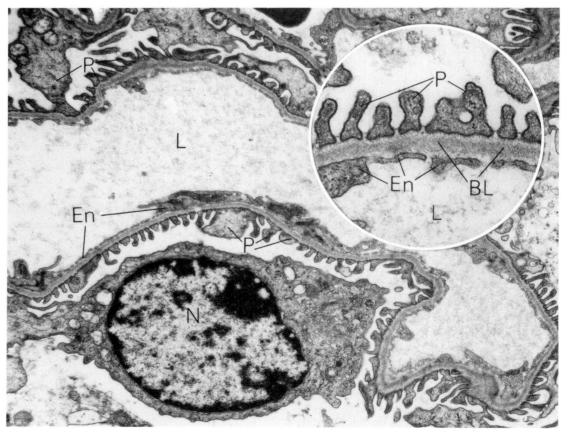

Figure 4.8. An electron micrograph of a kidney glomerular capillary. A basal lamina (BL) is seen interposed between the endothelial cell of the capillary (En) and the cytoplasmic processes (P) of the podocytes, which are located on the outer (abluminal) surface of the endothelial cell. The inset shows the relationship at higher magnification. Note that the two epithelial cells are separated by the basal lamina and no collagen fibrils are present. N, nucleus of podocyte; L, lumen of capillary. × 12,000; inset, × 40,0000.

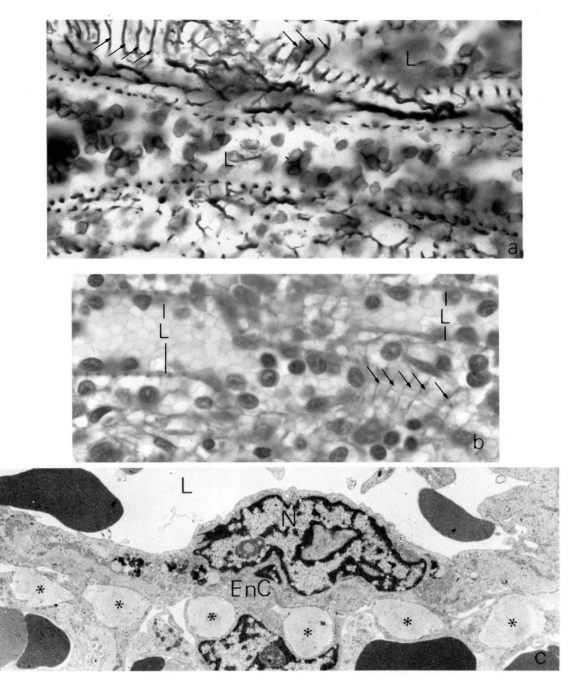

Figure 4.9(a). A photomicrograph of a silver preparation revealing two longitudinally sectioned venous sinuses of the spleen. These blood vessels are surrounded by a modified basement membrane, which takes the form of a ring-like structure much like the hoops of a barrel. The rings are blackened by the silver and appear as bands where the walls of the vessel have been tangentially sectioned (upper left, **arrows**). To the right the cut has penetrated deeper into the vessel, showing the lumen (L), and the cut edges of the rings are seen on both sides of the vessel. In the lower vessel, the cut rings have been sectioned in a virtual perpendicular plane, and the ring appears as a series of dots. × 400.

Figure 4.9(b). A photomicrograph of a PAS preparation of spleen. The basement membrane material is PAS-positive and shows the same structural configuration. Again, note the PAS-positive bands **(arrows)** where the section grazes the wall of the vessel **(arrows)** and the dot-like configuration where the cut has penetrated into the lumen (L). × 400.

Figure 4.9(c). An electron micrograph of the wall of a venous sinus showing a longitudinally sectioned endothelial cell **(EnC)**. The nucleus **(N)** of the cell is protruding into the lumen. The basal lamina material is identified by the **asterisks**. It has the same homogeneous appearance as seen in other sites, except it is aggregated into ring-like structures rather than into a flat layer or lamina. Moreover, its location and plane of section, as seen here, correspond to the silver and PAS-reactive dot-like material in Figure 4.9(a) and **(b)**. × 25,000.

thought to provide attachment of the epithelium to the underlying connective tissue and to influence the differentiation and proliferation of the epithelial cells that contact it.

Other proposed roles include providing a selective filtration barrier to substances moving between the interstitium and the parenchymal cell and possibly providing a scaffold during embryogenesis and regeneration. It is well known that under certain pathological conditions the basement membrane may undergo marked change. In diabetes, a disease that exacts a heavy toll on the vascular system, there is a striking thickening of the basement membrane of the small blood vessels. The capillaries of diabetics are more leaky to plasma proteins than normal, despite the increased thickness of the basement membrane. Increased production of type IV collagen and laminin appears to be responsible for the thickening of the basement membrane. However, diabetics demonstrate a decreased synthesis and accumulation of heparin sulfate proteoglycan, which may contribute to the increased permeability of the capillaries. It has also been suggested that thickening may be caused, in part, by the enhanced binding of proteins to the basement membrane. Also, in membrane glomerulonephritis, as well as in certain other nephritic syndromes, there is a thickening of the basal lamina of the kidney glomerular capillaries. The significance of these changes and their specific effect on tissue function is unclear. This is a reflection of our poor understanding of the role of the basement membrane.

CELL ADHESION AND INTERCELLULAR CONTACTS

Epithelial cells are not only characteristically in close apposition, but, with few exceptions, they are also extremely adherent to one another. Prior to the advent of electron microscopy it was thought that this property of adhesion was due to the presence of a viscous adhesive substance, referred to as "intercellular cement." It was also noted that the cement substance stained deeply at the apical-lateral margin of the cells of most cuboidal and columnar types of epithelium. When viewed in a plane perpendicular to the epithelial surface, the stainable material gives the appearance of a dot-like structure. However, when the plane of section passes parallel to and includes the epithelial surface, the dot-like component (described above) is seen as a dense bar or line between the apposing cells (Fig. 4.10). The bars, in fact, form a polygonal structure (or band) around the periphery of each cell. Because of its location in the terminal or apical portion of the cell and its bar-like configuration, the stainable material was designated **terminal bar.**

It is now evident that intercellular cement, as such, does not exist. The terminal bar, however, does represent a significant structure. Electron mi-

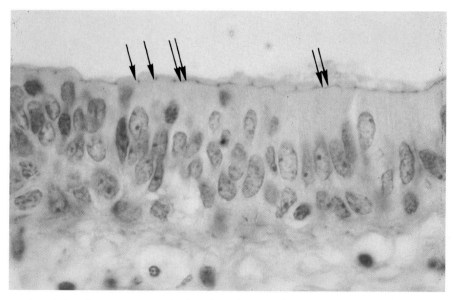

Figure 4.10. Photomicrograph showing the terminal bar in a pseudostratified epithelium. The bar appears as a dot **(single arrows)** when it is seen on its cut edge. When the bar is coursing parallel to the cut surface, and lying within the thickness of the section, it is seen as a linear or bar-like profile **(double arrows).**

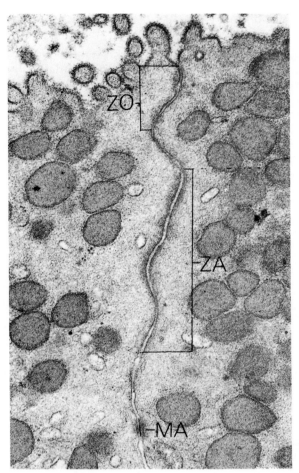

Figure 4.11. Electron micrograph of the apical portion of two adjoining epithelial cells of the gastric mucosa showing their junctional complex. ZO, zonula occludens; ZA, zonula adherens; and MA, macula adherens. × 30,000.

croscopy has shown it to be the site of specialized attachment devices for the adherence of adjoining epithelial cells (see Fig. 4.11). It is also the site of a barrier to the diffusion of substances between the epithelial cells. The specific structural components that make up the barrier and the attachment devices are readily identified in the electron microscope and are collectively referred to as the

junctional complex (see Table 4.1). The junctional complex is comprised of (1) the zonula occludens, the barrier device, (2) the zonula adherens, a continuous, band-like adhesion device that completely surrounds the cell joining it to its neighbors, and (3) the macula adherens, a spot contact adhesion device that also participates in joining the cell to its neighbors.

Zonula Occludens

The *zonula occludens,* also frequently referred to as a *tight junction,* is located at the most apical part of the lateral surface of the cell and represents a ring or circumferential band (thus, zonula) of plasma membrane union between neighboring cells. In the electron microscope, the zonula occludens appears as a narrow region in which the outer leaflets of the plasma membranes of the adjoined cells come in contact at close intervals resulting in multiple sites where the membranes appear to converge and fuse and from which intercellular fluid is excluded (Figs. 4.11 and 4.12). In relatively leaky epithelia, such as in certain kidney tubules, there are few points of membrane contact, whereas in highly impermeable epithelia, such as intestinal and urinary bladder epithelia, there are many points of contact. The more points of membrane contact, the more impervious the junction. Freeze fracture studies reveal that the points of contact are anastomosing linear bands between the cells (Fig. 4.13). The bands seen in freeze fracture are interpreted as being comprised of linear arrays of protein particles integral to each of the opposing cell membranes that bind to each other and, thus, obliterate the intercellular space. It is important to recognize that the zonula occludens, by limiting the passage of substances between adjacent cells, places energy demands upon the epithelial cells. In order to exchange solutes across epithelia, such as capillary endothelium or the intestinal absorptive epithelium, tremendous amounts of metabolic energy must be expended in transporting molecules across the plasma membrane and through the cell (via transmembrane transport and transcytosis systems).

TABLE 4.1. Terminology of Intercellular Contacts

LIGHT MICROSCOPY	ELECTRON MICROSCOPY
Terminal bar = Junctional complex =	Zonula occludens = tight junction Zonula adherens Macula adherens
Desmosome = Macula adherens	

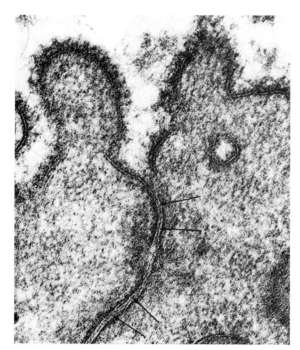

Figure 4.12. Zonula occludens from Figure 4.11 shown at higher magnification. Note the intimate contact of the outer lamellae of adjoining plasma membranes, which appear as a single line **(arrows)**. × 100,000.

Zonula Adherens

The *zonula adherens,* the second component, also exhibits a continuous circumferential configuration. It lies at a level just below the zonula occludens and is characterized by a uniform 15 to 20 nm space between opposing cell membranes (Fig. 4.14). The intercellular space is of low electron density, almost appearing clear, but evidently occupied by a material through which the two membranes maintain their adherence to one another. In the confines of the adherens, a moderately electron-dense material is found along the cytoplasmic side of the membrane of each cell. Associated with this electron-dense material is an array of 6-nm microfilaments (comprised of actin) that appear to anchor in the electron-dense material. In those epithelia that have an extensive microvillus border, such as intestinal epithelium, the filaments are particularly numerous and contribute to the terminal web as seen in light microcopy. These structures will be described shortly under epithelial cell surface modifications.

Macula Adherens (Desmosome)

The *macula adherens* represents an additional adhesion device that is typically located just below

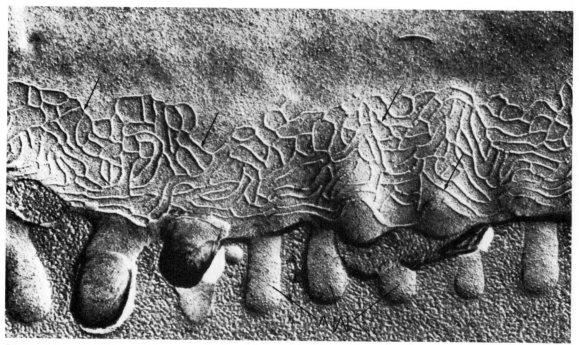

Figure 4.13. A freeze fracture preparation of intestinal epithelium. The zonula occludens appears as an anastomosing network of ridges **(arrows)** seen here on the P-face of the membrane. (The E-face of the fractured membrane would show a complementary pattern of grooves.) The strands or ridges are interpreted as linear arrays of integral protein particles within the membrane. The membrane of the opposing cell contains a similar network, which is in register and is firmly bonded to the first cell. The actual sites of fusion between cells is thus along the anastomosing network. × 100,000. (B. Hull and A. Staehelin, 1976.)

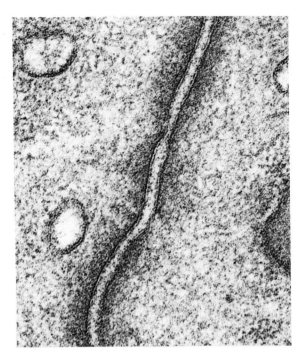

Figure 4.14. Zonula adherens, from Figure 4.11 at higher magnification. The plasma membranes are separated here by a relatively uniform space. The intercellular space appears clear, showing only a sparse amount of diffuse punctate substance. The cytoplasmic side of the plasma membrane exhibits a moderately electron-dense material. × 100,000.

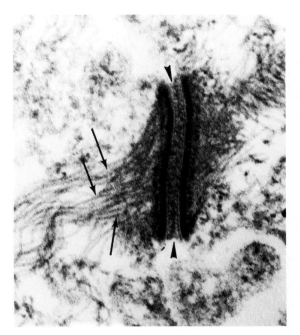

Figure 4.15. Electron micrograph of a macula adherens. The tonofilaments **(arrows)** attach into a dense material or plaque located on the cytoplasmic side of the plasma membrane. The intercellular space is also occupied by a dense material **(arrowheads)**, presumably the adhesion substance. The intercellular space above and below the macula adherens is not well defined due to extraction of the plasma membrane in order to define the integral components of the macula adherens. × 40,000. (Courtesy of Dr. E. Kallenbach.)

the level of the zonula adherens, although it is not necessarily limited just to that site. In many epithelia these attachments are found at different levels along the lateral cell surface, thus strengthening a cell's bond to its neighbors. The macula adherens is a particularly strong attachment structure, as shown by microdissection studies, and differs from the zonula adherens in several important respects. First, it is a disc-shaped structure, occurring as a row of spot attachments around the periphery of the cell, rather than as a continuous band. Second, it has a more complex structural appearance than the zonula adherens. On the cytoplasmic side of the plasma membrane there is an electron-dense plaque in which a multitude of 10-nm intermediate filaments are anchored (Fig. 4.15). The filaments, also referred to as **tonofilaments** when found in epithelial cells, probably play a role in dissipating physical forces throughout the cell from the attachment site. The intercellular space of the macula region measures just slightly more than that of the zonula adherens and is occupied by a dense intermediate line, presumably a component of the intercellular adhesive material of the junction.

The macula-type attachment structure is conspicuously present in epithelia subject to abrasion and physical stress. For example, in the epidermis and other stratified squamous epithelia, there are numerous focal attachment points between neighboring cells. The attachment sites are present around the entire periphery of the cells. Because of shrinkage artifacts in preparation of the tissue, the cells tend to pull away from one another and thus give the appearance of possessing numerous spinous processes. These processes are referred to as **intercellular bridges.** The bridges exhibit a dark-staining, thickened area which was given the name **desmosome** (connecting body). Originally the bridges were thought to represent cytoplasmic continuity between the cells. However, early studies with the electron microscope revealed that the desmosome of the bridge is actually an attachment device joining the pulled cytoplasmic strands of opposing cells and that, in fact, the desmosome is identical to the macula adherens of a junctional complex. The term desmosome, consequently, is now sometimes used interchangeably for macula adherens. However, it is worth remembering that the word desmosome was derived relative to light microscopy, whereas the term macula adherens was derived from electron microscopy to identify one of a series of structures of the junctional complex. Also, on the basis of staining characteristics, it is probably the macula adherens of the junctional complex that is the main contributor to the appearance of the terminal bar since desmosomes of the intercellular bridge take up sufficient stain to be recognized in the light microscope.

Hemidesmosome

Hemidesmosomes are, as the name implies, half desmosomes. They are found at the basal surface of some stratified squamous epithelia, and they make "contact" with the adjacent basal lamina. The cytoplasmic portion of the hemidesmosomes consists of an attachment plaque to which 10 nm filaments are attached; the attachment plaque is separated by a less dense layer of about 10 nm from the dense inner leaflet of the plasma membrane. Structurally, the cytoplasmic unit of the hemidesmosome resembles the equivalent components of a desmosome, except that instead of facing the same structure in an adjacent cell, the hemidesmosome faces a portion of the basal lamina. In some epithelia the basal lamina that faces the hemidesmosome is thickened as it is in Figure 4.16 and connecting

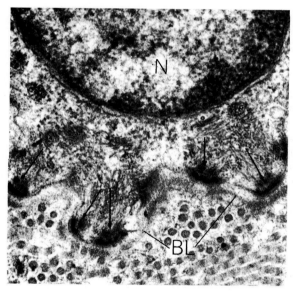

Figure 4.16. Electron micrograph of the basal aspect of a gingival epithelial cell. Below the nucleus (N) tonofilaments are seen converging on the dense attachment plaques **(arrows)** of the hemidesmosome. Below the plasma membrane are the basal lamina (BL) and collagen fibrils (most of which are cut in cross-section) of the connective tissue. × 40,000.

strands join the plasma membrane of the hemidesmosome to the basal lamina.

Gap Junction

At the electron microscope level, *gap junctions* (discussed in Chapter 2) are also visible structures that interconnect epithelial cells and occur between other types of cells (such as smooth and cardiac muscle). Gap junctions probably do not provide a strong physical support or attachment, but do function in the electrical coupling of cells and serve as passageways for the diffusion of metabolites and ions between cells.

Fascia Adherens

Physical attachments that occur between cells in tissues other than epithelia are usually not prominent, but there are a few notable exceptions. In cardiac muscle, the cells are arranged end to end forming thread-like contractile units. The attachment is by a combination of typical desmosomes or maculae adherentes and broad adhesion plates morphologically like the zonula adherens of epithelial cells. Since attachment is not a ring-like configuration, but rather a broad face, these attachments are designated *fascia adherens.*

In some instances, the contact between cells may be at a molecular level, involving individual membrane glycoproteins, which cannot be visualized with conventional microscopic techniques. These glycoproteins project out into the cell coat and link with individual specific glycoproteins expressed on neighboring cells. The type of glycoprotein varies from cell type to cell type and is believed to help confer a "social identity" onto cells. These molecular-scale contacts have the potential to be reversible and, thus, are employed embryologically as well as in adult tissues. Such interactions of cells occur during embryonic development to direct the migration and association of cells as organ systems develop or in the adult to direct the function of the cells of the immune system.

In summary, there is a requirement for attachments within certain populations of cells. In epithelium, the junctional complex is particularly significant because it serves to create a long-term barrier allowing the cells to compartmentalize and restrict the free passage of substances across its surfaces. While it is the zonula occludens of the junctional complex that principally effects this function, it is the adhesive properties of the zonulae and maculae adherentes that guard against physical disruption of the barrier. Also important is the requirement of strong attachment sometimes

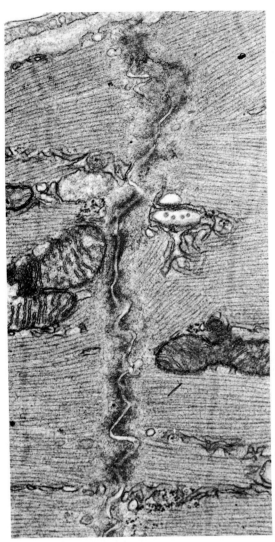

Figure 4.17. Electron micrograph showing the end-to-end apposition of two cardiac muscle cells. The intercellular space appears as a clear undulating area. On the cytoplasmic side of the plasma membrane of each cell there is a dense material similar to that seen in a zonula adherens. Since the attachment site here involves a portion of the end face of the two cells, it is a fascia adherens. × 38,000.

required in other sites. In the stratified epithelial cells of the epidermis it is the macula adherens that maintains cell adhesion. In cardiac muscle, where there is a similar need for strong adhesion, a combination of the macula adherens and fascia adherens provides this feature (Fig. 4.17).

CELL SURFACE MODIFICATIONS

Epithelial cells exhibit modifications of their cell surfaces that relate to function. Those surface modifications that will be dealt with are (1) microvilli, (2) stereocilia, (3) cilia, and (4) lateral and basal cell surface folds.

Microvilli

Microvilli are cytoplasmic finger-like protrusions from a cell surface. They are present on the apical surface of most epithelia. Observed in the electron microscope, they are seen to vary in appearance from small, irregular, bleb-like projections in some cell types to tall, closely packed, uniform projections that provide an enormous increase in the free surface area in other cell types. In general, the number and shape of the microvilli in a given cell type correlate with its absorptive capacity. Thus, cells whose principal function is the transport of fluid exhibit many closely packed, tall microvilli, while cells whose requirement for absorption is associated with other functional activities exhibit the smaller, more irregular microvilli. Among the fluid-transporting epithelia, for example, intestinal and kidney tubule epithelia, a distinctive border of vertical striations is readily detectable in the light microscope. This surface structure was originally given the name *striated border* for the intestinal absorptive cell and *brush border* for the kidney tubule cell. In locations where there is no apparent surface modification based on light microscope observations, microvilli, if present, are usually not numerous and, thus, not resolved with the light microscope.

The degree to which microvilli may vary among different types of epithelia is illustrated in Figure 4.18. The microvilli (striated border) of the intestinal epithelium are the most highly ordered, being even more uniform in appearance than those that constitute the brush border of kidney cells. They also contain a conspicuous core of microfilaments (actin) that are anchored to the plasma membrane at the tip and sides of the microvillus and extend down into the apical cytoplasm where they interact with a horizontal network of filaments, the terminal web, that lies just below the base of the microvilli (Fig. 4.19). The actin filaments primarily provide support and give rigidity to microvilli to help maintain their parallel array. It has been proposed that some of the microfilaments of the zonula adherens and the terminal web have a contractile ability, which could have the effect of decreasing the diameter of the apex of the cell causing the microvilli, whose stiff actin cores are anchored into the terminal web, to spread apart at their tips and increase the intervillous space. Actin filaments are also present in the microvilli of other cell types, but they are usually

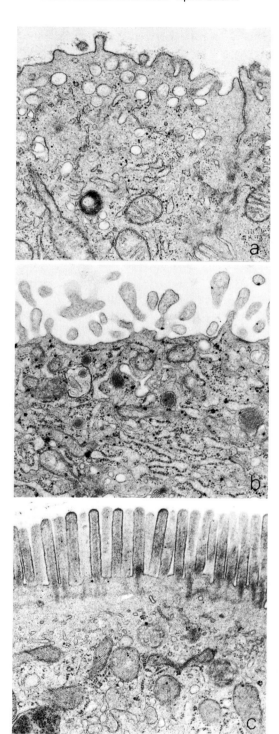

Figure 4.18. Electron micrographs showing variation in microvilli of different cell types. **(a)** Cell of uterine gland; very small projections. **(b)** Placenta; irregular, branching microvilli. **(c)** Intestinal absorptive cell with very uniform and regularly arranged microvilli. All figures, × 20,000.

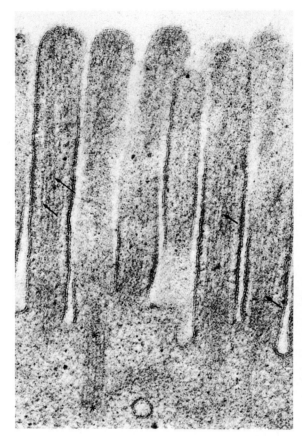

Figure 4.19. A higher power view of the microvilli seen in Figure 4.18(c). Note the presence of the microfilaments in the microvilli **(arrows)**, which extend into the apical cytoplasm **(asterisks)**. × 80,000.

much less well developed and often are so sparse in number that they are difficult to detect.

Stereocilia

Stereocilia are included in this section not because of their wide distribution among epithelia, but because of the traditional treatment of this unusual surface modification as a separate structural entity. They are, in fact, limited to the epididymis of the male reproductive system and to the sensory (hair) cells of the ear.

Stereocilia of the epididymis are exceedingly long and slightly irregular cytoplasmic processes that extend from the apical surface of the cell (Fig. 4.20). Electron microscopic examination reveals them to be very long microvilli. They lack notable internal structural features. In the light microscope these processes frequently give the superficial appearance of the hairs of a coloring brush due to the way the processes aggregate into a pointed bundle.

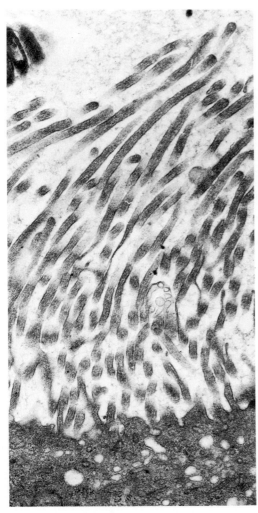

Figure 4.20. Electron micrograph of stereocilia from the epididymis. The cytoplasmic projections are similar to microvilli, but they are extremely long. × 20,000.

Stereocilia of the sensory epithelium of the ear are uniform in diameter and possess an internal filamentous structure. They serve as a receptor device rather than as an absorptive structure.

Cilia

When viewed in the light microscope *cilia* appear as short, fine, hair-like structures emanating from the free surface of the cell (Fig. 4.21). A thin, dark-staining band is usually seen extending across the cell at the base of the cilia. This dark-staining-band is due to structures, known as **basal bodies,** which take up stain and, when viewed in the light microscope, collectively appear as a band. However, each cilium is associated with a single basal body that is separate and distinct from those of

adjacent cilia. In the electron microscope the basal body is recognized as a modified centriole (Fig. 4.22).

In most ciliated epithelia, as in the trachea, bronchi, or oviducts, there may be several hundred cilia to a cell. In some epithelia only a single cilium may be present on a cell. In these instances, the cilia are thought to have a sensory role.

Structure of the Cilium. Each cilium, when examined in cross-section, reveals nine doublets of circularly arranged microtubules surrounding two central microtubules (Fig. 4.23). The microtubules comprising each doublet are constructed so that the wall of one microtubule, designated the B tubule, is actually incomplete; it shares a portion of the wall of the other microtubule of the doublet, the A tubule. The two central microtubules are separate from one another; each is a singlet. This 9 + 2 microtubule array courses from the tip of the cilium to its base where the outer paired microtubules join the **basal body.** The basal body is a modified centriole consisting of nine short microtubule triplets arranged in a ring. Each of the paired microtubules of the cilium is continuous with two of the triplet microtubules of the basal body. The central two microtubules of the cilium end at the level of the top of the basal body. Therefore, a cross-section of the basal body would reveal nine circularly arranged microtubule triplets, but not the two central singlet microtubules of the ciliary process.

The process of ciliary formation in newly differentiating cells involves the replication of the centriole to give rise to multiple procentrioles, one for each cilium that is destined to form. The procentrioles grow and migrate to the apical surface of the cell where each becomes a basal body. From each of the nine triplets that make up the basal body a microtubule doublet grows upward creating a projection containing the nine doublets found in the mature ciliary process. Simultaneously, the two singlet central microtubules form de novo within the ring of doublet microtubules, thus yielding the characteristic 9 + 2 arrangement.

Movement of the Cilium. Cilia undergo a regular and synchronous undulating movement. Each cilium in the living state exhibits a rapid forward movement in a rigid state (effective stroke), but becomes flexible and bends on the slower return movement (recovery stroke). The plane of movement of a cilium is perpendicular to a line joining the central pair of microtubules. Through sequential timing, the cilia in successive rows start their beat so that each is slightly more advanced in its cycle than the preceding row, thus creating a wave that sweeps across the epithelium. This metachronal rhythm is capable of moving mucus over

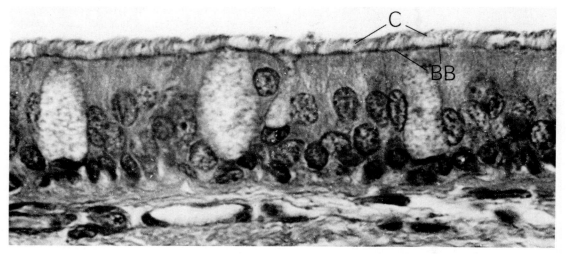

Figure 4.21. A photomicrograph of the pseudostratified ciliated epithelium of the trachea. The cilia (C) appear as hair-like processes extending from the apical surface of the cells. The dark line immediately below the ciliary processes is produced by the basal bodies (BB). × 750.

epithelial surfaces or facilitating the flow of fluid and other substances through tubular organs and ducts.

Ciliary activity is based on the movement of the doublet microtubules in relation to one another. Each doublet, when seen in cross-section at high resolution, exhibits a pair of "arms" that contain dynein and ATPase activity (see Fig. 4.23). The dynein arms extend from the A microtubule to form temporary cross-bridges with the B tubule of the adjacent doublet. Addition of ATP produces a sliding movement of the bridge along the B tubule and as a result the cilium bends.

A structural abnormality involving absence of dynein arms has been found in some individuals with Kartagener's syndrome, a hereditary disease associated with chronic respiratory difficulty (including bronchitis and sinusitis) and visceral asymmetry. Ciliary motility is severely impaired or absent in afflicted individuals and, as a consequence, there is reduced or no ciliary transport of mucus in the tracheobronchial system. As was indicated above, individuals afflicted with the disease often demonstrate complete situs inversus, transposition of the viscera, or some degree of visceral asymmetry. Inversion of the viscera may be related to the lack of ciliary activity during the developmental process. Another possibility is that microtubules that designate a form of polarity within cells may also indirectly influence the polarity of organ systems. Inversion of the viscera may occur resulting from abnormal microtubular structure. Males with Kartagener's syndrome are sterile. The flagellum of the sperm, which is similar in structure to the cilium, is immotile. In contrast, some women af-

flicted with the syndrome may be fertile. In such individuals, the ciliary movement may be sufficient, though impaired, to still permit transport of the ovum through the oviduct.

Lateral and Basal Cell Surface Folds

The lateral surface of certain epithelial cells may show a tortuous boundary due to infoldings or interdigitations of each cell with its neighbor (Fig. 4.24). These infoldings increase the lateral surface of the cell and are particularly prominent in cells that transport fluid rapidly, as in the intestinal epithelium. Under a fluid load water leaves the cell at the lateral surface by osmotically following sodium ions that are actively transported across the membrane. The intercellular space becomes distended (see Atlas Section, Plate 4) by the accumulation of fluid as it moves across the epithelium. In effect, the space may be likened to a cylinder. The concentration pressure gradient established within the "cylinder," provides a driving force to move the fluid from the intercellular space into the adjoining connective tissue. Since the cells possess an occluding junction at the luminal or free surface, the fluid can move only in the direction of the connective tissue.

Other cells known to transport fluid show infoldings at the basal cell surface. These basal surface modifications are prominent in proximal and distal tubules of the kidney (Fig. 4.25) and in certain ducts of the salivary glands. Mitochondria are typically concentrated at this basal site to provide the energy requirements for active transport and they are usually oriented within the folds. The ori-

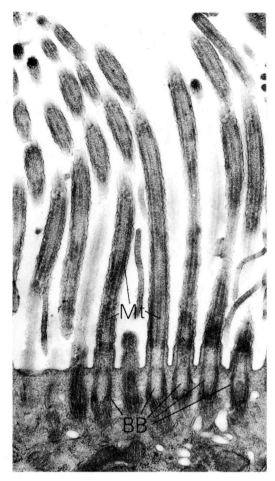

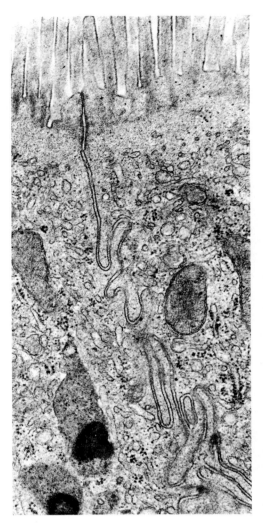

Figure 4.22. Electron micrograph of longitudinally cut cilia from the oviduct. The internal structures within the ciliary process are the microtubules (Mt). The basal bodies (BB) have an "empty" appearance due to the absence of the central pair of microtubules in this portion of the cilium. The other two basal bodies have been sectioned peripherally through the outer microtubule doublets. × 20,000.

Figure 4.24. Electron micrograph showing infoldings or interdigitations at the lateral surfaces of two adjoining intestinal absorptive cells.

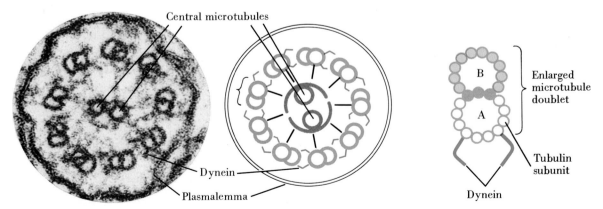

Figure 4.23. Electron micrograph of a cross-section of a cilium and a corresponding diagram showing the two central microtubules and the nine surrounding microtubule doublets. The dynein arms extend from the microtubule and make temporary bridges with the B microtubule of the adjacent doublet. The substructure of a microtubule doublet is shown in the adjacent diagram on the right. Note that the A microtubule of the doublet is comprised of 13 tubulin dimers arranged in a side-by-side configuration, whereas the B microtubule is comprised of 10 tubulin dimers and shares the remaining units with those of the A microtubule. (The length of the microtubules is dependent on the end-to-end addition of the tubulin dimer units. See Fig. 2.19.) (Electron micrograph, × 180,000, courtesy of Dr. K. Selman; diagram based on Junqueira LC, Carneiro J: *Basic Histology,* 3rd ed. Los Altos, CA, Lange, 1980.)

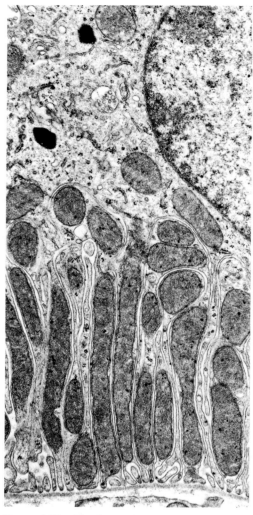

Figure 4.25. Electron micrograph of the basal portion of a kidney tubule cell showing the infolding of the plasma membrane with mitochondria contained within the cytoplasmia folds.

entation of the mitochondria combined with the basal membrane infoldings results in a striated appearance along the basal aspect of the cell when observed with the light microscope. Indeed, certain salivary gland ducts are referred to as **striated ducts.**

HISTOGENESIS OF THE EPITHELIUM

Each of the three germ layers in the developing embryo contributes to the formation of epithelial and epithelioid structures. Figure 4.26 illustrates the derivatives of the three germ layers.

Ectodermal Derivatives

The derivatives of the *ectoderm* may be divided into two major classes—*surface ectoderm* and *neuroectoderm.*

Surface ectoderm gives rise to: (1) the epidermis and its derivatives (hair, nails, sweat glands, sebaceous glands, and the parenchyma and ducts of the mammary gland), (2) the adenohypophysis, (3) cornea and lens epithelia of the eye, (4) the enamel organ and enamel of the teeth, and (5) components of the inner ear.

Neuroectoderm gives rise to: (1) the **neural tube** and its derivatives (the central nervous system including ependyma, pineal body, and neurohypophysis and the sensory epithelium of the eye, ear, and nose) and (2) the **neural crest** and its derivatives (components of the peripheral nervous system including ganglia, nerves, and glial cells, medullary cells of the adrenal gland, the amine precursor uptake and decarboxylation (APUD) cells of the diffuse neuroendocrine system (see Chapter 20), and melanoblasts, which are the precursors of melanocytes).

Mesodermal Derivatives

Mesoderm gives rise to: (1) the epithelium of the kidney and the gonads; (2) mesothelium, the epithelium lining the pericardial, pleural, and peritoneal cavities; (3) endothelium, the epithelium lining the cardiovascular and lymphatic vessels; and (4) the adrenal cortex. It might be noted that many of the more atypical epithelia arise from mesoderm. For example, the adrenal cortical cells, the Leydig cells of the testis, and the lutein cells of the ovary, all endocrine components, lack a free surface, a feature not characteristic of most epithelia. These secretory cells, which are derived from progenitor mesenchymal cells (nondifferentiated cells of embryonic origin found in connective tissue), are referred to as epithelioid. Although the differentiation process may involve a transient exposure of progenitor mesenchymal cells at a free surface, the differentiated cells do not acquire a surface location. Endothelium and mesothelium differ from epithelia derived from the other two germ layers in that they have no continuity or communication with the exterior of the body.

Entodermal Derivatives

Entoderm (or endoderm) gives rise to: (1) the epithelium of the respiratory system; (2) the epithelium of the alimentary canal (excluding the epithelium of the oral cavity and anal region, which are of ectodermal origin); (3) the epithelium of all

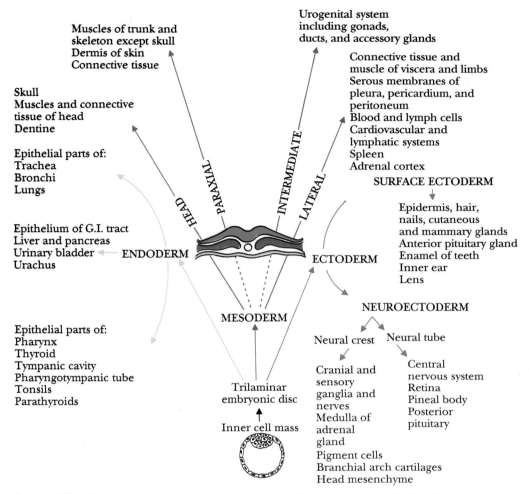

Muscles of trunk and
skeleton except skull
Dermis of skin
Connective tissue

Skull
Muscles and connective
tissue of head
Dentine

Epithelial parts of:
Trachea
Bronchi
Lungs

Epithelium of G.I. tract
Liver and pancreas
Urinary bladder
Urachus

ENDODERM

Epithelial parts of:
Pharynx
Thyroid
Tympanic cavity
Pharyngotympanic tube
Tonsils
Parathyroids

HEAD

PARAXIAL

INTERMEDIATE

LATERAL

MESODERM

Trilaminar
embryonic disc

Inner cell mass

Urogenital system
including gonads,
ducts, and accessory glands

Connective tissue and
muscle of viscera and limbs
Serous membranes of
pleura, pericardium, and
peritoneum
Blood and lymph cells
Cardiovascular and
lymphatic systems
Spleen
Adrenal cortex

SURFACE ECTODERM

Epidermis, hair,
nails, cutaneous
and mammary glands
Anterior pituitary gland
Enamel of teeth
Inner ear
Lens

ECTODERM

NEUROECTODERM

Neural crest   Neural tube

Cranial and
sensory
ganglia and
nerves
Medulla of
adrenal
gland
Pigment cells
Branchial arch cartilages
Head mesenchyme

Central
nervous system
Retina
Pineal body
Posterior
pituitary

Figure 4.26. Derivatives of the three germ layers. (Based on Moore KL: *The Developing Human,* 2nd ed. Philadelphia, WB Saunders, 1977.)

of the organs and glands associated with these systems, including the liver, pancreas, and gall bladder; (4) the epithelial components of the thyroid, parathyroid, and thymus glands; and (5) the epithelial lining of the tympanic cavity and auditory (eustachian) tubes. Thyroid and parathyroids develop as epithelial outgrowths from the pharyngeal wall and then lose their attachments from their sites of original outgrowth. Similarly, the thymus originates as an epithelial outgrowth of the pharyngeal wall, grows into the mediastinum, and then loses its original connection.

Neural Crest Cells and Ectomesenchyme

A special class of cells, called *ectomesenchyme,* which are derived from neural crest cells in the head region, which requires special mention. At about the time that the neural folds close to form a tube, some of the neuroectodermal cells at the lateral edges of the neural plate separate and are not incorporated into the tube. These cells migrate and form the *neural crest* over the neural tube. As was explained previously, these cells migrate extensively in the developing embryo and give rise to components of the peripheral nervous system, including Schwann and other glial cells, all sensory cells, sympathetic and parasympathetic autonomic ganglia and neurons, medullary cells of the adrenal gland, the APUD cells of the diffuse neuroendocrine system, and melanoblasts, which are the precursors of melanocytes. In the cranial region, neural crest cells also form the connective tissue, bone, cartilage, and some muscle of the face, and components of the tooth, but not the enamel.

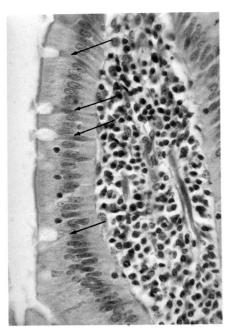

Figure 4.27. Photomicrograph of the intestinal epithelium showing single goblet cells **(arrows)** dispersed among absorptive cells.

These neural crest cells that give rise to connective and other tissues of the face are also called *ectomesenchyme.*

GLANDS

Glands of the body are classified into two major groups according to how their products are distributed through the body. *Exocrine glands* secrete their products onto a surface, usually through ducts or tubes. *Endocrine glands* secrete their products into the bloodstream and are ductless. The products of endocrine glands are called *hormones.* The structure and function of endocrine glands will be considered in later chapters.

Exocrine glands are further classified into structural types. If the glandular component consists of a single cell among other cells that are not glandular, the gland is called *unicellular.* The usual example of a unicellular gland is the *goblet cell.* These cells are positioned among other columnar (Fig. 4.27) or pseudostratified columnar cells and they produce mucus. Goblet cells are located in the lining and glands of the intestines and in certain passages of the respiratory tract.

Multicellular glands are glands in which the glandular component consists of more than one cell. They are further subclassified according to the arrangement of the gland cells and the presence or absence of branching of the duct elements. The simplest arrangement of a multicellular gland is a cellular sheet in which each surface cell is a secretory cell. For example, the entire lining of the stomach and its gastric pits is a sheet of mucus secreting cells (Fig. 4.28). Other multicellular glands typically form tubular invaginations from the surface (Fig. 4.29). The end-piece of the gland contains the secretory cells; the portion of the gland connecting the secretory cells to the surface serves as a duct. If the duct is unbranched, the gland is called *simple;* if the duct is branched, it is called *compound.* If the secretory portion is shaped like a tube, the gland is *tubular;* if it is flasklike, the gland is *alveolar,* or *acinar;* if the tube ends in a

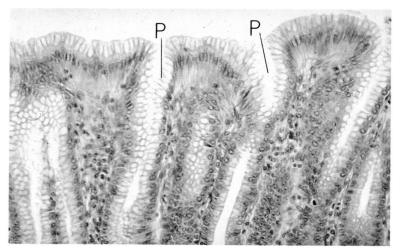

Figure 4.28. Photomicrograph of the stomach surface. The epithelial cells lining the surface are all mucus-secreting cells, as are the cells lining the gastric pits (P).

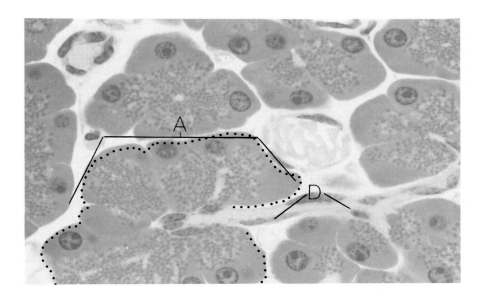

Figure 4.29. Photomicrograph of pancreatic acinus (A) with its duct (D). The small round objects within the acinar cells represent the stored secretory precursor material.

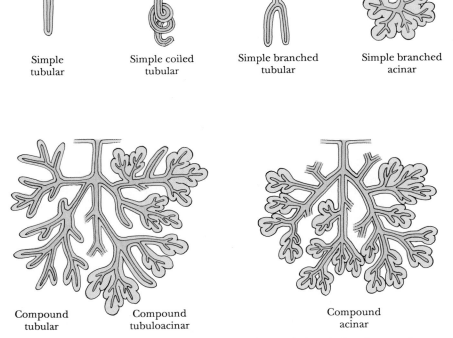

Figure 4.30. Schematic diagram of various types of glands showing configuration of the duct and secretory cells. (Based on Weiss L, Greep RO: *Histology,* 4th ed. New York, McGraw-Hill, 1977.)

sac-like dilation, the gland is **tubuloalveolar.** Tubular secretory portions may be straight, branched, or coiled; alveolar portions may be single or branched. Various combinations of duct and secretory portion shapes are found in the body. Thus, exocrine glands may be **simple straight tubular, simple coiled tubular, simple alveolar, compound tubular, compound alveolar,** or **compound tubuloalveolar** (Fig. 4.30).

The secretory cells of glands associated with the alimentary canal and with the respiratory passages are usually described as being **mucous** or **serous** according to whether their secretions are thick or watery, respectively. Goblet cells, secretory cells of the sublingual salivary glands, and surface cells of the stomach are examples of mucus-secreting cells. The mucous nature of the secretion is the result of extensive O-glycosylation of the constituent proteins with anionic oligosaccharides. Their mucous product is water soluble and is lost during the routine preparation of the tissues, and thus, the apical cytoplasm of mucous cells appears to be empty in the H&E-stained paraffin section. The nucleus of a mucous cell often appears to be flattened against the base of the cell. Acini containing serous cells are found in the parotid glands and in the pancreas. The nucleus of a serous cell is typically rounded or oval in appearance and the apical cytoplasm is often intensely stained with eosin if the secretory granules are well preserved. Acini of some glands, such as the submaxillary glands, contain both mucous and serous cells. In these cases, the serous cells are more removed from the lumen of the alveolus and are shaped as crescents or demilunes at the periphery of the mucous acinus or tubule. Their secretions reach the duct of the gland by means of small intercellular canaliculi between the mucous cells (Fig. 4.31). Similar intercellular channels can occur between cells in serous acini.

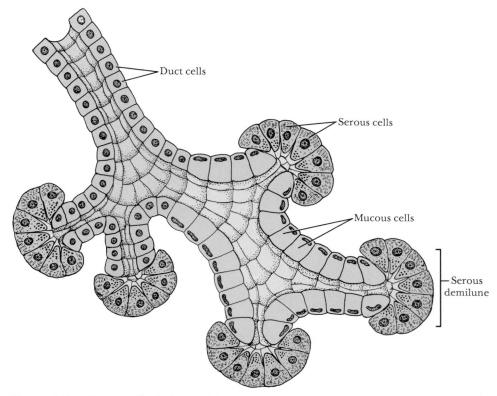

Figure 4.31. Diagram illustrating a tubuloalveolar gland. Both tubular and acinar regions are comprised of mucous secretory cells (note the flattened nuclei that are characteristic of these cells). The alveolus is depicted with a single serous cell forming a demilune (typically a number of serous cells form the demilune). The thin, watery serous secretion of the demilune cells makes its way into the alveolar lumen via a narrow canaliculus, or channel, between mucous cells. (Based on Weiss L, Greep RO: *Histology,* 4th ed. New York, McGraw-Hill, 1977.)

Labels in figure: Duct cells; Serous cells; Mucous cells; Serous demilune

MUCOUS AND SEROUS MEMBRANES

In two general locations within the body, surface epithelium and its underlying connective tissue form a functional unit called a *membrane.* The term membrane as used here is not to be confused with biological membranes that surround cells. The two types of membrane are mucous membrane and serous membrane.

The *mucous membrane,* also called the *mucosa,* lines those cavities that connect with the outside of the body, namely, the alimentary canal, the respiratory tract, and the genitourinary tract. It consists of surface epithelium (with or without glands); a supporting connective tissue, called the *lamina propria;* a *basal lamina* separating the epithelium from the lamina propria; and sometimes a layer of smooth muscle, called the *muscularis mucosae,* as the deepest layer.

The *serous membrane,* also called the *serosa,* lines the peritoneal, pleural, and pericardial cavities. These cavities are usually described as closed cavities of the body, although in the female the peritoneal cavity communicates with the exterior by way of the uterine tubes. Structurally, the serosa consists of a lining epithelium, called *mesothelium;* a supporting connective tissue; and a basal lamina between the two. Serous membranes do not contain glands; the fluid on their surface is watery.

PLATE 1. Simple Squamous and Simple Cuboidal Epithelia

Selected examples of epithelia are depicted here and on the next several pages. For each example, note the shape and arrangement of the epithelial cells, the location of their free surfaces, and the location of the underlying or adjacent connective tissue.

Figure 1 shows the *simple squamous epithelium* (mesothelium) covering the outer surface of the intestine. The epithelium overlies a well-defined layer of connective tissue **(CT)** containing several small blood vessels **(BV)** and deeper is a layer of smooth muscle **(SM)**. The epithelial cells are very flat, as judged by the shape of their nuclei **(N)**. Note that cell boundaries are not evident and that the nuclei are unevenly spaced. The uneven spacing is because the sectioning knife passes through some cells without including the nucleus. This phenomenon can be better understood and visualized in **Figure 2,** which is a nonsectioned (whole mount), silver-impregnated preparation of a piece of a very thin mesentery (the structure that holds the intestines in place). The mesentery is lying on the slide and the microscope is focused on the upper surface of the mesentery to reveal the surface epithelial cells. The epithelial cell boundaries are revealed by a deposition of reduced silver along the intercellular spaces. The nuclei **(N)** appear oval or round when viewed from the surface, as opposed to flat or elongate when seen on edge, as in a section. If one were to draw a line representing a knife cut across the cells as revealed in this figure, it is possible to envision why the epithelial nuclei are unevenly spaced in sectioned material; the knife would pass through the cytoplasm of each cell, but would not necessarily cut across the nucleus of each cell. Some of the more ovoid nuclei in the preparation belong to fibroblasts **(F)** located in the underlying connective tissue. They are in the same focal plane as the epithelial cells and are thus superimposed.

Another example of a *simple squamous epithelium* is shown in **Figure 3.** The micrograph reveals a sectioned renal corpuscle and adjacent kidney tubules. The renal corpuscle consists of a special capillary bed, the glomerulus, which is enclosed by Bowman's capsule, part of which (the visceral layer) is directly adjacent to the capillaries and part of which (the parietal layer) forms a thin-walled spherical structure comprised of simple squamous epithelium. The nuclei **(N)** of the cells forming the parietal layer appear as flattened bodies which

---

KEY

AV, arteriole vessel supplying glomerulus
BV, blood vessel
CT, connective tissue
Ep, epithelium
F, fibroblast nucleus
N, nucleus

SM, smooth muscle
arrow, site of bile canaliculus
asterisk, tubule possessing simple cuboidal epithelium

Fig. 1, monkey, × 640
Fig. 2, monkey, × 640
Fig. 3, human, × 640

Fig. 4, monkey, × 640
Fig. 5, human, × 400

---

show the same uneven spacing as in **Figure 1.** The free surface of the epithelium faces Bowman's space. The tubules marked with an **asterisk** (lower left) provide a good example of a *simple cuboidal epithelium.* The single layer of cells that comprise the tubules are cuboidal in shape. Although cell boundaries are not evident, one can assess that the height of each cell approximates its width by the spacing of the nuclei. Thus, it is a cuboidal epithelium.

Figure 4 represents another example of a simple cuboidal epithelium **(Ep);** it shows the cells which cover the surface of the ovary. The epithelium rests on a highly cellular connective tissue **(CT).** The surface epithelial cells are approximately square, or cuboidal in three dimensions. The free surfaces of these cells face the abdominal cavity and are a modification of the simple squamous epithelium or mesothelium shown in **Figures 1** and **2.**

The cells of the liver, **Figure 5,** are a somewhat unusual example of a simple cuboidal epithelium. In terms of shape the liver parenchymal cell approximates a cube; these cells are arranged in sheets separated by blood vessels **(BV)** known as sinusoids. The epithelium is unusual in that several surfaces of the cell possess a groove which represents the free surface. Where a grooved surface is present on one cell, the adjoining cell possesses an identical grooved surface. The two opposing grooves, thus, form a small lumen or canaliculus, allowing the bile produced by the liver cells to reach a bile duct. Though not visible at the magnification shown, the canaliculi are located at the exact point of the **arrows** (see bile canaliculus, Plate 84).

PLATE 1

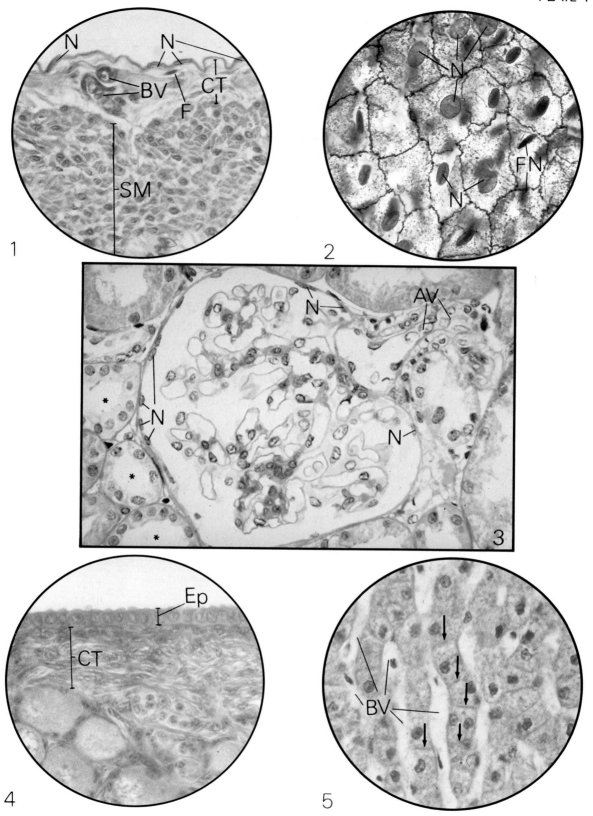

PLATE 2. Simple and Stratified Epithelia

The exocrine pancreas shown in **Figure 1** reveals three epithelial forms. First, within the **circle** is a well-oriented acinus, a functional group of secretory cells, each of which is pyramidal in shape. The secretory cells form a spherical or tubular structure. The free surface of the cells and lumen are located in the center of the circle. (The lumen is not clearly evident, but in a similar cell arrangement in **Figure 4** (see circle) the lumen and secretory surface can be seen.) Since the height of the cells (the distance from the edge of the circle to the lumen) is greater than the width, the epithelium is *simple columnar*. The second epithelial type is represented by a small, longitudinally sectioned duct (**arrows**) extending across the field. It is comprised of flattened cells (note the nuclear shape), and on this basis the epithelium is *simple squamous*. Finally, there is a larger cross-sectioned duct (**asterisk**) into which the smaller duct enters. The nuclei of this larger duct tend to be round and the cells square in profile. Thus, these duct cells are a *simple cuboidal epithelium*.

Figure 2, a section of kidney, reveals cross-sectioned tubules of several types. Those that are labeled with the **arrows** provide another example of a simple cuboidal epithelium. The arrows point to the lateral cell boundaries; note that cell width approximates cell height. The cross-sectioned tubules marked with **asterisks** are another type; they are smaller in size, but are also comprised of a simple cuboidal epithelium.

Figure 3 shows the lining epithelium of the stomach, forming a sheet of mucus-secreting cells. The epithelial cells are extremely tall with a mucus-containing apical region just above the elongated nuclei. The cells are like tall pegs that extend down to the highly cellular connective tissue (**CT**). The two round cells or lymphocytes (**arrows**) at the base of the epithelium have wandered into the simple columnar epithelium from the underlying connective tissue, a frequent finding in the digestive tract.

Figure 4 shows a columnar epithelium from the trachea. However, in addition to the tall columnar cells (**CC**) there is also a definite layer of basal cells (**BC**). The columnar cells, which contain the elongate nuclei and possess cilia (**C**), extend from the surface to the basement membrane (clearly evident in the trachea as a thick, homogeneous region that is part of the connective tissue [**CT**]). The basal cells are interspersed between the columnar

KEY	
BC, basal cell	boundaries of
C, cilia	cuboidal tubule cells;
CC, columnar cell	Fig. 3, lymphocytes in
CT, connective tissue	epithelium
arrows, Fig. 1, tubule	**asterisk,** duct or tubule
comprised of simple	of simple cuboidal
squamous epithelium;	epithelium
Fig. 2, lateral	

Fig. 1, monkey, × 450	**Fig. 4,** monkey, × 450
Fig. 2, human, × 450	**Fig. 5,** human, × 450
Fig. 3, monkey, × 450	**Fig. 6,** human, × 225

cells. Since all of the cells rest on the basement membrane, they are regarded as a single layer as opposed to two discrete layers, one over the other. Because the epithelium appears to be stratified, but is not, it is called *pseudostratified columnar epithelium*. The **circle** in the micrograph delineates a tracheal gland, similar to the acinus circled in Figure 1. Note that the lumen of the gland is clearly visible and the cell boundaries are also evident. The gland epithelium is simple columnar.

Figure 5 shows a portion of the wall of the epididymis and provides another example of pseudostratified columnar epithelium. Again, two layers of nuclei are evident, those of basal cells (**BC**) and columnar cells (**CC**). However, as in the previous example, although not evident, the columnar cells rest on the basement membrane; thus, the epithelium is pseudostratified. Note that where the epithelium is vertically oriented on the right of the micrograph, there appear to be more nuclei and the epithelium is thicker. This is a result of a tangential plane of section. As a rule, always examine the thinnest area of an epithelium to visualize its true organization.

Figure 6 reveals the *stratified squamous epithelium* of the vaginal wall. The deeper cells, particularly those of the basal layer, are small, with little cytoplasm, and thus the nuclei appear closely packed. As the cells become larger, they tend to flatten out, forming disc-like squames. Because the surface cells retain this shape, the epithelium is stratified squamous.

PLATE 2

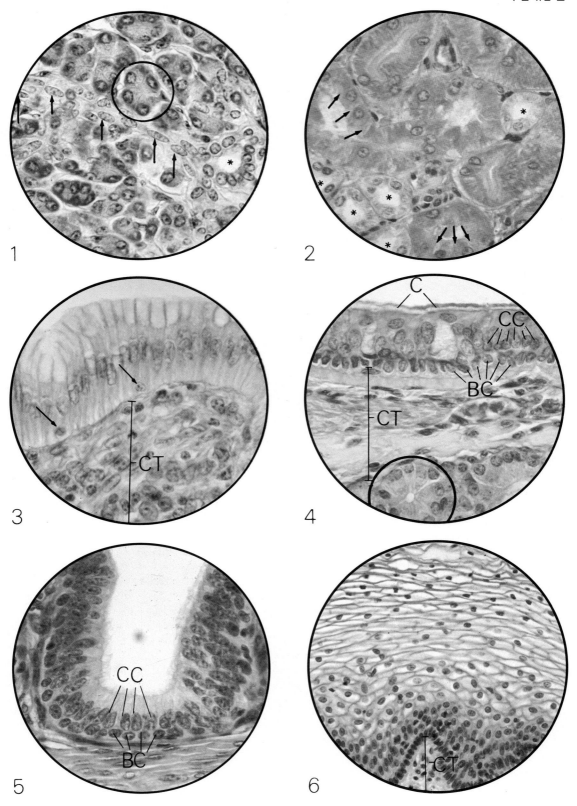

PLATE 3. Stratified Epithelia and Epithelioid Tissues

The micrograph of part of the wall of the esophagus in **Figure 1** reveals two different epithelia. On the left of the figure is the lining epithelium of the esophagus. It is multilayered with squamous surface cells; therefore, it is a *stratified squamous epithelium*. On the right is a duct of an esophageal gland, cut in varying planes due to its tortuous path through the connective tissue. By examining a region where the plane of section is at a right angle to the surface, usually the thinnest area, the true character of the epithelium is apparent. In this case the epithelium consists of two cell layers with cuboidal surface cells; thus, it is *stratified cuboidal* **(SC).**

Figure 2 reveals a portion of the duct of a sweat gland just before entering the stratified squamous epithelium (epidermis) of the skin. (The **dotted line** traces an obscured portion of the duct within the epidermis.) This duct is also comprised of a stratified cuboidal epithelium **(SC).** Note the arrangement of the duct cells—two layers; the cells of the inner layer (the surface cells) appear more or less square. Since the epidermal surface cells are not included in the field, the designation stratified squamous cannot be determined from the information offered by the micrograph.

Figure 3 reveals a crypt or fold at the anorectal junction, the terminal portion of the intestine. The area shows a transition where the epithelium changes from a *stratified cuboidal* **(SC)** to a *stratified columnar* **(SCol)** epithelium. Note how the surface cells along the lower part of the fold change in shape. Neither the cuboidal cells nor the columnar surface cells reach the basement membrane, but rather each represents a distinct cell layer occupying a surface position; therefore, the epithelia are stratified. Continuing along the columnar surface toward the right and just beyond the field would reveal a further change to a stratified squamous epithelium at the anal opening. (See Atlas Plate 82 for an orientation micrograph of this area.)

Figure 4 reveals the epithelium of the urinary bladder. It is actually a stratified epithelium, but it changes in appearance according to the degree of distension of the bladder; thus it is called *transitional epithelium.* In the nondistended state, as in **Figure 4,** the epithelium is about four or five cells deep. The surface cells are large and dome-shaped **(asterisks);** occasionally two nuclei are present in a single cell. The cells immediately under the surface

KEY

C, capillary
CT, connective tissue
En, endocrine cells
Ex, exocrine cells
IC, interstitial (Leydig) cells
SC, stratified cuboidal

epithelium
SCol, stratified columnar epithelium
SS, stratified squamous epithelium
asterisks, dome-shaped cells

Fig. 1, monkey, × 250
Fig. 2, human, × 450
Fig. 3, monkey, × 450
Fig. 4, monkey, × 450
Fig. 5, monkey, × 300
Fig. 6, human, × 450

cells are pear-shaped and slightly smaller. The deepest cells are the smallest and the nuclei appear more crowded. When the bladder is distended, the superficial cells are stretched into squamous cells and the epithelium is reduced in thickness to about three cells deep. It should be noted, however, that a specimen of the bladder wall is usually in a contracted state when it is removed, unless special steps have been taken to preserve it in a distended state. Because of this, its appearance is usually like that seen in **Figure 4.** Transitional epithelium is also present on the surface of the renal pelvis, the ureters, and part of the urethra.

Figure 5 shows the interstitial (Leydig) cells of the testis. They are present in clumps between the seminiferous tubules. These cells **(IC)** possess certain epithelial characteristics. However, they do not possess a free surface nor do they develop from a surface; instead they develop from mesenchymal cells. They are referred to as *epithelioid* cells because they contact similar neighboring cells much the same as epithelial cells contact each other. The Leydig cells are endocrine in nature.

The endocrine islet of Langerhans cells **(En)** of the pancreas are shown in **Figure 6.** They also have an epithelioid arrangement, that is, the cells are in contact, but lack a free surface. In contrast, the surrounding alveoli of the exocrine pancreas **(Ex)** are made up of cells with a free surface onto which the secretory product is discharged. Note that capillaries **(C)** are prominent in the endocrine tissues. Similar examples of epithelioid tissue are seen in the adrenal, parathyroid, and pituitary glands, all of which are endocrine glands.

PLATE 3

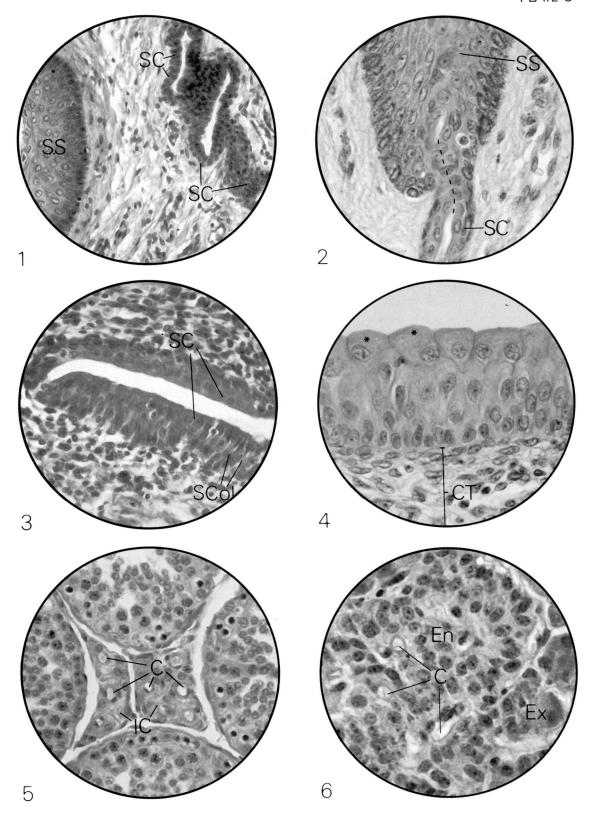

PLATE 4. Columnar Epithelium, Electron Microscopy

This electron micrograph of the small intestine illustrates some of the salient features of epithelium, particularly as they relate to the light microscopic image. It includes some of the underlying connective tissue, which in this instance is almost entirely occupied by a capillary containing a number of red blood cells (**RBC**).

The epithelium is simple columnar. All of the cells are absorptive; no goblet cells are included. The two round cells at the base of the epithelium are lymphocytes (**Lym**) that migrated from the connective tissue. Similar lymphocyte invasion of the epithelium, a typical occurrence, is also seen in **Figure 3,** Plate 2.

In appraising the electron micrograph, note first the relationship between the cells above the level of the nuclei. The cytoplasm of each cell comes into intimate apposition with its neighbors and consequently the cell boundaries at this magnification are difficult to discern. Below this level prominent intercellular spaces are present (**asterisks**). Here it is easy to define the limits of the individual cells. Next, examine the very basal aspect of the epithelium. Note that each cell extends by means of lateral cytoplasmic processes (**arrows**) to meet with its neighbors, thus again providing intimate cell apposition. At some sites, these basal processes are discontinuous (**circles**). This is probably due to the recent migration of the lymphocytes from the connective tissue into the epithelium. The basal cytoplasmic extensions rest on the basal lamina. (The basal lamina is not recognizable at this low magnification, but can be seen in the next plate.) The intercellular spaces, in effect, form a continuous compartment between the epithelial cells; the compartment is bounded above by the apical cytoplasm, where adjoining cells meet, and below by the lateral basal processes, which also join with one another. The visualization of this intercellular space is also possible with the light microscope (see Atlas Plate 78, Fig. 3). The presence of intercellular spaces of this type is characteristic of epithelia actively engaged in fluid transport, i.e., the active movement of fluid across an epithelium from lumen to the underlying connective tissue, and thus may be observed not only in the intestine,

KEY

Lym, lymphocyte
RBC, red blood cell
arrows, basal lateral
 process
asterisks, intercellular
 spaces

circles, discontinuity
 between basal
 processes
curved arrows,
 junctional complexes

Fig. × 4100

but in many other epithelia where fluid is actively transported. The essential point, however, is that despite the intercellular spaces, these cells, as an epithelium, do maintain intimate apposition with one another and, in this way, function as a selective barrier.

Two other features pertinent to epithelial cells as they relate to light microscopy are also evident in this micrograph. One concerns the apical contacts between neighboring cells, namely, the junctional complexes (**curved arrows**). Each complex appears as a short, thin, dark line in the electron micrograph. The complexes provide strong adhesion between adjoining cells and serve as a permeability barrier. Their unit structure and functional aspects are dealt with on the next text page. The junctional complexes are comparable to the fine, dot-like structures seen in the light microscope where they are referred to as terminal bars (see Fig. 4.10).

The other feature worthy of mention here relates to the microvilli that extend from the apical surface of the epithelial cells. In the small intestine the microvilli appear as closely packed, finger-like cytoplasmic projections, extremely uniform in size and shape. Because of their uniformity, at the light microscope level, they have a finely striped or striated appearance, hence the term *striated border*. Examination of Atlas Plate 78, **Figure 3** reveals the striated border as seen at medium power magnification in the light microscope.

PLATE 4

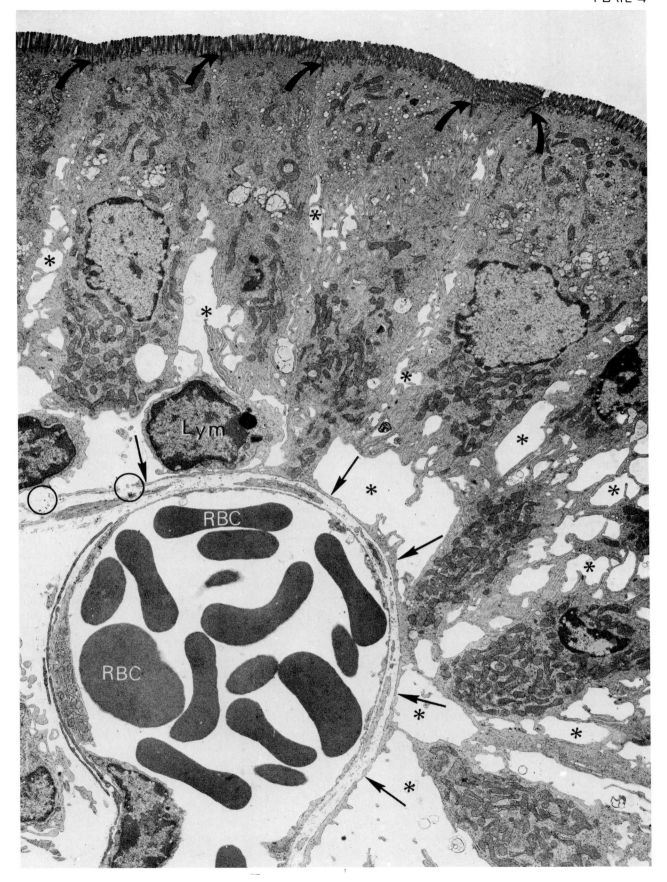

Figure 1 shows a portion of the apical cytoplasm of two epithelial cells from the same specimen as in Plate 4. The micrograph reveals the microvilli **(M)**, the junctional complex **(JC)**, and below this, the nonspecialized region of cell apposition **(NS)**.

Microvilli of the intestinal absorptive cell are uniform in size and shape. They display numerous fine, core filaments **(arrows)** that course the length of the microvilli and enter the underlying cytoplasmic region of the cell to become part of the terminal web **(TW)**. The latter is a filamentous component that extends across the breadth of the cell as a narrow band in the most apical region of the cell. Other cell organelles are excluded from the terminal web (or may only transiently pass through, as in the case of pinocytotic vesicles that originate from the plasma membrane at the base of adjacent microvilli). At the light microscope level the terminal web appears as a slightly darker-staining region in contrast to the striated border above and the cytoplasm immediately below. The staining of the terminal web is undoubtedly due to the numbers of filaments **(double arrows)** aggregated in this region of the cell.

Two of the three functionally important components of the junctional complex can be seen in **Figure 1.** One is the zonula occludens **(ZO)**, a surface specialization involving the membranes of adjacent cells. The outer leaflets of the opposing cell membranes within this specialization are in very close contact, essentially eliminating the intercellular fluid from the area. (The points of contact are actually in the form of rows or lines of membrane particles that can be seen in freeze fracture preparations.) The contact between the cells results in a narrow zone in which the intercellular space is functionally obliterated. The contact zone forms a band around the cell, thus preventing the free passage of substances across the epithelium via the intercellular space.

Immediately below the zonula occludens is the second structural component of the junctional complex, namely, the zonula adherens **(ZA)**. It, too, is a modification of the cell surface. Here the plasma membranes of the adjacent cells diverge slightly, leaving a uniform intercellular space of 15 to 20 nm. The fine filaments of the terminal web converge and insert into dense material bordering the cytoplasmic side of the plasma membrane of the zonula adherens. It is probable that the zonula adherens is the main element that contributes to

KEY	
CL, capillary lumen	**arrows,** Fig. 1, core
F, fibroblast process	filaments of microvilli;
JC, junctional complex	Fig. 2, basal lamina
M, microvilli	**arrowheads,** capillary
RBC, red blood cell	endothelium
TW, terminal web	**asterisk,** oblique cut of
ZA, zonula adherens	plasma membrane
ZO, zonula occludens	**double arrows,** filaments
NS, nonspecialized	of terminal web
region of cell	
apposition	
Fig. 1, × 26,000	**Fig. 2,** × 15,000

the visualization of the terminal bar seen in the light microscope. Although the zonula adherens appears relatively electron lucent, with no apparent structural content, as the name implies, it is thought to serve as a zone of strong adhesion between adjacent cells. Core filaments of the microvilli are regarded to be actin. There is evidence indicating that these filaments are functionally joined by myosin to constitute a contractile apparatus. (Myosin is usually lost during the routine preparation of the tissue.)

The macula adherens also serves as a strong attachment site, but occurs as focal or spot-like (macula) attachments between adjacent cells in contrast to the band-like zonula adherens that rings the cell. The macula adherens is not present in **Figure 1** but may be seen in Figure 4.11. The macula adherens corresponds to the desmosome of the light microscopist. When discernible in the light microscope, it appears as a fine dot or fusiform thickening.

Figure 2 shows the basal portion of the epithelium. The epithelial compartment extends as far as the basal lamina **(arrows)**. The lamina has been cut on edge and it appears as a delicate linear structure, so thin, that it cannot be resolved with the light microscope. Note that the basal processes of adjacent epithelial cells meet and in effect "close off" the intercellular epithelial space. The basal closure is simply a close approximation of the basal processes of adjacent cells without the presence of a junctional complex.

The figure also shows a small part of a red blood cell **(RBC)**, a capillary lumen **(CL)**, and the capillary endothelium **(arrowheads)**.

PLATE 5

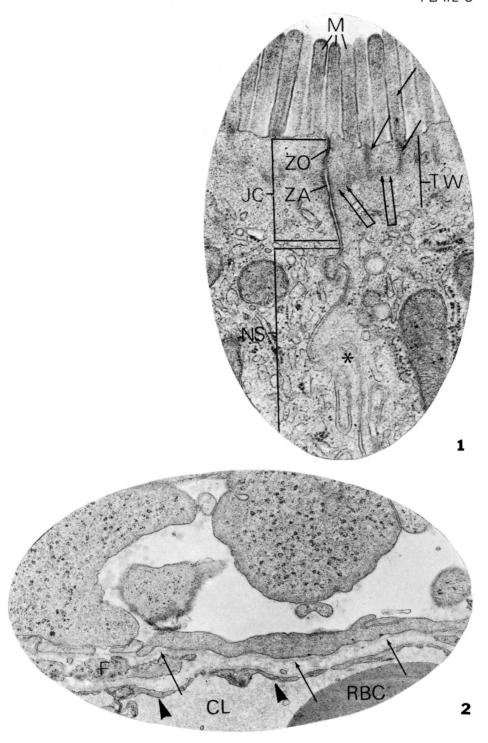

Connective Tissue

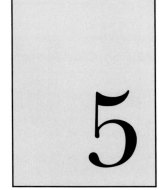

The term **connective tissue** is a general heading for a diverse group of tissues with a variety of functions. It includes tissues traditionally known as **connective tissue proper** and a subgroup of **specialized connective tissues** with highly specialized functions. In general, connective tissue consists of cells and extracellular fibers embedded in a matrix of coextensive ground substance and tissue fluid.

Connective tissue proper develops from **mesenchyme,** the embryonic connective tissue. It ultimately forms a vast and continuous compartment throughout the body, bounded at its peripheral reaches by the basal lamina of the various surface epithelia and by the basal lamina of the glands that secrete onto the surfaces. The connective tissue immediately under the surface epithelia serves as a supporting structure for the overlying epithelium. The support goes beyond simple mechanical support in that the connective tissue contains the blood vessels and nerves that serve the needs of the epithelium. More removed from the body surfaces, this vast continuous connective tissue compartment contains the larger blood vessels and nerves that course throughout the body.

Specialized connective tissues also develop from mesenchyme (except in the head where certain progenitor cells are derived from the ectoderm by way of the neural crest cells as was described in Chapter 4 in the section on neural crest cells and ectomesenchyme). The type of development followed by the mesenchyme derived cells reflects the function served by the tissue. If the functions of these specialized connective tissues are mechanical, the extracellular fibers and ground substance are the major features of the tissue. This is the case with ligaments, tendons, cartilage, and bone. In bone and some cartilage, the extracellular constituents become mineralized. If the specialized functions are protective (inflammatory and immune reactions) or the maintenance of energy reserves, the cells are the major features of the tissue. This is the case with lymphatic tissue, which participates in the immune response, and adipose tissue, which functions in energy storage. Another highly specialized tissue, usually classified as being related to the connective tissues, is blood. In this tissue, the extracellular material, namely, the plasma, is liquid.

CLASSIFICATION OF CONNECTIVE TISSUE

Classifications of connective tissues are difficult to formulate. They have changed through the years as new information uncovers significant relationships or minimizes the presumed significance of others. Thus, the following classification should not be regarded as definitive, but rather as an aid in learning and grouping. The classification is shown in Table 5.1. The dense connective tissue classified as connective tissue proper is **irregularly arranged,** that is, the fiber bundles are interwoven and have no regular orientation. (The fiber bundles of **dense regular connective tissue,** one of the specialized tissues, are arranged in parallel and, thus, are adapted for bearing tension in one direction.)

CONNECTIVE TISSUE PROPER

Connective tissue proper is divided into two general subtypes. **Loose connective tissue** contains aggregates of loosely arranged fibers and many cells. **Dense connective tissue** contains more numer-

TABLE 5.1. Classification of Connective Tissue

Connective tissue proper
  Loose connective tissue
  Dense (irregular) connective tissue
Specialized connective tissue*
  Dense regular connective tissue (ligaments and
    tendons)
  Adipose tissue (Chapter 6)
  Blood (Chapter 9)
  Bone (Chapter 8)
  Cartilage (Chapter 7)
  Hemopoietic tissue (Chapter 9)
  Lymphatic tissue (Chapter 13)
Embryonic connective tissue
  Mesenchyme
  Mucous connective tissue

*The designations *elastic tissue* and *reticular tissue,* in the past, have been listed as separate categories of specialized connective tissue. The tissues usually cited as examples of elastic tissues are certain ligaments associated with the spinal column and the tunica media of elastic arteries. The identifying features of reticular tissue is the presence of reticular fibers and reticular cells together forming a three-dimensional stroma. This reticular tissue serves as the stroma for hemopoietic tissue (specifically the red bone marrow) and lymphatic tissue organs (lymph nodes, spleen, but not the thymus gland).

thicker fibers, but considerably fewer cells (Fig. 5.1). The cells in dense connective tissue are chiefly of a single type, namely, the fibroblast, which is responsible for producing and maintaining the fibers. Loose connective tissue contains not only the fibroblast, but also a variety of other cells, most of which participate in the body's defense mechanisms. Since the primary location of loose connective tissue is beneath those epithelia that cover the surfaces and line the internal cavities of the body, it represents the initial site in which antigens and other foreign substances, such as bacteria, can be challenged and destroyed. The majority of the cell types present in loose connective tissue are transient wandering cells that migrate from the local blood vessels in response to specific stimuli. In many areas, however, the continued presence of invasive foreign substances results in constantly large populations of these cells. This is particularly true of the lamina propria of certain mucous membranes.

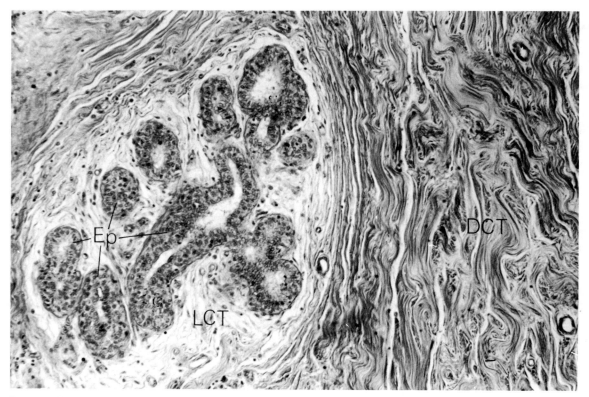

Figure 5.1. Light micrograph comparing loose and dense connective tissue from the mammary gland stained with H&E. On the left, surrounding the epithelium of the gland (Ep), is loose connective tissue. On the right and upper left of the figure is dense irregular connective tissue (DCT). The loose connective tissue (LCT) is comprised of a wispy arrangement of collagen fibers with many cells. Note the large number of nuclei as seen at this low magnification. In contrast, the dense connective tissue reveals a relative paucity of nuclei. However, the collagen is considerably more abundant and is comprised of very thick fibers. × 200.

CONNECTIVE TISSUE FIBERS

Collagen Fibers

The fibers of connective tissue are of three types: collagen, elastic, and reticular. *Collagen,* or *collagenous fibers* are the principal and most abundant fibers of connective tissue. They are also the most abundant fibers of bone and the dentin of teeth. Collagen fibers are flexible and have a high tensile strength. With the light microscope, they typically appear as wavy structures of variable width and indeterminant length (Fig. 5.1). They stain readily with eosin and other acid dyes, and they can be colored differentially with the dye aniline blue, used in Mallory's connective tissue stain, or the dye light green in Masson's stain.

When examined in the electron microscope, the collagen fiber is seen to consist of a bundle of fine, thread-like subunits, the collagen fibrils (Fig. 5.2). The collagen fibrils within a bundle are relatively uniform in diameter. However, in different locations and in different stages of development, the fibrils differ in size. In developing or immature tissues, the fibrils may be as small as 15 to 20 nm in diameter, while those in dense regular connective tissue of tendons or in other tissue that undergoes stress may measure up to 200 nm.

Collagen fibrils exhibit a sequence of closely spaced transverse bands which repeat every 68 nm along the length of the fibril (Fig. 5.2 inset). The banding is a reflection of the arrangement of the collagen molecules that constitute the fibril (Fig. 5.3). These molecules measure about 300 nm long by 1.5 nm thick. They are aligned end-to-end in overlapping rows with a gap between the molecules within each row. The gap and overlap of the collagen molecules account for the 68 nm periodicity.

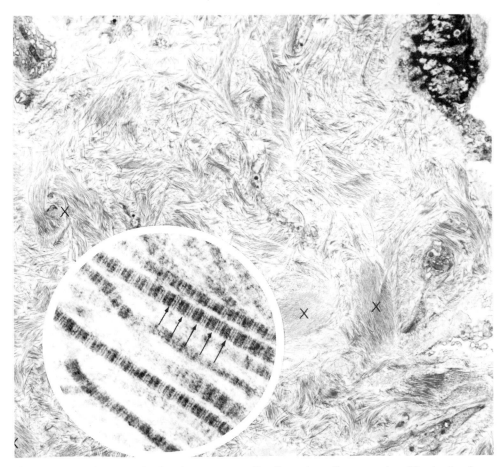

Figure 5.2. Electron micrograph of a dense connective tissue from the capsule of the testis of a young boy. The thread-like collagen fibrils are aggregated in some areas (X) to form relatively thick bundles, whereas in certain other areas the fibrils are more dispersed. The **inset** shows a higher magnification longitudinal arrays of collagen fibrils from the same specimen. Note the banding pattern. The spacing of the **arrows** indicates the 68-nm repeat pattern.

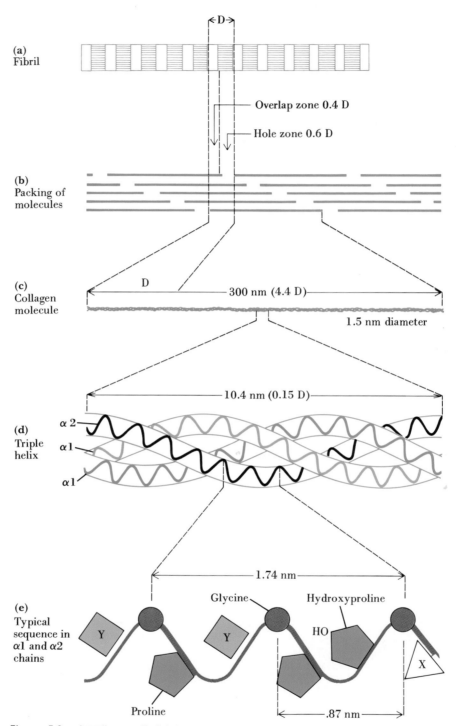

Figure 5.3. A collagen fibril **(a)** displays periodic banding with a distance (D) of 68 nm between repeating bands .It is made up of staggered collagen molecules **(b)**, each of which is about 300 nm long and 1.5 nm in diameter **(c)**. The collagen molecule consists of a triple helix **(d)**; the three components of the triple helix consist of alpha chains. Each third amino acid of the alpha chain is a glycine. The X position following glycine is frequently a proline, and the Y position preceding the glycine is frequently a hydroxyproline **(e)**. (Based on Prockop DJ, Guzman NA: *Hospital Practice* 12:2, Dec. 1977.)

TABLE 5.2. Types of Collagen

TYPE	COMPOSITION*	LOCATION	FUNCTIONS
I	$[\alpha1(I)]_2\alpha2(I)*$ or $[\alpha1(I)]_3$	Connective tissue of skin, bone, tendon, ligaments, dentine, sclera, fascia, and organ capsules (account for 90% of body collagen)	Provide resistance to force, tension, and stretch
II	$[\alpha1(II)]_3$	Cartilage (hyaline and elastic), notochord, and intervertebral disc	Provide resistance to pressure
III	$[\alpha1(III)]_3$	Connective tissue of organs (uterus, liver, spleen, kidney, lung, etc.), smooth muscle, endoneurium, blood vessels, and fetal skin	Provide structural support and elasticity
IV	$[\alpha1(IV)]_3$ or $[\alpha2(IV)]_3$	Basal laminae of epithelial and endothelial cells; kidney glomeruli, and lens capsule	Provide support and filtration barrier
V	$[\alpha1(V)]_2\alpha2(V)$	Basal laminae (external laminae) of smooth and skeletal muscle cells, Schwann and glial cells, and placental epithelium (also found in very small quantities with other types of collagen)	Provide support and may be involved in other roles not yet defined

* Each collagen fibril is composed of three polypeptide chains intertwined in helical configuration. The Roman numerals in column 2 indicate that the alpha chains (α) have a distinctive structure that differs from the chains with different numerals. Thus, collagen type I has two $\alpha1$ chains and one $\alpha2$ chain.

The *collagen* molecule is made up of three polypeptide chains, called alpha chains, arranged as a triple helix. The alpha chains are not all alike, and according to the differences in alpha chains, 15 different types of collagen molecules have been described to date. The five most common and best characterized types of collagen, designated type I through type V, are listed in Table 5.2. In type I collagen, one of the alpha chains differs from the other two; the other types are each composed of three similar alpha chains. Except at the ends of the alpha chains, every third amino acid is a gly-

---

HERITABLE DISORDERS OF CONNECTIVE TISSUE

There are a number of diseases that are associated with errors in collagen synthesis. For example, Ehlers-Danlos syndrome is an hereditary disorder characterized by hypermobility of joints and hyperextensibility of the skin, which is very thin. These individuals are predisposed to sudden death from rupture of large blood vessels or the large intestine. There are several forms of the disease. In some of them, the specific molecular defect is known. In individuals with one of the type IV variants of the disease, the defect is associated with the synthesis and structure of type III collagen, which is the collagen type associated with skin and blood vessels (see Table 5.2). The skin of affected individuals may lack type III collagen. There is no effective treatment for the disease.

A second example of a hereditary disease, which results from abnormal collagen synthesis, is osteogenesis imperfecta. Individuals suffering from this disorder have increased fragility of bones. In some individuals, the sclera of the eye is colored blue instead of the normal white. They may also have hearing loss, abnormalities of the teeth, or a combination of these features. There are several variants of the disease. All appear to be associated with the synthesis of type I collagen. Some of the genetic defects result in the production of shortened polypeptides of type I collagen; others may result in the abnormal assembly and maintenance of bone and other connective tissue elements. There is no effective treatment for this disease either. Since type I collagen is a major component of bones, the features of the disease are usually most evident during infancy and childhood when the individual is growing.

cine. The glycine, proline, and hydroxyproline are essential for the triple helix conformation (other amino acids in Fig. 5.3 are designated as X or Y). Associated with the collagen molecule are sugar groups which are joined to hydroxylysyl residues. Because of the sugar groups, collagen is properly designated as a glycoprotein. The sugar groups, however, are not sufficiently numerous or of a reactive type to give a positive reaction with the periodic acid-Schiff (PAS) procedure. The collagen of reticular fibers has more sugar groups, thereby allowing these fibers to exhibit a positive PAS reaction.

Reticular Fibers

Reticular fibers are closely related to collagenous fibers in that they both consist of collagen fibrils. However, the fibrils in reticular fibers are always of narrow diameter (about 20 nm); they do not form large bundles; in many locations they are dispersed singly in a more extensive matrix of ground substance; and they contain a higher content of sugar groups. In routinely stained hema-

toxylin and eosin (H&E) paraffin sections, reticular fibers are not identifiable. However, reticular fibers are readily displayed by means of the PAS reaction. They are also displayed with special silver staining procedures. After silver treatment, the fibers appear black (and, thus, they are said to be **argyrophilic**); the thicker collagen fibers are colored brown with the same treatment (Fig. 5.4).

Reticular fibers are typically arranged in a network or mesh-like pattern. In loose connective tissue, networks of reticular fibers are found at the boundary of connective tissue with epithelium and around adipocytes, small blood vessels, and nerves. In addition to their location in loose connective tissue, reticular fibers are present in the adult as a supporting stroma in the hemopoietic and lymphatic tissues, in the liver and certain other glands, and around smooth muscle cells. They are present in embryonic connective tissue (mesenchyme), but are replaced by collagen fibers as the tissue matures.

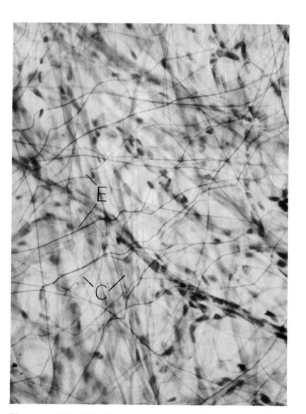

Figure 5.5. Photomicrograph of a mesentery spread stained with resorcin fuchsin. The mesentery is very thin and the microscope can be focused through the entire thickness of the tissue. The delicate thread-like branching strands are the elastic fibers (E). Collagen fibers (C) are also evident. They are much thicker, and while they cross one another, they do not branch.

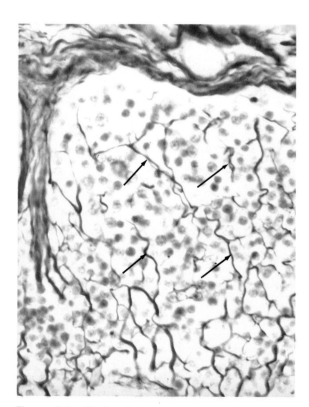

Figure 5.4. Photomicrograph of a lymph node silver preparation showing the connective tissue capsule at the top and trabeculum extending from it at the left. The reticular fibers **(arrows)** form an irregular anastomosing network.

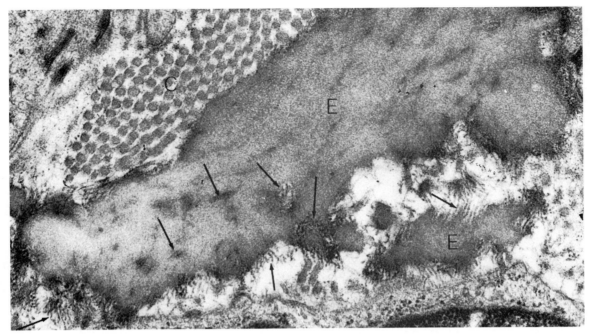

Figure 5.6. Electron micrograph of an elastic fiber. The elastin (E) has a relatively amorphous appearance. The microfibrils **(arrows)** are present at the periphery and within the substance of the fiber. A number of collagen fibrils (C) are also present in the micrograph.

Elastic Fibers

As the name implies, ***elastic fibers*** have elastic properties. These fibers are typically thinner than collagenous fibers, and they are arranged in an apparently random fashion, branching to form networks. Elastic fibers stain with eosin, but not well, and, thus, they cannot usually be distinguished from collagenous fibers of the connective tissue proper in routine H&E preparations. Since elastic fibers become somewhat refractile with certain fixatives, they may be distinguished from collagenous fibers in H&E preparations when they display this characteristic. However, elastic fibers can be selectively stained with special dyes such as resorcin fuchsin, as shown in Figure 5.5. Other special dyes and methods that color elastic material selectively include Weigert's Elastic Tissue Stain, purple-violet; Gomori's Aldehyde Fuchsin Stain, blue-black; Verhoeff Haematoxylin Elastic Tissue Stain, black; and Modified Taenzer-Unna Orcein Stain, red-brown. With the electron microscope, the elastic fibers are seen to consist of an amorphous component called ***elastin*** and a fibrillar component called ***microfibrils***[1] (Fig. 5.6). The microfi-

brils are relatively straight and thin (12 nm in diameter). In young, developing elastic material, the microfibrils predominate over the amorphous component; in adult elastic material, the amorphous component predominates.

Elastic material is the major extracellular substance in two major locations: in elastic ligaments associated with the spinal column and in elastic arteries. In the elastic ligaments, the elastic material is in the form of fibers. In the elastic arteries the elastic material is in the form of fenestrated lamellae. The lamellae are arranged as concentric layers within the vessel wall.

GROUND SUBSTANCE

The ***ground substance*** surrounds the cells and fibers of connective tissue. This is histologically unstructured or amorphous and consists of proteoglycans (PG) and glycosaminoglycans (GAG) of various types. A glycosaminoglycan consists of repeating disaccharide units, one of which is a sulfated hexosamine. An exception to this general pattern is hyaluronic acid, the largest glycosaminoglycan, in which the hexosamines are not sulfated. However, some of the sugars attached to the molecule are negatively charged uronic acids. A proteoglycan is comprised of a glycosaminoglycan chain covalently bound to a core protein. The

---

[1] The microfibril, an extracellular fibrillar component, should not be confused with the microfilament, an intracellular component composed of actin.

TABLE 5.3. Glycosaminoglycans

NAME	APPROXIMATE MOLECULAR WEIGHT (IN DALTONS)	DISACCHARIDE COMPOSITION
Hyaluronic acid	10^6	D-Glucuronic acid + N-Acetylglucosamine
Chondroitin 4-sulfate	20,000	D-Glucuronic acid + N-Acetylgalactosamine 4-sulfate
Chondroitin 6-sulfate	20,000	D-Glucuronic acid + N-Acetylgalactosamine 6-sulfate
Dermatan sulfate	55,000	L-Iduronic acid + N-Acetylgalactosamine 4-sulfate
Keratan sulfate	7,000	Galactose (or galactose 6-sulfate) + N-Acetylglucosamine 6-sulfate

major kinds of glycosaminoglycans, along with their approximate molecular weights and disaccharide compositions, are given in Table 5.3.

The ground substance of cartilage has been subject to considerable investigation, and the current understanding of how proteoglycans are organized and related to collagen fibrils in the ground substance of cartilage is illustrated in Figure 5.7. The proteoglycan monomer (molecule) consists of a central core protein (mol wt = 300,000) to which about 80 to 100 chondroitin sulfate chains are attached like bristles of a test tube brush. The proteoglycan monomers are joined to a hyaluronic acid molecule, which is extremely long,

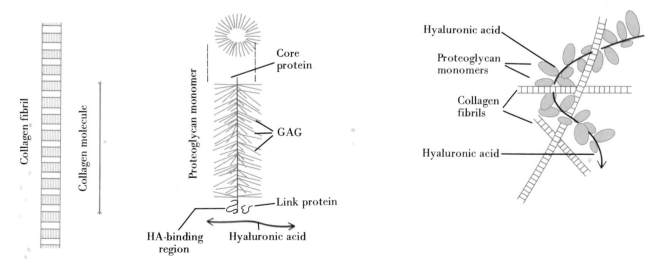

Figure 5.7. Schematic diagram showing a model for the organization of ground substance of cartilage. On the left, a collagen fibril and a collagen molecule are depicted for reference. The next item shows a proteoglycan monomer, hyaluronic acid (HA), and a link protein. The proteoglycan monomer consists of approximately 100 glycosaminoglycan units (GAG) joined to a core protein. The end of the core protein contains an HA-binding region; interaction with the HA is strengthened by a link protein. On the right, an HA molecule forming a linear aggregate with many proteoglycan momomers is interwoven with a network of collagen fibrils. (Based on Hascall VC, Lowther DA: In Nancollas GH, et al: *Biological Mineralization and Demineralization*. New York, Springer, 1982, p. 181.)

thereby forming a large proteoglycan-hyaluronic acid (PG-HA) aggregate. The attachment of each proteoglycan to the hyaluronic acid is reinforced by a "link protein." On the right side of the figure, a portion of a PG-HA aggregate is shown with several adjacent collagen fibrils. The PG-HA aggregate is intertwined through the spaces between the collagen fibrils and joined at certain points to the collagen fibrils.

The ground substance of cartilage is extremely rich in proteoglycans and is extremely hydrated. In tissues where there is much less ground substance and considerably less water (as in the cornea), the proteoglycans contain only one or two glycosaminoglycans per core protein as compared to the 80 to 100 found in cartilage.

When present in high concentration, as in cartilage, the proteoglycans can be stained with hematoxylin and with basic dyes. The staining is due chiefly to the presence of sulfate groups. Moreover, with certain basic dyes, such as toluidine blue, the ground substance of cartilage displays metachromasia. When present in lower concentrations, proteoglycans can be displayed with colloidal iron or with the dye alcian blue.

CONNECTIVE TISSUE CELLS

The resident or regularly present cells of loose connective tissue are the *fibroblast, connective tissue macrophage* (*histiocyte*), *mast cell,* and *plasma cell.* Loose connective tissue also contains a large number of transient cells that migrate from the blood, namely, *neutrophils, eosinophils, monocytes,* and *lymphocytes.* In addition, it may contain *adipocytes, myofibroblasts,* and *undifferentiated mesenchymal cells.*

The Fibroblast and Fiber Synthesis

The fibroblast is the cell that produces the extracellular fibers and ground substance of connective tissue. Where active production of these extracellular materials is in progress, as in wound repair, the cytoplasm of the fibroblast displays a slight basophilia due to the presence of increased amounts of rough endoplasmic reticulum (rER). In the usual sample of adult connective tissue, the fibroblast cytoplasm is somewhat more attenuated and less conspicuous. It stains slightly with eosin, but it is usually difficult to distinguish it from the extracellular fibers, which also stain with eosin (Fig. 5.8). In addition, the fibroblast typically possesses long, thin cytoplasmic processes, but they cannot be distinguished from the extracellular fibers in routinely stained paraffin sections. The nu-

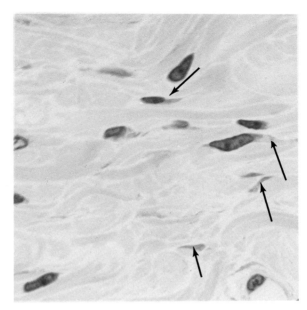

Figure 5.8. A light micrograph of a connective tissue specimen fixed with glutaraldehyde, embedded in plastic and stained with H&E. Thin strands of fibroblast cytoplasm **(arrows)** belonging to a few preferentially oriented cells can just barely be recognized between collagen fibers. In routine H&E paraffin preparations, it is usually impossible to distinguish the attenuated and poorly preserved fibroblast cytoplasm from the collagen fibers. Typically, only the nuclei of these cells are evident.

cleus of the fibroblast is typically ovoid and somewhat flattened. In face view, it displays finely granular chromatin (heterochromatin) and a small nucleolus. With the electron microscope, the most conspicuous organelles of the fibroblast cytoplasm are the rER, mitochondria, and the Golgi apparatus (Fig. 5.9).

Collagen Synthesis. The production of collagen fibers involves a series of events, some of which occur inside the cell and others outside. Three basic events occur in the cytoplasm of the fibroblast in association with vesicles (Fig. 5.10):

(1) Polypeptide chains are produced by polyribosomes of the rER from information provided by messenger RNA (translation) and are simultaneously discharged into the cisternae of the rER.

(2) Within the cisternae of the rER and the Golgi, a number of post-translational modifications of the polypeptide chains occur. These include: (a) cleavage of the signal peptide (see Chapter 2); (b) hydroxylation of prolysine and lysine residues, while the polypeptides are still in the nonhelical conformation; (c) addition of O-linked sugar groups (glycosylation) to some hy-

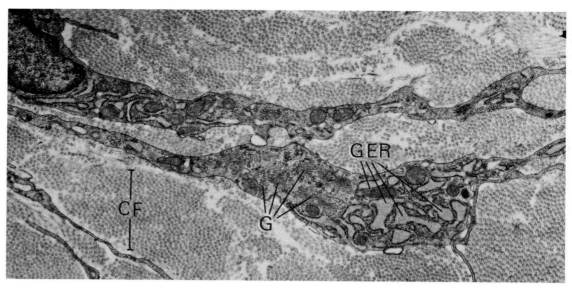

Figure 5.9. Electron micrograph of processes of several fibroblasts. The nucleus of one is the upper left of the micrograph. The cytoplasm shows conspicuous profiles of granular (or rough) endoplasmic reticulum (GER). The cisternae of the reticulum are distended, a reflection of active synthesis. In proximity to the reticulum is a Golgi profile (G). Surrounding the cells are collagen fibrils (CF); almost all have been cut in cross-section and, thus, appear as small dots at this magnification.

droxylysine residues and N-linked sugars to the two terminal portions; (d) formation of a triple helix by three polypeptide chains except at the terminals where the polypeptide chains remain uncoiled; and (e) formation of intrachain and interchain disulfide bonds that influence the shape of the molecule and stabilize the interactions of the polypeptides. The resultant molecule is called procollagen. (It might be noted that ascorbate, or vitamin C, is among the requirements for post-translational changes in the structure of procollagen; this explains why in vitamin C deficiency wounds fail to heal and bone formation is impaired.)

(3) The procollagen moves to the exterior of the cell by means of secretory granules. Microtubules are involved in the movement of the secretory granules from the region of the Golgi to the cell surface; if the microtubules are disrupted with agents such as colchicine or vinblastine, the secretory granules accumulate in the Golgi region.

After the procollagen is secreted into the extracellular space,[2] enzymes cleave most of the un-

coiled amino acid residues from the terminals of the procollagen, thereby forming a molecule called *tropocollagen* (Fig. 5.11). The tropocollagen molecules aggregate to form the collagen fibril (see Fig. 5.2). The development of the tensile strength of the collagen fibril is due to the formation of cross-links between lysine and hydroxylysine residues on the polypeptides of the neighboring row of collagen molecules after they have aggregated. The formation of cross-links with time also makes the older molecules more stable.

Cells other than fibroblasts that produce collagen are mesenchymal cells, myofibroblasts, perineurial cells, cementoblasts, odontoblasts, osteoblasts, cartilage cells, and some smooth muscle cells. In addition, epithelial cells, muscle cells, adipocytes, and Schwann and glial cells produce type IV and V collagen that are components of their basal laminae (see Table 5.2).

Elastin Synthesis. Elastin is synthesized by the fibroblast and modified by means of the same basic cellular pathway involved in the formation of collagen. Both processes can occur simultaneously in a cell. The orderly modification and assembly of procollagen and proelastin, and later of tropocolla-

---

[2] The cell appears to utilize multiple mechanisms to localize collagen fiber assembly at a site near its surface. First, secretory vesicles containing procollagen are concentrated at the pole of the cell where assembly is to occur. Second, the surface of the cell at this pole is indented to create a protective extracellular region, or "cove" where assembly is to occur. The cove surrounds the nascent end of a growing collagen fiber. Third, collagen self-assembles from tropocollagen in a concentration-dependent fashion. Therefore, all that is required for collagen to assemble in an orderly fashion is for the cell to create a zone of high tropocollagen concentration and migrate in a direction to facilitate the linear growth of the collagen filament(s).

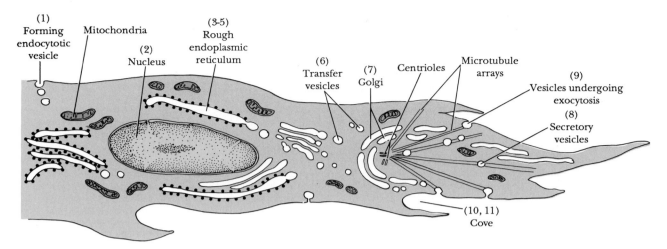

(1) Forming endocytotic vesicle Mitochondria (2) Nucleus (3-5) Rough endoplasmic reticulum (6) Transfer vesicles (7) Golgi Centrioles Microtubule arrays (9) Vesicles undergoing exocytosis (8) Secretory vesicles (10, 11) Cove

EVENTS IN COLLAGEN SYNTHESIS

Intracellular Events

(1) Uptake of amino acids (proline, lysine, etc.) by endocytosis

(2) Formation of mRNA

(3) Synthesis of alpha chains with registration peptides by ribosomes

(4) Hydroxylation of proline and lysine residues and cleavage of signal sequence in rER

(5) Glycosylation of specific hydroxylysyl residues in rER

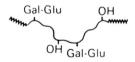

(6) Formation of procollagen triplet helix molecules in rER and movement into transfer vesicle

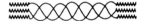

(7) Packaging of the procollagen by the Golgi into secretory vesicles

(8) Movement of vesicles to plasma membrane assisted by microfilaments and microtubules

(9) Exocytosis of procollagen

Extracellular Events

(10) Cleavage of registered, nonhelical ends of the procollagen to form tropocollagen

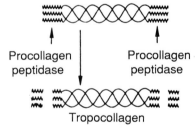

Procollagen peptidase   Procollagen peptidase

Tropocollagen

(11) Polymerization of tropocollagen into collagen fibril (in coves initially)

Figure 5.10. Schematic representation of the biosynthetic events and the organelles participating in collagen synthesis (Modified from Junqueira L, Carneiro J, Long J: Basic Histology, 5th Ed., Los Altos, CA, Lange, 1986).

gen and tropoelastin, involves elements of regulation and self-assembly built into the precursor proteins themselves. These coding or signal regions direct the movements of the polypeptide chains through metabolic machinery of the cell and their interactions with other molecules.

Like airline tags on luggage, the signal regions ensure that the components of procollagen and proelastin remain separate and properly identi-

fied, as they pass one another during their transit through the organelles of the cell where a series of synthetic events occur and then ultimately arrive at their proper destination.

Mast Cell

The mast cell is an ovoid connective tissue cell with a spherical nucleus. Its cytoplasm is filled with

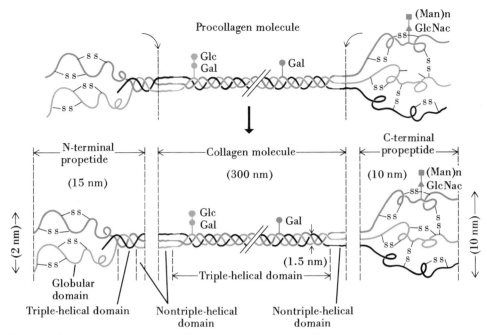

Figure 5.11. Illustration showing procollagen molecule with N- and C- terminals. **Small curved arrows** in upper part of illustration show where terminals are split from the procollagen molecule to form the collagen molecule (tropocollagen molecule). On the C-terminal (right side of the diagram), the sugar subunit is GlcNac$_2$ attached to [Man]$_n$. (Based on Prokop DJ, et al: *N Engl J Med* 30:18, 1979.)

large, membrane-limited granules (Fig. 5.12). The mast cell is related to, but not identical to, the basophil of the blood, which contains similar large granules in its cytoplasm. In small laboratory animals, the granular contents are more or less homogeneous; in humans, the granules also contain lamellar and paracrystalline material. The mast cell cytoplasm displays only small amounts of rER, smooth endoplasmic reticulum (sER), mitochondria, and a Golgi.

Mast cells are not easily identified in human tissue sections unless special fixatives are used to preserve the granules. After the use of special fixatives, such as glutaraldehyde, mast cell granules can be displayed with basic dyes, such as toluidine blue, which stain the mast cell granules intensely due to their high content of sulfate in heparin, a sulfated proteoglycan (Fig. 5.13). In the rat, routine fixatives are sufficient to preserve the mast granules.

It is not evident, from the view afforded by microscopy, whether the fibroblasts passively rest in spaces in the matrix (that is, ground substances and fibers) or are mechanically attached and integrated with it. Our understanding of the role of the fibroblast in forming, maintaining, and turning over the extracellular matrix does not require a physical attachment to it. However, tissue culture studies reveal that fibroblasts are anchored tightly to matrix elements and that these attachments are important to the cell as it extends cytoplasmic processes and moves. The attachments made by the fibroblasts involve several mechanisms that may be divided into two classes (some of the mechanisms are understood better than others). The first class of mechanisms requires the presence of receptors for proteins of fibrils, such as collagen, and receptors for glycoproteins, such as fibronectin, which are attached to the fibrils. A second class appears to involve the covalent association of GAGs with specific integral plasma membrane proteins. The attachments established between the fibroblasts and the matrix involve proteins, that are distinct from proteins that mediate cell-cell contacts. In terms of function, these proteins are similar to those involved in attachments of epithelial cells to the basal lamina. Small variation in the structure of the proteins involved in these contacts confer an individuality to the different cell and matrix types with which they are associated. These differences may establish molecular specificity and presumably assist in specialization of function found in different tissue sites.

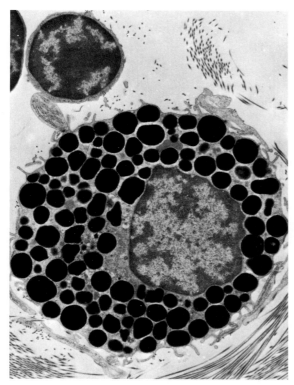

Figure 5.12. An electron micrograph of a mast cell. The cytoplasm is virtually filled with granules. Note a small lymphocyte is present in the upper left of the figure. × 6,000.

Several active substances are contained in mast cell granules. These are released from the cell upon appropriate stimulation, such as exposure to an antigen to which the individual has already been sensitized. (Sensitization develops when an individual is exposed to a foreign substance, desig-

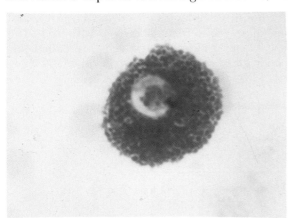

Figure 5.13. A photomicrograph of a mast cell stained with toluidine blue. The granules stain intensely and, because of their numbers, tend to appear as a solid mass in some areas. The nucleus of the cell is represented by the pale-staining area.

nated an antigen, which the body recognizes as "nonself" and against which the body produces antibodies.) Upon initial exposure to the antigen, cells of the immune system, which express on their surface antibody molecules that recognize and are specific for the antigen (cognate antibodies), are induced to proliferate, thereby resulting in the production of more antibody specific to the original antigen. Several major classes of antibodies, referred to as immunoglobulins, are produced (see Chapter 13). The mast cells do not produce antibodies but are dependent upon plasma cells to produce antibodies that bind to their surface. When stimulated by the presence of "foreign" antigen, the plasma cells produce antibodies that are released into the connective tissue. Immunoglobulins of the IgE class, which are specific to individual antigens, bind to receptors located in the plasma membrane of the mast cells. Upon subsequent exposure to the same antigen, an antigen-antibody reaction occurs that causes the discharge of mast cell granules.) The discharge of mast cell granules can result in immediate hypersensitivity reactions—allergy and anaphylaxis.

Four substances known to be released by mast cells are: **histamine,** the **slow-reacting substance of anaphylaxis;** the **eosinophil chemotactic factor of anaphylaxis,** and **heparin.** In the immune response, histamine and slow-reacting substance of anaphylaxis increase the permeability of small blood vessels, thereby causing edema of the surrounding tissues. Heparin is an anticoagulant. The eosinophil chemotactic factor of anaphylaxis stimulates eosinophils to migrate to the sites where mast cells have released their agents (the eosinophils counteract the effects of the histamine and slow-reacting substance of anaphylaxis.

Mast cells are especially numerous in the connective tissues of the skin and mucous membranes. They are distributed chiefly in the vicinity of small blood vessels, a target of histamine and SRS-A. Mast cells are also present in the capsules of organs and to a lesser degree within the organs, for example, in the connective tissue that surrounds the blood vessels of the organ. A notable exception is the central nervous system. While the meninges (sheets of connective tissue that surround the brain and spinal cord) contain mast cells, the connective tissue around the small blood vessels within the substance of the brain and spinal cord is devoid of mast cells, thereby protecting the brain and spinal cord from the potentially disrupting effects of the edema characteristic of allergic reactions. Mast cells are also numerous in the thymus and to a lesser degree in other lymphatic organs, but they are not present in the spleen.

The Macrophage and the Mononuclear Phagocytic Spleen (MPS)

There is a system of cells, widely distributed throughout the body, that have the ability to phagocytize avidly vital dyes, such as trypan blue, and India ink. These cells engulf and accumulate the vital dyes so that they are visible with the light microscope. Classical histologists described these cells as constituting the reticuloendothelial system (RES). Certain cells not belonging to this system (for example, fibroblasts) can also engage in phagocytosis, but such activity is not avid nor is it enhanced by immunological stimulation. It is now known that cells that engage in the avid phagocytosis of injected vital dyes are derived from monocytes. This common origin serves as the major distinguishing feature of the system as it is currently perceived, and the system is now called the *mononuclear phagocytic system* (MPS). The cells of the MPS are listed in Table 5.4.

Macrophage (Histiocyte)

Connective tissue *macrophages,* also known as *histiocytes,* have been traditionally described as *fixed* or *wandering.* The two designations refer to different states of the same cell. The wandering macrophage is slightly ovoid in shape; the fixed macrophage contains long cytoplasmic processes, as revealed by scanning and transmission electron microscopy.

The surface of the cell is thrown into numerous folds and finger-like projections (Fig. 5.14). The surface folds are active in phagocytosis in that they engulf substances to be phagocytosed. In the case of large objects, such as other cells, the folds spread over and surround the object to be phagocytosed. The cytoplasm of the macrophage contains relatively large Golgi, rER, sER, mitochondria, secretory vesicles, and lysosomes. The

lysosomes are the structures most indicative of the specialized phagocytic capability of the cell. In addition, there may be endocytotic vacuoles, secondary lysosomes, and other evidence of phagocytosis. The rER and Golgi support the synthesis of proteins of the phagocytotic and lysosomal systems as well as of the secretory system. The secretory products leave the cell by both the constitutive and regulated exocytotic pathways (see Chapter 2). Regulated secretion can be activated by phagocytosis, immune complexes, complement, and signals from lymphocytes (which include the release of *lymphokines,* biologically active molecules that influence the activity of other cells). The secretory products released by the macrophage include a wide variety of substances related to the immune response, anaphylaxis, and inflammation. The release of neutral proteases and GAGases (enzymes able to break down GAG) facilitates the migration of the macrophages through the connective tissue.

With conventional stains, the light microscope tissue macrophages are difficult to identify unless they display obvious evidence of phagocytic activity. Lysosomes can be demonstrated by virtue of their acid phosphatase activity (both at the light and electron microscope level) and such special staining procedures aid in the identification of the macrophage. A feature, not always evident, but one that is often useful in identifying the macrophage, is indentation of the nucleus.

While the main function of the macrophage is phagocytosis, either as a defense activity (as in phagocytosis of bacteria) or as a cleanup operation (as in phagocytosis of cell debris), the macrophage appears also to play a role in immune reactions by presenting lymphocytes with concentrations of antigens from phagocytosed foreign cells or proteins. Also, when macrophages encounter large foreign bodies, they fuse to form large cells with up to 100 nuclei. These multinucleated cells are called *foreign body giant cells.*

TABLE 5.4. Mononuclear Phagocytic System

NAME OF CELL	LOCATION
Macrophage (histiocyte)	Connective tissue
Kupffer cell	Liver
Alveolar macrophage	Lungs
Macrophage	Spleen, lymph nodes, bone marrow, and thymus
Pleural and peritoneal macrophage	Serous cavities
Osteoclast	Bone
Microglia	Central nervous system
Langerhans cell	Epidermis

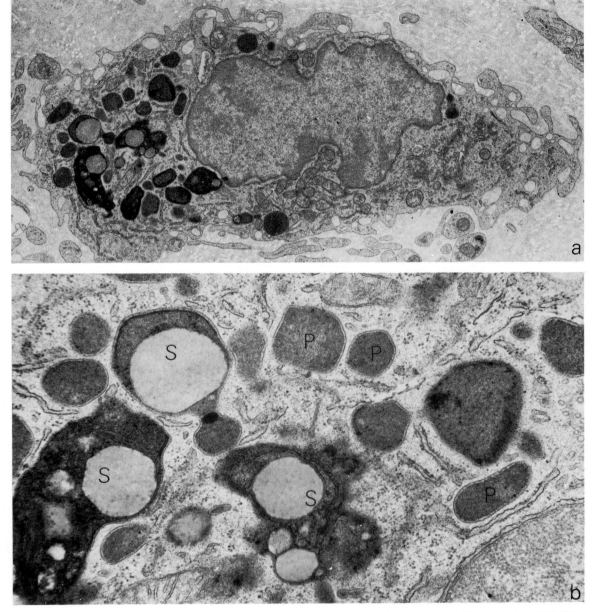

Figure 5.14(a). An electron micrograph of a macrophage. The most distinctive feature is the population of granules. Those that have a homogeneous matrix are primary lysosomes. Those that have a heterogeneous appearance represent secondary lysosomes. The surface of the cell reveals a number of finger-like projections, some of which may be sections of extensive surface folds. × 10,000. **(b)** A higher magnification of the lysosomes. P, primary lysosomes, S, secondary lysosomes. × 45,000.

Plasma Cells

Plasma cells are derivatives of B lymphocytes; they are active in the production and secretion of antibodies. Antibodies are proteins, and accordingly, the cytoplasm of the plasma cell contains large amounts of rER and a large Golgi apparatus (Fig. 5.15). These are the predominant organelles within the cell and they occur in sufficient amounts so that their presence can be ascertained with the light microscope. The cytoplasm of the plasma cell displays strong basophilia due to the presence of rER; the Golgi is unstained or only lightly tinged with eosin and appears as a clear area adjacent to the nucleus (see Fig. 2.11). The nucleus of the plasma cell is spherical and typically offset or ec-

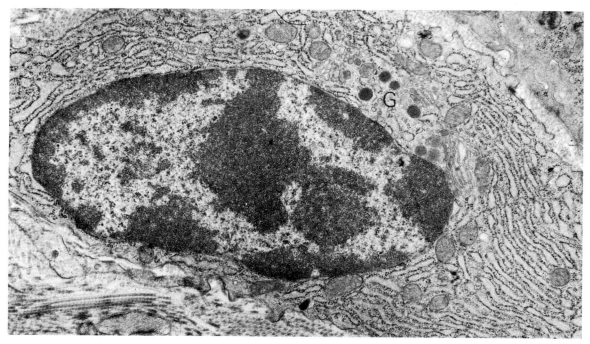

Figure 5.15. Electron micrograph of a plasma cell. The cytoplasm exhibits a very extensive rER, occupying much of the cytoplasm. The Golgi apparatus (G) is also relatively large, a further reflection of the cell's secretory activity. × 15,000.

centrically positioned. It is relatively small, not much larger than the nucleus of the lymphocyte. It contains large clumps of peripheral heterochromatin alternating with clear areas of euchromatin. The nucleus in histological sections has traditionally been described as resembling a "cart wheel."

The cell is typically ovoid in shape, but when the cells are crowded or closely packed, their profiles appear angulated, conforming to the pressures of close packing.

Plasma cells are regularly found in the lamina propria of the gastrointestinal tract. They also ap-

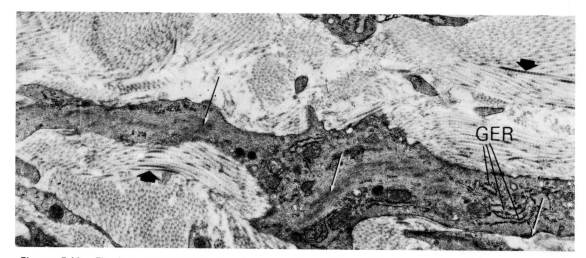

Figure 5.16. Electron micrograph showing a portion of the cytoplasm of a myofibroblast. The cell exhibits certain features of fibroblast, such as areas with a moderate amount of granular, or rough endoplasmic reticulum (GER). (Compare with Fig. 5.9.) However, there are other areas that contain aggregates of fine filaments and cytoplasmic densities (**arrows**), features characteristic of smooth muscle cells. The **arrowheads** indicate longitudinal profiles of collagen fibrils. A low power micrograph of this cell is shown in the Atlas Section, Plate 8, in relation to other connective tissue cells.

pear in other sites, such as connective tissue of the respiratory tract, salivary glands, and elsewhere, according to the demand for local antibody production.

Lymphocytes

Connective tissue lymphocytes are the smallest of the free cells in the connective tissue, having a diameter of 6 to 8 μm (see Fig. 5.12). Their functional role in the immune response is discussed in Chapters 9 and 13. Normally, small numbers of lymphocytes are found in the connective tissue throughout the body. However, the number increases dramatically at sites of tissue inflammation and repair. Lymphocytes are most numerous in the lamina propria of the respiratory and gastrointestinal tracts where they are involved in the immunosurveillance against pathogens and foreign substances that enter the body through these routes.

Lymphocytes appear as cells having a thin rim of cytoplasm surrounding a deeply staining, heterochromatic nucleus. (In many incidences, the cytoplasm of connective tissue lymphocytes may not be visible.) Lymphocytes are a heterogenous population of two functional cell types: (1) *T lymphocytes,* which have a long life-span and are involved in cell-mediated immunity and (2) *B lymphocytes,* which have variable life-spans and are involved in the production of antibodies. In response to the presence of antigens, B lymphocytes may divide

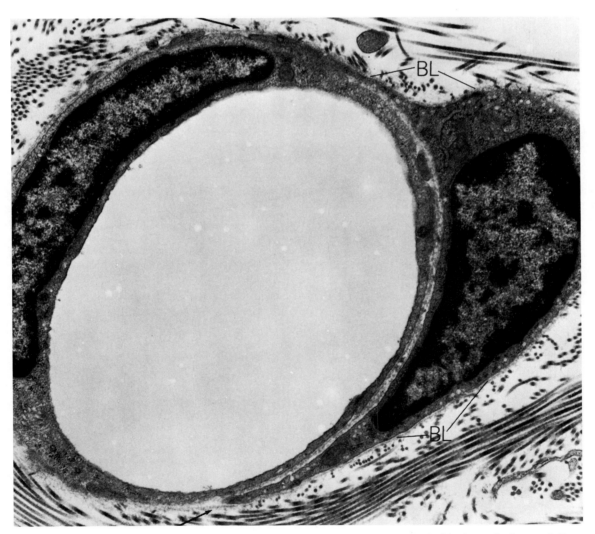

Figure 5.17. Electron micrograph of a small blood vessel. The nucleus at the left belongs to the endothelial cell, which forms the wall of the vessel. At the right is another cell, a pericyte, which is in intimate relation to the endothelium. Note that the basal lamina (BL) covering the endothelial cells divides **(arrows)** also to surround the pericyte.

several times producing more B lymphocytes and large clones of cells that mature into *plasma cells.* The plasma cell is short-lived (only 2 or 3 days) and highly specialized for antibody production and secretion.

Myofibroblast

The myofibroblast is a connective tissue cell that is not readily identifiable in routine H&E preparations. However, in the electron micro-scope, it displays properties of both the fibroblast and the smooth muscle cell (Fig. 5.16). In addition to the rER and Golgi profiles (characteristic of the fibroblast), the myofibroblast contains relatively large bundles of myofilaments (characteristic of the smooth muscle cell). The myofibroblast differs from the smooth muscle cell in that there is no basal lamina surrounding it (smooth muscle cells are surrounded by a basal (or external) lamina), and it is usually seen as an isolated cell, though its processes may contact other myofibroblasts

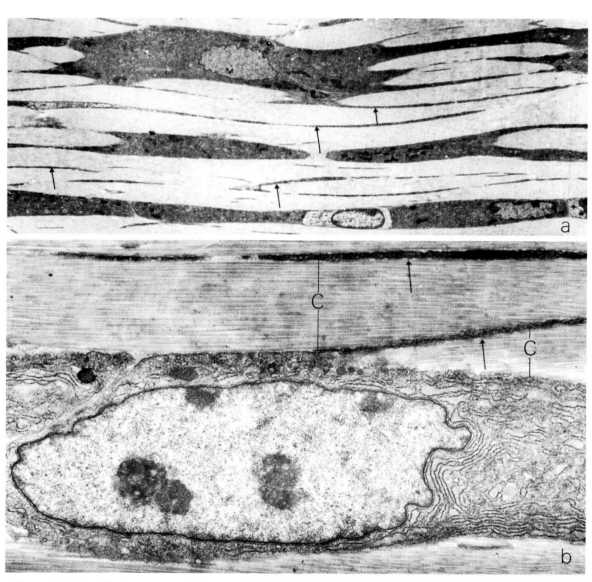

Figure 5.18(a). Electron micrograph of a tendon at low power showing the fibroblasts and their thin processes **(arrows)** lying between the collagen bundles. × 1,600. **(b)** A tendon fibroblast with prominent profiles of rER shown at higher magnification. The collagen fibers (C) can be resolved as consisting of very tightly packed collagen fibrils. × 9500. (From Rhodin J: *Histology.* New York, Oxford University Press, 1974.)

(smooth muscle cells are typically seen next to other smooth muscle cells).

Undifferentiated Mesenchymal Cells

Classical histologists postulated the existence of cells in loose connective tissue of the adult that retain the multipotentials of the embryonic mesenchymal cells. These cells were called undifferentiated mesenchymal cells. Such cells would give rise to differentiated cells that would be utilized for large-scale repair and formation of new tissue, such as new blood vessels or new or ectopic bone and cartilage. One postulated precursor for such newly differentiated cells is the *pericyte*, also called the *adventitial cell* and the *perivascular cell*. Pericytes are found around capillaries (Fig. 5.17) and venules. They are surrounded by basal lamina material that is directly continuous with the basal lamina of the capillary endothelium. The pericyte is typically wrapped, at least partially, around the capillary and its nucleus takes a corresponding shape, that is, flattened but curved to conform to the tubular shape of the capillary. Electron micrographs of the pericyte reveal little evidence of differentiation: a few small mitochondria, numerous free ribosomes, some vesicles, and occasionally, short profiles of rER. The pericyte contains lateral processes that extend from the cell body and partially encircle the capillary. This morphology argues against the suggestion based on the location of the pericytes that they function in regulating the dimensions of the capillaries. Except for the shape and location of the nucleus, the above features require electron microscopy for their visualization; thus, it is difficult to identify the pericyte with certainty in paraffin section.

The identification of the so-called undifferentiated mesenchymal cell remains a difficult problem to solve and will probably remain so until immunocytochemical approaches can be developed so that the precursor cells can be distinguished. Only then will it be possible to determine whether the processes of ongoing tissue renewal and reconstruction use as their sources the so-called undifferentiated stem cell or, alternatively, the dedifferentiated derivatives of the mature cells described in this chapter.

DENSE REGULAR CONNECTIVE TISSUE

Tendons

Dense regular connective tissue is the main functional component of *tendons* and *ligaments*.

Tendons are cord- or band-like structures that join muscle to bones. Histologically, a tendon consists of parallel bundles of collagenous fibers between which are rows of fibroblasts (Fig. 5.18). The fibroblasts appear stellate when the tendon is cut in cross-section; the cytoplasmic projections seen in cross-section are thin cytoplasmic sheets. In longitudinal H&E-stained paraffin sections of a tendon, the fibroblasts are seen to occupy rows and they are identified by the staining of the nucleus and the immediately surrounding cytoplasm. The nuclei are typically flattened. When seen on edge, they appear as a densely stained bar; when seen in face view, they appear as less intensely stained oval profiles. The cytoplasmic sheets that extend from the body of the fibroblasts are not evident in longitudinal sections because they are so thin, and although they stain with eosin, they cannot be distinguished from the collagen fibers that also stain with eosin. The substance of the tendon is surrounded by a thin connective tissue capsule in which the collagen fibers are not nearly as orderly. This connective tissue is continuous with the connective tissue associated with the blood vessels that pass into the interior of the tendon organ.

Ligaments

A ligament is similar to a tendon in that it also consists of parallel extracellular fibers and fibroblasts. The fibers, however, are less regularly arranged than those of tendon. A ligament joins bone to bone and, in some locations, such as in the spinal column, this requires some degree of elasticity. Thus, while collagen is the major extracellular fiber of most ligaments, some of the ligaments associated with the spinal column contain mainly elastic fibers and lesser amounts of collagen fibers. These ligaments are called *elastic ligaments*.

Capsules

Capsules of organs are sometimes described as dense regular connective tissue. While it is true their extracellular fibers are more organized than fibers in dense irregular connective tissue, the variety of cells typically found in capsules more closely resembles the cell profile of connective tissue proper (dense irregular connective tissue) than the cell profile of dense regular connective tissue. Capsules almost always contain mast cells, macrophages, and sometimes fat cells in addition to fibroblasts; the regular connective tissue of tendons and ligaments typically contains only fibroblasts.

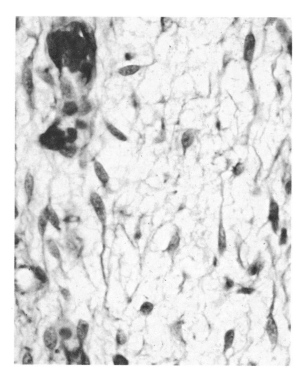

Figure 5.19. Photomicrograph of mesenchymal tissue from a developing fetus. Structurally, the mesenchymal cells comprise a homogeneous population, even though some of the cells may be committed to give rise to cells that differentiate into specific cell types. They exhibit cytoplasmic processes, which often give the cell a tapering or stellate appearance. The extracellular component of the tissue contains a sparse arrangement of reticular fibers and abundant ground substance.

EMBRYONIC CONNECTIVE TISSUE

Mesenchyme is the embryonic connective tissue. It originates from mesoderm and neural crest ectoderm. Mesenchyme consists of stellate cells, delicate reticular fibers, and usually considerable ground substance (Fig. 5.19). Mesenchyme itself develops directly into loose connective tissue; the reticular fibers are gradually replaced by collagenous fibers and the relative amount of ground substance is diminished. Mesenchymal cells give rise to most of the connective tissue cells. Mesenchymal cells also migrate to form cell aggregates in the development of other tissues and organs (such as cartilage, bone, and muscle). For the most part, the mesenchyme develops into the connective tissue elements of the organ; however, in some instances, the mesenchymal cells give rise to epithelium, as in kidney tubules, and epithelioid tissues, as in the adrenal cortex and the interstitial (Leydig) cells of the testis.

Mucous connective tissue is a form of mesenchyme in which the amount of ground substance is especially abundant. While it is present in certain parts of the embryo, it is not easily distinguished from regular mesenchyme. The usual example of mucous connective tissue is Wharton's jelly, present in the umbilical cord. Histologically, it consists of stellate cells, collagenous fibers, and very abundant ground substance. Much of the ground substance is extracted during preparation of the slide and it is difficult to distinguish remaining precipitates of ground substance from collagenous fibers and cytoplasmic processes.

ATLAS PLATES

6–10

PLATE 6. Loose and Dense Connective Tissue

The tissues surrounding the epithelial elements of inactive mammary gland lobules serve as an excellent example of loose and dense connective tissue, particularly for the purpose of comparing them within the same field of view. **Figure 1** reveals at low magnification loose connective tissue **(LCT)** immediately surrounding the gland epithelium **(Ep).** It is relatively less stained with eosin compared to the dense connective tissue **(DCT)** that occupies much of the field. The dense connective tissue with its numerous thick fibers is in contrast to the loose connective tissue that has a relative paucity of fibers. **Figure 2** shows one of the lobules at higher magnification and more clearly reveals the typical wispy nature of the collagen fibers found in loose connective tissue.

The most conspicuous components of loose connective tissue are the numerous cells interspersed singly and in small groups between the delicate collagen fibers and the small blood vessels **(BV)** that supply the connective tissue and adjacent epithelium. Although the magnification of **Figure 2** is not sufficiently high to explore cytological detail, two general cell types are recognized based on nuclear shape. One population of cells contains elongate nuclei **(arrows)**; these most likely belong to fibroblasts. The other population contains round nuclei; most of these nuclei represent lymphocytes **(L)**; although some are of plasma cells. The significant feature, however, is that this loose connective tissue is highly cellular, considerably more so than the surrounding dense connective tissue. Typically, the cells of dense connective tissue are fibroblasts. They are usually not present in appreciable numbers; and under normal conditions, few if any other cell types are present.

Figure 3 is another example of loose connective tissue from the wall of the vagina, just below the epithelial surface. Again, note the myriad nuclear profiles. The area immediately to the right of the upper marked blood vessel **(BV)** is shown at higher magnification in **Figure 4.** Here the wispy nature of the fine collagen fibers is evident and the variation of nuclear profiles is even more apparent. Identification of the cell type represented by each nucleus is not possible; however, certain cells of the total population can be identified with assurance. Thus, the small, dense, round nuclei without visible surrounding cytoplasm belong to lympho-

cytes **(L)**. Some of the round nuclei exhibit a surrounding but eccentric mass of cytoplasm. These are plasma cells **(PC)**. Sometimes the cytoplasm of a plasma cell may be obscured partially by the nucleus, making identity less assured. Such is the case of the cell indicated by the question mark **(?)**. Since the size, density, and chromatin pattern of its nucleus are similar to those of the more readily identifiable plasma cells, it too is probably a plasma cell. With respect to the fibroblasts, the nuclei are typically elongate. Two fibroblast nuclei **(F)** are indicated in the micrograph; both are elongate but one appears quite narrow. It is being viewed on edge, whereas the broader nucleus profile represents a fibroblast in face view. Typically, the cytoplasm of the fibroblasts is obscured by blending in with the collagen. Some of the nuclei seen here may represent macrophages or mast cells, but without identifiable cytoplasmic inclusions, these cells cannot be identified.

To summarize, the light microscopic appearance of loose connective tissue includes the presence of several cell types; the cells are not organized in any special pattern; the collagen fibers are fine and wispy; and the tissue usually stains lightly with eosin due to the relative paucity of collagen fibers and loss of ground substance. In contrast, dense connective tissue is comprised of thick collagen bundles that stain deeply with eosin and has relatively few cells, most of which are fibroblasts. It should also be pointed out that both connective tissues contain elastic fibers, but the fibers are not discernible without special staining methods (see Plate 10).

KEY

AT, adipose tissue
BV, blood vessel
DCT, dense connective
   tissue
Ep, epithelium
F, fibroblast nucleus

L, lymphocyte
LCT, loose connective
   tissue
PC, plasma cell
arrow, elongate nucleus

Fig. 1, human, × 160
Fig. 2, human, × 250

Fig. 3, human, × 250
Fig. 4, human, × 480

PLATE 6

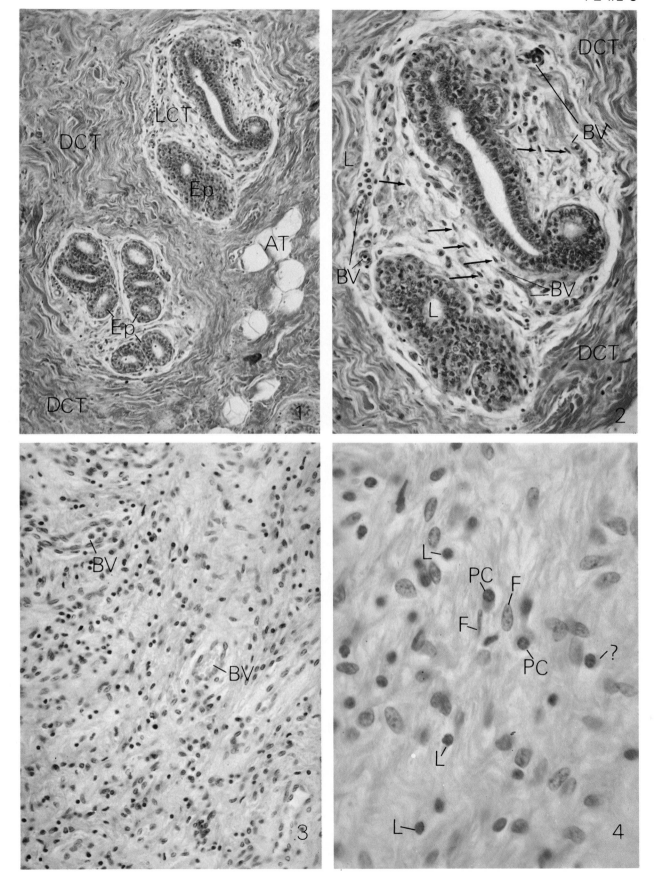

PLATE 7. Connective Tissue, Electron Microscopy

The formed elements that constitute a connective tissue, namely, the fibers and cells, are readily characterized at the ultrastructural level. The specimen shown here is from a section through the wall of an oviduct. The tissue is rather cellular, but it also contains a considerable amount of fibrous material. In terms of its constituent elements, it is comparable to the connective tissue shown in **Figure 3** of Plate 6. With the electron microscope, the morphological character of the tissue constituents becomes immediately apparent. The fibroblasts **(F)**, which constitute the bulk of the connective tissue cell population, usually exhibit long cytoplasmic processes that pass between the collagen bundles. The processes extend for indeterminant distances and may become so attenuated **(arrowheads)** that their thinness precludes the possibility of being visualized with the light microscope.

In addition to the fibroblast population, there are at least two other connective tissue cell types present in this specimen (see **rectangles**). One is a cell with both myoid and fibroblast-like features. This we refer to as a myofibroblast **(My).** The other is a cell which has certain features that suggest it is a monocyte **(M)** or a closely related cell type. These two cell types, along with a fibroblast, are illustrated at higher magnification in Plate 8.

The collagen fibers **(CF),** between which the fibroblast processes pass, have a stippled appearance at this relatively low magnification. This is due to the cut, end-on profiles of the individual collagen fibrils. It is these thread-like units, the fibrils that, when aggregated in bundles form the fiber that is visualized at the light microscope level.

KEY

Cap, capillary
CF, collagen fiber
F, fibroblast
M, monocyte
My, myofibroblast

RBC, red blood cell
V, venule
arrowhead, attenuated
  fibroblast process

Electron micrograph,
  × 4100

In the specimen shown here, almost all of the collagen fibers have been cross-sectioned, and consequently it is possible to discern their variable size and shape. In the routinely prepared light microscopic specimen, during the fixation and dehydration stages of its preparation, there may be considerable initial hydration and then, with subsequent dehydration, shrinkage of the tissue occurs. One consequence of this is the artificial separation of the collagen fibers. The fibers are then discerned in the light microscope as wispy, isolated, thread-like elements, rather than the more even distribution seen in the electron microscope.

Typically one finds small blood vessels passing through the substance of the connective tissue and, in this view, there is a capillary **(Cap)** as well as a longitudinally sectioned venule **(V)**. The latter contains a number of red blood cells **(RBC).**

PLATE 7

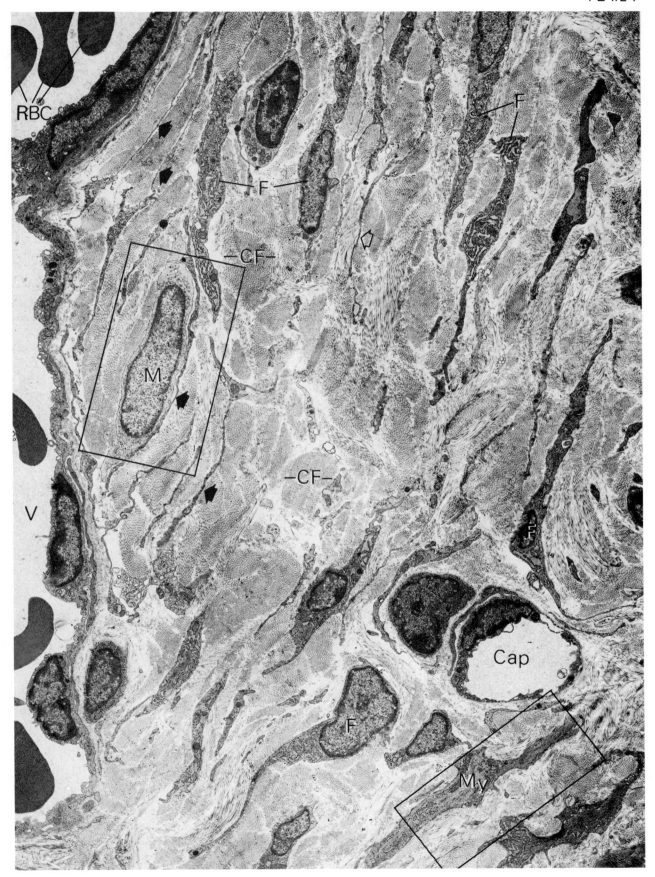

PLATE 8. Connective Tissue Cells, Electron Microscopy

As noted previously, the cytological features displayed by the various connective tissue cell types at the ultrastructural level serve as an accurate "fingerprint" that allows one, with few exceptions, to identify readily the cell type in question. For example, **Figure 1** reveals portions of two adjacent fibroblasts. Despite the fact that only a small portion of each cell is evident, they can be immediately identified as fibroblasts on the basis of the presence of a moderate amount of granular endoplasmic reticulum **(GER)** and by the elongate processes which both cells exhibit.

The cisternae of the endoplasmic reticulum are notable dilated, as seen in the lower cell, and contain a homogeneous substance of moderate density. This substance is a product of the synthetic activity of the ribosomes on the surface of the reticulum and, having been released into the cisternae, represents for the most part a precursor of the collagen seen in the extracellular space. In this same cell, the section reveals a portion of the Golgi apparatus **(G).** The Golgi consists of a multitude of small vesicles and flattened sac-like profiles.

The portion of the cell shown in **Figure 2** is in many respects similar to the fibroblasts just described and, at the light microscopic level, it would probably be indistinguishable from them. Note that in one area profiles of granular endoplasmic reticulum are evident **(GER)** and their contents exhibit the same texture and density as that of the fibroblast. However, the cell differs from the fibroblast in that the cytoplasm reveals an extensive filamentous component, just barely visible at this magnification. Associated with these filaments are "cytoplasmic densities" **(arrows);** the combination of these dense areas and a high concentration of cytoplasmic filaments is a feature characteristic of smooth muscle cells. It is evident that this cell type, designated as a myofibroblast, functions both as a fibroblast and a contractile cell. Other examples of this kind of cell can be found in the testis, ovary, spleen, and nerve (perineurium).

KEY

CF, collagen fiber
GER, granular
  endoplasmic reticulum
G, Golgi apparatus
SER, smooth
  endoplasmic reticulum

arrow, cytoplasmic
  densities
arrowhead,
  longitudinally
  sectioned collagen
  fibrils

All electron
  micrographs, × 11,000

The last cell type, on this plate, **Figure 3,** is one that would probably also be recognized as a fibroblast if viewed in the light microscope. As seen here, the cell exhibits a flattened nucleus and a little cytoplasm about it. The cytoplasm is somewhat nondescript, the most notable feature being the small vesicular profiles of smooth endoplasmic reticulum **(SER).** Presumably this cell is a monocyte that may be in transition to a tissue macrophage. Again, the essential point here is that we are viewing a cell type cytologically different from a fibroblast, although with the light microscope, in a routinely stained H&E section, the distinction between these two cells is not possible.

In all three figures, the collagen fibrils can be clearly identified as the subunits of the collagen fibers **(CF).** In most locations, the fibrils have been cross-sectioned and appear as closely packed circular profiles; in locations where the fibrils have been sectioned more longitudinally **(arrowheads),** the typical cross-banded pattern is evident. Again, it is indicated that individual fibrils cannot be identified with the light microscope; rather, one sees a bundle of fibrils and this bundle is then referred to as a collagen fiber. One can also ascertain from these illustrations that the diameter of the collagen fiber depends on how many fibrils are within the bundle.

PLATE 8

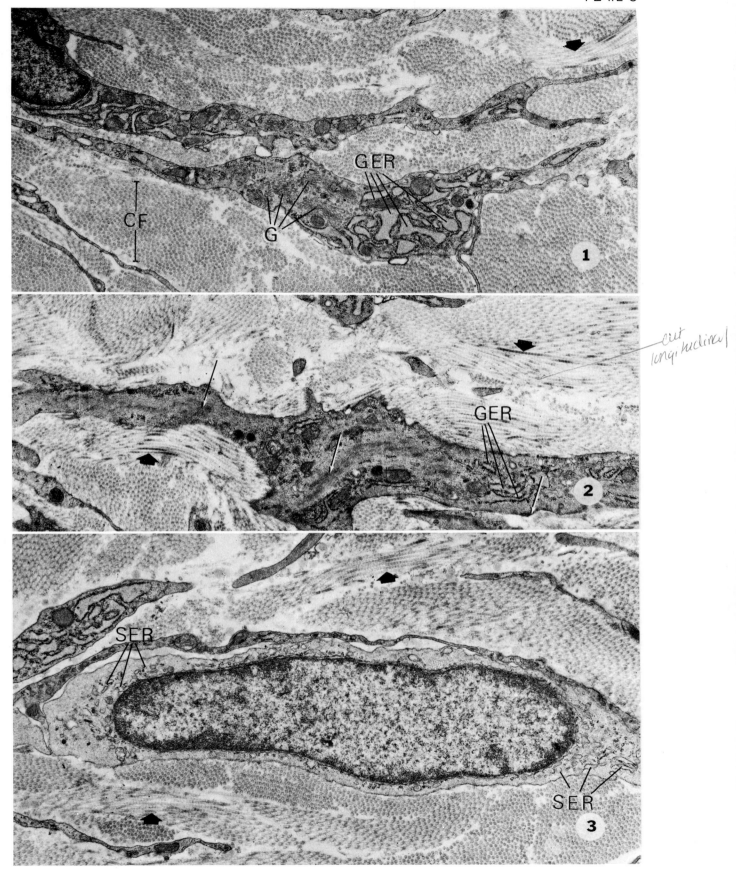

crit longitudinal

PLATE 9. Regular Connective Tissue

Regular connective tissue is connective tissue in which the fibrous elements are organized in a parallel array. This is epitomized in ligaments and tendons.

Figure 1 is a longitudinal section of a ligament. It shows rows of collagen fibers separated by rows of cells, practically all of which are fibroblasts. The nucleus of the fibroblast is conspicuous, but the cytoplasm is difficult to discern. The lateral extent of the collagen bundles is not always clear; however, it is suggested by the location of the cells (as evidenced by their nuclei). One regularly sees folds and even cracks in routine H&E preparations of ligaments (and also tendons). These folds are frequently at right angles to the long axis of the collagen bundles. They are considered to be the result of the vibrational impact of the cutting knife. Indeed, even smaller cross-directional markings may be present, and these should not be confused with the cross-striations of striated muscle.

Examinations of **Figure 2,** a higher magnification of a ligament, indicates that the cells between the collagen bundles are of one type; they are fibroblasts. The nuclei of these cells are shaped like oval plates. Therefore, when the broad face of the nucleus is viewed, it appears oval, and when the nucleus is viewed on edge, it appears flat. Ligaments are described as being less regularly organized than tendons.

A tendon is illustrated in **Figure 3.** It also consists of parallel bundles of collagen fibers that are separated by rows of fibroblasts. The nuclei of

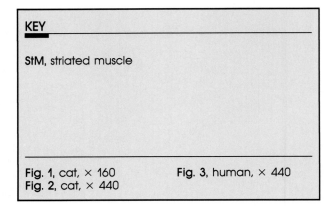

KEY

StM, striated muscle

Fig. 1, cat, × 160   **Fig. 3,** human, × 440
Fig. 2, cat, × 440

these cells are viewed on edge and they appear as the thin, dark-staining profiles. A small amount of striated muscle **(StM)** is shown where it connects to the tendon. Although both tendon and muscle appear as oriented fibers and nuclei, the muscle contains cross-striations, but the tendon does not.

The capsules of organs also contain rather well-organized bundles of collagen fibers. These are more likely to be disposed in sheets rather than cords. Therefore, the term "lamellated" is sometimes applied to this form of dense regular connective tissue. Capsules almost always contain mast cells, macrophages, and sometimes fat cells in addition to fibroblasts; the regular connective tissue of ligaments and tendons typically contains only fibroblasts.

PLATE 9

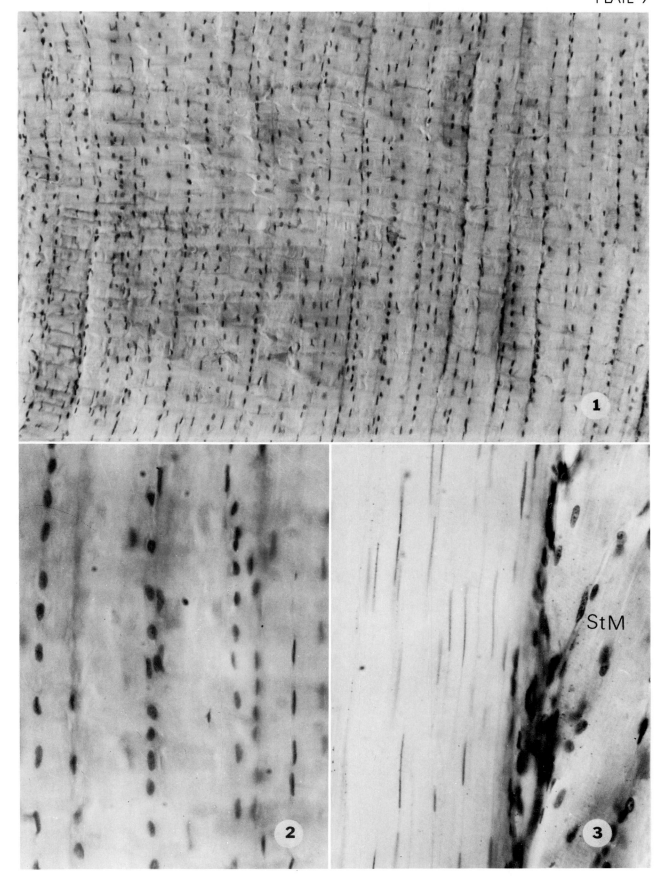

StM

PLATE 10. Elastic Fibers and Elastic Lamellae

Elastic fibers are present in loose and dense connective tissue throughout the body, but in lesser amounts than collagenous fibers. Elastic fibers are not conspicuous in routine H&E sections, but may be readily visualized with special staining methods. (The following selectively color elastic material: Weigert's Elastic Tissue Stain, purple-violet; Gomori's Aldehyde Fuchsin Stain, blue-black; Verhoeff Haematoxylin Elastic Tissue Stain, black; and Modified Taenzer-Unna Orcein Stain, red-brown.) By a combination of the special elastic stains and counterstains, such as H&E, not only the elastic fibers, but the other tissue components are revealed. **Figure 1** shows the connective tissue of the skin, referred to as the dermis, stained to show the nature and distribution of the elastic fibers **(E),** which appear purple. The collagen fibers **(C)** have been stained by the eosin and the two fiber types are easily differentiated. The connective tissue at the top of the figure, close to the epithelium (the papillary layer of the dermis), contains thin elastic fibers (see upper left of figure) as well as less coarse collagen fibers. The lower portion of the figure shows considerably heavier elastic and collagen fibers. Also note that many of the elastic fibers appear as short rectangular profiles. These profiles simply represent fibers traveling through the thickness of the section at an oblique angle to the path of the knife. Careful examination will also reveal a few fibers that appear as dot-like profiles. They represent cross-sectioned elastic fibers. Overall, the elastic fibers of the dermis have a three-dimensional interlacing configuration, thus the variety of forms.

Figure 2 is a whole mount specimen of mesentery, similar to **Figure 2** in Plate 1, but prepared to show the connective tissue elements and differentially stained to reveal elastic fibers. The elastic fi-

---

KEY

BV, blood vessel
C, collagen fibers

D, duct of sweat gland
E, elastic fibers

Fig. 1, monkey, × 160
Fig. 2, rat, × 160

Fig. 3, monkey, × 80

---

bers **(E)** appear as thin, long, criss-crossing and branching threads without discernible beginnings or endings and a somewhat irregular course. Again, the collagen fibers **(C)** are contrasted by their eosin staining and appear as long, straight profiles that are considerably thicker than the elastic fibers.

Elastic material also occurs in sheets, or lamellae, as opposed to string-like fibers. **Figure 3** shows the wall of an elastic artery (pulmonary artery) that was stained to show the elastic material present. Each of the wavy lines is a lamella of elastic material that is organized in the form of a fenestrated sheet or membrane. The plane of section is such that the elastic membranes are seen "on edge." This specimen was not subsequently stained with H&E. The empty-appearing spaces between elastic layers contain collagen and cellular elements, namely, smooth muscle cells, but they remain essentially unstained.

Tissues of the body containing large amounts of elastic material are limited in distribution to the walls of elastic arteries and some ligaments that are associated with the spinal column.

PLATE 10

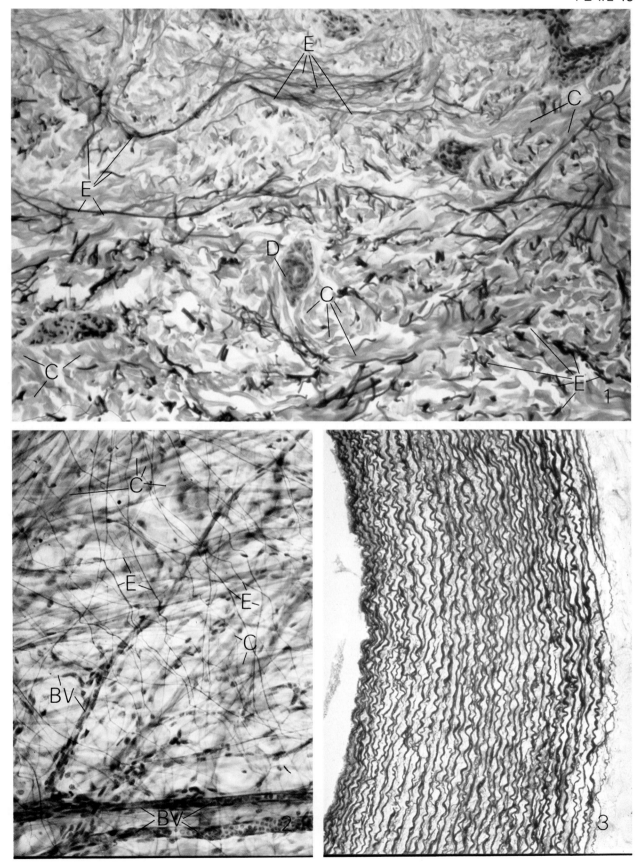

Adipose Tissue

6

Adipose tissue is a specialized form of connective tissue consisting of fat-storing cells, called *adipocytes,* in association with a rich blood supply. The body has a limited capacity to store carbohydrate and protein, and the fat contained within the adipocytes represents the storage of nutritional calories in excess of what is utilized. Fat is an efficient form of calorie storage since it has about twice the calorie density of carbohydrate and protein. There are two types of adipose tissue: *white,* or *unilocular,* and *brown,* or *multilocular.* In humans, brown adipose tissue is present during fetal development, but diminishes from birth through the first decade of life. White adipose tissue, also present during fetal development, persists as the adipose tissue of the adult.

WHITE ADIPOSE TISSUE

In well-nourished individuals, unilocular adipose tissue forms a more or less continuous layer, called the *panniculus adiposus,* in the connective tissue under the skin. Histologically, the subcutaneous layer of connective tissue is also referred to as the *hypodermis.* Generally, adipose tissue is preferentially located in the connective tissue under the skin of the lower part of the abdomen, buttocks, axilla, and thigh. Sex differences in the thickness of the fatty layer in different parts of the body account, in part, for the difference in body contour between the male and the female. Adipose tissue is also preferentially located in the omentum, mesentery, and retroperitoneal space and is usually well developed around the kidneys. It is also found in bone marrow and between other tissues where it appears to fill in the spaces. In the palms of the hands, the soles of the feet, and the orbits around the eyeballs, the adipose tissue evidently serves a structural function as a cushion. During reduced caloric intake, when the adipose tissue elsewhere becomes depleted of lipid, this structural adipose tissue remains undiminished.

Origin of Fat Cells

Early histologists were undecided as to whether adipose tissue was a specific organ, distinct from connective tissue, or whether it was merely ordinary connective tissue in which fibroblasts stored fat globules. The current consensus is that adipocytes are a specific cell type that derive from mesenchymal cells and from pericytes, the cell associated with the wall of small blood vessels (see Fig. 5.17). In most mammals, including humans, white adipose tissue begins to develop in miduterine life. The adipocytes develop from groups of undifferentiated cells along small blood vessels where the adipose tissue will be. These islands of cells are fat-free at this time. They have been called primitive fat organs because they consist of cells that are committed to become adipocytes. The primitive fat organ is characterized by the presence of proliferating preadipocytes and proliferating capillaries. Lipid deposition in preadipocytes transforms the cells into adipocytes. Small lipid droplets first accumulate in the cytoplasm of the cell and then fuse to form a large droplet. The droplet continues to enlarge until the cell, now an adipocyte, is a thin rim of cytoplasm around the lipid droplet. In some rodents, for example, mice and rats, adipose tissue starts to form at about the time of birth. Moreover, the formation of preadipocytes and conversion into adipocytes can take place simultaneously without the preformation of a distinctive primitive fat organ.

Structure of Adipocytes and Adipose Tissue

Unilocular fat cells are large; they can be 100 μm or more in diameter. Fat cells are spherical when isolated, but are polyhedral or oval when crowded together in adipose tissue. The large size of the fat cell is due to the presence of a single large droplet of lipid. It causes the nucleus to be flattened and displaced to one side of the cytoplasm to form a thin rim around it. In routine histological sections, the lipid is lost through dissolution in fat solvents, such as xylene, and consequently the adipose tissue has the appearance of a delicate meshwork of polygonal profiles (Fig. 6.1a and b).

The thin strand of meshwork separating two adjacent adipocytes represents the cytoplasm of both cells and a small amount of extracellular space. However, the strand is usually so thin that it is not possible to resolve its component parts with the light microscope. The adipose tissue is richly supplied with blood vessels; capillaries are found at many of the angles of the meshwork where three adjacent adipocytes meet. Silver stains show that the adipocytes are surrounded by reticular fibers.

Special stains also show that there are unmyelinated nerve fibers and numerous mast cells in adipose tissue.

A curious feature of the fat cell, revealed with the electron microscope, is that the fat droplet is not surrounded by a membrane. It is possible that the fat droplet is actually enclosed by a monomolecular leaflet (a structure representing half of the lipid bilayer of a typical cell membrane) at its periphery. This layer would provide an interface between the hydrophobic contents of the fat droplet and the hydrophilic cytosol. The electron microscope also shows that the fat cell is surrounded by a basal lamina. The cytoplasm of the fat cell contains a small Golgi complex, free ribosomes, short profiles of rough endoplasmic reticulum, filaments, and mitochondria near the nucleus. Filaments, mitochondria, and profiles of smooth endoplasmic reticulum are in the thin rim of cytoplasm (Fig. 6.2).

Regulation of Adipose Tissue

The amount of adipose tissue in an individual is determined by heredity and environmental factors, chief of which is caloric intake. Identical twins

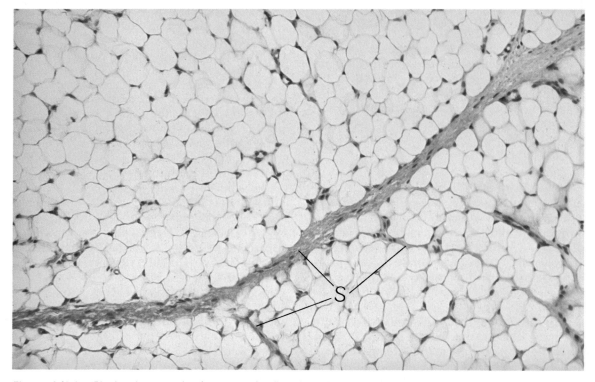

Figure 6.1(a). Photomicrograph of a mass of unilocular adipose tissue showing its characteristic meshwork appearance in an hematoxylin and eosin preparation. Each space represents the site of the single large drop of lipid before its dissolution from the cell during preparation of the tissue. The surrounding eosin-stained material represents the cytoplasm of the adjoining cells and some intervening connective tissue. Heavier connective tissue septa (S) creates lobules of varying size.

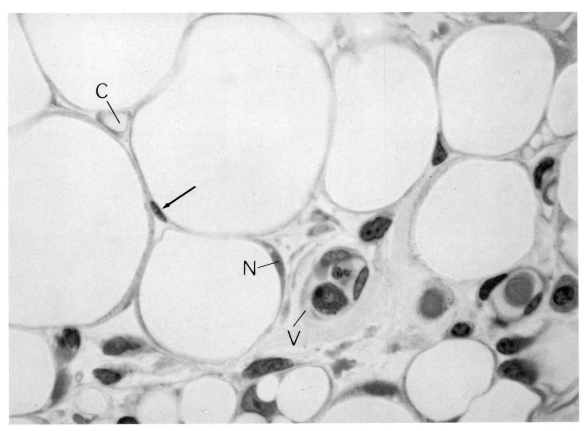

Figure 6.1(b). High-power photomicrograph of a well-preserved plastic-embedded specimen of unilocular adipose tissue. The cytoplasm of the individual adipose cells is recognizable in some areas, and part of the nucleus (N) of one of the cells is included in the plane of section. A second nucleus **(arrow)**, which appears intimately related to one of the adipose cells, may actually belong to a fibroblast; it is difficult to tell with assurance. Because of the large size of the adipose cells, the nucleus is infrequently observed in a given cell. A capillary (C) and a venule (V) are also evident in the micrograph.

usually have the same, or close to the same, amount of body fat. While the amount of body fat in identical twins may vary somewhat, the patterns of distribution are always the same. Studies with genetically obese rodents show that the obesity is associated with an increased efficiency of food utilization. Obese rodents use a larger proportion of their food calories for the formation of adipose tissue, that is, the body weight per gram of food consumed is greater in obese rodents than in littermate controls. The factors that account for the positive caloric balance in the obese rodents are probably diminished heat production and diminished activity.

Mobilization and deposition of lipid is influenced by neural and hormonal factors. Early investigations on the influence of nerves on adipose tissue showed that, during the initial stages of starvation, cells in a denervated fat pad continue to deposit fat, while cells in the intact contralateral fat pad mobilize fat. It is now known that norepinephrine (which is liberated by the endings of nerve cells of the sympathetic nervous system) initiates a series of metabolic steps that lead to the activation of lipase. This enzyme splits triglycerides, which constitute over 90 percent of the lipid in the fat droplets; the enzymatic activity is an early step in the mobilization of the lipid. The neural mobilization of lipid is particularly important during periods of fasting and exposure to severe cold. On the other hand, insulin enhances the conversion of glucose into triglycerides of the fat droplet by the adipocyte. Other hormones also modify various steps in the metabolism of adipose tissue. These include thyroid hormone, glucocorticoids, and hormones of the pituitary gland.

A form of obesity of special interest to the medical and veterinary student is that due to injury of the hypothalamus. While clinical manifestations of hypothalamic obesity are associated with increased food consumption, experiments with laboratory animals subjected to hypothalamic injury

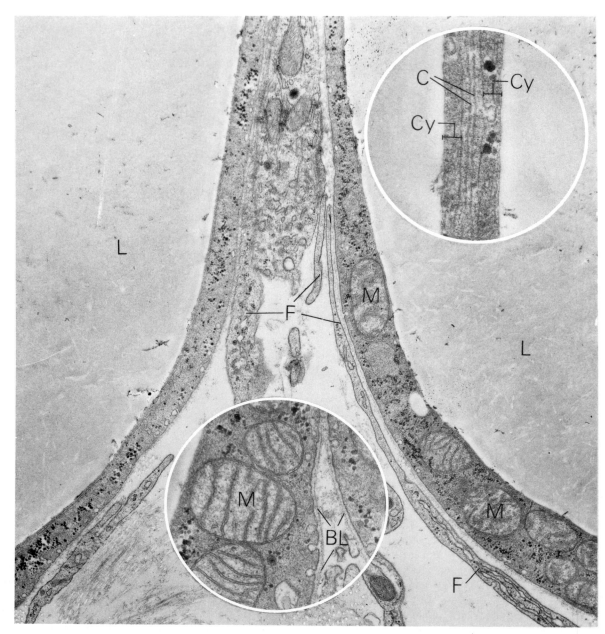

Figure 6.2. Electron micrograph shows portions of two adjacent adipose cells. The cytoplasm and thin processes of several fibroblasts (F) are present between the adipose cells. The cytoplasm of the adipose cells reveals mitochondria (M) and glycogen, the latter appearing as the very dark particles. The **upper inset** shows the attenuated cytoplasm (Cy) of two adjoining adipose cells. Each cell is separated by a narrow space containing basal lamina material and an extremely attenuated process of a fibroblast (C). The **lower inset** shows the basal lamina (BL) of the adipose cells as a discrete layer where the cells are adequately separated from one another. × 15,000; **upper inset,** × 65,000; **lower inset,** × 30,000.

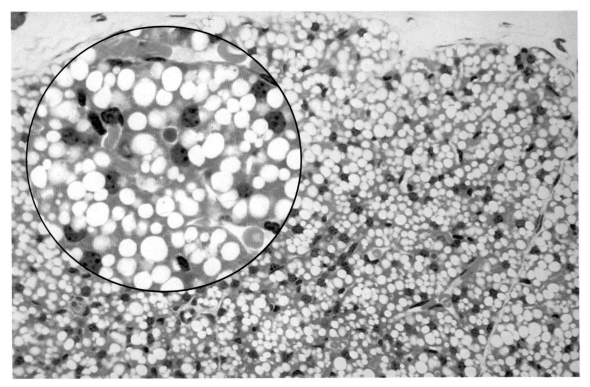

Figure 6.3. Photomicrograph of brown adipose tissue from a newborn. The cells contain fat droplets of varying size. The **inset** shows the cells and their populations of droplets at a higher magnification. The cells are closely packed and the cell boundaries are difficult to discern.

show that caloric intake is not the only factor leading to obesity. Lesioned rats deposit more body fat than control animals fed similar amounts of food.

BROWN ADIPOSE TISSUE

Brown adipose tissue is called multilocular because the fat cells contain numerous fat droplets rather than the large single droplet of cells of white adipose tissue. The cells of brown adipose tissue are smaller than those of white adipose tissue. The nucleus of a mature multilocular adipocyte is typically in an eccentric position within the cell, but it is not flattened as is the nucleus of a unilocular adipocyte. In routine hematoxylin and eosin-stained sections, the cytoplasm of the multilocular adipocyte appears to consist largely of empty vacuoles because the lipid that ordinarily occupies the vacuolated spaces is lost during preparation (Fig. 6.3). The multilocular adipocyte contains numerous mitochondria, a small Golgi, and only small amounts of rough and smooth endoplasmic reticulum. The mitochondria are unique in that they do not contain elementary particles (which contain many of the enzymes for ATP production), that is, the energy produced by the mitochondria is dissipated as heat rather than stored as ATP.

Brown adipose tissue is subdivided into lobules by partitions of connective tissue, but the connective tissue stroma between individual cells within the lobules is sparse. The tissue has an exceedingly rich supply of blood capillaries and numerous unmyelinated nerve fibers are demonstrable among the fat cells. Multilocular adipocytes depleted of their lipid bear a closer resemblance to epithelial cells than to connective tissue cells.

Brown adipose tissue is present in large amounts in hibernating animals. It serves as a ready source of lipid-heating fuel that is utilized by the animal upon arousal from hibernation. It is also present in nonhibernating animals, again, serving as a source of lipid-heating fuel. In humans, multilocular adipose tissue is present in large amounts in the newborn. The amount gradually decreases, but it remains widely distributed through the first decade of life. It then disappears from most sites except for regions around the kidney and aorta and regions in the neck and mediastinum. As in the mobilization of lipid in white fatty tissue, lipid is mobilized and heat is generated by multilocular adipocytes upon stimulation of the sympathetic nervous system.

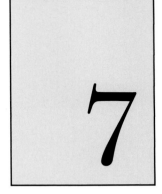

Cartilage

Cartilage is a form of connective tissue composed exclusively of cells called chondrocytes and a highly specialized extracellular matrix. Like the dense regular connective tissue of the tendon and ligament, it is an avascular tissue and the matrix serves as the route for the diffusion of substances between the blood vessels in the surrounding connective tissue and the chondrocytes. The matrix of cartilage is solid and firm though somewhat pliable and this accounts for the special resilient properties of cartilage. It is well adapted to serve in a weight-bearing capacity, especially at points of movement as in synovial joints (see below). Because it is able to do this even during internal growth of the cartilage itself, cartilage is a key tissue in growing bones.

Traditionally, three different kinds of cartilage are distinguished on the basis of characteristics of the matrix: (1) *hyaline cartilage,* (2) *fibrocartilage,* and (3) *elastic cartilage.*

HYALINE CARTILAGE

Hyaline cartilage is distinguished by the presence of a glassy, homogeneous, amorphous matrix. (Its name is derived from the Greek word *hyalos:* "glass.") Spaces, called *lacunae,* are located throughout the cartilage and within the lacunae and the cartilage cells. The matrix surrounds the lacunae; it consists of two components, collagen (predominantly type II) fibrils and ground substance.

Cartilage Matrix

The collagen fibrils of hyaline cartilage are relatively thin, about 20 nm in diameter. They do not display the characteristic 68-nm banding. (In certain locations, the collagen fibrils are thicker and the thicker fibrils may display the typical banding.) The collagen fibrils of hyaline cartilage are generally arranged in a three-dimensional felt-like pattern.

Chemical analysis of the ground substance of hyaline cartilage reveals the presence of three kinds of glycosaminoglycans: *hyaluronic acid, chondroitin sulfate,* and *keratan sulfate.* The chondroitin and keratan sulfates are joined to a core protein to form a *proteoglycan monomer* (Fig. 7.1). Within the tissue, the hyaluronic acid is associated with about 80 proteoglycan units to form large aggregates whose structure are reinforced by *link proteins.* The large hyaluronate proteoglycan aggregates are bound to the thin collagen fibrils by electrostatic interactions and cross-linking glycoproteins. The cartilage matrix also contains other proteoglycans that do not form aggregates, and noncollagenous and nonproteoglycan glycoproteins.

Like other matrices, cartilage matrix is highly hydrated. From 60 to 78 percent of the net weight of hyaline cartilage is water. Much of this water is bound, which explains the resiliency of cartilage. However, some of the water is bound loosely enough to allow the diffusion of small solutes. In articular cartilage, there are regional changes in water content. These changes occur during joint movement and when the joint is subjected to pressure. The high degree of hydration and the movement of water are factors that allow the cartilage matrix to respond to varying pressure loads and contribute to cartilage's weight-bearing capacity.

Although the matrix of hyaline cartilage is described as being amorphous and homogeneous, the components of the ground substance are not uniformly distributed. Because of the large num-

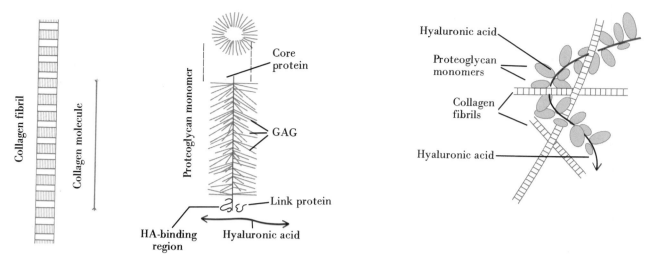

Figure 7.1. Schematic diagram showing a model for the organization of ground substance of cartilage. On the left, a collagen fibril and a collagen molecule are depicted for reference. The next item shows a proteoglycan monomer, hyaluronic acid (HA), and a link protein. The proteoglycan monomer consists of approximately 100 glycosaminoglycan units (GAG) joined to a core protein. The end of the core protein contains an HA-binding region, which is joined to the HA by a link protein. On the right, an HA molecule forming a linear aggregate with many proteoglycan monomers is interwoven with a network of collagen fibrils. (Based on Hascall VC, Lawther DA: In Nancollas et al (eds): *Biological Mineralization and Demineralization.* New York, Springer, 1982, p. 181.)

bers of sulfate groups, the proteoglycans stain with basic dyes and with hematoxylin and, thus, the basophilia seen in stained sections of cartilage provides information on the distribution of sulfated proteoglycans. The highest concentration of these substances is immediately around the lacuna. This ring of intensely staining matrix has been designated as the *capsule* by classical histologists (Fig. 7.2). There is also a somewhat lesser concentration of sulfated proteoglycans in the vicinity of cell clusters, an area designated as the *territorial matrix.* Sulfated proteoglycans are in their lowest concentration in regions of the matrix furthest removed from the cells. These areas are designated as the *interterritorial matrix.* Aside from these regional differences in the distribution of proteoglycans, there are also differences related to age in that the amount of proteoglycans diminishes as cartilage ages.

Cartilage Cells

In routine hematoxylin and eosin (H&E) preparations, cartilage cells typically display considerable distortion. This is because they normally contain glycogen and lipid, both of which are lost during the preparation of the tissue. In cartilage cells that are active in matrix production, the cytoplasm displays areas of basophilia (indicative of protein synthesis) and clear areas (due to the presence of the Golgi apparatus) (Fig. 7.3). In older, less active cells, the Golgi is reduced in size, but

lipid droplets and accumulated glycogen stores may also be evident as clear areas. WIth the electron microscope, the active cartilage cell is seen to contain numerous profiles of rough endoplasmic reticulum (rER), a large Golgi, secretory granules, vesicles, intermediate filaments, microtubules, and actin microfilaments (Fig. 7.4). In old cartilage cells, there are numerous intermediate filaments.

Location of Hyaline Cartilage

Hyaline cartilage is the initial skeleton of the fetus (Fig. 7.5). It is the precursor to bones that will develop by the process of endochondral ossification. While endochondral bone development is in progress, hyaline cartilage serves as the *epiphyseal growth plate,* and this cartilagenous plate remains functional as long as the bone grows in length (Fig. 7.6). In the adult long bone, hyaline cartilage is present only at the articular bone surface (Fig. 7.7). Hyaline cartilage is also present in the adult as the skeletal unit in the trachea, bronchi, larynx, nose, and the ends of the ribs (costal cartilages).

Perichondrium

Hyaline cartilage is generally surrounded by a firmly attached connective tissue called the *perichondrium* (see Fig. 7.2). However, this does not apply where the cartilage forms a free surface as in joint cavities and where the cartilage makes direct contact with bone. The perichondrium consists of

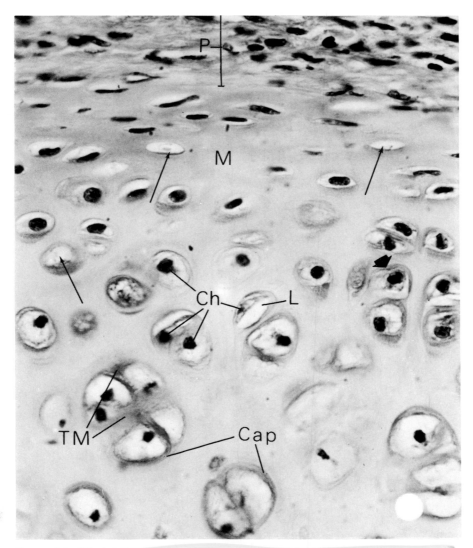

Figure 7.2. Photomicrograph of hyaline cartilage stained with H&E. The chondro-cytes (Ch) are poorly preserved and display little more than the nucleus residing in an empty-appearing lacuna (L). In some instances, the cells have dropped out of the lacunae (**arrows**). The cartilage matrix, however, shows the darker-staining cap-sule (Cap) immediately around the lacunae and the territorial matrix (TM) between chondrocytes in a cluster. The upper portion of the figure shows the perichondrium (P), from which new cartilage cells are derived (appositional growth). Growth from within the cartilage (interstitial growth) is reflected by the chondrocyte pairs and clusters in the lower part of the micrograph. × 640.

dense connective tissue whose cells are indistin-guishable from fibroblasts and, in many respects, the perichondrium resembles a capsule. However, it is more than a covering capsule because it serves as the source of new cartilage cells. The perichon-drium is divided into an inner cellular layer, which gives rise to cartilage cells, and an outer, more fi-brous layer. This division is not always evident, es-pecially in perichondrium that is inactive with re-spect to producing new cartilage. The changes that

occur during the differentiation of new chondro-cytes in a growing cartilage are illustrated in the Atlas section, pages 000 and 000.

Calcification

The matrix of hyaline cartilage undergoes cal-cification as a regular occurrence in three well-de-fined situations: first, that portion of articular car-tilage that is in contact with the bone is calcified;

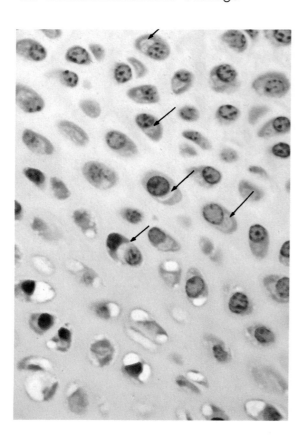

Figure 7.3. Photomicrograph of a young, growing cartilage from a plastic-embedded specimen, stained with H&E. The cartilage cells are well preserved. The cytoplasm is deeply stained, exhibiting a distinct and relatively homogeneous basophilia. The clear areas **(arrows)** represent sites of the Golgi apparatus. × 500.

Note Scalloped edges!

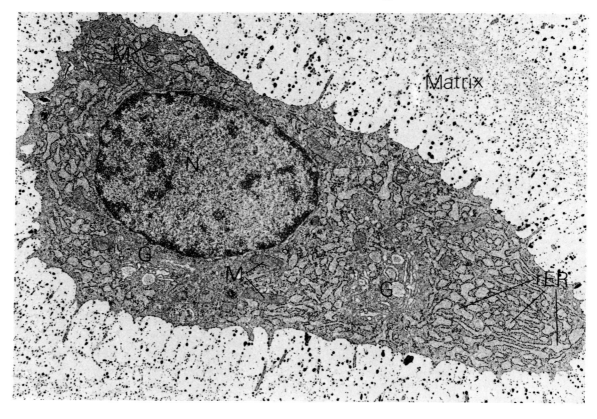

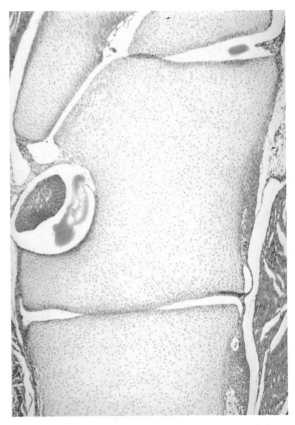

Figure 7.5. Photomicrograph of several of the cartilages forming the initial skeleton of the foot. The hyaline cartilage of the fetal skeleton will be replaced by bone as development proceeds (endochondral ossification). A developing tendon is evident in the indentation of the cartilage seen on the left side of the micrograph.

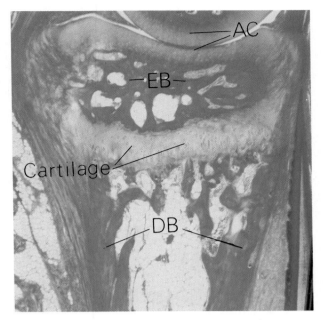

Figure 7.6. Photomicrograph of a portion of a growing long bone. The spaces in the bone are occupied by marrow. A disc of cartilage—the epiphyseal disc—separates the epiphyseal bone (EB) from the diaphyseal bone (DB). The articular surface of the bone is also comprised of cartilage (AC). Whereas the epiphyseal cartilage disappears with the cessation of lengthwise growth of the bone, the articular cartilage remains throughout life.

second, calcification always occurs in cartilage that is about to be replaced by bone during the growth period of the individual; third, hyaline cartilage throughout the body calcifies as part of the aging process.

ELASTIC CARTILAGE

Elastic cartilage is a form of cartilage in which the matrix contains elastic fibers and sheets of elastic material in addition to collagen fibrils and ground substance. The elastic fibers are best demonstrated in paraffin sections with special stains such as resorcin fuchsin and orcein. The elastic material gives the cartilage increased elasticity as evidenced by the pliability of the cartilage in the external ear.

Elastic cartilage is found in the external ear, in the walls of the external auditory canal and the auditory (eustachian) tube, and in the larynx. In all of these locations there is surrounding perichondrium, like that found round most hyaline cartilage. Unlike hyaline cartilage, the matrix of elastic cartilage does not calcify.

FIBROCARTILAGE

Fibrocartilage is a form of cartilage in which the matrix contains obvious bundles of thick colla-

Figure 7.4. Electron micrograph of a young, active chondrocyte and surrounding matrix. The nucleus of the chondrocyte is eccentrically located and the cytoplasm displays numerous and somewhat dilated profiles of rER, Golgi profiles (G), and mitochondria (M). The large amount of rER and the extensive Golgi area indicate that the cell is actively engaged in the production of cartilage matrix. Within the matrix, there are numerous dark particles. They contain proteoglycans of the matrix. The particles adjacent to the cell are particularly large. They are in the region of the matrix that is identified as the capsule of the lacuna with the light microscope. (Courtesy of Dr. H. Clarke Anderson, 1984.)

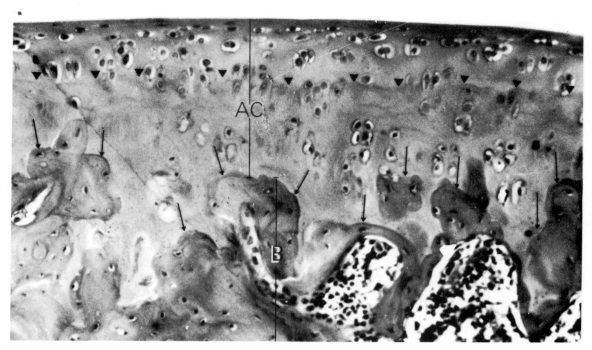

Figure 7.7. Photomicrograph of the epiphysis of a long bone. The articular surface is comprised of hyaline cartilage. The **arrows** indicate the boundary between the articular cartilage (AC) and the underlying bone (B). The deeper part of the articular cartilage—the portion below the **arrowheads**—appears darker than the more superficial portion. This deeper portion is characteristically calcified. Although the calcium salt has been removed from the specimen, its previous existence is marked by a deeper staining than the noncalcified matrix.

gen fibers, mostly of the type I variety. The bundles of collagen are sufficiently large to be seen with the light microscope in H&E sections. Fibrocartilage is typically present in the intervertebral discs, the symphysis pubis, the articular discs of the sternoclavicular and temporomandibular joints, the menisci of the knee joints, and certain places where tendons attach to bones. Usually, the presence of fibrocartilage indicates that resistance to both compression and shear are required of the tissue.

HISTOGENESIS OF CARTILAGE

Cartilage arises from mesenchyme (with the exception of some of the cartilage in the head, which is derived from ectomesenchyme by way of neural crest cells). In the area where cartilage is to develop, mesenchymal cells become rounded and form a mass of cells with relatively little intercellular material. This mass of precartilage cells is called a **blastema.** The cells of the blastema, still in close apposition, begin to produce cartilage matrix. At this time, the cells are referred to as **chondroblasts.** They progressively move apart as they continue to deposit matrix. When they are completely sur-

rounded by matrix material, the cells are called **chondrocytes.** The mesenchymal tissue immediately surrounding the chondrogenic mass ultimately becomes the perichondrium.

GROWTH

Cartilage is capable of two kinds of growth, appositional and interstitial (see Fig. 7.2). Appositional growth is the formation of cartilage onto the surface of pre-existing cartilage. The cells engaging in appositional growth derive from the perichondrium. Interstitial growth is within the cartilage mass. This is possible because the chondrocytes are still capable of cell division and because the matrix is distensible. Although the daughter cells temporarily occupy the same lacuna, they become separated as they secrete new matrix material. As some of the matrix is secreted, a partition is formed between the cells and, at this point, each cell occupies its own lacuna. With continued secretion of matrix, the cells become even further removed from each other.

In adult cartilage, chondrocytes are frequently situated in compact groups or they may be aligned in rows. These groups of chondrocytes are formed as a consequence of several successive divisions during the last phase of development. There is little additional matrix production and the chondrocytes remain in close apposition. Such groups of chondrocytes are called *isogenous groups.*

The ability of damaged cartilage to repair itself is limited. When repair does occur, it is due mainly to activity of the perichondrium and only to a limited degree to interstitial growth of the cartilage itself.

Cartilage is a tissue that is associated with low oxygen tensions. First, it is avascular and, by virtue of their distance from blood vessels, the cells are considered to exist in a climate of low oxygen concentration. Second, in tissue culture systems that would ordinarily lead to the development of bone, cartilage develops if the oxygen tension is lowered.

CARTILAGE CANALS

Although cartilage is described as being an avascular tissue, many cartilages are penetrated by small canals containing blood vessels. The blood vessels are surrounded by connective tissue. Although these canals are variable in terms of their location, appearance, and disappearance, nevertheless they do persist until old age in some cartilages (for example, in laryngeal and nasal cartilages). The significance of cartilage canalas has not yet been clarified.

PLATE 11. Cartilage I, Light and Electron Microscopy

Hyaline cartilage is found in the adult as the structural framework for the larynx, trachea, and bronchi; it is found on the anterior ends of the ribs and on the surfaces of synovial joints. In addition, cartilage constitutes much of the fetal skeleton and plays an important role in the growth of many bones.

Figure 1 shows hyaline cartilage from the trachea. It appears as an avascular expanse of a matrix material and a population of cells referred to as chondrocytes **(Ch)**. The chondrocytes produce the matrix; the space they occupy is called a lacuna **(L)**. Surrounding and in immediate apposition with the cartilage is a cover of connective tissue, the perichondrium **(P)**. The perichondrium is more than a simple capsule in that it also serves as a source of new chondrocytes during the appositional growth of the cartilage. Often the perichondrium reveals two layers: an outer, more fibrous, layer and an inner, more cellular, layer. It is this inner, more cellular, layer that is chondrogenic.

Cartilage matrix contains collagenous fibrils masked by the ground substance and, thus, the fibrils are not evident in routine H&E preparations. The matrix also contains, among other components, sulfated glycosaminoglycans that impart a basophilia with hematoxylin or other basic dyes. However, if the sulfated material is not adequately retained, as is usually the case in routine H&E preparations, then the matrix stains predominately with eosin and to a minimal extent with hematoxylin. Also, the matrix material immediately surrounding a lacuna tends to stain more intensely with basic dyes. This region is referred to as a capsule **(Cap)**. Not uncommonly, the matrix may stain deeply in localized areas **(asterisks)** and appear much like capsule matrix. This is the result of the capsule being included within the thickness of the section, but not the lacuna.

Frequently two or more chondrocytes are extremely close, separated only by a thin partition of matrix. These are said to be isogenous cell clusters because they arise from a single predecessor cell. The proliferation of cells by this means, with the consequent addition of matrix, results in *interstitial growth* of the cartilage, that is, growth within the substance of the cartilage. The perichondrium provides for another kind of growth on the surface of the cartilage known as *appositional growth.*

Figure 2, a low-power electron micrograph, shows to advantage the nature and relationship of the cartilage and perichondrium. The perichondrial cells **(P)** extend long, flat cytoplasmic pro-

cesses between the collagen fibers. Their nuclei are flattened and are surrounded by scant cytoplasm. While these cells constitute the cellular component of the perichondrium, and thus are referred to as perichondrial cells, morphologically they are typical fibroblasts. In contrast, the fully differentiated, mature chondrocytes exhibit round to ovoid nuclei with a moderate amount of cytoplasm. Not being subject to the shrinkage encountered in routine light microscopic preparations, the chondrocyte in electron microscopic preparations does not separate from its surrounding matrix. Consequently, one does not see an empty or partially empty lacuna.

Since the cartilage shown is in a growing state, it is possible to point to the changes that occur during the process of appositional growth. The cells labeled **A, B,** and **C** represent transitional stages in the differentiation of a fibroblast to a chondrocyte. Cell **A** is already in the process of transforming into a chondrocyte. Cell **B** is similar to **A** in shape, but it exhibits a slightly scalloped surface on its upper left side (this is just barely discernible at the low magnification of the micrograph). In addition, the matrix along this surface shows a greater density than that seen on the opposite side of the cell. The more dense material represents cartilage matrix. Cell **C** represents a further transition; this cell is now a young chondrocyte. The entire surface of the cell is scalloped and is completely surrounded by cartilage matrix. Also, the nucleus of the cell has become ovoid and the cell has become more polygonal in shape. With time, the nucleus will assume the more rounded shape of the mature cartilage cells.

KEY

A, B, C, progression chondrocyte differentiation
Ca, calcium deposits
Cap, Capsule
Ch, chondrocytes
G, glycogen
L, laucuna
Li, lipid

P, perichondrium
asterisk, capsule of a lacuna, but with lacuna and contained chondrocyte not included within the thickness of the section

Fig. 1, human, × 450;   **Fig. 2,** mouse, × 3000

PLATE 11

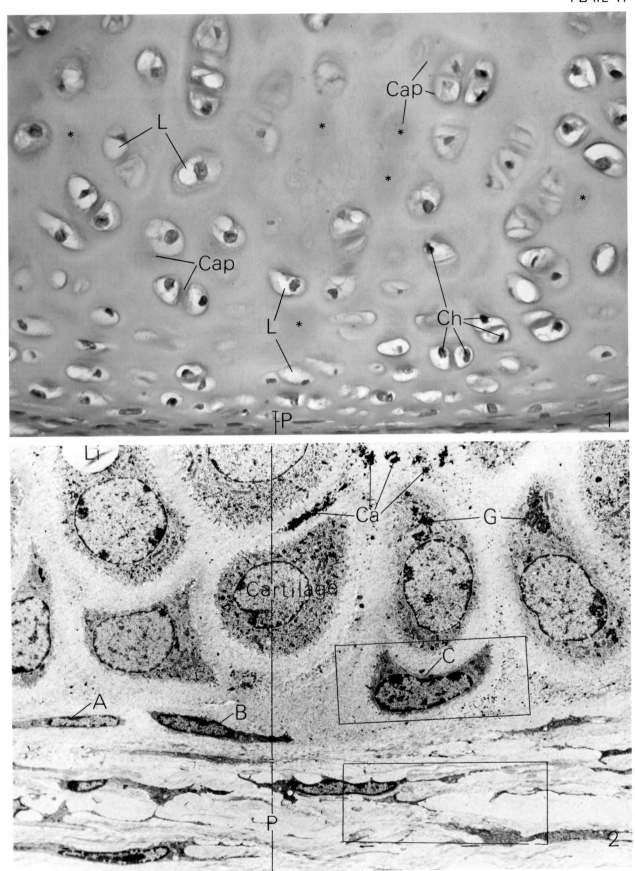

PLATE 12. Cartilage II, Electron Microscopy

Figures 1 and **2** are higher powers of the cells and extracellular matrices from the rectangles in the preceding plate. They allow for a more detailed comparison of the perichondrium and cartilage. The perichondrium in **Figure 1** reveals portions of two fibroblasts or perichondrial cells. One of the cells displays multiple arrays of rough-surfaced or granular endoplasmic reticulum **(GER),** a feature characteristic of the fibroblast. The surface of the cell is relatively smooth. Also characteristic of the fibroblast are the long, tenuous cytoplasmic processes **(F)** that extend between the bundles of collagen fibrils **(CF).** During the process of its differentiation and maturation into a chondrocyte, the fibroblast changes from a flat elongate cell to one that is ovoid to round. Small, irregular projections on the surface of the differentiated chondrocyte **(Figure 2)** give the cell a ruffled or scalloped appearance **(arrowheads).** These projections first appear when cartilage matrix formation is initiated. Other than the accumulation of lipid and glycogen, the cytoplasm of the cartilage cell does not appear appreciably different from the cytoplasm of the fibroblast. The chondrocyte in **Figure 2,** because of the particular region through which the cell was sectioned, does not reveal its granular endoplasmic reticulum. This organelle is particularly well developed in the active chondrocyte. However, the cell does display a fairly prominent portion of its Golgi apparatus **(GA).** Also, note that the glycogen **(G)** within the cell can be just resolved as a particulate component at this magnification. The other very electron dense, extracellular material represents calcium deposits **(Ca).**

The extracellular formed elements of the perichondrial matrix consists mostly of collagen fibrils that are aggregated into bundles, that is, collagen fibers **(CF),** oriented in varying directions. The **upper inset** shows bundles of cross and obliquely sectioned collagen fibrils from the area included

within the circle of **Figure 1.** These collagen fibers belong to the perichondrium. Note the very tight packing of the fibrils. Elastic fibers **(E)** are also evident in the perichondrium. They are comprised of an electron-lucent core material and numerous surrounding, electron-dense microfibrils. The microfibrils **(arrows)** are just perceptible at this magnification. In contrast to the perichondrial connective tissue matrix, the cartilage matrix **(Figure 2),** exclusive of the calcium deposits, appears almost homogeneous, particularly when observed at lower magnifications. It contains extremely fine (5 to 20 nm) matrix fibrils. These fibrils consist primarily of type II collagen, which forms a fibril with a smaller diameter and a less discernible periodic banding pattern, as compared with type I collagen. The **lower inset** shows the cartilage matrix from the area included in the circle of **Figure 2.** Note the fineness of the fibrils and the absence of typical banded collagen fibrils. The relative homogeneity of the cartilage matrix, as seen here, accounts for its amorphous appearance when observed in the light microscope.

KEY

Ca, calcium deposits
CF, collagen fibrils
E, elastic fibers
F, fibroblast process
G, glycogen
GA, Golgi apparatus
GER, granular endoplasmic reticulum

arrowheads, scalloped surface of chondrocyte
arrows, microfibrils of elastic fibers

Fig. 1–2, mouse,
× 16,000 (insets,
× 31,000)

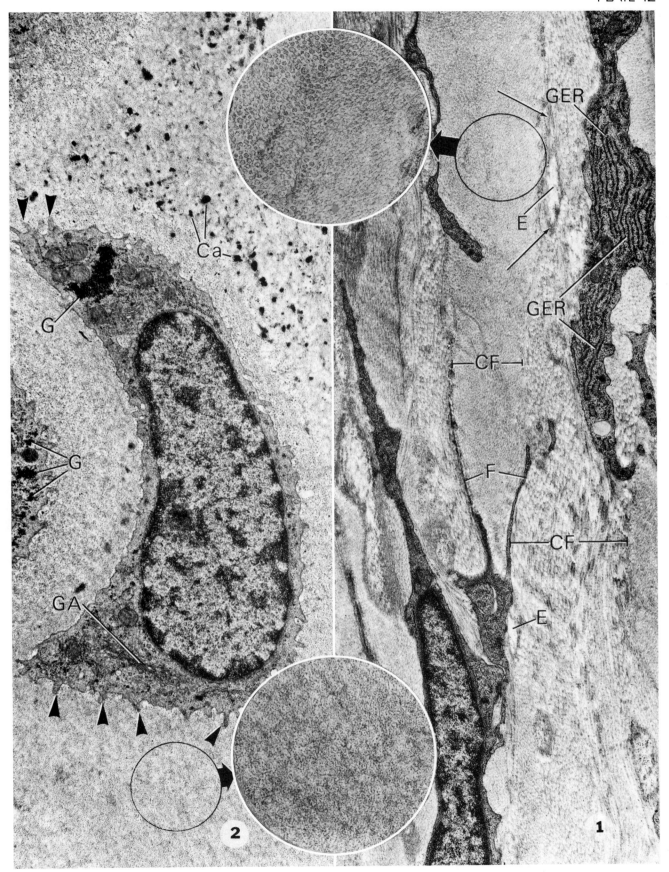

PLATE 12

PLATE 13. Cartilage and the Developing Skeleton

Hyaline cartilage is present as a precursor to bones in the fetus. This cartilage is replaced by bone tissue, except where one bone contacts another bone, as in a joint. In these locations, cartilage persists and covers the bone as articular cartilage. In addition, cartilage, being capable of interstitial growth, persists in weight-supporting bones as a "growth plate" as long as growth in length occurs. The role of hyaline cartilage in bone growth is considered below.

Figure 1 is a section through a fetal foot and shows the cartilages that ultimately will become the bones of the foot. In several places, developing ligaments (**L**) can be seen where they join the cartilages. The nuclei of the fibroblasts within the ligaments are just barely perceptible. They are aligned in rows and are separated from other rows of fibroblasts by collagenous material. The hue and intensity of color of the cartilage matrix, except at the periphery, is due to the combined uptake of the H&E. As already noted, the presence of sulfated glycosaminoglycans results in staining by hemotoxylin. However, the matrix of cartilage that is about to be replaced by bone, such as that shown here, becomes impregnated with calcium salts, and the calcium is receptive to staining with hematoxylin. It should be noted that the many enlarged lacunae (seen as light spaces within the matrix where the chondrocytes have fallen out of the lacunae) are due to hypertrophy of the chondrocytes, an event associated with calcification of the matrix. Thus, where these large lacunae are present, that is, in the center region of the cartilage, the matrix is heavily stained.

Figure 1 also shows that the cartilage is surrounded by perichondrium, except where it faces a joint cavity (**JC**). Here the bare cartilage forms a surface. Note that the joint cavity is a space between the cartilage whose boundaries are completed by connective tissue (**CT**). The connective tissue at the surface of the cavity is special. It will constitute the synovial membrane in the adult and contribute to the formation of a lubricating fluid (synovial fluid) that is present in the joint cavity. Therefore, all the surfaces that will enclose the adult joint cavity are derived originally from mesenchyme. This is an apparent exception to the general principle that epithelium is found on surfaces. Synovial fluid is a viscous substance, containing,

among other things, glycoaminoglycans; it can be considered an exudate of interstitial fluid. The synovial fluid might be considered an extension of the extracellular matrix, since the joint cavity is not lined by an epithelium.

Figure 2 shows a developing long bone of the finger and its articulation with the distal and proximal bones. Before the stage shown here, each bone consisted entirely of a hyaline cartilagenous structure similar to the cartilages seen in **Figure 1**, but shaped like the long bones into which they develop. Here only the ends, or epiphyses, of the bone remain as cartilage, the epiphyseal cartilage (**C**). The shaft, or diaphysis, has become a cylinder of bone tissue (**B**) surrounding the marrow cavity (**MC**). The dark region at the ends of the marrow cavity is calcified cartilage (**arrowheads**) that is being replaced by bone. (The bone at the ends of the marrow cavity constitutes the metaphysis.) The specimen has been stained by the thionine-picric acid method and the calcified cartilage appears dark brown. The newly formed metaphyseal bone, which is admixed with this degenerating calcified cartilage and difficult to define at this low magnification, has the same yellow-brown color as the diaphyseal bone. By the continued proliferation of cartilage, the bone grows in length. Later the cartilage becomes calcified; bone is then produced and occupies the site of the resorbed cartilage. With the cessation of cartilage proliferation and replacement by bone, growth of the bone stops and only the cartilage at the articular surface remains. The details of this process are explained under endochondral bone formation (Plates 19 and 20).

KEY

B, bone
C, cartilage
CT, connective tissue
JC, joint cavity

L, ligament
MC, marrow cavity
arrowhead, calcified cartilage

Fig. 1, rat, × 85;

Fig. 2, human, × 30

PLATE 13

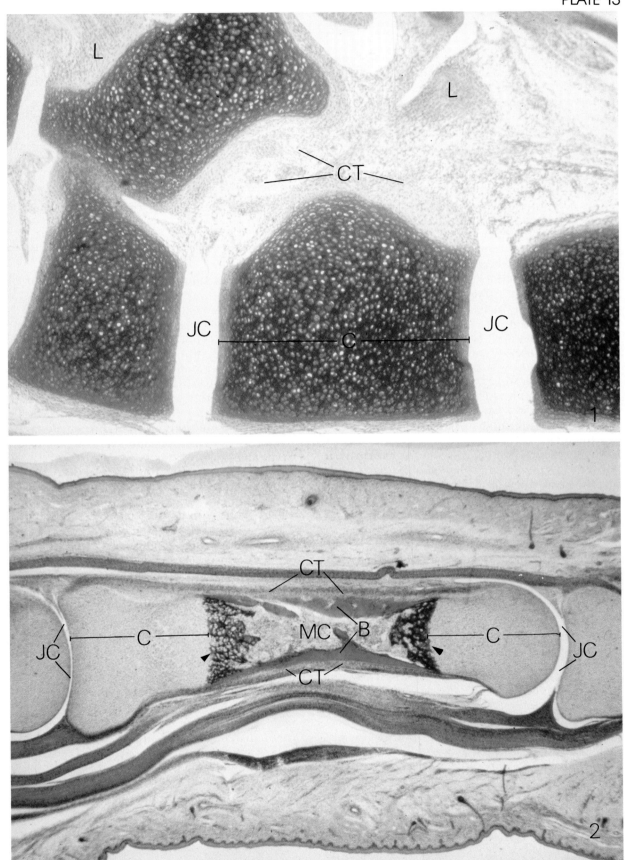

PLATE 14. Elastic Cartilage

Elastic cartilage is found in the auricle of the external ear, in the auditory tube, and in part of the larynx. It differs from hyaline cartilage in that the matrix contains elastic material either as fibers or as interconnecting sheets in addition to the other constituents of cartilage matrix. The elastic material imparts properties of elasticity to the cartilage that are not shared by hyaline cartilage.

A section of the epiglottis containing elastic cartilage (**EC**) as the centrally located structure is shown in **Figure 1.** The essential components of the cartilage, namely, the matrix that stains deep blue, and the light, unstained lacunae, surrounded by matrix, are readily evident in the low-magnification illustration. The perimeter of the cartilage is covered by perichondrium; its fibrous character is just barely evident in **Figure 1.** Also to be noted is the adipose tissue (**AT**) within the boundaries of the elastic cartilage.

Both above and below the elastic cartilage there is connective tissue and each surface of the epiglottis is formed by stratified squamous epithelium. Mucous glands (**MG**) are in the connective tissue in the bottom of the figure.

Figure 2 shows an area of the elastic cartilage at higher magnification. The elastic fibers appear as the blue, elongate profiles within the matrix. They are most evident at the edges of the cartilage, but they are obscured in some deeper parts of the matrix where they blend with the elastic material that forms a honeycomb about the lacunae. Elastic fibers (**E**) are also in the adipose tissue (**AT**) between the adipocytes.

Some of the lacunae in the cartilage are arranged in pairs separated by a thin plate of matrix. The plate of matrix appears as a bar between the adjacent lacunae. This is a reflection of interstitial

growth by the cartilage in that the adjacent cartilage cells are derived from the same parent cell. They have moved away from each other and secreted a plate of cartilage matrix between the two lacunae. Most chondrocytes shown in **Figure 2** occupy only part of the lacuna. This is due, in part, to shrinkage, but also to the fact that older chondrocytes contain lipid in large droplets that is lost during the processing of the tissue. The shrinkage of chondrocytes within the lacunae, or their loss due to dropping out of the section during preparation, causes the lacunae to stand out as light unstained areas against the darkly stained matrix.

The circular **inset** shows the elastic cartilage at still higher magnification. Here, the elastic fibers (**E**) are again evident as elongate profiles chiefly at the edges of the cartilage. Most of the chondrocytes in this part of the specimen show little shrinkage. Many of the cells display a typically rounded nucleus and the cytoplasm is evident. Note again that some lacunae contain two chondrocytes indicative of interstitial growth.

KEY

AT, adipose tissue
E, elastic fiber

EC, elastic cartilage
MG, mucous gland

Fig. 1, × 80;

Fig. 2, × 250 (inset, × 400)

PLATE 14

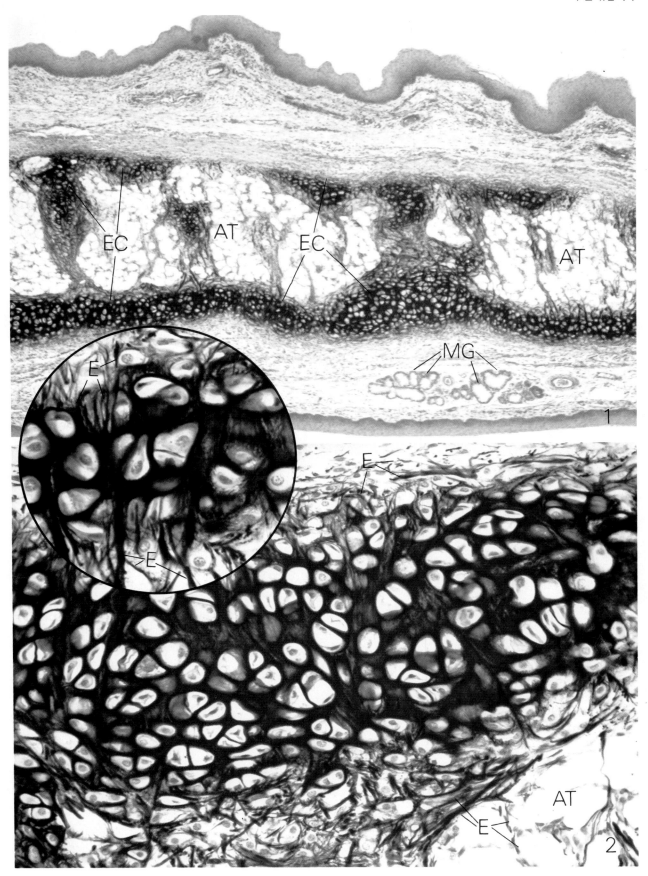

PLATE 15. Fibrocartilage

Fibrocartilage is a combination of dense connective tissue and cartilage. The amount of cartilage varies, but in most locations, the cartilage cells and their matrix occupy a lesser portion of the tissue mass. Fibrocartilage is found at the intervertebral discs, the symphysis pubis, the knee joint, the mandibular joint, the sternoclavicular joint, and the shoulder joint. It may also be present along the grooves or insertions for tendons and ligaments. Its presence is associated with sites where a degree of resiliency is required to help absorb sudden physical impact. Histologically, fibrocartilage appears as small fields of cartilage blending almost imperceptibly with regions of fibrous tissue. No perichondrium is present.

A low-magnification view of fibrocartilage is shown in **Figure 1.** The specimen has been treated using the Mallory method, which stains collagen light blue. The tissue has a fibrous appearance and, at this low magnification, the nuclei of the fibroblasts **(F)** appear as small, elongate or spindle-shaped bodies. There are relatively few fibroblasts present as is characteristic of dense connective tissue. The cartilage cells **(C)** are more numerous and exhibit close spatial groupings, that is, isogenous groups. Some of the cartilage cells appear as elongate clusters of cells, while others appear in single-file rows. The matrix material immediately surrounding the cartilage cells has a homogeneous appearance and is thereby distinguishable from the fibrous connective tissue.

KEY

C, cartilage   **arrow,** lacuna
F, fibroblast

Fig. 1, human, Mallory   **Fig. 2,** human, Mallory
method, × 160;   method, × 700

Figure 2 shows at higher magnification the area circumscribed by the rectangle in **Figure 1.** The cartilage cells are contained within lacunae **(arrows),** and their cytoplasm stains deeply. The surrounding cartilage matrix material is scant and blends into the fibrous tissue. The presence of cartilage matrix material can be detected best by observing the larger group of cartilage cells at the left of **Figure 2** and then observing this same area in **Figure 1.** Note the general light homogeneous area around the cell nest in the lower power view. This is the region of cartilage matrix. In the higher power of **Figure 2** it is possible to see that some of the collagen fibers are incorporated in the matrix where they appear as wispy bundles.

PLATE 15

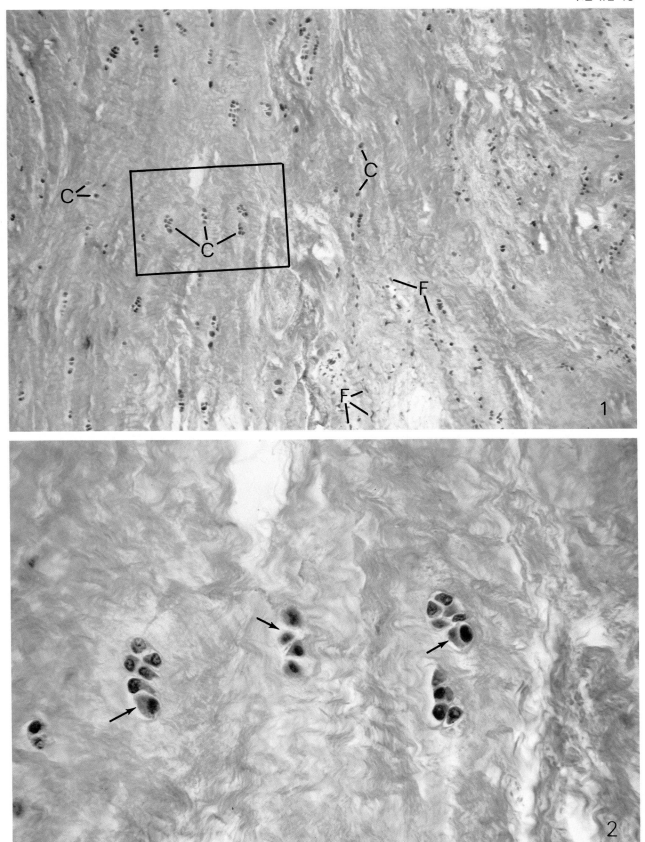

Bone

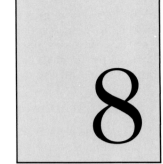

Bone is a specialized form of connective tissue that, like the other connective tissues, consists of cells and intercellular material. The feature that distinguishes bone is the mineralization of the intercellular matrix[1] material, resulting in an extremely hard tissue capable of providing support and protection. The mineral is calcium, in the form of hydroxyapatite crystals [$Ca_{10}(PO_4)_6(OH)_2$]. The calcium of the matrix can be mobilized and taken up by the blood as needed to maintain appropriate levels thoughout the tissues of the body. Thus, it has an important secondary role in the homeostatic regulation of calcium blood levels.

The bone matrix consists of collagen fibers and ground substance (proteoglycans), both of which are mineralized. Within the substance of the bone tissue are spaces, called *lacunae,* which harbor the bone cells. Typically, there is one bone cell, called an *osteocyte,* within the lacuna. The osteocyte possesses numerous processes contained within little tunnels called *canaliculi.* These extend from the lacunae into and through the substance of the mineralized matrix. The canaliculi extending from one lacuna connect with the canaliculi

from neighboring lacunae. In this manner, a continuous network of canaliculi and lacunae is formed throughout the entire mass of mineralized tissue. Electron micrographs have shown contacts, namely, gap junctions, between processes of different osteocytes within the canaliculi, indicating that the bone cells are in communication with one another.

In addition to the osteocyte, three other cell types are identified with bone tissue: *bone lining cells, osteoblasts,* and *osteoclasts.* Each of these cells, including the osteocyte, will be discussed later in detail. For the moment, they may be defined very briefly as follows. *Osteoblasts* are present on surfaces of developing bone; they are bone-forming cells. *Osteoclasts* are large, multinucleated cells found on bone surfaces during the early stages of bone remodeling. They are bone-resorbing cells. Remodeling is an important process that also will be described later. *Bone lining cells,* also known as *osteoprogenitor cells,* are located on internal bone surfaces. They may be resting cells or cells about to be called on to produce bone, therefore, the name osteoprogenitor cell. None of these three cell types is surrounded by mineralized bone matrix. However, once the osteoblast completes the process of forming bone in its immediate environs, that is, after it surrounds itself with bone matrix, it then is referred to as an *osteocyte.*

BONE TISSUE AND BONES

A distinction must be made between bone tissue and bones, which are the organs of the skeletal system. Like other organs, bones are comprised of a number of tissues. Typically, a bone consists of bone tissue, other connective tissues of various sorts, including hemopoietic tissue, fat tissue,

---

[1] Because of its mineral content, special methods are employed in preparing a bone sample for microscopic examination. It is possible to sacrifice the organic material by removing as much as possible and allowing the bone to dry. The bone is then cut into thin slices with a saw and further reduced in thinness on a grinding stone. When the bone specimen is sufficiently thin, it is mounted on a slide for microscopic examination. Such a specimen is called a ground specimen; it is anorganic, or essentially so. It is also possible to remove the mineral component of bone with demineralizing solutions (acids or chelating agents). After the mineral has been removed, the tissue is treated in the same manner as other tissue being prepared for microscopic observation. Obviously, the ground section reveals the mineralized component of the tissue and it is not suitable for the study of cellular elements, whereas the demineralized sample reveals the soft tissue components (cells, matrix, etc.) but not the mineral.

blood vessels, nerves, and, if the bone forms a freely movable (synovial) joint, hyaline cartilage, and, in some cases, fibrocartilage. The ability of the bone to perform its skeletal function is due to the bond tissue and the cartilage.

Classification of Bone Tissue

There are several ways to classify bone tissue. At this time, it is appropriate to begin with a classification that requires simply the unaided eye or, at most, a hand lens. On this basis, upon the examination of a cut face of a dry bone (Fig. 8.1), one can identify **compact** (or **dense**) **bone** and **spongy** (or **cancellous**) **bone.** The cut face of compact bone appears to be solid, whereas the cut face of spongy bone has the appearance of a sponge. In spongy bone, there are **trabeculae** (or **spicules**) of minera-

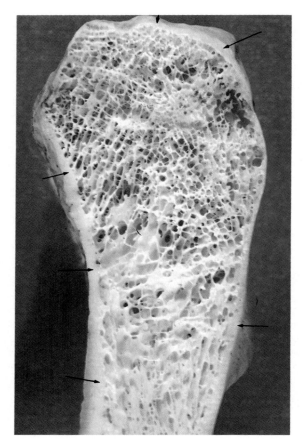

Figure 8.1. Gross specimen of a longitudinally sliced long bone. The outer portion of the bone has a solid structure (**arrows**) and represents compact bone. The interior of the bone exhibits a spongy configuration and consists of numerous interconnecting marrow spaces bounded by bony traveculae.

lized tissue; empty spaces between the trabeculae occupy a considerable but variable volume. In the intact living bone, the regions between the trabeculae are filled with bone marrow.

Classification and General Structure of Bones

Spongy and compact bone tissue are located in specific parts of bones. It is useful, then, to outline briefly the kinds of bones and survey where the two kinds of bone tissue are located. On the basis of shape, bones can be classified into four groups: long, short, flat, and irregular. **Long bones** are longer in one dimension and consist of a shaft and two ends; examples are the tibia and the metacarpals. A schematic diagram of a long bone sectioned longitudinally through the shaft, called the **diaphysis,** and its two expanded ends, each called an **epiphysis,** is shown in Figure 8.2. The flared portion of the epiphysis that is directly contiguous to the diaphysis is called the **metaphysis.** It extends from the diaphysis to the epiphyseal line. A large cavity filled with bone marrow, called the **marrow** or **medullary cavity,** forms the inner portion of the bone and is surrounded by bone tissue. In general, the outermost part of the bone tissue is compact and the innermost part is spongy. In the shaft, almost the entire thickness of the bone tissue is compact; at most, only a small amount of spongy bone faces the medullary cavity. At the ends of the bone, the reverse is true. Here the spongy bone is thick and the compact bone is little more than a thin outer shell.

Short bones are nearly equal in length, depth, and width, for example, the carpal bones. They possess a shell of compact bone on the outside and spongy bone on the inside. Short bones usually form movable joints with their neighbors, and, as with long bones, the articular surfaces are covered with hyaline cartilage. Elsewhere, periosteum covers the outer surface of the bone.

Flat bones are thin and plate-like and include, for example, the bones of the calvaria (the skull cap) and the sternum. They consist of two layers of relatively thick compact bone with an intervening layer of spongy bone.

Irregular bones have a shape that does not fit into any one of the three groups just described; the shape may be complex, for example, the vertebra, or the bone may contain air spaces or sinuses, as in the ethmoid. (Because of the unique character of these bones with their air spaces, they are sometimes referred to as **pneumatic bones.**) Irregular bones are, to a large degree, combinations of the above types.

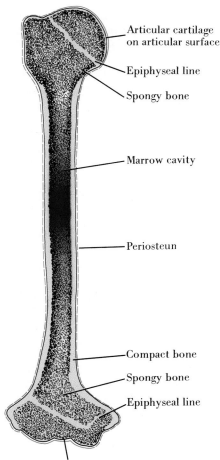

Articular cartilage on articular surface

Epiphyseal line

Spongy bone

Marrow cavity

Periosteun

Compact bone

Spongy bone

Epiphyseal line

Articular cartilage on articular surface

Figure 8.2. Structure of a typical long bone. The shaft of the long bone, the diaphysis, contains a large marrow or medullary cavity surrounded by a thick-walled tube of compact bone. A small amount of spongy bone may line the inner surface of the compact bone. The ends, or epiphyses, of the long bone consist chiefly of spongy bone with a thin outer shell of compact bone. An additional term, the metaphysis, refers to the expanded or flared part of the bone at the extremities of the diaphysis. Except for the articular surfaces that are covered by hyaline (articular) cartilage, indicated by the **blue line**, the outer surface of the bone is covered by a fibrous connective tissue capsule called the periosteum, indicated by the **dashed blue line**.

Surfaces of Bone

External Surface. Typically, at its extremities, a bone articulates with a neighboring bone to form a movable (synovial) joint. The contact area of the bone, referred to as the **articular surface,** is covered with hyaline cartilage, also called **articular cartilage** because of its location and function. The articular cartilage is exposed to the joint cavity without a covering. Elsewhere, the bone is covered by **periosteum,** a membrane of dense connective tissue. The periosteum is composed of an outer fibrous layer and an inner cell-rich layer containing osteoblasts (if bone formation on the surface is in progress) and other cells indistinguishable from fibroblasts that are capable of becoming active as osteoblasts in response to the appropriate stimulus. If active bone formation is not in progress on the bone surface, the fibrous layer is the main component of the periosteum and few cells are seen in the inner layer. However, the relatively few cells that are present are capable of becoming osteoblasts under appropriate stimulus.

Generally, the collagenous fibers of the periosteum are parallel to the surface of the bone in the form of a capsule. The character of the periosteum is different where ligaments and tendons attach to the bone. Collagen fibers from these structures extend directly, but at an angle, into the bone tissue. These collagen fibers are called **Sharpey's fibers.**

Lining Surfaces of Bone Cavities. Few bones are solid structures. Like the long bone that has already been described, most bones, despite their shape, have a medullary cavity with at least some spongy bone present. The lining tissue of both the bone facing the medullary cavity, and the trabeculae of the spongy bone, is referred to as **endosteum.** The endosteum, often only one cell thick, contains bone-forming and bone-resorbing cells, or resting forms of these cells that are capable of becoming active in response to appropriate stimuli. The resting form of an osteoblast in the endosteum is flat and has a squamous shape; it is called a **bone lining cell** or **endosteal** cell.

During the early stages of growth of the individual, the medullary cavity and the spaces in the spongy bone contain **red bone marrow.** This is the tissue in which blood cells develop. Thus, the red marrow consists of developing blood cells in different stages of development and a network of reticular cells and fibers that serve as a supporting framework for the developing blood cells. In later stages of growth and in the adult, when the rate of blood cell formation has diminished, the tissue in the medullary cavity consists mostly of fat cells; it is then called **yellow marrow.** Under the appropriate stimuli, the yellow marrow can revert to red marrow. The spaces of the spongy bone generally retain the red marrow and continue to function in blood cell formation throughout the life of the individual.

Blood Supply. The blood supply to the shaft of a long bone is chiefly by arteries that enter the marrow cavity through nutrient foramina in the diaphysis and in the epiphysis. Additional vessels may provide a supplementary supply to the metaphysis (metaphyseal arteries). Drainage of the bone is by veins that leave through the nutrient foramina or through the bone tissue of the shaft and out through the periosteum (see Fig. 8.3). The blood supply to the bone tissue is essentially centrifugal, from marrow cavity through the bone tissue and out via periosteal vessels. Periosteal arteries do enter bone tissue but almost exclusively at the epiphysis and at sites where tendons and ligaments attach to the bone. The nutrient arteries that supply the diaphysis and epiphysis arise developmentally as the principal vessel of a periosteal bud from which the primary and secondary centers of ossification develop (see page 154). The metaphyseal arteries, in contrast, developmentally arise from periosteal vessels that become incorporated into the metaphysis during the growth process, that is, through the widening of the bone.

With respect to nourishment of the bone tissue itself, the Volkmann's canals provide the major route and anastomosis within the compact bone. The smaller blood vessels enter into the Haversian canals wherein one may find a single arteriole and a venule, and others, only a single capillary. A considerably lesser supply to the bone tissue arises from the periosteal vessels, but these usually provide for only the very outermost portions of the compact bone. It might be noted also that the bone tissue lacks lymphatics and only the periosteal tissue is provided with lymphatic drainage.

STRUCTURE OF ADULT BONE

Adult Compact Bone—The Haversian System (Secondary Osteon)

The shaft of an adult human bone, such as the femur or tibia, contains numerous units of bone structure called a **Haversian system** or a **secondary osteon.** In its fully developed form, the Haversian

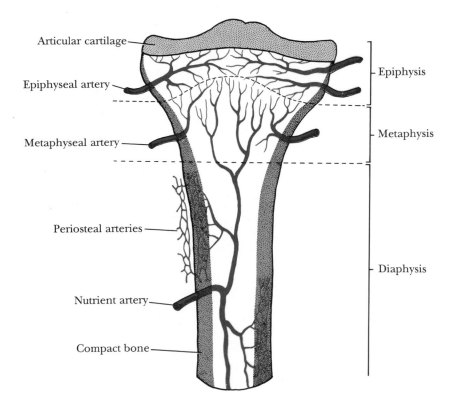

Figure 8.3. Diagram showing blood supply of a mature long bone. The nutrient artery and the epiphyseal arteries enter the bone through nutrient foramina that arose developmentally as the principal vessel of a periosteal bud during early development. Metaphyseal arteries arise from periosteal vessels that become incorporated into the metaphysis as the bone grows in diameter.

system is somewhat cylindrical in shape with its long axis distributed in domains, and fibrils in a particular domain of a layer are parallel and oriented in a direction different from the direction of fibrils in domains of adjacent lamellae. The lacunae for the cells and, thus, the cells themselves, appear to be slightly flattened between the lamellae and, consequently, they have their long axis parallel to the lamellae of mineralized matrix. Canaliculi containing the processes of osteocytes are arranged mostly in a radial pattern with respect to the canal. The system of canaliculi, which open to the Haversian canal, also serves for the passage of substances between the bone cells and the blood vessels.

In addition to the concentric lamellae that make up the Haversian system, other lamellar patterns of bone occur in a sample of compact adult long bone. Some of these are lamellar territories between the Haversian systems. These are referred to as *interstitial lamellae* (Fig. 8.4). Other lamellae constitute the outer portion of the compact bone. These are called *circumferential lamellae* or, more specifically, *outer circumferential lamellae.* Circumferential lamellae also may be present in the inner region of the compact bone. The interstitial lamellae are remnants of older osteons or of circumferential lamellae.

Another kind of vascular canal is also found in adult compact bone and this is the *Volkmann's canal* (Fig. 8.4). It contains blood vessels that join with those of the Haversian canal. The Volkmann's canal is not surrounded by concentric lamellae, a key feature to its histological identification.

Haversian systems are replacement bone; they were formed by the internal remodeling of pre-

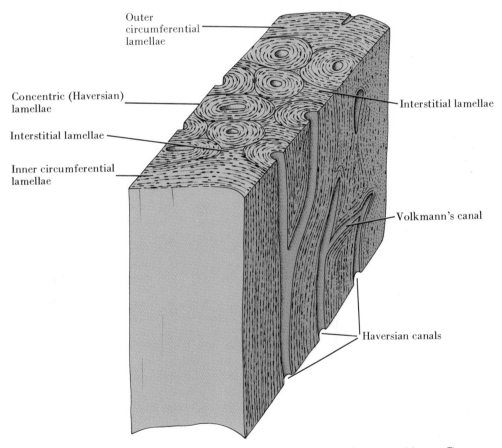

Figure 8.4. Three-dimensional diagram of a dried sample of compact bone. The concentric lamellae and the Haversian canal that they surround constitute a Haversian system. Between the Haversian systems are lamellae, remnants of old Haversian systems. They are designated as interstitial. The inner and outer surfaces of the compact bone in the figure show additional lamellae—the outer and inner circumferential lamellae— which are arranged in broad layers. (Based on Tandler J: *Lehrbuch der Systematischen Anatomie.* Leipzig, Vogel, 1926.)

existing compact bone (see below). It is for this reason that the Haversian system is called a secondary osteon.

Adult Spongy Bone

Adult spongy bone is very similar to adult compact bone except that mineralized tissue is arranged as trabeculae or spicules and numerous interconnecting marrow spaces of various size are present between the bone tissue located there. The matrix of the bone is lamellated and, if the trabeculae are sufficiently thick, they display profiles indicative of Haversian systems.

MATURE AND IMMATURE BONE

Most samples of compact and spongy bone from an adult skeleton display the patterns of lamellar bone as described above. Such bone may also be classified as *adult* or *mature bone*. On the other hand, the bone tissue initially deposited in the skeleton of the developing fetus is called *immature bone*. It differs from adult bone in several respects (Fig. 8.5).

First, immature bone does not display an organized lamellated appearance and, on the basis of

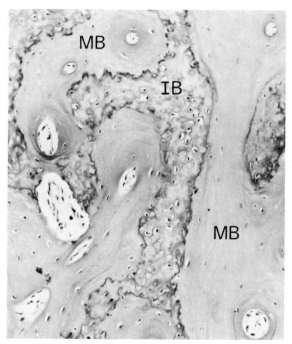

Figure 8.5. Low-power photomicrograph showing immature bone (IB) and mature bone (MB) in an H&E section of decalcified bone. The immature bone has more cells and the matrix is not layered in regular patterns. (From Ham AW, Cormack DH: *Histology*, 8th ed. Philadelphia, JB Lippincott, 1979.)

collagen fiber arrangement, such bone is designated as *nonlamellar*. Nonlamellar bone may also be referred to as *bundle* or *woven bone* because of the interlacing arrangement of the collagen fibers.

Second, immature bone contains relatively more cells per unit areas than does mature bone. The cells in immature bone tend to be randomly arranged, whereas cells in mature bone tend to have their long axis in the same direction as the lamellae.

Third, the matrix of immature bone has more ground substance than the matrix of mature bone has. Furthermore, the matrix in immature bones stains more intensely with hematoxylin, whereas the matrix of mature bone stains more intensely with eosin.

Fourth, although not evident in typical histological sections, immature bone is more completely mineralized when it is initially formed, whereas mature bone undergoes a prolonged secondary mineralization. The secondary mineralization of mature bone is evident in microradiographs of ground sections that show younger Haversian systems to be less mineralized than older Haversian systems.

Fifth, immature bone forms more rapidly than mature bone.

Although mature bone is clearly the major bone form in the adult and immature bone is the major bone forming in the developing fetus, areas of immature bone are regularly seen in the adult, especially where bone is being remodeled. Areas of immature bone also are seen regularly in the alveolar sockets of the adult oral cavity and where tendons insert into bones.

CELLS OF BONE TISSUE

As noted earlier in this chapter, four types of cells are associated with bone tissue: the osteoprogenitor or bone lining cell; the osteoblast; the osteocyte; and the osteoclast. With the exception of the osteoclast, each of these cells may be regarded as a modulated form of the same cell type because each undergoes transformation from one form to the other in relation to functional activity. In contrast, the osteoclast has as its origin a different cell line and is responsible for bone resorption, an activity associated with bone remodeling.

Osteoprogenitor Cell

The *osteoprogenitor cell* is generally regarded as a resting or reserve cell that can be stimulated to transform into an osteoblast and produce bone matrix. Osteoprogenitor cells are found on the surfaces of bone during normal growth and in the adult during bone remodeling. They comprise the population of cells in the innermost layer of the periosteum, the endosteal lining cells of the marrow cavities, and the lining cells of the Haversian and Volkmann's canals. The osteoprogenitor cells also have the capacity to divide and proliferate as evidenced by autoradiographic studies. In growing bones, the osteoprogenitor cells appear as flattened cells with lightly staining, elongate, or ovoid nuclei and inconspicuous acidophilic or slightly basophilic cytoplasm. Electron micrographs reveal profiles of rough endoplasmic reticulum (rER) and free ribosomes as well as a small Golgi area and other organelles. The morphology of the osteoprogenitor cell is consistent with the findings that their stimulation leads to the more active secretory cell, the osteoblast.

In the mature individual where remodeling of bone is not occurring, the bone surfaces are covered by a layer of extremely flat cells with very attenuated cytoplasm and a paucity of organelles beyond the perinuclear region (Fig. 8.6). They do not form a complete lining on the bone surface, but where the lining cells contact one another, gap junctions can be found. These cells, designated simply as **bone lining cells,** are analogous to the osteoprogenitor cells, but are probably a more quiescent state than those located at sites where bone growth is occurring. They are also thought to function in the maintenance and nutritional support of the osteocytes embedded in the underlying bone matrix. This role is based on the observation that the cell processes of the bone lining cells extend into the canalicular channels of the adjacent bone and communicate by means of gap junctions with processes of the osteocyte.

The degree of differentiation of the osteoprogenitor cell is not entirely clear. Although they derive from mesenchymal cells, their capability to transform into three kinds of cells, (such as adipose cells, chondroblasts, or fibroblasts), has not yet been clarified. This question is of importance because the healing of fractures of bone involves the formation of new connective tissue and cartilage in the callus that develops around the bone as part of the repair process. The origin of these cells is unclear.

Osteoblast Cell

The *osteoblast* is the differentiated bone-forming cell responsible for the production of bone matrix. It secretes both the collagen and the ground

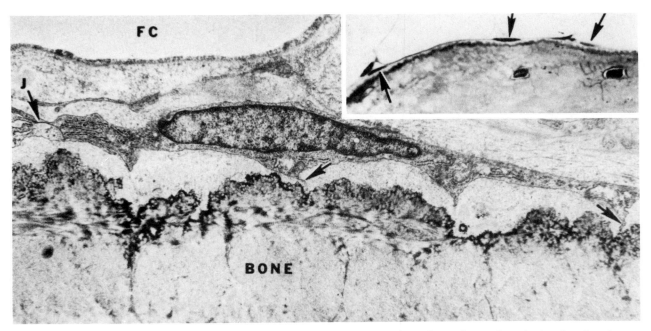

Figure 8.6. Electron micrograph showing portions of two bone-lining cells on the surface of a spicule of mature bone. The cytoplasm is very attenuated and contains small amounts of rER and free ribosomes. A gap junction (J) is seen between the two bone-lining cells. In addition, cytoplasmic processes (**arrows**) are clearly seen where they pass through the noncalcified bone matrix (osteoid). A fat cell of the marrow is also present (FC). The **inset** is a high-power light micrograph of a similar bone spicule and included for orientation purposes. The bone-lining cells on the surface of the spicule are indicated by the **arrows.** Electron micrograph, ×8900; light micrograph, ×700.

substance that constitutes the initial unmineralized bone or *osteoid.* The osteoblast is also associated with the calcification of the matrix. The calcification process appears to be initiated by the osteoblast through the secretion into the matrix of small 50- to 250-nm membrane-bound *matrix vesicles.* The vesicles are rich in alkaline phosphatase and are actively secreted only during the period that the cell is producing the bone matrix. The role of these vesicles is discussed on page 159 under biological mineralization.

In the light microscope, osteoblasts are recognized by their cuboidal or polygonal shape and their aggregation as a single layer of cells lying in apposition to the forming bone (Fig. 8.7). Because the newly deposited matrix is not immediately calcified, it stains much lighter (or not at all) compared to the mature mineralized matrix that stains prominently with eosin. Because of this staining property, the osteoblasts appear to be separated from the bone by a light band. This is referred to

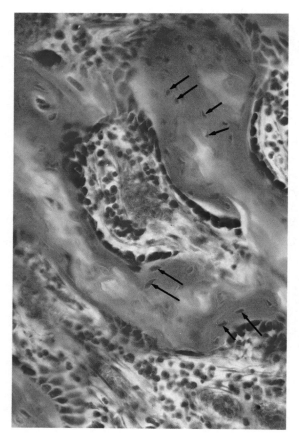

Figure 8.7. Photomicrograph of growing bone spicules. The osteocytes are the small, relatively inconspicuous cells within the bone matrix (**arrows**). The osteoblasts are larger and are on the surfaces of the bone tissue.

as osteoid; it is the nonmineralized matrix. The cytoplasm of the osteoblast is markedly basophilic and the Golgi complex, because of its size, is sometimes observed as a clear area adjacent to the nucleus. With periodic acid-Schiff (PAS) staining, small positive-reacting granules are observed in the cytoplasm. Also, a strong alkaline phosphatase reaction, associated with the cell membrane, can be detected by appropriate histochemical staining.

At the electron microscope level, the osteoblast exhibits very thin cytoplasmic processes that penetrate through the adjacent osteoid that the cell has produced and joined by gap junctions to similar processes of those cells. These cells most recently have become osteocytes within the mineralizing bone. It is by this method, that is, by the early establishment of junctions between the osteoblast and the adjacent osteocyte (as well as between adjacent osteoblasts), that the neighboring cells within the bone tissue communicate.

The cytoplasm of the osteoblast is characterized by adundant rER and free ribosomes (see Atlas section, Plate 23). This is consistent with their basophilia, as observed in the light microscope, as well as with their role in the production of collagen and proteoglycans for the extracellular matrix. The Golgi and surrounding regions of the cytoplasm contain numerous vesicles with a flocculent content, which is presumed to contain the matrix precursors. It is these vesicles that are seen as the PAS-staining granules by light microscopy. [The matrix vesicles (see page 159), which are produced by the osteoblast, appear to arise by a different pathway, originating as sphere-like outgrowths that pinch off from the plasma membrane to become free in the matrix]. Other cell organelles of note are the numerous rod-shaped mitochondria and occasional dense bodies and lysosomes.

Osteocyte

The *osteocyte* is the mature bone cell. It is enclosed by the bone matrix that it had previously laid down as an osteoblast; thus, the osteocyte represents a transformed osteoblast. The osteocytes are responsible for maintaining the bone matrix. They have the capacity to synthesize, as well as resorb matrix, at least to a limited extent. Such activities are important in contributing to the homeostasis of blood calcium. Death of the osteocytes either through trauma, e.g., a fracture, or cell senescence results in resorption of the bone matrix by osteoclast activity, followed by repair or remodeling of the bone tissue by osteoblast activity.

Each osteocyte occupies a space, or *lacuna,* that conforms to the lenticular shape of the cell.

The osteocytes extend their cytoplasmic processes through fine tunnels or canaliculi in the matrix to contact, by means of gap junctions, processes of neighboring cells. In H&E sections, the canaliculi and the processes they contain are not discernable, but in ground sections, the canaliculi are readily evident. Unlike its former state as an osteoblast, the osteocyte is typically smaller due to its reduced perinuclear cytoplasm. Often in prepared microscopic specimens, the cell is highly distorted due to shrinkage and other artefacts resulting from decalcification of the bone matrix. In such instances, the

nucleus may be the only prominent feature. In well-preserved specimens, the osteocytes usually exhibit reduced cytoplasmic basophilia, but little additional cytoplasmic detail can be ascertained. By means of electron microscopy, variations in the functional state of the cell are recognized. Indeed, there is evidence that the osteocyte is able to modify the surrounding bone matrix through synthetic and reabsorptive activities. The quiescent osteocyte exhibits a paucity of rER and a markedly diminished Golgi complex (Fig. 8.8a). An osmiophilic lamina representing mature calcified matrix is seen

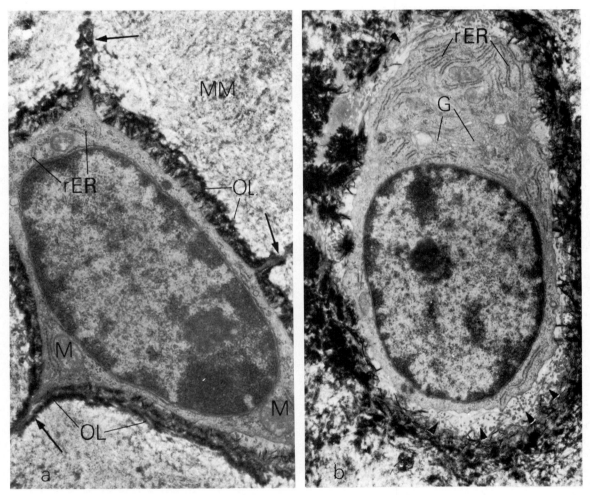

Figure 8.8. Electron micrographs of three osteocytes depicting different functional states. In (a) the osteocyte is relatively quiescent. It exhibits only a few profiles of rER and a few mitochondria (M). The cell virtually fills the lacunae that it occupies; the **arrows** indicate where cytoplasmic processes extend into canaliculi. Apatite crystals have been lost from the matrix, which is ordinarily mineralized (MM), but some apatite crystals fill the pericellular space. The apatite crystals obscure the other substances within the pericellular space. The dark band marking the boundary of the lacuna is the osmiophilic lamina (OL). The cell is (b) is a formative osteocyte. It shows larger amounts of rER and a large Golgi profile (G). Of equal importance is the presence of a small amount of osteoid in the pericellular space within the lacuna. The osteoid shows profiles of collagen fibrils (**arrowheads**) not yet mineralized. The lacuna of a formative osteocyte is not bounded by an osmiophilic lamina.

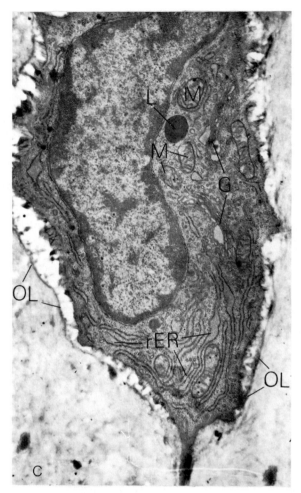

Figure 8.8(c). This cell is a resorptive osteocyte. It contains a substantial amount of rER, a large Golgi (G), mitochondria (M), and lysosomes (L). The pericellular space is devoid of collagen fibrils and may contain some flocculent material. The lacuna containing a resorptive osteocyte is bounded by an osmiophilic lamina (OL).

in close apposition to the cell membrane. In contrast, the formative osteocyte shows evidence of matrix deposition and exhibits certain characteristics similar to the osteoblast. Thus, the rER and Golgi are more abundant and there is evidence of osteoid in the pericellular space within the lacuna (Fig. 8.8b).

The resorptive osteocyte, like the formative osteocyte, contains numerous profiles of endoplasmic reticulum and a well-developed Golgi. Moreover, lysosomes are often observed (Fig. 8.8c). The concept that the resorptive osteocyte is removing matrix is supported by the observation that the pericellular space is devoid of collagen fibrils and may contain a flocculent material suggestive of a breakdown product. The more peripheral nonre-

sorbed matrix is bounded by an osmiophilic lamina, which presumably represents the boundary of the intact mature calcified matrix. It is believed by many investigators, though not all, that resorption of bone by this mechanism, a process designated as *osteocytic osteolysis,* with the concomitant release of calcium ions into the plasma allows for increase of blood calcium to maintain appropriate levels. The stimulus for the resorption of bone is parathyroid hormone.

Osteoclast

The *osteoclast* is a large multinucleated cell whose function is to resorb bone. When active, the osteoclast rests directly on the surface of the bone where resorption is to take place (Fig. 8.9). As a result of its activity, a shallow bay, called *Howship's lacuna* or *resorption bay,* is formed in the bone

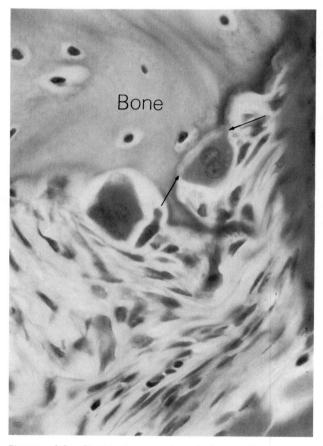

Figure 8.9. Photomicrograph of bone tissue where resorption is taking place. Two osteoclasts are evident. Note that each cell exhibits several nuclei. One of the osteoclasts is in close apposition to the bone and the site of ruffled border (**arrows**) can be seen. Also note the osteocytes in the bone tissue.

directly under the osteoclast. The cell is conspicuous not only because of its size, but also because of its marked eosinophilia. Using histochemical techniques, it also exhibits a strong reaction for acid phosphatase due to the numerous lysosomes that it contains.

The portion of the cell directly in contact with the bone can be divided into two parts: a central region containing numerous plasma membrane infoldings forming microvillous type structures, called the *ruffled border,* and a lesser ring-like perimeter of cytoplasm, the *clear zone,* which more or less demarcates the limits of the bone area being resorbed. The clear zone contains abundant microfilaments, but is essentially lacking in other organelles. The ruffled border stains less intensely than the remainder of the cell and often appears as a light band adjacent to the bone at the resorption site (Fig. 8.9). At the electron microscopic level, apatite crystals from the bone substance are observed between the processes of the ruffled border (see page 178). Beyond the ruffled border, but in close proximity, are numerous mitochondria and lysosomes. The nuclei are typically in the part of the cell more removed from the bone surface. In this same region are profiles of rER, multiple stacks of Golgi saccules, and many vesicles arising from the Golgi.

Some, if not most, of the vesicles are lysosomes, which appear to be released into the extracellular space at the bottom of the clefts between the cytoplasmic processes of the ruffled border. This is an example of lysosomal hydrolases functioning outside of the cell. Once liberated, the hydrolytic enzymes, which include collagenase, result in the extracellular digestion of the organic components of the bone matrix. However, before this event, or at least concomitantly, it is necessary to decalcify the bone matrix. Current evidence strongly suggests that decalcification, that is, the dissolution of the calcium salts, occurs through secretion of organic acids by the membranes of the ruffled border. Moreover, a low pH favors the action of acid hydrolyses. Accordingly, a local acidic environment is created in the extracellular space between the bone and the osteoclast. The clear zone adjacent to the ruffled border seems to create a seal against the bone, thus, creating a compartment at the site of the ruffled border where the focal decalcification and degradation of the matrix occurs. Support for this concept of acid secretion by the osteoclast comes, in part, from the finding that carbonic anhydrase, an enzyme associated with carbonic acid production, is present in the region of the ruffled border.

In addition to the ruffled border being the site of hydrolytic enzyme release and acid secretion, numerous coated pits and coated vesicles are also present at this site, thus, suggesting endocytic activity. It is not clear whether or not the osteoclast engages in the endocytic uptake of degraded matrix products or if other cells, such as the fibroblasts, are responsible. From a practical point, osteoclasts are generally observed at sites where bone remodeling is in progress. (The process or remodeling will be described shortly.) Thus, in sites where osteons are being altered or where a bone is undergoing change during the growth process, osteoclasts are relatively numerous and are easily found. As already noted, an increase in the parathyroid hormone level promotes bone resorption and has a demonstrable effect on osteoclast activity. In contrast, calcitonin has a counterbalancing effect, reducing osteoclast activity. Little is known, however, relative to the mechanism of bone remodeling and endocrine activity.

Lastly, in considering the osteoclast, it is important to recognize that these cells are unrelated to the bone-forming cells contrary to what was once thought. They arise from monocytes and acquire their multinucleate form either by repeated DNA replications and nuclear divisions without substance cell divisions, or by the fusion of many monocytes.

BONE FORMATION

Bone formation is a complex process that is sometimes difficult to understand if an adequate distinction is not made between development of the bone as an organ and histogenesis of bone tissue. The development of a bone is traditionally classified as *endochondral* or *intramembranous,* according to whether a cartilage model serves as the precursor of the bone (endochondral ossification) or whether the bone is formed by a simpler method, without the intervention of a cartilage precursor (intramembranous ossification). The bones of the extremities and those parts of the axial skeleton that bear weight (for example, vertebrae) develop by endochondral ossification. The flat bones of the skull and face, the mandible, and the clavicle develop by intramembranous ossification. The separate labels for types of bone or bone tissue should not be taken to mean existing bone is either membrane bone or endochondral bone. It is emphasized that these names refer only to the mechanism by which a bone is initially formed. Because of the rapid remodeling that occurs during bone development, the initial bone tissue that was laid down by endochondral formation or by intramembranous formation is quickly replaced. The replacement bone is established on the pre-existing bone by appositional growth and is identical in both cases. Although the long bone is classified as forming by endochondral formation, its development involves the histogenesis of endochondral bone and also the histogenesis of membrane bone, the latter occurring through the activity of the periosteal (membrane) tissue.

Intramembranous Ossification

This is the process whereby bone is formed through the differentiation of mesenchymal cells into osteoblasts. The first evidence of intramembranous ossification occurs around the eighth week of gestation in the human. The pale-staining elongate mesenchymal cells within the loose mesenchyme migrate and aggregate in specific areas, the sites where bone is destined to form. This condensation of cells within the mesenchymal tissue is the "membrane" referred to in the term intramembranous ossification. As the process continues, the newly organized tissue at the presumptive bone site becomes more vascularized and the aggregated

mesenchymal cells become larger and rounded. Moreover, the cytoplasm of the mesenchymal cells changes from eosinophilic to basophilic, and a clear Golgi area becomes evident. These cytological changes result in the differentiated osteoblast, which then secretes the collagen and proteoglycans of the bone matrix (osteoid). The osteoblasts within the bone matrix become increasingly separated from one another as the matrix is produced, but they remain attached by the thin cytoplasmic process (Fig. 8.10). Because of the abundant collagen content, the bone matrix appears more dense than the surrounding mesenchyme in which the intercellular spaces reveal only delicate connective tissue fibers.

The newly formed bone matrix appears in histological sections as small, irregularly shaped spicules. With time, the matrix becomes calcified and the interconnecting cytoplasmic processes of the bone-forming cells, now termed osteocytes, are contained within canaliculi. Concomitantly, the surrounding primitive cells in the "membrane" proliferate giving rise to a population of what may now be regarded as osteoprogenitor cells. Some of

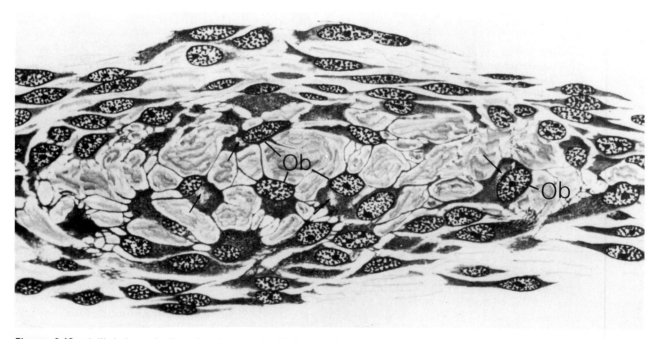

Figure 8.10. Initial stage in the development of intramembranous bone as seen in the skull of a cat embryo. The central area shows densely aggregated collagenous fibers (osteoid) that will become the bone matrix upon later calcification. The cells in the midst of this matrix are osteoblasts (Ob). They are relatively large cells that exhibit basophilic cytoplasm and a large Golgi area (**arrows**). The osteoblasts exhibit fine cytoplasmic processes that join with the processes of their neighbors. Peripheral to these cells are other more elongate cells that are in the process of differentiating into osteoblasts. At the very periphery are those cells that have much smaller elongate nuclei with very thin cytoplasmic processes extending from each end of the nucleus of the cell. They are the least differentiated cells and appear much like a fibroblast. The extracellular fibers in the vicinity of these cells are delicate and sparse. (Modified from a drawing by A. A. Maximow.)

the osteoprogenitor cells come into apposition with the initially formed spicules, transform into osteoblasts, and add more matrix. By this method (appositional growth), the spicules enlarge and become joined in a trabecular network having the general shape of the developing bone. Through continued mitotic activity, the osteoprogenitor cells maintain their numbers and, thus, provide a constant source of osteoblasts for growth of the bone spicules (osteoblasts are differentiated cells and do not divide). The new osteoblasts, in turn, lay down bone matrix in successive layers giving rise to woven bone. This immature bone, which has already been discussed (page 146), is characterized internally by interconnecting spaces occupied by connective tissue and blood vessels. Bone tissue formed by the method just described is sometimes referred to as *membrane bone* or *intramembranous bone.*

Endochondral Ossification

The process begins with the proliferation and aggregation of mesenchymal cells at the site of the future bone. The mesenchymal cells differentiate into chondroblasts that, in turn, produce cartilage matrix. The hyaline cartilage produced at this early stage acquires the general shape and appearance of the specific bone that will be formed. This "cartilage model," once established, grows by interstitial as well as appositional growth. Most of the increase in the length of the cartilage model can be attributed to interstitial growth occurring near the ends of the model. The increase in its width is largely by addition of cartilage matrix produced by new chondrocytes arising from the chondrogenic layer of perichondrium surrounding the cartilage mass. Illustrations 1 and 1a of Figure 8.11 show the very early cartilage model.

The first sign of ossification occurs with a change in activity of the perichondrium. The perichondrial cells no longer give rise to chondrocytes. Instead, bone-forming cells are produced. Thus, the connective tissue surrounding the cartilage model is no longer functionally a perichondrium, but instead, because of its altered role, it is now called periosteum. Moreover, we may now describe an osteogenic layer within the periosteum since the cells within this layer are differentiating into osteoblasts. As a result of these changes, a thin layer of bone is formed around the cartilage model. We may further describe this bone as periosteal bone because of its location or as intramembranous bone because of its method of development. In this case of a long bone, a distinctive cuff of periosteal bone is established around the cartilage model in what

can be described as the diaphyseal portion of the developing bone. This is shown in illustrations 2 and 2a of Figure 8.11.

With the establishment of the periosteral bone tissue, the chondrocytes in this mid-region of the cartilage model become hypertrophic. As these cells enlarge, their surrounding cartilage matrix becomes compressed forming thin irregular cartilage plates between the hypertrophic cells. The hypertrophic cells begin to synthesize alkaline phosphatase and, concomitantly, the cartilage matrix undergoes calcification. See illustrations 3 and 3a of Figure 8.8. (The calcification of the cartilage matrix is not to be confused with calcification that occurs in bone tissue.) The matrix, when calcified, inhibits diffusion of nutrients, ultimately causing the death of the chondrocytes. With the death of the chondrocytes, much of the matrix breaks down and neighboring lacunae become confluent producing an increasingly large cavity. While these events are occurring, one or several blood vessels grow through the thin, diaphyseal bony collar to vascularize the cavity (see illustrations 4 and 4a of Figure 8.11). As the blood vessels penetrate and grow into the cavity, other cells from the periosteum migrate along with the blood vessels. Some of these primitive cells become osteoprogenitor cells. Other primitive cells also gain access to the cavity via the new vasculature and give rise to the marrow. As the calcified cartilage breaks down and is partially removed, some remains as irregular spicules. When those osteoprogenitor cells come in apposition with the remnant-calcified cartilage spicules, they become osteoblasts and begin to lay down bone (osteoid) on the spicule framework. Thus, the bone formed in this manner is endochondral bone. The combination of the bone, which is initially only a thin layer, and the underlying calcified cartilage is described as a *mixed spicule.* Histologically, these mixed spicules can be recognized by virtue of their staining characteristics. Calcified cartilage tends to be basophilic while bone is distinctly eosinophilic. Such spicules persist for a short time before the calcified cartilage component is removed. The remaining bone component of the spicule may continue to grow by appositional growth, thus becoming larger and stronger, or it may undergo resorption as new spicules are being formed.

Growth of Endochondral Bone

The events described above represent the early stage of endochondral bone formation as seen in the fetus. The nature by which these bones develop requires the continued presence of carti-

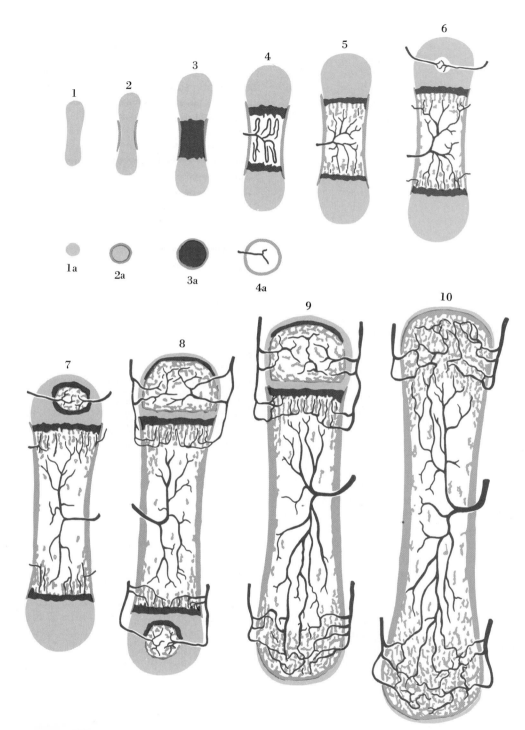

Figure 8.11. Schematic diagram of development of a long bone. Numbers **1** to **10** depict longitudinal sections; numbers **1a** to **4a** depict cross-sections through the shaft of the bone. The process begins with the formation of a cartilage model (**1** and **1a**); next, a periosteal (perichondrial) collar of bone forms about the diaphysis (shaft) of the cartilage model (**2** and **2a**); and then, the cartilaginous matrix in the diaphysis begins to calcify (**3** and **3a**). Blood vessels and perivascular connective tissue cells then erode and invade the calcified cartilage (**4** and **4a**), creating a primitive marrow cavity in which remnant spicules of calcified cartilage remain at the two ends of the cavity. Endochondral bone forms on these spicules of calcified cartilages. The bone at the ends of the developing

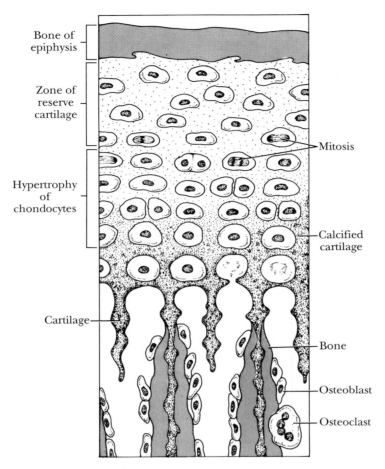

Bone of
epiphysis

Zone of
reserve
cartilage

Mitosis

Hypertrophy
of
chondocytes

Calcified
cartilage

Cartilage

Bone

Osteoblast

Osteoclast

Figure 8.12. A light micrograph showing the zonation in the epiphyseal cartilage of a growing long bone. The various zones of reserve cartilage (RC), the zone of proliferation (PC), the zone of hypertrophy (HC), the zone of calcified matrix (C), and finally, the zone of resorption, which is represented by eroded cartilage that is in direct contact with the connective tissue.

lage during the entire growth period: a process that extends throughout fetal life and continues for a period of more than a decade and a half, the growing period of the average individual into early adulthood. This continuing growth process will now be described. With time, as the diaphyseal marrow cavity enlarges (see illustration 5 of Fig. 8.11), a distinct zonation can be recognized in the cartilage at either end of the cavity.

The zonation of the cartilage, which is referred to as the epiphyseal cartilage, can be described as follows (Fig. 8.12). The epiphyseal cartilage in the region most distal to the diaphyseal center of ossification appears as typical hyaline cartilage. There is no suggestion of cellular proliferation or active matrix production. This area is referred to as the ***zone of reserve cartilage.*** Adjacent to this zone, in the direction of diaphysis, the carti-

marrow cavity constitutes the metaphysis. Periosteal bone continues to form; the periosteal bone is intramembranous bone. It can be recognized histologically because it is not accompanied by local cartilage eosin, nor is the bone deposited on spicules of calcified cartilage. In **6**, blood vessels and perivascular cells invade the upper epiphyseal cartilage, and a secondary center of ossification is established in the upper epiphysis (**7**). A similar epiphyseal ossification center forms at the lower end of the bone (**8**), and an epiphyseal disc, or plate, is thus formed between each epiphysis and the diaphysis. With continued growth of the long bone, the lower epiphyseal plate disappears (**9**), and finally with cessation of growth the upper epiphyseal plate disappears (**10**). The metaphysis then becomes continuous with the epiphysis. Epiphyseal "lines" remain where the epiphyseal plate last existed. (From Bloom W, Fawcett DW: *A Textbook of Histology, 10th ed. Philadelphia, WB Saunders, 1975.)*

lage cells undergo division and become organized into distinct columns. This is the *zone of proliferation.* The cartilage cells here are larger than those in the reserve zone and are actively producing matrix. Next is the *zone of hypertrophy.* The cartilage cells are greatly enlarged; their cytoplasm is clear, a reflection of the glycogen that they accumulate, and the matrix is compressed into linear bands between the columns of hypertrophied cartilage cells. In the next zone, the cartilage cells begin to degenerate and the matrix becomes calcified. Thus, it is referred to as the *zone of calcified matrix.* The last zone of the *zone of resorption.* The cartilage here is in direct contact with the connective tissue of the marrow cavity. Small blood vessels and connective tissue invade the site occupied by the dying chondrocytes as a series of spearheads leaving the calcified cartilage as longitudinal spicules, at least as seen in a longitudinal section of the bone. Actually the cartilage would appear as a honeycomb in a cross-section of the bone since the invasion of the vessels and accompanying connective tissue migrates into the sites previously occupied by the cartilage cells. Bone deposition then occurs on the cartilage matrix spicules in the same manner as described for the formation of the initial ossification center. As the bone is laid down in the calcified spicules, the cartilage is resorbed ultimately leaving a primary spongy bone. This spongy bone undergoes reorganization through osteoclastic activity and addition of new bone tissue, thus accommodating to the continued growth and physical stresses placed on the bone.

Shortly after birth, a secondary ossification center develops in the upper epiphysis. The cartilage cells hypertrophy and degenerate. As in the diaphysis, calcification of the matrix occurs and blood vessel and osteogenic cells from the perichondrium invade the region, creating a new marrow cavity (see illustrations 6 and 7 of Fig. 8.11). Later, a similar epiphyseal ossification center forms at the lower end of the bone (see illustration 8 of Fig. 8.11). This too is regarded as a secondary center though it develops later. With the development of the secondary ossification centers, the only cartilage that remains from the original model is the articular cartilage at the ends of the bone and a transverse disc, known as the *epiphyseal plate,* which separates the epiphyseal and diaphyseal cavities. The cartilage of the epiphyseal plate is responsible for maintaining the growth process; its proliferative zone giving rise to the cartilage upon which bone is later laid down. The thickness of the plate remains rather constant. Thus, the amount of new cartilage produced (zone of proliferation)

equals the amount resorbed (zone of resorption). The resorbed cartilage is, of course, substituted by spongy bone.

In reviewing the growth process, it is important to realize that the actual lengthening of the bone occurs when new cartilage matrix is produced. This has the effect of pushing the epiphysis away from the diaphysis, thus, the elongation of the bone. The events that follow simply involve the mechanism by which the newly formed cartilage is ultimately substituted by bone tissue during the developmental process.

It should be noted that external remodeling of the bone occurs as it grows in length and, at the same time, retains its overall shape. The external remodeling consists in preferential resorption of bone in some areas and deposition of bone in other areas, as outlined in Figure 8.13. The histological features of intramembranous and endochondral bone formation are considered in the Atlas Section, Plates 19–23.

Cessation of Growth

When the individual achieves maximal growth, proliferation of new cartilage within the growing bones terminates. The cartilage that has already been produced continues to undergo the changes that lead to the deposition of new bone and, finally, there is no remaining cartilage. At this point, the epiphyseal and diaphyseal marrow cavities become confluent. The elimination of the epiphyseal plate is referred to as epiphyseal closure. Illustration 9 of Figure 8.11 shows the lower epiphyseal cartilage no longer present and lastly, in illustration 10, both epiphyseal cartilages are gone. Growth is now complete and the only remaining cartilage is found on the articular surfaces of the bone. Vestigial evidence of the site of the epiphyseal plate is reflected by an "epiphyseal line," comprised of bone tissue.

Development of the Haversian System

Haversian systems develop in compact bone. The compact bone might have formed from "fetal" spongy bone (for example, by the compaction[2] of primary spongy bone), it might have been deposited directly as adult compact bone (for example,

---

[2] Spongy bone can be converted into compact bone by the continued deposition of bone onto the surface of spongy bone spicules. As the spicules increase in size, the marrow space decreases. The process continues until the spicules have been converted into a large mineralized mass with little intervening soft (marrow) tissue. It is then compact bone.

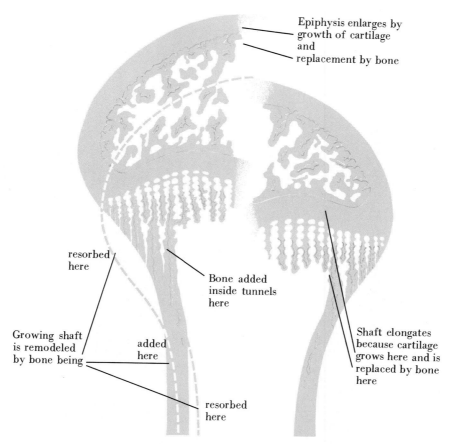

Epiphysis enlarges by growth of cartilage and replacement by bone

resorbed here

Bone added inside tunnels here

Growing shaft is remodeled by bone being

added here

Shaft elongates because cartilage grows here and is replaced by bone here

resorbed here

Figure 8.13. Diagram of external remodeling of a long bone, showing two periods during the growth of the bone. The younger bone profile is shown on the right, the older on the left. Superimposed on the left side of the figure is the shape of the bone (left half only) as it appeared at the earlier time. The bone is now longer, but it has retained its general shape. In order to grow in length and retain the general shape of the particular bone, bone resorption occurs on some surfaces and bone deposition occurs on other surfaces as indicated in the diagram. (Based on Ham AW: *J Bone Joint Surg* 34A:701, 1952.)

the circumferential lamellae of an adult bone), or it might be older compact bone consisting of Haversian systems and interstitial lamellae. In any event, a tunnel is bored through the compact bone by osteoclasts. As the tunnel is formed, bone deposition on its walls begins almost immediately. The two aspects of cellular activity are organized as a ***bone remodeling*** unit (Fig. 8.14).

There are two distinct parts to the bone remodeling unit: an advancing ***cutting cone*** (also called a ***resorption canal***) and a ***closing cone.*** The cutting cone consists of active osteoclasts followed by an advancing capillary loop and pericytes. It also contains numerous cells in mitosis. These presumably give rise to osteoblasts, additional pericytes, and endothelial cells. (It should be recalled that the osteoclasts derive from blood-borne mono-

cytes.) The osteoclasts cut a canal about 200 μm in diameter. This canal establishes the diameter of the future Haversian system. The cutting cone constitutes only a small fraction of the bone remodeling unit, and thus, it is seen much less frequently than the closing cone of the developing Haversian system. After the diameter of the future Haversian system is established, osteoblasts begin to deposit the organic matrix (osteoid) of bone on the walls of the canal in successive lamellae. With time, the bone matrix in each of the lamellae becomes mineralized. As the successive lamellae of bone are deposited, from the periphery inward, the canal ultimately attains the relatively narrow diameter of the adult Haversian canal. This process in which new Haversian systems are formed is referred to as ***internal remodeling.***

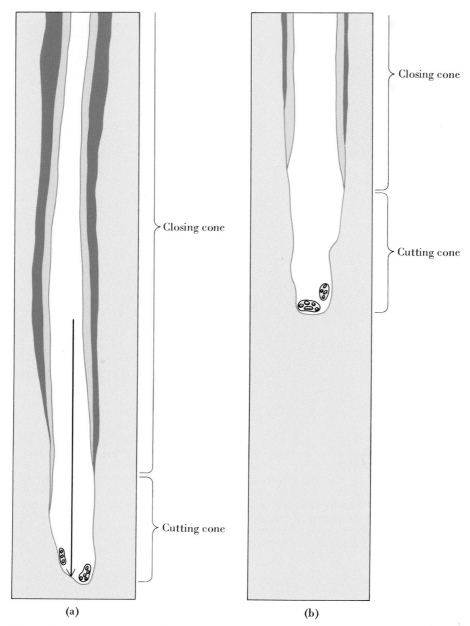

Figure 8.14. Diagram of the formation of a Haversian system based on a longitudinal section of the radius of an adult dog. A tunnel is being bored downward by the action of osteoclasts at the blind end—the cutting cone—of the tunnel (**a**). Osteogenesis follows in the wake of the bone destruction, thereby narrowing the diameter of the tunnel with the addition of new bone lamellae. Ultimately, the tunnel becomes the Haversian canal. The brown bands represent new bone; the pink bands internal to the bone represent osteoid. Osteoblasts (not shown) line the surface of the osteoid. Together the osteoblasts and adjacent osteoid serve to identify the closing cone. Seventeen days before sacrifice, the dog received an injection of tetracycline, which binds to sites of mineralization. Examination of the section with an ultraviolet light source at a later time enables one to visualize the tetracycline and draw what the histologic picture would have been on the day of injection (**b**). Thus, at a glance, it is possible to assess the length of the tunnel [**arrow** in (**a**)] that was bored during a 17-day period. (After P. Lacroix, 1976.)

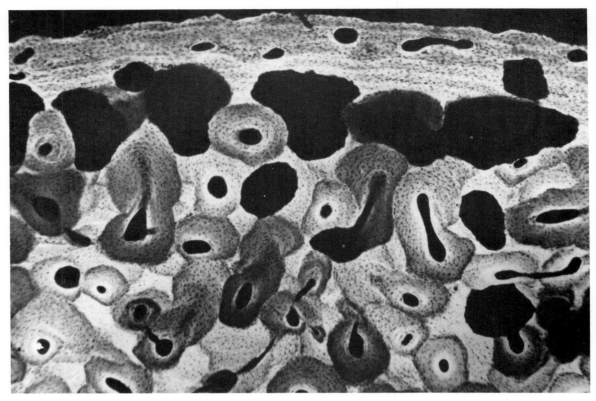

Figure 8.15. Microradiographs of a 200-μm thick cross-section of bone from a normal 19-year-old male. Secondary Haversian bone is actively replacing non-Haversian bone, which is seen on the periosteal (upper) surface. The degree of mineralization is reflected by the shade of light and dark in the microradiograph. Thus, very light areas represent the highly mineralized tissue, which deflect the x-rays and prevent them from striking the photographic film. Conversely, dark areas contain less mineral and, thus, are less effective in deflection of the x-rays. Note how the interstitial areas (the older bone) are very light, whereas some of the Haversian systems are very dark (these are the most newly formed). The Haversian canals appear black since they represent only soft tissue. ×57. (Courtesy of Dr. J. Jowsey.)

Compact adult bone contains Haversian systems of varying age and usually, according to the age of the individual, some resorption tunnels. If a ground section of bone is examined microradiographically, it can be seen that younger Haversian systems are less completely mineralized than older systems (Fig. 8.15). They undergo a progressive secondary mineralization which continues (up to a point) even after the Haversian system has been fully formed. Figure 8.15 also illustrates the dynamic internal remodeling of compact bone. In the adult, deposition balances resorption. In the aged, resorption often exceeds deposition. If this imbalance becomes excessive, a condition known as osteoporosis develops (see below).

BIOLOGICAL MINERALIZATION AND MATRIX VESICLES

Biological mineralization is an extracellular event. It occurs in the extracellular matrices of bone, cartilage, and the dentin, cementum and enamel of teeth. All of these, except enamel, contain collagen fibrils and ground substance within the matrix, and mineralization occurs both within the collagen fibrils and external to the collagen fibrils, presumably with the ground substance. (Enamel mineralization occurs within the extracellular organic matrix secreted by the enamel organ). Despite the extracellular location of biological mineralization and the fact that physiochemical factors are operational, nevertheless biological mineralization is a cell-regulated event.

In places where mineralization of immature bone, cartilage, dentin, and cementum is initiated, small vesicles, called *matrix vesicles,* are seen in the matrix. These vesicles are typically located at some distance from the cells where mineralization is to occur. The vesicles measure about 100 nm in diameter; they are formed by a pinching off of plasma membrane from the cells producing the mineralized tissue (osteoblasts, chondrocytes, odonto-

NUTRITIONAL AND HORMONAL FACTORS IN BONE FORMATION

Both nutritional and hormonal factors affect the degree of bone mineralization. It has been known for a long time that calcium deficiency during growth causes *rickets,* a condition in which the bone matrix does not calcify normally. Rickets may be due to insufficient amounts of dietary calcium or to insufficient vitamin D (a steroid prohormone), which is needed for absorption of calcium by the intestines. In the adult, the same nutritional or vitamin deficiency leads to *osteomalacia.*

Although rickets and osteomalacia are no longer major problems where nutrition is adequate, another form of insufficient bone mineral is regularly seen in the condition known as *osteoporosis.* As already noted, in this condition bone tissue (both mineral and matrix) is diminished, presumably because resorption by osteoclasts exceeds deposition by osteoblasts. Osteoporosis develops as a consequence of immobilization (as in a bedridden patient) and in postmenopausal women. The factors that bring on the imbalance in cellular activity are not known, although some re-lief appears to result from maintaining hormonal (estrogen) levels and dietary fluoride levels.

In addition to its influence on intestinal absorption of calcium, vitamin D is also needed for normal calcification. Other vitamins known for a long time to affect bone are A and C. Vitamin A deficiency results in a suppression of endochondral growth of bone: vitamin A excess leads to fragility and subsequent fractures of long bones. Vitamin C is essential for synthesis of collagen and its deficiency leads to scurvy. The matrix produced in scurvy is not calcifiable.

Several hormones affect bone directly. Parathyroid hormone increases the number of osteoclasts and osteoclastic activity, thereby promoting bone resorption. Calcitonin enhances deposition of calcium. Pituitary growth hormone stimulates growth in general and especially growth of epiphyseal cartilage and bone. Oversecretion of growth hormone during childhood leads to giantism and abnormal increase in the length of bones; oversecretion in adults leads to acromegaly, an abnormal thickening of the bones.

blasts, and so on). The matrix vesicles contain alkaline phosphatase and other enzymes that are considered to load the membrane of the vesicle and then the vesicle itself with calcium (and phosphate?). In turn, the loaded matrix vesicle ruptures and presumably effects an increase in local concentration of mineral sufficient to initiate mineralization. Matrix vesicles have not been seen where adult bone forms or in enamel formation.

ATLAS PLATES

16–24

PLATE 16. Bone, Ground Section

Blood vessels reach the Haversian canals from the marrow through other tunnels called Volksmann's canals. In some instances, Volkmann's canals travel from one Haversian canal to another, as shown in the **lower right** of **Figure 1** where a Volksmann's canal **(VC)** is communicating between two Haversian canals. Volksmann's canals can be distinguished from Haversian canals in that they pass through lamellae, whereas Haversian canals are surrounded by concentric rings of lamellae.

Figure 2 shows a higher power of the labeled osteon from the **upper left** of **Figure 1**. It includes some of the circumferential lamellae **(CL)** that are now seen at the bottom of the micrograph (the micrograph has been reoriented). Note the lacunae **(L)** and also the fine thread-like profiles emanating from the lacunae. These thread-like profiles represent the canaliculi, spaces within the bone matrix that contained cytoplasmic processes of the osteocyte. The canaliculi by their communication with canaliculi of neighboring lacunae form a three-dimensional channel system throughout the bone.

Figure 3 provides a still higher magnification of the circumferential lamellae. These lamellae are found around the shaft of the long bone at the outer as well as the inner surface of the bone. (The osteoblasts that contribute to the formation of circumferential lamellae at these sites come from the periosteum and endosteum, respectively, whereas the osteons are constructed from osteoblasts in the canal of the developing Haversian system.) **Figure 3** reveals to advantage not only the canaliculi, but also the lamellae of the bone. The latter are just barely defined by the faint lines **(arrows)** that extend across the micrograph. Collagenous fibers in neighboring lamellae are oriented in different directions. This change in orientation accounts for the faint line or interface between adjacent lamellae.

The micrographs shown on the accompanying plate show lamellar bone. They were obtained from a ground bone section.[3] Specimens prepared

---

[3] Ground sections are prepared by removing as much soft tissue and organic matter from the bone as possible and allowing the bone to dry. Thin slices of bone are then cut with a saw. The slices are ground to adequate thinness to be viewed through the microscope. The specimen may be treated with India ink to define the spaces that were formerly occupied by organic matter, for example, cells and other soft tissue components. A simpler method involves mounting the ground specimen on the slide with a viscous balsam medium that keeps air imprisoned in the spaces. The result is similar to that seen in a good India ink preparation. In the accompanying specimen prepared by this method some of the Haversian canals and the Volkmann's canal are filled with the mounting medium making them translucent instead of black.

KEY	
CL, circumferential lamellae	**arrow**, lamellar boundary
	L, lacuna
HC, Haversian canal	O, osteon
IL, interstitial lamellae	VC, Volkmann's canal

Fig. 1, × 80	Fig. 3, × 400, human.
Fig. 2, × 300	

in this manner are of value chiefly to display the architecture of compact bone.

Figure 1 reveals a cross-sectioned area of a long bone at low power and includes the outer or peripheral aspect of the bone, which can be identified by the presence of circumferential lamellae **(CL)**. (The exterior or periosteal surface of the bone is not included in the micrograph.) To the right of the circumferential lamellae are the osteons **(O)** or Haversian systems that appear as circular profiles. Between the osteons are interstitial lamellae **(IL)**, the remnants of previously existing osteons.[4]

Osteons are essentially cylindrical structures. In the shaft of a long bone, the long axes of the osteons are oriented parallel to the long axis of the bone. Thus, a cross-section through the shaft of a long bone would reveal the osteons in cross-sections, as in **Figure 1**. At the center of each osteon is a Haversian canal **(H)**, which contains blood vessels, connective tissue, and cells lining the surface of the bone material. Because the organic material is not retained in ground sections, the Haversian canals and other spaces will appear black if filled with India ink, or air, depending on the method used. Concentric layers of mineralized substance, the concentric lamellae, surround the Haversian canal and appear much the same as growth rings of a tree. The canal is also surrounded by concentric arrangements of lacunae. These appear as the small, dark, elongate structures.

---

[4] During the period of bone growth and during the adult life, there is constant internal remodeling of bone. This involves the destruction of osteons and formation of new ones. However, the breakdown of an osteon is usually not complete; part of the osteon may remain intact. Moreover, portions of adjacent osteons may also be partially destroyed. The space created by the breakdown process is reoccupied by a new osteon. The remnants of the previously existing osteons become the interstitial lamellae.

PLATE 16

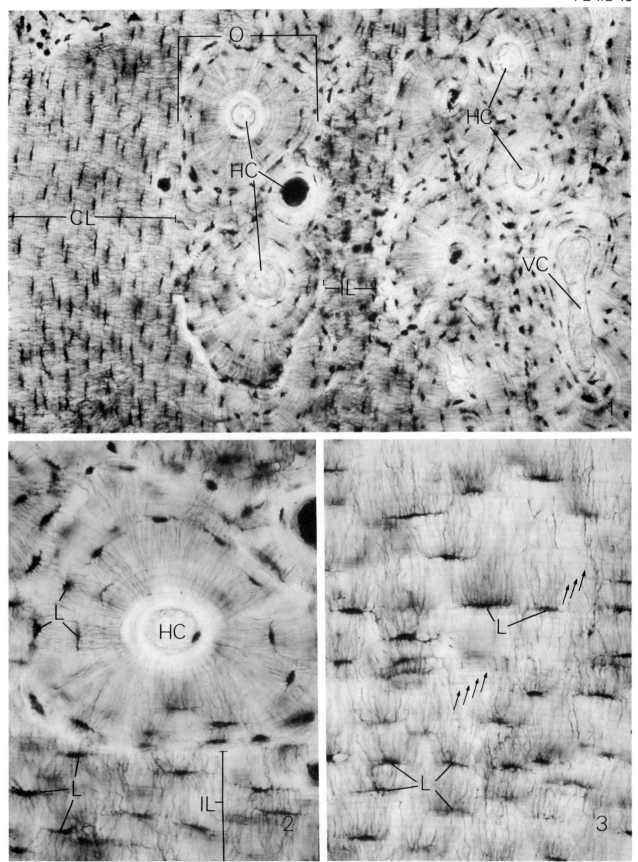

PLATE 17. Cortical Bone, Electron Microscopy

This electron micrograph shows, at low magnification, an osteon from the femur of a young rabbit. The bone was decalcified leaving the cells and extracellular soft tissue components (collagen) essentially intact. The particular osteon illustrated here consists of three complete lamellae, numbered **1** to **3** and, immediately surrounding the Haversian canal **(HC),** a fourth lamella that is incomplete **(asterisks).** The outer limit of the osteon is marked by a cement line **(CL),** and beyond this is an interstitial lamella **(IL).**

The most apparent structures in the Haversian canal are the blood vessels. Both are capillaries **(Cap).** The smaller vessel is surrounded by pericytes, whereas the larger one does not possess this additional cellular investment. It should be noted that the closely packed preosteoblasts around the capillaries can be mistaken easily for smooth muscle cells of larger blood vessels with the light microscope. However, the electron microscope shows that veins and arteries are not present in Haversian canals, but rather there are two types of capillaries. The cells within the Haversian canal (other than those associated with the capillaries) are either osteoblasts or preosteoblasts. The osteoblasts **(Ob)** line the Haversian canal. The remainder of the cells are regarded as preosteoblasts **(POb).** They are less differentiated cells, but are in the process of transforming into osteoblasts in order to replace those that will become incorporated into the bone matrix that they produce. In examining the osteo-

blasts, it should be noted that one of them exhibits a process extending into a canaliculus **(double arrow)** of the incomplete lamella. Similarly, the osteocyte **(Oc)** in the lower portion of the figure also shows cytoplasmic processes entering canaliculi **(arrows).**

The canaliculi **(C)** within the lamellae, and those extending across the lamellae appear less numerous than the number in a light micrograph (see Plate 16). The difference is a reflection of the thickness of the section, more canaliculi being included in the relatively thick light microscope section than in the thin section utilized in electron microscopy.

KEY

Cap, capillary	**Oc,** osteocyte
C, canaliculus	**POb,** preosteoblast
CL, cement line (of Ebner)	**double arrow,** osteoblast process in canaliculus
IL, interstitial lamella	**arrow,** osteocyte process in canaliculus
HC, Haversian canal	
L, lacuna	**1, 2, 3,** lamellae
Ob, osteoblast	

Fig. × 3,000 (Electron micrograph, courtesy of S. C. Luk, C. Nopajaroonsri, and G. T. Simon, *J Ultrastruct Res* 46:184, 1974.)

PLATE 17

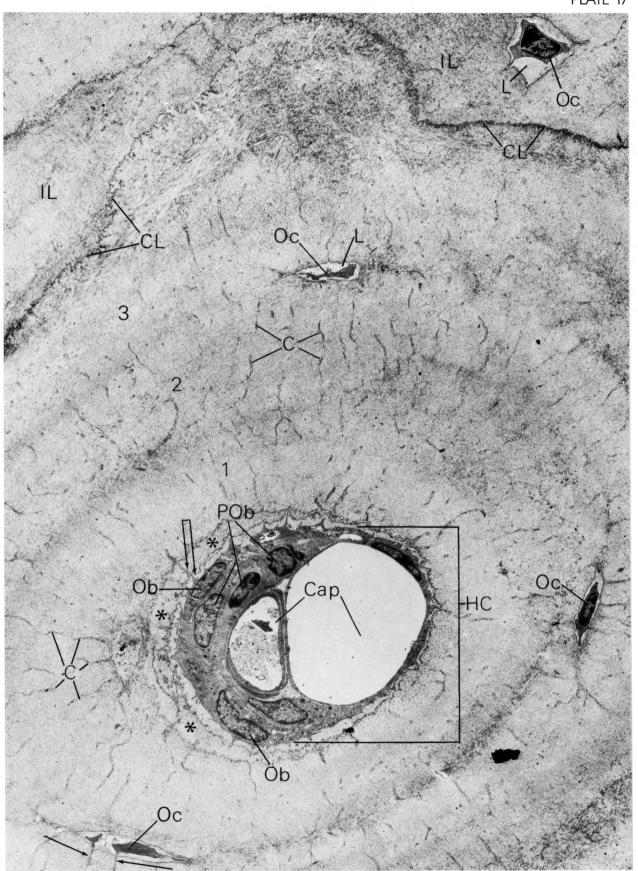

PLATE 18. Spongy and Compact Bone

The second method for viewing bone with the light microscope is the examination of demineralized tissue sections. (Ground sections were considered in Atlas section, Plate 16.) This procedure involves steps that are essentially similar to those employed for the routine preparations of histological sections, except that after fixation the tissue is placed in a demineralizing solution (acid or chelating agent). Once the mineral has been removed, the tissue is treated just as any other tissue sample (as described in Chapter 1). The demineralized section retains all of the formed soft tissue components that are normally seen in an H&E section.

Figure 1 shows a demineralized section of two bones forming a joint cavity. Articular cartilage **(AC)** covers bare surfaces in contact with the neighboring bone. The free surface of each cartilage presents a relatively smooth contour, whereas the junction between the cartilage and the bone **(SB)** is more irregular.

The articular cartilage is hyaline **(upper inset).** It shows the characteristic features of hyaline cartilage as outlined in Atlas section, Plate 11, namely, chondrocytes in lacunae, a homogeneous avascular matrix (homogeneous in that it presents no formed elements visible with the light microscope), and variable staining of the matrix. At least some of the cartilage cells are in lacunae that are close to each other, suggesting that they are daughter cells from the same parent cell.

The bone under the articular cartilage is spongy bone. It consists of spicules or trabeculae of bone tissue as well as marrow spaces **(M).** In this sample, the marrow consists primarily of adipose tissue. In addition to the marrow spaces, the bone tissue also contains space, or tunnels, for blood vessels **(BV);** in this respect, bone differs fundamentally from the hyaline cartilage on the articular surface, which is avascular. The essential features of the bone tissue are seen at higher magnification in the **upper circular inset.** These are: osteocytes **(Oc)** in lacunae; an eosinophilic matrix; and blood vessels **(BV).** The spongy bone depicted in Figure 1 is nonlamellar, that is, the matrix is not organized as lamellae, but rather the collagen fibers are in the form of interwoven bundles. Certain features of woven nonlamellar bone are also displayed in the **inset,** namely, the cells are unevenly and randomly dispersed and they are not arranged in an oriented pattern around the blood vessels. For purposes of

KEY

AC, articular cartilage   M, marrow
BV, blood vessel   Oc, osteocyte
CB, compact bone   Po, periosteum
Eo, endosteum   SB, spongy bone

Fig. 1, × 80   Fig. 2, × 80 (upper inset, × 175; lower inset, × 350).

comparison, note how the lacunae (and, therefore, also the osteocytes) display an oriented pattern about the Haversian canal in **Figure 2** of Atlas section, Plate 16.

The shaft of a long bone is shown in **Figure 2.** The center of the bone consists of a large marrow cavity **(M)** filled chiefly with adipose tissue; surrounding the marrow cavity is the bone tissue of the shaft. It is compact bone **(CB).** Although the compact bone tissue contains tunnels for blood vessels **(BV),** it does not contain marrow spaces. On its outer surface, the bone tissue is covered by a periosteum **(Po)** and its inner surface is covered by endosteum **(Eo, lower inset).** The endosteum consists of several layers of cells (nuclei of these cells are clearly evident) and collagenous fibers. The endosteal cells have the potential to develop into osteoblasts (as do periosteal cells) if the need should arise, for example, in fracture repair.

Histologically, the compact bone shown in **Figure 2** displays three characteristics: an eosinophilic matrix; lacunae in which osteocytes are located; and vascular tunnels **(BV).** The osteocytes **(Oc)** are identified chiefly by virtue of their nuclear staining that stands out in contrast to the surrounding eosinophilic matrix. The boundaries of the lacunae and the canaliculi radiating from them (see Atlas section, Plate 16) are not evident.

In the adult human, compact bone is organized chiefly as Haversian systems or as other forms of lamellar bone. While this form of bone tissue is readily evident in well-oriented ground sections, it is not always easy to identify in decalcified sections. It is particularly difficult to make this identification in longitudinal decalcified sections of a long bone as shown in **Figure 2.**

PLATE 18

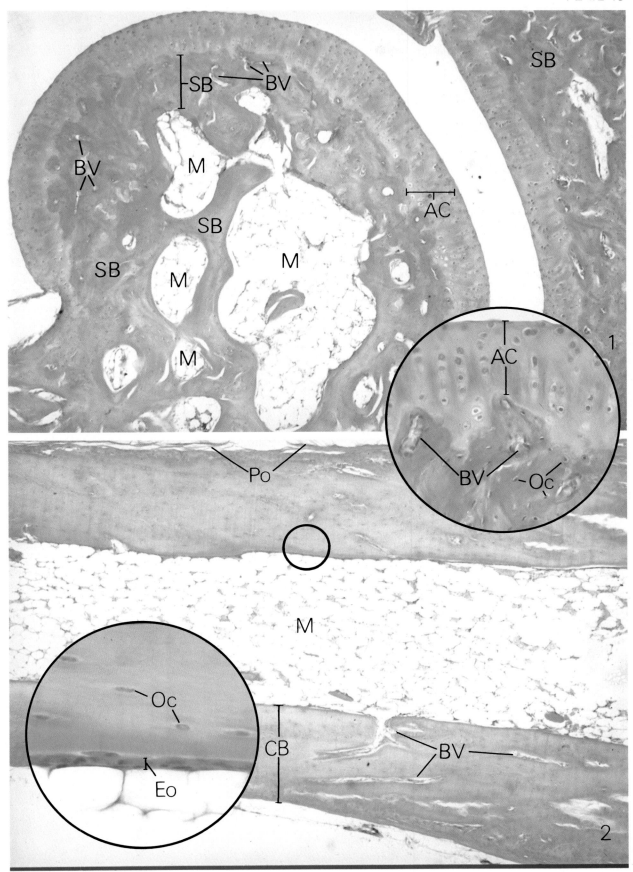

PLATE 19. Endochondral Bone Formation I

Endochondral bone formation involves a cartilage precursor, which serves as a fetal skeleton, and the simultaneous removal of the cartilage and its replacement with bone tissue. In addition, as a bone grows, some of the bone tissue is removed while newer bone tissue is being laid down, a process called remodeling.[5] Two specialized cell types have been identified with the process of bone growth and remodeling. The osteoblast is engaged in the formation of bone. Although the removal of bone is not as well understood, it has been established that multinucleated cells, called osteoclasts, are engaged in the removal of bone. (Osteocytes can alter and resorb bone in their immediate vicinity. The process is called osteocytic osteolysis; its role in bone remodeling, if any, is not clear.)

The early steps of endochondral bone formation are evident in **Figure 1.** The structure seen here is the cartilage model of the bone about to be formed. The steps of bone formation are as follows. (1) The cartilage cells in the center of the cartilage model become hypertrophic (**HC**). (2) The matrix of the cartilage becomes calcified (**CM**). (The calcified matrix stains with hematoxylin and appears as the darker condensed matrix material between the enlarged cartilage cells.) (3) A collar of bone forms around the circumference of the center of the cartilage model. This bone is called *periosteal bone* (**PB**) because the osteoblasts that have produced the bone material develop from the periosteum. (It should be noted that the periosteal bone is, in fact, intramembranous bone because it develops within the connective tissue membrane that immediately surrounds the developing bone and not on a spicule of calcified cartilage.)

The bone in **Figure 2** shows later events and a continuation of the earlier ones just described. A vascular bud (not shown) and accompanying perivascular cells from the periosteum have invaded the shaft of the cartilage model and brought about its dissolution, thereby forming a cavity (**Cav**). Examination at higher power would reveal that the cavity contains fat cells, developing blood cells, and other connective tissue elements. While the new steps occurs, the earlier steps continue. (1) The

---

[5] Remodeling which alters the shape of the bone is called *external remodeling;* that which does not alter the shape of the bone, as in the formation of Haversian systems, is called *internal remodeling.*

cartilage cells proliferate at the epiphyses (**C**), thereby increasing the length of the developing bones. (2) The periosteal bone (**PB**) continues to form. (3) The cartilage cells facing the cavity become hypertrophic. (4) The cartilage matrix becomes calcified. (5) Erosion of cartilage occurs creating spicules of cartilage. (6) Bone forms on the spicules of the calcified cartilage at the erosion front; this bone is *endochondral bone* (**EB**).

As these processes continue, one end of the cartilage model (the epiphysis) is invaded by blood vessels and connective tissue from the periosteum (periosteal bud), and it undergoes the same changes that occurred in the shaft except that no periosteal bone forms. This same process then occurs at the other end of the bone. Consequently, at each end of the developing long bone, a cartilaginous plate (epiphyseal plate) is created that lies between two sites of bone formation. **Figure 3** shows an early stage after the invasion of the epiphysis. A secondary ossification center (**OS°**) has formed and, along with this event, the head of the long bone will develop a cavity similar in its content to that of the diaphysis. The cartilage separating the two cavities is the epiphyseal plate (**EP**). At the early stage shown in **Figure 3,** the plate is not well defined. Despite the enlargement of the epiphyseal cavity, the remaining cartilage between the two cavities persists as a disc or plate until growth ceases. The **inset** shows come calcified cartilage (**CC**) as well as the early deposition of endochondral bone (**EB**) within the secondary ossification center.

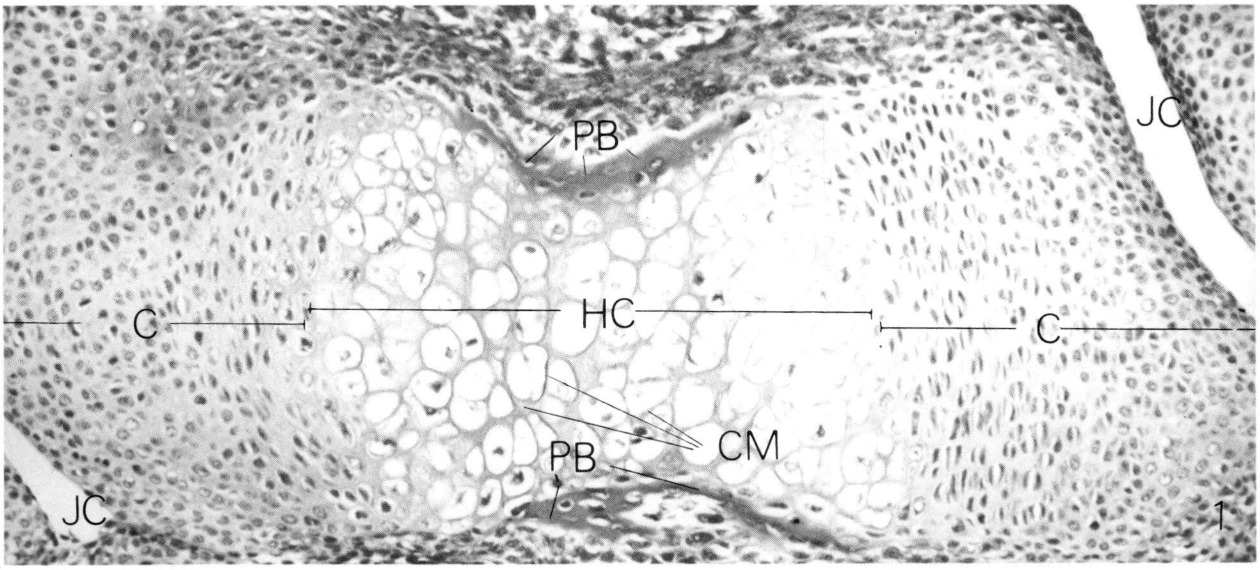
PB
JC
C
HC
C
CM
PB
JC
1

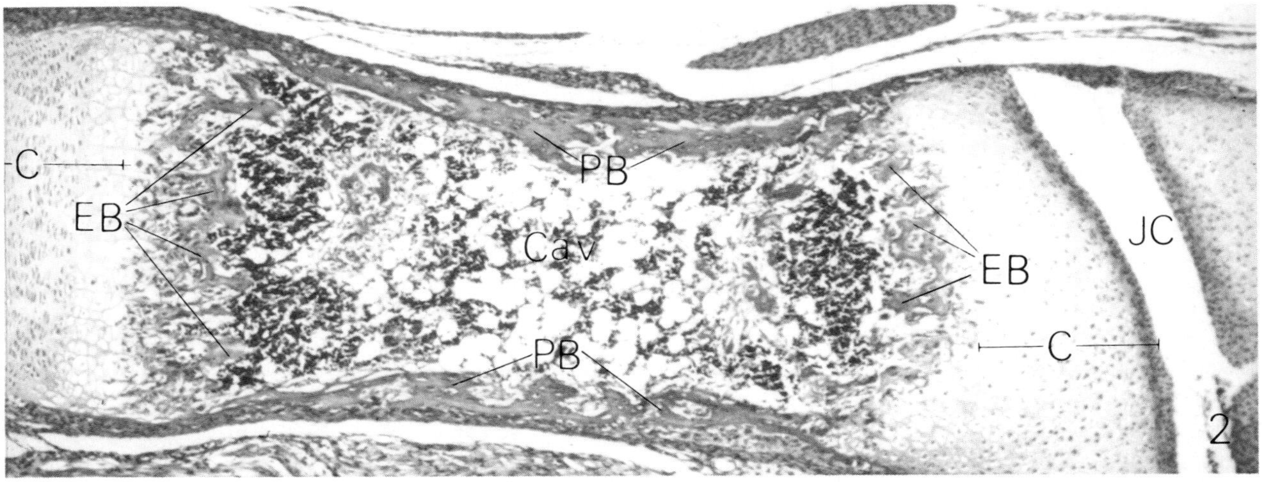
C
PB
EB
Cav
JC
EB
PB
C
2

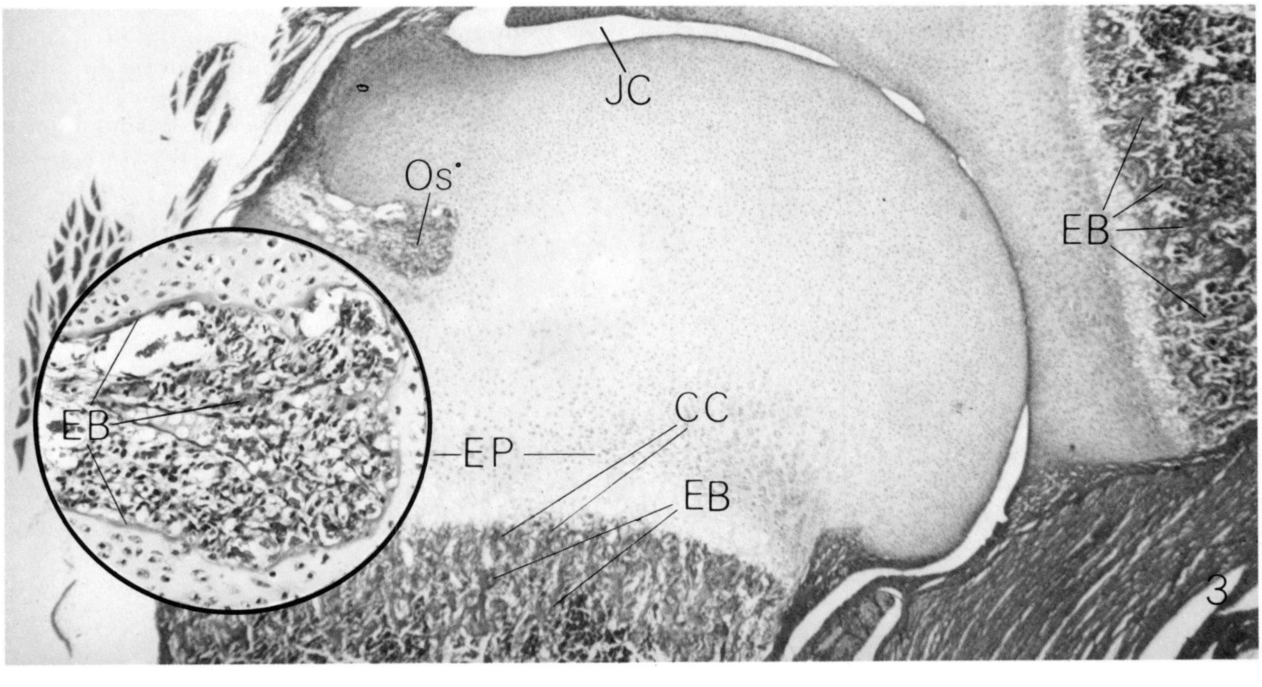
JC
Os
EB
EB
CC
EP
EB
3

PLATE 20. Endochondral Bone Formation II

A magnification of an epiphysis higher than that seen in **Figure 3** of the preceding plate is shown as **Figure 1.** Different zones of the cartilage of the epiphyseal plate reflect the progressive changes that occur in active growth of endochondral bone. These zones are not sharply delineated and the boundaries between them are somewhat arbitrary. They lead toward the marrow cavity (**M**), so that the first zone is furthest from the cavity. The zones are: *(1) The zone of reserve cartilage* (**RC**): The first zone is furthest from the cavity. The cartilage cells of this zone have not yet begun to participate in the growth of the bone; they are reserve cells. These cells are small, usually only one to a lacuna, and not grouped. At some time, some of these cells will proliferate and undergo the changes outlined for the next zone. *(2) Zone of proliferating cartilage* (**PC**): The cells of this zone are increasing in number; they are slightly larger than the reserve cells and close to their neighbors; they begin to form rows. *(3) Zone of hypertrophic cartilage* (**HC**): The cells of this zone are aligned in rows and are significantly larger than the cells in the preceding zone. *(4) Zone of calcified matrix* (**C**): In this zone the cartilage matrix is impregnated with calcium salts. *(5) Zone of resorption:* This zone is represented by eroded cartilage that is in direct contact with the connective tissue. Spicules (actually a honeycomb at the level of the advancing blood vessels) of cartilage are formed because the pericapillary cells invade and resorb in spearheads rather than along a straight front. Specifically, the pericapillary cells break into the rows of hypertrophied chondrocytes temporarily leaving the calcified cartilage between the rows of cells. In this manner, spicules of calcified cartilage are formed. Bone deposition (**EB**) then occurs on the surfaces of these calcified cartilage spicules.

Figure 2 is a higher power of the lower middle area of **Figure 1.** It shows calcified cartilage spi-

cules on which bone has been deposited. In the lower portion of **Figure 2,** the spicules have already grown to create anastomosing bone trabeculae. These initial trabeculae still contain remnants of calcified cartilage as evidenced by the pale blue color of the cartilage matrix (compared to the red staining of the bone). Osteoblasts (**Ob**) are aligned on the surface of the spicules where bone formation is active.

The **upper inset** shows the surface of several spicules from the **left circle** in **Figure 2** at higher magnification. Note the osteoblasts (**Ob**), some of which are just beginning to produce bone in apposition to the calcified cartilage (**C**). The **lower right of the inset** shows bone (**EB**) with an osteocyte (**Oc**) already embedded in the bone matrix.

The **lower inset,** representing the **circled area on the right** in **Figure 2,** reveals several osteoclasts (**Ocl**). They are in apposition to the spicule, which is mostly cartilage. A small amount of bone is evident based on the red-staining material in this inset. Note the light area (**arrow**) representing the ruffled border of the osteoclast. Examination of **Figure 2** reveals a number of other osteoclasts (**Ocl**).

KEY

C, calcified cartilage matrix	Ocl, osteoclast
EB, endochondral bone	Oc, osteocyte
HC, hypertrophic cartilage	PC, proliferating cartilage
M, marrow	RC, reserve cartilage
Ob, osteoblast	arrow, ruffled border of osteoclast

Fig. 1, human, × 80	**Fig. 2,** human, × 150 (insets, × 380).

PLATE 20

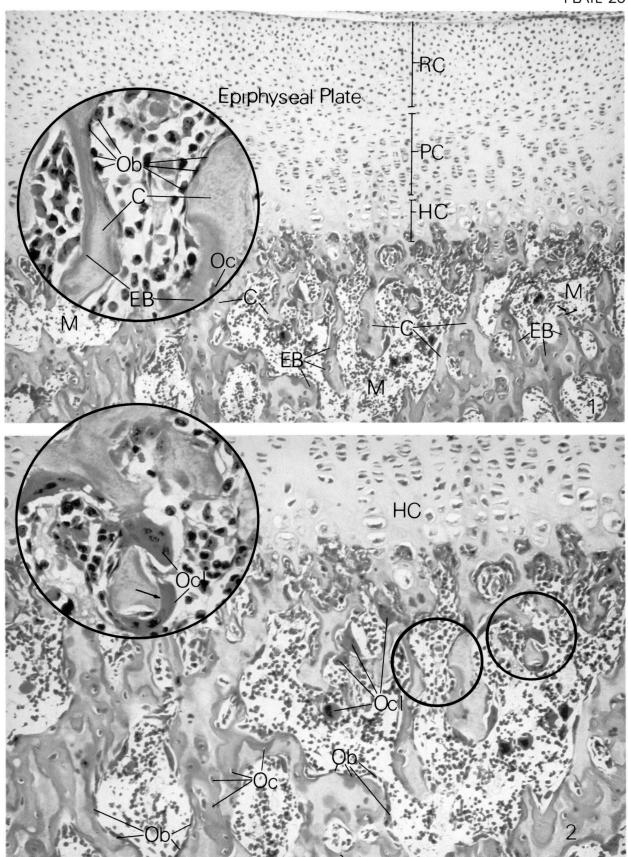

Epiphyseal Plate

RC

PC

HC

Ob

C

Oc

EB

M

C

C

EB

M

EB

M

1

HC

Ocl

Ocl

Ob

Oc

Ob

2

PLATE 21. Intramembranous Bone Formation

The flat bones of the skull, the mandible, and the clavicle ossify, at least in part, via an intramembranous route. The bones that form via an intramembranous route do not provide structural support as do the bones that ossify via an endochondral route.

The formation of intramembranous bone in the mandible is shown in **Figure 1.** This is a low power panoramic view that shows some developing spicules of bone and their relationship to the surface of the face. The bone spicules (**BS**) appear as the elongated irregular dark profiles in the connective tissue. The oval structure is Meckel's cartilage (**MC**).

The sequence of events in intramembranous bone formation can be studied by examining a spicule (**rectangle**) at higher magnification (**Figure 1, inset**). The earliest steps are illustrated at the top and later events at the bottom. Cells of the connective tissue aggregate at the site where the bone is to be laid down and differentiate into osteoblasts (**Ob**). The osteoblasts engage in the production of osteoid (**Os**), which contains collagenous fibrils and ground substance. Osteoid can be recognized because it is situated on the surface of bone spicules; osteoblasts are usually seen in contact with it, and it stains less intensely with eosin than does the "matrix" of the bone. Osteoid becomes calcified and is then bone. When osteoblasts have surrounded themselves with their product and come to lie in lacunae, they are called osteocytes.

Intramembranous bone formation and the remodeling of the skull are illustrated in **Figure 2.** Note that osteoblasts and osteoid are present along almost the entire surface of bone on the skin side. Lines can be seen in the spicules (**BS**) that reflect the general contours and pattern of bone deposition. These lines are intact on the side of the spicule upon which bone is being deposited, but they are interrupted where bone is being resorbed (**arrow**).

Figure 3 shows developing intramembranous bone at higher magnification. The nuclei of the osteocytes (**Oc**) stain with hematoxylin and stand

KEY	
BS, bone spicule	Ocl, osteoclast
BV, blood vessel	Os, osteoid
MC, Meckel's cartilage	**arrow**, edge where
Ob, osteoblast	bone was resorbed
OC, osteocyte	

Fig. 1, pig, × 65	**Fig. 3**, human, × 160
Fig. 2, human, × 65	**Fig. 4**, rabbit, × 640.

out against the pink-staining matrix. The osteoblasts (**Ob**) are located on the surface of the bone spicule, immediately adjacent to the lightly staining osteoid (**Os**) that they have just formed. Two osteoclasts (**Ocl**) can be seen on the undersurface of one of the spicules. Loose connective tissue is between the bone spicules; the bone vessels (**BV**) are located within this connective tissue at approximately equal distance from the neighboring bone spicules.

Osteoclasts are multinucleated cells that engage in the removal of bone. They are immediately adjacent to the bone that is actually being removed (**Fig. 4**). A ruffled border is present at the cell-bone junction, but this can be seen only in the most favorable preparations. After osteoclasts have been at work for some time, they form a slight concavity on the surface of the bone. This concavity is called Howship's lacuna.

Notice in these figures the blood vessels are located at approximately equidistant points from the advancing fronts of bone formation. The bone at this point of development resembles spongy bone and it is designated primary spongiosa. Most of this bone will continue to develop into compact bone. With continued bone formation, the bone trabeculae will become thicker and, ultimately, bone will replace most of the connective tissue surrounding the blood vessels. This will then be compact woven bone.

PLATE 21

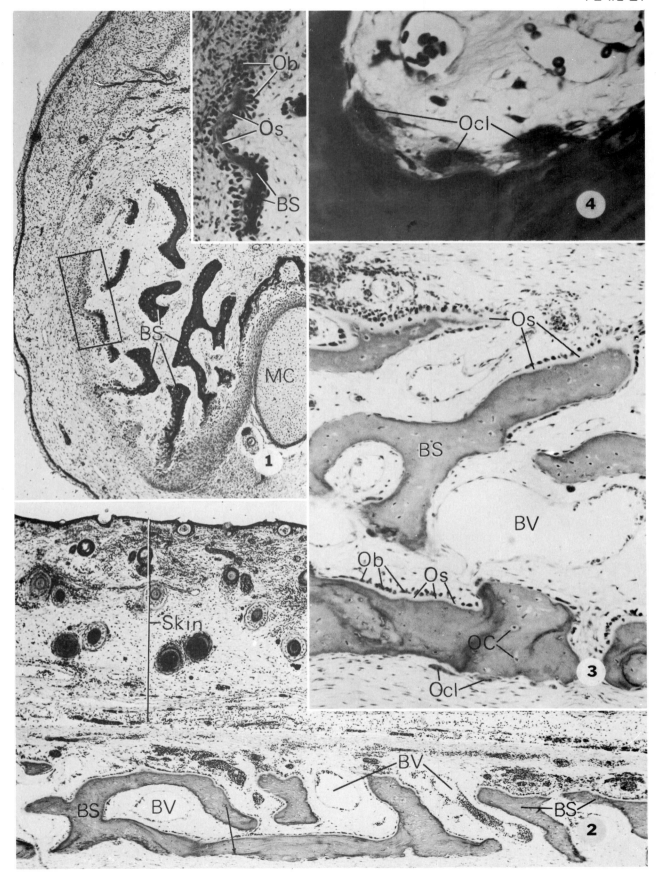

PLATE 22. Developing Bone I, Electron Microscopy

This electron micrograph reveals the periosteal surface of a growing long bone. It is from the midportion of the shaft, a region of the bone that develops by intramembranous ossification. Accordingly, no cartilage is present. The upper part of the illustration reveals typical fibroblasts **(Fib)** and bundles of collagen fibers **(CF).** This constitutes the layer that, with the light microscope, is referred to as the fibrous portion of the periosteum **(FP).** Below is the cellular layer of the periosteum that contains the preosteoblasts **(POb)** and osteoblasts **(Ob).**

The osteoblasts are aligned on the surface of the developing bone. They appear more or less cuboidal in shape. The lateral boundaries of adjacent osteoblasts are not very conspicuous, but the distinction between adjacent cells is somewhat enhanced by differences in electron density of the cytoplasmic matrix. The osteoblasts contain large amounts of rough-surfaced endoplasmic reticulum **(RER)** and an extensive Golgi apparatus (see Atlas section, Plate 23), features indicative of cells highly active in protein synthesis and secretion. Note that the preosteoblasts possess more cytoplasm than the fibroblasts, but the preosteoblast's rough-surfaced endoplasmic reticulum **(RER)** is not yet as extensive as the reticulum in the osteoblasts.

Below the osteoblasts is the osteoid **(Os),** the material that in the light microscope simply appears as the poorly staining homogeneous band between the osteoblasts and the bone. The osteoid consists principally of collagen, ground substance, and some processes from the osteoblasts that extend between the collagen fibrils. These are shown at higher magnification in Atlas section, Plate 23.

In order to understand the biology of bone growth it is necessary to realize that the osteoblasts move away from the bone as they secrete their product, the osteoid. Shortly after the osteoid is produced, it becomes calcified by a wave of mineralization that follows the movement of the osteo-

blasts, with the osteoid always intervening. The calcium is in the form of hydroxyapatite crystals. In this specimen, most of the calcium salts have been lost from the bone **(B);** consequently, it has a relatively electron-lucid appearance. However, calcium salts remain at the mineralization front where it appears as the black electron-opaque material **(asterisks).**

At intervals, certain osteoblasts no longer continue to move away from the bone and, as a consequence, the cell is surrounded by the osteoid it has produced. As the mineralization front progresses, the cell becomes surrounded by bone. It is then contained within a lacuna and referred to as an osteocyte. A recently formed osteocyte **(Oc)** can be seen in the micrograph. Note that the bone matrix that borders the lacuna has retained its calcium salts. The processes of the osteocyte are contained in canaliculi **(C).**

Other osteocytes also arise in the same manner as just described. Thus, as the bone thickens, the osteoblast layer tends to become depleted as the osteoblasts become transformed into osteocytes. However, the depletion is balanced by the proliferation of connective tissue cells that differentiate first into preosteoblasts and then into osteoblasts.

KEY

B, bone
C, canaliculus
CF, collagen fibers
Fib, fibroblast
FP, fibrous periosteum
Ob, osteoblast
Oc, osteocyte

Os, osteoid
POb, preosteoblast
RER, rough-surfaced endoplasmic reticulum
asterisk, mineralization front

Fig., × 5000.

PLATE 22

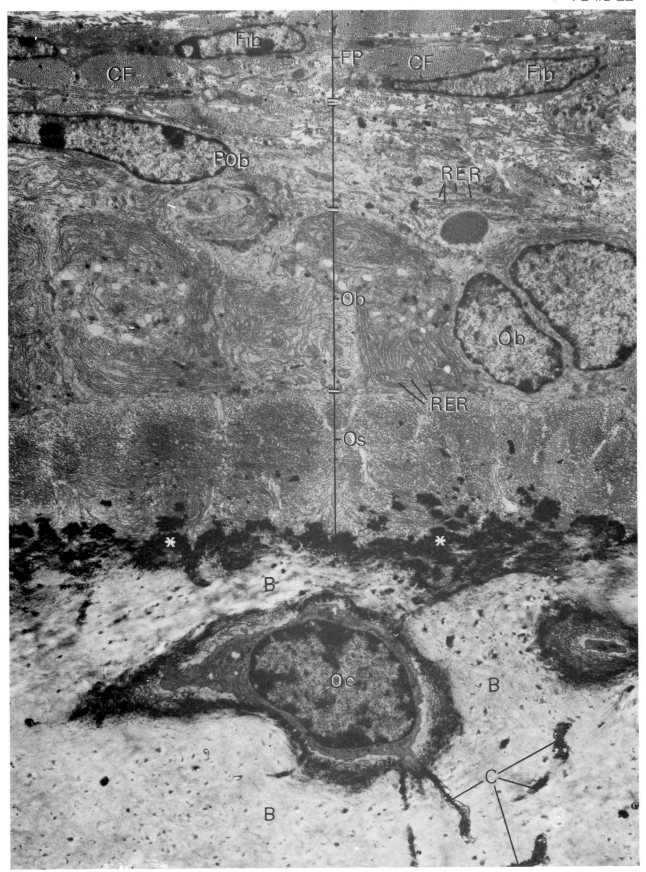

PLATE 23. Developing Bone II, Electron Microscopy

The osteoblasts shown in **Figure 1** are comparable to those seen in the preceding plate. The higher magnification shows to advantage the cytological detail of the cells.

In characterizing the osteoblast as well as understanding the nature of its product, it is important to realize that osteoblasts are derived from connective tissue cells that are indistinguishable from fibroblasts. They retain much of the cytological morphology of the fibroblasts and this is evident in the accompanying electron micrograph. In active fibroblasts, there is a large amount of rough-surfaced endoplasmic reticulum and an extensive Golgi apparatus. The osteoblasts pictured here also contain a large amount of rough-surfaced endoplasmic reticulum **(RER)** and a prominent Golgi apparatus **(GA),** indicative of their role in the production of osteoid. The Golgi apparatus shown in the osteoblast contains typical flattened sacs and transport vesicles. It also shows enlarged vesicles that contain material of various density. Two of the large elongated Golgi vesicles **(arrows)** contain a filamentous component. On the basis of special staining techniques for electron microscopy, such filaments are considered to be collagen precursor.

The osteoblasts in **Figure 1** (and those in the preceding plate) are cuboidal and, because of their close apposition, they bear a resemblance to cuboidal cells in an epithelial sheet. While the osteoblasts are indeed arranged on the surface of the developing bone in a sheet-like matter, they nevertheless exhibit properties of connective tissue cells, not epithelial cells. It should be noted that no basal lamina surrounds the osteoblasts. Moreover although none is pictured in **Figure 1,** collagen fibrils are occasionally observed between osteoblasts. The osteoblast is highly polar, secreting onto the bone surface. The surface of the osteoblast that faces the osteoid **(Os)** can be regarded to be the secretory face, or secretory pole of the cell.

The secretory face of the osteoblast is shown

KEY

C, collagen fibrils
GA, Golgi apparatus
N, nucleus of osteoblast
Os, osteoid
POb, preosteoblast
RER, rough-surfaced endoplasmic reticulum

arrows, Fig. 1, elongate Golgi vesicles with collagen precursor; Fig. 2, process of osteoblast
arrowhead, large collagen fibrils

Fig. 1, × 14,000   **Fig. 2,** × 30,000.

adjacent to the osteoid at higher magnification in **Figure 2.** Both the round and the somewhat larger, irregularly shaped profiles of the osteoid are collagen fibrils **(C).** Ground substance occupies the space between the collagen fibrils. It should be recalled that the osteoblast is moving away from the bone leaving its product behind. The collagen fibrils closest to the cell are of small diameter and represent the most recently formed fibrils. With time, as the cell recedes and as the mineralization front approaches, the collagen fibrils increase in diameter. This is thought to occur by the accretion of additional collagen onto the fibrils already present. It is not unlikely that some large, irregularly shaped fibrils **(arrowheads)** arise by a combination of accretion and the fusion of smaller fibrils. By the time the mineralization front reaches the fibrils, they have achieved their greatest diameter. Mineralization results in an impregnation of both the collagen fibrils as well as the ground substance with calcium hydroxyapatite.

The illustration also shows processes of the bone-forming cells **(arrow).** These processes will be contained in canaliculi after the osteoblast is transformed into an osteocyte.

PLATE 23

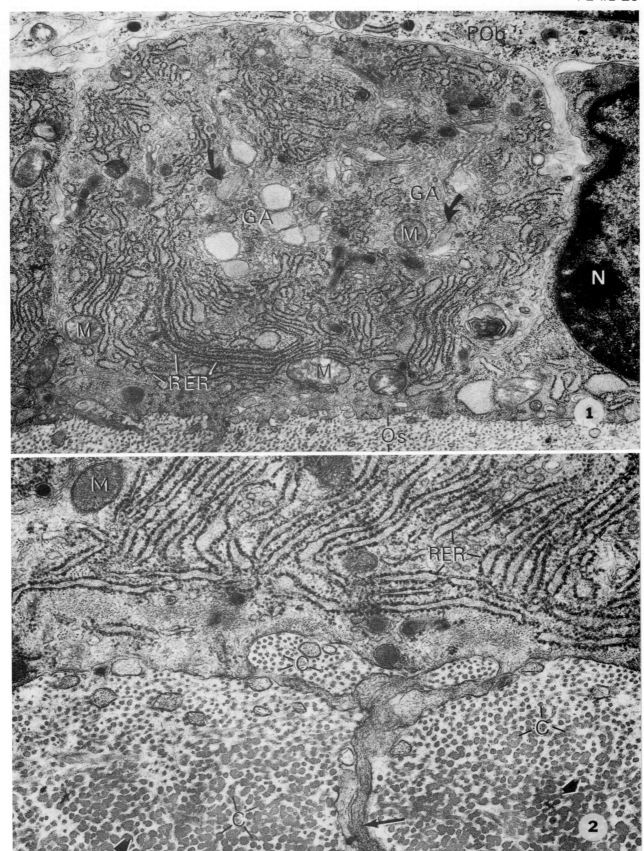

PLATE 24. Osteoclast, Electron Microscopy

This illustration shows a segment of bone surface **(B)** and, adjacent to the bone, portions of two cells, an osteoblast **(Ob)** and an osteoclast **(Oc)**. The difference between these two cell types is reflected not only in their cytological appearance but also in the character of the adjacent extracellular matrix. The osteoblast is typically separated from the mineralization front of the bone by osteoid **(Os)**. The portion of the cell seen in relation to the osteoid is readily identified as an osteoblast by its extensive rough-surfaced endoplasmic reticulum. Similarly, the osteoid is recognized by the presence of the numerous collagen fibrils.

In contrast, the osteoclast is adjacent to a mixture of collagen fibrils and hydroxyapatite crystals. In effect, at this site, bone is being broken down. The portion of the osteoclast that is in apposition with this partially digested bone possesses numerous infoldings of the plasma membrane **(inset)**. When viewed with the light microscope, the infoldings are evident as the ruffled border. When the plane of section is at right angles to the infoldings, they resemble microvilli. They are, however, folds, not finger-like microvillous projections, and when sectioned in a plane paralleling a fold **(asterisks)**, a broad nonspecialized expanse of cytoplasm is seen. This is the cytoplasm within the fold of the ruffled border **(Rb)**; it is free of organelles except for fine filaments. Apatite crystals **(arrowheads)** can often be seen in the extracellular space of the infoldings.

The cytoplasm of the osteoclast contains numerous mitochondria **(M)**, lysosomes, and Golgi profiles, all of which are functionally linked with the resorption and degradation of the bone substance. Electron micrographs show that the apatite

KEY	
B, bone	RF, resorption front
Ob, osteoblast	**arrows**, collagen fibrils
Oc, osteoclast	**arrowheads**, apatite
Os, osteoid	crystals
M, mitochondria	**asterisk**, cytoplasm
MF, mineralization front	within
RB, ruffled border	folds of ruffled border

Fig. × 10,000 (**inset,** × 25,000).

crystals are ingested by the cell. After the apatite crystals are ingested, the calcium is mobilized for passage into the bloodstream (in a manner not yet fully understood). The organic matrix (collagen and ground substance) is also resorbed by the osteoclast, but again the exact mechanisms are not clear. However, there is evidence that the osteoclast secretes hydrolytic enzymes into the area of bone where actual resorption is in progress.

As in Atlas section, Plate 22, the bone, except at the mineralization front **(MF)** and the resorption front **(RF)**, appears unusually light because the mineral component has been lost during the preparation of the specimen. In the lower part of the illustration, some collagen fibrils are evident; the **arrows** indicate where cross-banding is visible.

The proximity of osteoblasts and osteoclasts on the bone surface is not atypical. It highlights the fact that the bone surface is subject to continuous localized change, especially in growing individuals.

PLATE 24

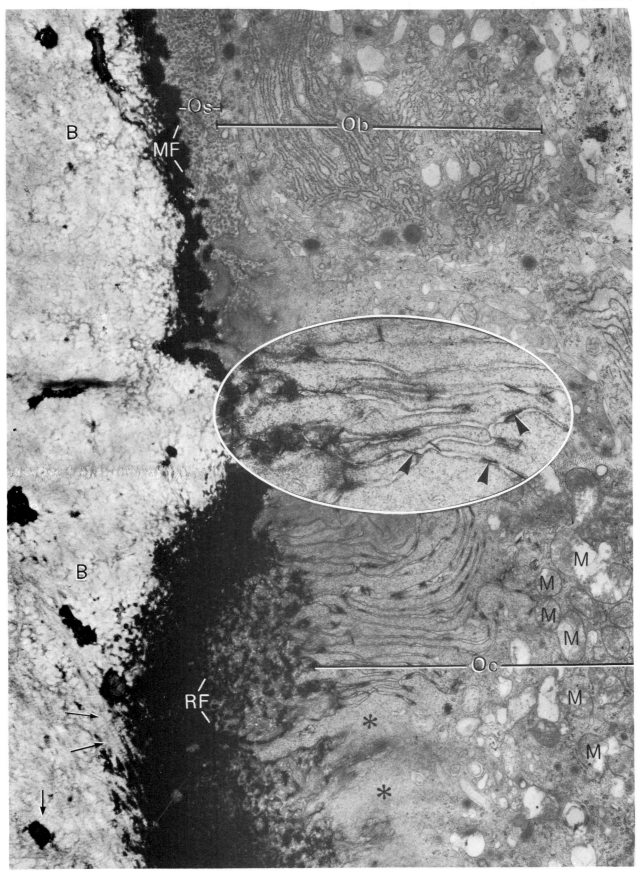

Blood

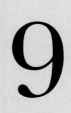

The blood belongs to the group of tissues designated as connective tissues. It is the fluid tissue that circulates through the cardiovascular system, being propelled chiefly by the pumping action of the heart. The blood plays many roles in the body. It conveys nutrients and oxygen to cells; it carries carbon dioxide and waste materials away from cells; it contains cellular and humoral agents that battle infection and "foreign cells" [those introduced through grafts or transfusions, as well as cells that have altered their normal state within the body (*transformed*) and have become cancer cells]; it delivers the humoral agents and specific cells to tissues as they are needed; it contains regulatory agents such as hormones that influence many activities within the body; it is thermoregulatory; and it maintains a delicate constancy of structure within certain limits, which is essential to the functional integrity of the body.

The blood consists of *formed elements* and *plasma.* The formed elements are red blood cells, white blood cells, and platelets. *Plasma* is the liquid intercellular material that imparts to the blood its fluid properties. The relative volume of cells and plasma is about 45 percent and 55 percent, respectively. This value is called a *hematocrit.* It is obtained by centrifuging a blood sample with anticoagulants added. The hematocrit value is then obtained by measuring the percent occupied by the cells and that occupied by the plasma. At the upper part of the cellular layer there is an additional narrow layer called the *buffy* coat. It consists of white blood cells and platelets. There are far more red blood cells (5×10^6/mm³ of blood) than white blood cells (6×10^3/mm³ of blood). Whereas the cells are the major object of interest in histology, it is also useful to examine briefly the plasma.

PLASMA

The composition of plasma is outlined in Table 9.1. As seen from the table, most of the plasma consists of water. It serves as the solvent for a variety of solutes including proteins, dissolved gasses, electrolytes, nutrients, waste materials, and regulatory substances.

The proteins are the largest of the dissolved substances. They can be subdivided by a number of procedures into three major groups designated as the fibrinogens, globulins, and albumins. *Fibrinogens,* the largest proteins, are made in the liver and function in blood clotting. *Albumins,* also made in the liver, are the smallest proteins. They are responsible for exerting the major osmotic pressure on the blood vessel wall. If albumins leak out of the blood vessels, as in the case of albumin being lost from the blood to the urine in the kidneys, the osmotic pressure of the blood decreases and fluid accumulates in the tissues. (This increase in tissue fluid is most readily noted by a swelling of the ankles at the end of a day.) The *globulins* include the *immunoglobulins,* by far the largest component of the globulin fraction. The immunoglobulins are antibodies, a class of functional molecules of the immune system. (Antibodies are discussed in Chapter 13.) Because they are large and usually retained within the blood vessels and because their reaction with fixatives tends to hold them in place, plasma proteins are often retained in hematoxylin and eosin-stained sections of tissues. Plasma proteins do not possess structural form above the molecular level; and, thus, when they are retained in the tissue block, they appear within some blood vessels as a homogeneous substance staining evenly with eosin.

TABLE 9.1. Composition of Blood Plasma

COMPONENT	PERCENT
Water	91–92
Protein (fibrinogens, globulins, albumin)	7–8
Other solutes	1–2
Electrolytes (Na⁺, K⁺, Ca²⁺, Mg²⁺, Cl⁻, HCO₃⁻, PO₄³⁻, SO₄²⁻)	

Nonprotein nitrogen substances (NPN) (urea, uric acid, creatine, creatinine, ammonium salts)

Nutrients (glucose, lipids, amino acids)

Blood gasses (oxygen, carbon dioxide, nitrogen)

Regulatory substances (hormones, enzymes)

Aside from these proteins and the regulatory substances, which are also proteins, most of the other plasma constituents are sufficiently small to pass easily through the blood vessel wall into the extracellular spaces of the adjacent connective tissue under physiological conditions. Thus, the interstitial fluid of the connective tissues is derived from blood plasma and it has an electrolyte composition reflective of blood plasma. The composition of extracellular fluid in nonconnective tissues is not entirely understood inasmuch as epithelium and special cell groups are separated from the connective tissue by a basal lamina and these cell groups appear to create special microenvironments according to their function. For example, it has long been known that a blood-brain barrier exists between the blood and nerve tissue. It is now known that "barriers" also exist between the blood and the parenchymal tissue in the testis, thymus gland, and certain other epithelial compartments.

CELLS

The formed elements of the blood and their relative numbers are given in Table 9.2. Red blood cells or erythrocytes perform their functions while they are within the bloodstream. However, the white blood cells regularly leave the blood through the walls of capillaries and venules to enter the connective tissues, lymphatic tissues, and bone marrow where they perform specific functions. Thus, while blood cells must be regarded as transients within the blood. That is, they use the bloodstream as a vehicle for transport to specific sites within the body.

TABLE 9.2. Formed Elements of the Blood

FORMED ELEMENT	NUMBER OR PERCENT
Red blood cells (erythrocytes)	4–5 million/mm³
White blood cells (leukocytes)	6000–9000/mm³
Agranulocytes	
Lymphocytes	30–35% (percentage of white cells)
Monocytes	3–7%
Granulocytes	
Neutrophils	55–60%
Eosinophils	2–5%
Basophils	0–1%
Platelets (thrombocytes)	200,000–400,000/mm³

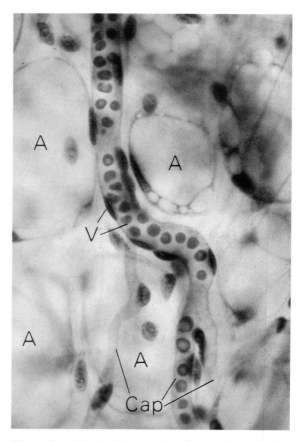

Figure 9.1. Photomicrograph of several capillaries (Cap) joining to form a venule (V) as observed in a full-thickness mesentery spread. The red blood cells appear in single file in one of the capillaries. The light center area of some of the red blood cells is due to their biconcave shape. Examination of in vivo preparations similar to this shows that the red blood cells are highly plastic and can fold on themselves when passing through very narrow capillaries. [The large round structures (A) are adipose cells.]

Blood Smears

The method that displays the cell types of peripheral blood to greatest advantage is the blood smear. This differs from the usual preparation seen in the histology laboratory in that the specimen is not embedded in paraffin and sectioned. Rather, a drop of blood is placed directly on a slide. The drop is spread thin with another slide, allowed to dry, and then stained. Another point of difference in the preparation of a blood smear is that instead of hematoxylin and eosin, special mixtures of dyes are used for staining blood cells. The resulting preparation may be examined with or without a coverslip.

Dyes used to stain blood smears are usually based on modifications of the Romanoswky-type stain. This consists of a mixture of methylene blue (a basic dye), related azures (also basic dyes), and eosin (an acid dye). On the basis of how they stain with Romanowsky-type dye mixtures, white blood cells are divided into granulocytes and agranulocytes. The granulocytes possess obvious, specific granules within their cytoplasm, whereas the agranulocytes do not. In principle, the basic dyes stain nuclei, granules of basophils, and RNA of the cytoplasm, whereasa the acid dye stains the red blood cells and the granules of eosinophils. It was originally thought that the neutrophil granules were staianed by a "neutral dye" that formed when methylene blue and its related azures were combined with eosin. However, the mechanism whereby neutrophil granules are stained is not clear. To complicate matters further, some of the basic dyes (the azures) are metachromatic and they may impart a violet-to-red color to the material they stain.

Red Blood Cells

Red blood cells, or erythrocytes, constitute the largest number of cells in the blood. Circulating erythrocytes are biconcave discs with a diameter of 7.8 μm, a thickness at the rim of 2.6 μm, a central thickness of 0.8 μm. In tissue sections erythrocytes range in size from 6 to 10 μm depending upon the conditions used in preservation of the tissue. In blood smears, erythrocytes measure about 7.5 μm in diameter. Circulating erythrocytes are rather unusual cells in that they do not possess a nucleus. They are shaped as biconcave discs and usually display this appearance, tending to give the impression that their form is rigid and inelastic (Fig. 9.1). However, the contrary is true. Erythrocytes are elastic and they readily deform, if necessary, in passing through small blood vessels. Red blood cells stain uniformly with eosin. In thin sections, viewed with the electron microscope, they are seen to be devoid of organelles, and the interior of the cell is seen to consist of a dense, finely granular material (Fig. 9.2). A plasma membrane surrounds the cell. This membrane is an enzyme-containing functional component of the red blood cell and not just a container. Although circulating red blood cells lack organelles, they are highly specialized and functional cells, engaged in the transport of respiratory gasses, oxygen, and carbon dioxide.

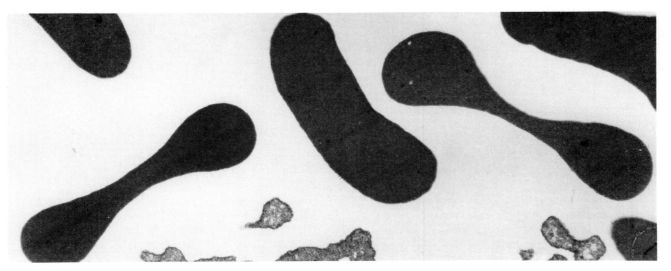

Figure 9.2. Electron micrograph of peripheral blood erythrocytes. Two of the cells have been sectioned vertically at or near their widest diameter and reveal the biconcave form. The cell in the center has been sectioned obliquely near its periphery. The cytoplasmic fragments at the bottom of the micrograph are portions of white blood cells. × 10,000. (Courtesy of Dorothea Zucker-Franklin.)

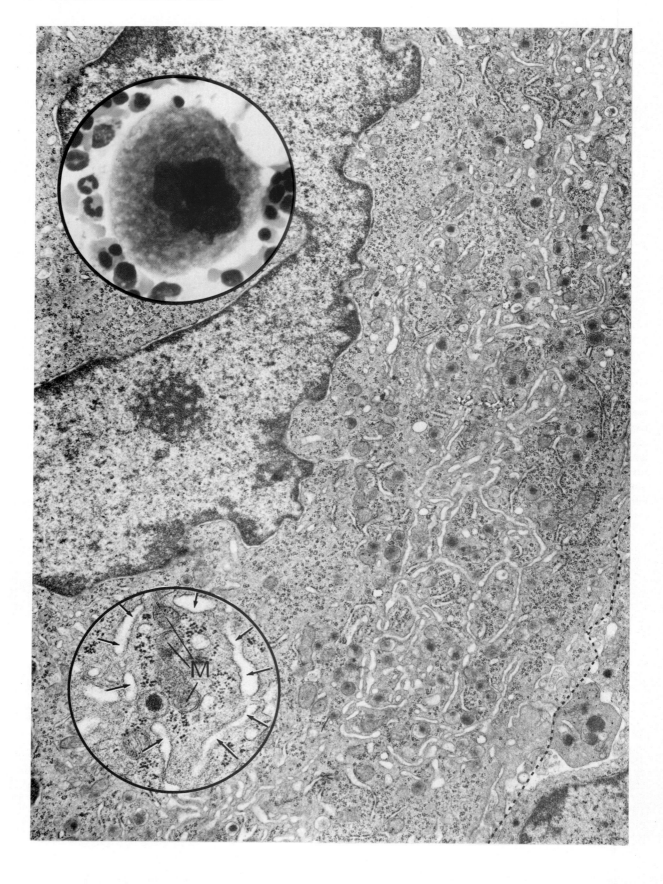

Hemoglobin. The specific component of the red blood cell that is essential for this function is **hemoglobin.** When hemoglobin is not present in sufficient amounts, either because the normal amount in each cell is decreased or the amount in each cell is sufficient, but the cells are reduced in number, the condition is manifest clinically as anemia. Anemia has a variety of causes including the loss of blood, insufficient iron for hemoglobin synthesis, and genetic factors.

Hemoglobin consists of four polypeptide chains complexed to iron-containing heme groups. The polypeptide chains are not all alike and, depending on the kinds of polypeptide chains present, hemoglobin is designated as HbA, HbA$_2$, and HbF. Adult hemoglobin is about 96 percent HbA, 2 percent HbA$_2$, and 2 percent HbF. HbF is the major form of hemoglobin in fetal blood. The persistence of high percentages of HbF in the adult is associated with certain types of anemia.

Platelets

Platelets are small cytoplasmic fragments within the circulating blood. They derive from large polyploid cells in the bone marrow called **megakaryocytes** (Fig. 9.3). In the formation of platelets, small bits of cytoplasm are separated from the peripheral regions of the megakaryocyte by extensive **platelet demarcation channels.** The membrane that lines these channels arises by invagination of the plasma membrane; therefore, the channels are in continuity with the extracellular space. The continued development and fusion of the platelet demarcation membranes results in the complete partitioning of cytoplasmic fragments to form individual platelets.

Platelets function in blood clotting, clot retraction, and clot dissolution, and they contain cytoplasmic constituents related to these functions (Fig. 9.4). These include two types of granules, **alpha lysosomal granules** and **very dense granules** (con-

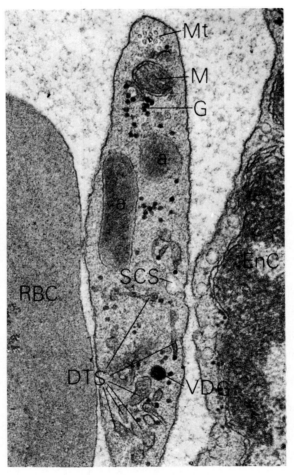

Figure 9.4. Higher-power electron micrograph of the platelet in Figure 9.2. The cell coat does not show to advantage, but the inclusions and organelles are revealed. They include a mitochondrion (M), microtubules (Mt), a single profile of the surface connecting system (SCS), profiles of the dense tubular system (DTS), the moderately dense alpha granules (a), a single very dense granule (VDG) and glycogen particles (G). The microfilaments are not evident against the background matrix of the platelet.

Figure 9.3. Electron and light micrographs of megakaryocytes. The **color inset** is a light micrograph revealing an entire megakaryocyte from a marrow smear. Its nucleus is multilobed and folded on itself giving an irregular outline. The "foamy" peripheral cytoplasm of the megakaryocyte represents areas in which segmentation to form platelets is occurring. The smaller surrounding cells are developing blood cells. The electron micrograph shows a portion of a megakaryocyte from a bone marrow section that includes two lobules of the nucleus and some of the surrounding cytoplasm. The limit of the cell is defined by the **dotted line, lower right.** The cytoplasm reveals evidence of platelet formation as evidenced by the extensive platelet demarcation channels. The higher power inset (**bottom of figure**) shows a segment of cytoplasm that is almost fully partitioned by the platelet demarcation channels (**arrows**). The inset also shows mitochondria (M), a maturing very dense granule, and glycogen particles. A mature circulating platelet is shown in Figure 9.4 for comparison. Light micrograph inset, × 1000; electron micrograph, × 15,000; electron micrograph inset, × 30,000.

taining serotonin); two systems of tubules, one connecting to the surface and another containing an electron-dense material; microtubules; and filaments.

When a blood vessel wall becomes broken, platelets adhere to the damaged tissue and release certain substances counteracting the injury. Among these substances are serotonin and thromboplastin. Serotonin is a vasoconstrictor that causes the vascular smooth muscle cells to contract, thereby diminishing local blood flow. Thromboplastin, also released by the cells of the damaged blood vessel, initiates a series of reactions leading to clot formation. Platelets then also bring about clot retraction and, finally, presumably after the clot has served its function, clot dissolution. Platelets, in the human, have a life-span of about 10 days.

In a blood smear, the platelets may be seen as individual units, but more often they adhere to each other, forming small clusters (see Atlas Section, Plate 25). Platelets are about 2 μm in diameter and they display a characteristic staining pattern. Part of the platelet stains more intensely with the dyes used in a blood smear; this part is called the *chromomere* or the *granulomere.* The less intensely stained region is called the *hyalomere.* The hyalomere contains predominantly the microtubules, which play a role in maintaining the shape of the platelet, and filaments, which participate in the contraction during the clot retraction. The granulomere contains the tubules, dense granules, and other components.

Neutrophils

In a blood smear, neutrophils are the most numerous of the white blood cells. They are named for their characteristic cytoplasmic staining, but they are also readily identified by the multi-lobed shape of their nucleus; on this basis, they are also called *polymorphonuclear neutrophils* and *polymorphs.* The mature neutrophil possesses three or four lobes of nuclear material joined by thinner nuclear strands. The arrangement is not static, but rather the lobes and connecting strands change their shape, position, and even number. The chromatin of the polymorph has a characteristic arrangement. Wide regions of heterochromatin are located chiefly at the periphery of the nucleus, in contact with the nuclear envelope, whereas regions of euchromatin are chiefly at the center of the nucleus, with relatively smaller regions contacting the nuclear envelope (Fig. 9.5).

The neutrophil is an active phagocyte and its cytoplasm contains numerous granules that reflect this function. There is sparse representation of other membrane-bound organelles. Small Golgi profiles are evident in the center of the cell; mitochondria are few and may not be evident in a section. Two kinds of granules are present in the neutrophil: *specific granules* and *azurophilic granules.* The specific granules are smaller and more numerous. They possess an antibacterial agent and they are alkaline phosphatase positive. The larger, less numerous azurophilic granules contain a dense core in addition to the other finely stippled material in the granule. The azurophilic granules are the lysosomes of the neutrophil and contain peroxidase and lysosomal enzymes.

The classical example of neutrophil function is their involvement in inflammation. The term *inflammation* refers to the local tissue response to injury. It is essentially a connective tissue response. Clinically, inflammation is characterized by heat, swelling, redness, pain, and loss of function. It involves an initial constriction of the blood vessels and an increase of vascular permeability, particularly the postcapillary venules. As a consequence, the amount of interstitial fluid increases and cells enter the inflammatory site from the blood. The neutrophils are the most numerous of the first wave of cells to enter the inflammatory site and they engage in phagocytosis, for example, the phagocytosis of bacteria. With the electron microscope, it is possible to follow the interaction of neutrophils and bacteria. After the neutrophil has ingested the bacterium, the specific granules fuse with and empty their antibacterial agent into the phagosomes. Then, the azurophilic granules fuse with the phagosome and pour their hydrolytic enzymes into the phagosome (now called a secondary lysosome). These enzymes bring on the lysis of the bacterium. Neutrophils perish in this process, and the accumulation of dead bacteria and neutrophils constitutes the thick yellowish substance called *pus.* Other white blood cells, especially monocytes, secondarily enter the inflammatory site. The monocytes transform into macrophages and phagocytose bacteria and tissue debris. With time, the character of the inflammatory cell population changes. Macrophages remain at the inflammatory site longer than neutrophils and, thus, they are the major cell type later on during the inflammation. The neutrophils and monocytes are attracted to the inflammatory site by chemical factors, a process referred to as *chemotaxis.* Lymphocytes, eosinophils, and basophils also play a role in inflammation. However, their role is more specifically directed toward the immunological aspect of the process (see Chapter 13).

An important property of neutrophils and other leukocytes is motility. Although while circulating through the blood vessels, the neutrophil is

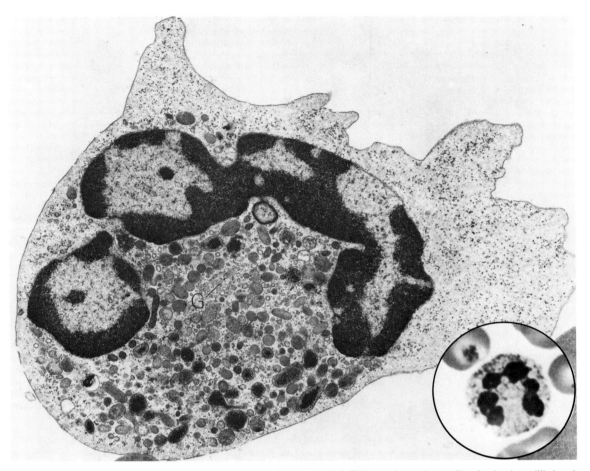

Fig. 9.5. Electron micrograph of a human mature neutrophil. The nucleus shows the typical multilobed configuration with heterochromatin at the periphery and the euchromatin more centrally located. A small Golgi apparatus (G) is present and other organelles are sparse. The punctate appearance of the cytoplasm adjacent to the convex aspect of the nuclear profile is due to glycogen particles. Adjacent to the concave aspect of the nuclear profile are numerous granules. Specific granules appear less dense and more rounded than the azurophilic granules. The latter are fewer in number and appear extremely electron dense. For comparative purposes, a neutrophil from a blood smear as observed in the light microscope is shown in the **inset.** (Electron micrograph courtesy Dorothea Zucker-Franklin.)

rounded, when it contacts a substratum, it tends to flatten somewhat and extend pseudopods from the main body of the cell. In thin sections, the cytoplasmic content of the pseudopod appears as an expanse of finely granular cytoplasmic matrix with no membranous organelles (see Fig. 9.5). The finely granular appearance is due to the presence of actin filaments, some microtubules, and glycogen. These are involved in the extension of the cytoplasm to form the pseudopod and then the contraction, which accounts for the motility of the cell.

Basophils

Basophils are the least numerous of the white blood cells and, often, several hundred white blood cells need to be examined in a blood smear before one is found. Basophils are so designated because large granules in their cytoplasm stain with basic dyes. The basophil nucleus is usually obscured in stained blood smears, but its characteristics are evident in electron micrographs (Fig. 9.6). It is a lobulated nucleus; heterochromatin is chiefly in a peripheral location and euchromatin is chiefly centrally located. The electron microscope also shows that typical cytoplasmic organelles are poorly represented except for the large membrane-bound granules that, as already mentioned, are also seen with the light microscope as are the basophilic granules. These large membrane-bound granules contain a granular substance and myelin figures. Biochemically, the granules contain hydrolytic enzymes, heparin, histamine, and slow react-

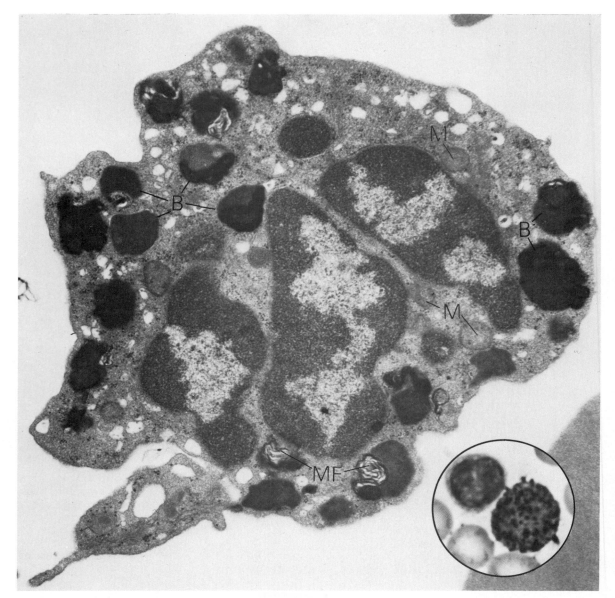

Figure 9.6. Electron micrograph of a human basophil. The nucleus appears as three separate bodies; the connecting strands are not in the plane of section. The basophil granules (B) are very large and have an irregular morphology. Some granules reveal myelin figures (MF). The small, spherical, less dense profiles are mitochrondria (M). **Inset:** A blood smear demonstrating the light microscope appearance of a basophil and an adjacent small lymphocyte. (Electron micrograph courtesy Dorothea Zucker-Franklin.)

ing substance (SRS). Histamine and SRS are vasoactive agents that, among other actions, bring on the dilation of small blood vessels.

Basophils are related, but not identical, to mast cells of the connective tissue. Both the mast cell and basophil bind an antibody, immunoglobin E (IgE), which upon subsequent exposure to, and reaction with, its allergen results in the release of the vasoactive agents from the basophil (and mast cell) granules. These substances cause the severe vascular disturbances associated with hypersensitivity and anaphylaxis (see Chapter 13).

Eosinophils

Eosinophils are so designed because of the large refractile granules in their cytoplasm that stain with eosin (Fig. 9.7). The nucleus of eosinophils is typically bilobed. As with neutrophils, the compact heterochromatin is chiefly adjacent to the

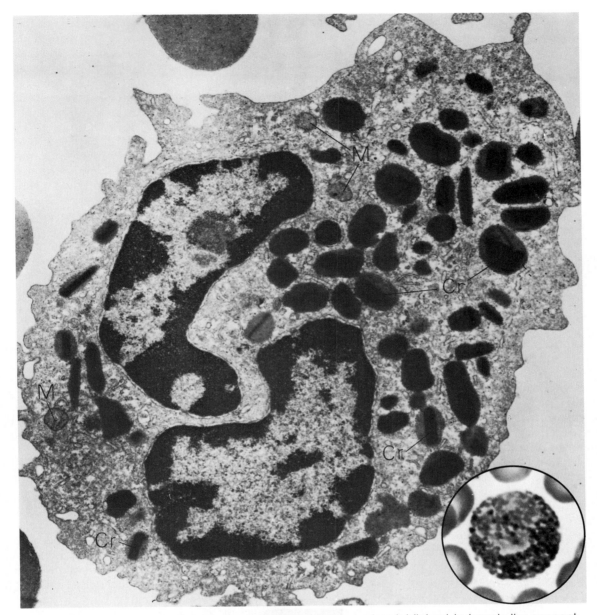

Figure 9.7. Electron micrograph of a human eosinophil. The nucleus is bilobed, but again the connecting segment is not within the plane of section. The granules are moderate in size compared to those of the basophil and show a crystalline body (Cr) within the substance of the granule. Careful examination shows the extreme density of a region within the granules to be due to the crystalline body; the remainder of the granule is less dense. A few mitochondria (M) are also evident. **Inset:** Light microscope appearance of an eosinophil from a blood smear. (Electron micrograph courtesy of Dorothea Zucker-Franklin.)

nuclear envelope, whereas the euchromatin is chiefly in the center. The cytoplasm of the eosinophil contains only sparse representation of membranous organelles, except for numerous large elongated granules, measuring 1 μm and even more in their largest dimension. The center of the granule contains a crystalline body that is readily seen with the electron microscope. These large granules with their crystalline bodies are the lysosomes of the eosinophil. They contain peroxidase, histaminase, arylsulfatase, and other hydrolytic enzymes. Histaminase neutralizes the activity of histamine, and arylsulfatase neutralizes the action of SRS.

The eosinophil is known to release arylsulfatase and histaminase at sites of allergic reaction, thereby diminishing the deleterious effects of these vasoactive agents. The eosinophil is also known to participate in other immunological responses. It engages in the phagocytosis of antigen-antibody complexes. Thus, the count of eosinophils in blood samples of individuals suffering from allergies and parasitic infections are high.

Lymphocytes

Lymphocytes are the main functional cells of the *lymphatic* or *immune system* (see Chapter 13). In the tissues associated with the immune system, three groups of lymphocytes can be identified according to size: small, medium, and large, ranging in size from 6 to 18 μm. In contrast, in the bloodstream, only small and medium lymphocytes, 6 to 12 μm in diameter, are present; the vast majority being small lymphocytes. In understanding the function of the lymphocytes, it is important to realize that the majority of the lymphocytes found in blood or lymph represent *recirculating immunocompetent cells,* which have developed the capacity to recognize and respond to foreign antigen and are in transit from one site of lymphatic tissue to another.

In blood smears, the small lymphocyte has an intensely staining, slightly indented, spherical nucleus surrounded by a thin rim of pale blue cytoplasm. Electron microscopy has revealed that the cytoplasm primarily contains free ribosomes and a few mitochondria. Other organelles are so sparse that they are not usually seen in a thin section. Small, dense lysosomes that correspond to the azurophil granules are occasionally seen, and a pair of centrioles and a small Golgi complex are located in the area of the indentation of the nucleus, known as the cell center. In the medium lymphocyte, the cytoplasm is more abundant, the nucleus is larger and less heterochromatic, and the Golgi complex is somewhat more developed (Fig. 9.8). Greater numbers of mitochondria and polysomes and small profiles of rough endoplasmic reticulum are also seen in these medium-sized cells. The ribosomes are the basis for the slight basophilia displayed by lymphocytes in stained blood smears.

T- and B-Lymphocytes. As was described in Chapter 2, lymphocytes can be assigned to two functional categories: (1) *T-lymphocytes* or *T-cells,* which have a long life-span and are involved in cell-mediated immunity and (2) *B-lymphocytes,* or *B-cells,* which have variable life-spans and are involved in the production of antibodies. All lymphocytes are involved in the phenomenon of immunological memory and are primed during their maturation to respond to a specific antigen. When

the lymphocytes first encounter the specific antigen, which they have been "programmed" to recognize through the molecules on their plasma membranes, they are stimulated to undergo several mitotic cell divisions. Some of the resulting lymphocytes differentiate into *effector cells* (i.e., cells that have specific functions), for example, a B-lymphocyte may divide several times producing more B-lymphocytes and large clones of cells that differentiate into *plasma cells* involved in the production of antibodies, or a T-lymphocyte may undergo several rounds of cell division producing cells that differentiate into *cytotoxic lymphocytes* (see below) capable of lysis of foreign or viral infected cells. Other B- and T-cells do not undergo differentiation into effector cells but serve as long-lived *memory cells,* which are primed to respond more rapidly and to a greater extent to subsequent exposure to their specific antigen.

Although the T- and B-cells cannot be distinguished on the basis of their morphology, they do have distinctive surface proteins that can be used to identify the cells by using immunolabeling techniques. B-cells have intramembrane immunoglobulin molecules that function as antigen receptors. T-cells have unique cell surface proteins (not antibodies), which appear during discrete stages in the maturation of the cells within the thymus. These surface molecules mediate or augment specific T-cell functions and are required to facilitate the recognition or binding of T-cells to foreign antigens. In human blood, it has been found that approximately 70 to 80 percent of the lymphocytes are mature T-cells and 10 to 15 percent are mature B-cells. Approximately 5 percent of the cells are identified as *null lymphocytes* and do not demonstrate the presence of the surface markers associated with T- or B-cells. The null lymphocytes are believed to be circulating stem cells. The size differences described above may have functional significance in that, in the large lymphocytes there may be cells that have been stimulated to divide. There may be plasma cell precursors that are undergoing differentiation in response to the presence of antigen.

Cytotoxic, Helper, and Suppressor T-Lymphocytes. Three fundamentally different types of T-lymphocytes have been identified: *cytotoxic lymphocytes, helper lymphocytes,* and *suppressor lymphocytes.* The activities of these cell types are mediated by molecules located on their surface. By employing immunolabeling technique, it has been possible to identify specific type of T-cells and study their function.

Cytotoxic Lymphocytes. The *cytotoxic T-lymphocytes* or *killer T-cells* (CTL) serve as the pri-

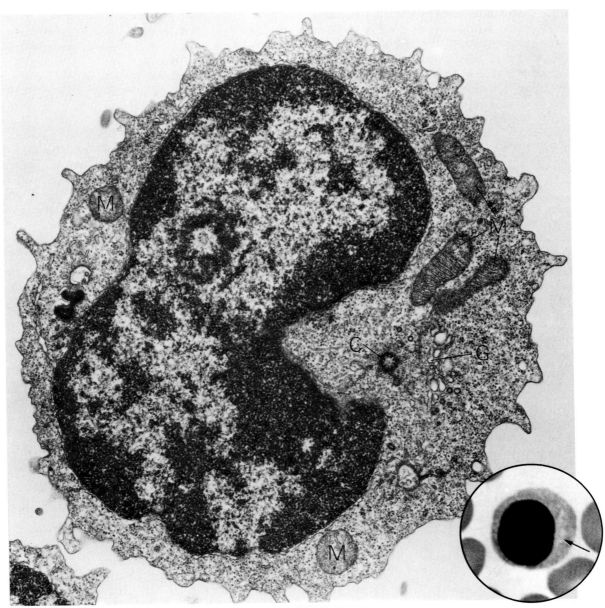

Figure 9.8. Electron micrograph of a medium-sized lymphocyte. The punctate appearance of the cytoplasm is due to the presence of numerous free ribosomes. Several mitochondria (M) are evident. The cell center or centrosphere region of the cell (the area of the nuclear indentation) also shows a small Golgi apparatus (G) and a centriole (C). **Inset:** Light microscope appearance of a medium-sized lymphocyte from a blood smear. The Golgi-containing centrosphere region is indicated by the **arrow.** (Electron micrograph courtesy of Dorothea Zucker-Franklin.)

mary effector cells in cell-mediated immunity. The CTLs recognize other cells that have foreign antigens on their surfaces and kill the cells by causing them to lyse (by creating holes in the plasma membrane). A classic target of a CTL is a virus-infected cell that displays viral glycoproteins on its surface.

Helper Lymphocytes. The *helper T-lymphocytes (T_H cells)* assist B-cells as well as other T-cells in their response to antigens. The interaction between most antigens and the antibodies on the surface of B-cells is insufficient to stimulate B-cell growth, differentiation, and secretion of soluble antibody. Only multivalent antigen molecules can stimulate the B-cells by themselves. A major function of the T_H cell is to recognize foreign antigens and then secrete factors (such as lymphokines) that stimulate B-cells or others that participate in immune reactions, such as CTLs or macrophages.

Suppressor Lymphocytes. The *suppressor T-cells (T$_S$ cells)* suppress the activity of B-cells. They appear to dampen the response to foreign antigens and may play a role in suppressing the immune response to self molecules (those normally present in an individual). The T$_S$ cells may also function in the regulation of erythroid cell maturation in the bone marrow.

Monocytes

Monocytes are the largest of the white cells in a blood smear. Monocytes are the precursor cells of a system of cells designated as the *monocuclear phagocyte system.* They are in passage from the bone marrow to the body tissues, where they will differentiate into the various phagocytes, for example, tissue macrophages (histocytes). Monocytes remain in the blood for about only 3 days. The nucleus of the monocyte is typically more indented than that of the lymphocyte (Fig. 9.9). The indentation is the site of the cell center where there are a well-developed Golgi apparatus and centrioles. The monocyte also contains smooth and rough endoplasmic reticulum and small mitochondria. Although classified as agranular, there are often numerous small, dense granules (lysosomes) in the cytoplasm of the monocyte.

As already indicated, during inflammation, the monocyte leaves the blood vessel at the site of inflammation, transforms into a tissue macrophage, and participates in the phagocytosis of bacteria and other tissue debris. The monocyte-macrophage also plays a role in immune responses by concentrating antigen and presenting this to lymphocytes (see page 186).

FORMATION OF BLOOD CELLS (HEMOPOIESIS)

The first phase of *hemopoiesis* or *hematopoiesis* in the developing individual occurs in "blood islands" in the wall of the yolk sac. In the second,

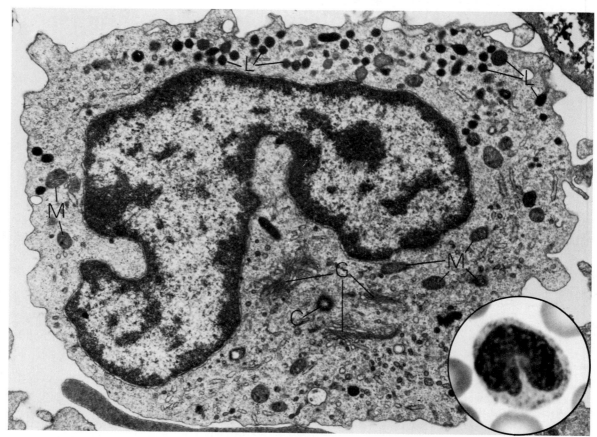

Figure 9.9. Electron micrograph of a human mature monocyte. The nucleus is markedly indented, and the cell center shows several Golgi profiles (G) as well as a centriole (C). The small dark granules are the lysosomes (L) of the cell. The slightly larger and less dense profiles are mitochondria (M). **Inset:** Light microscopic appearance of a monocyte from a blood smear. (Electron micrograph courtesy of Dorothea Zucker-Franklin.)

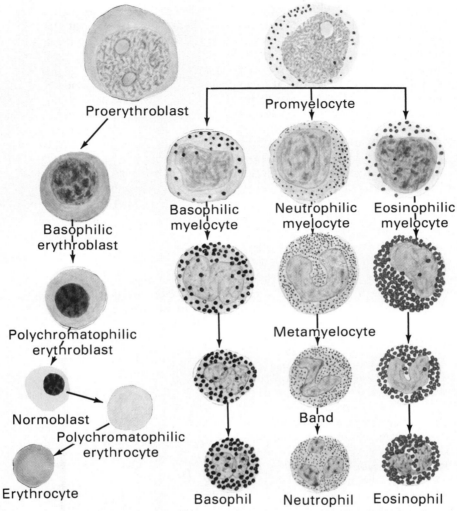

Proerythroblast

Promyelocyte

Basophilic erythroblast

Basophilic myelocyte

Neutrophilic myelocyte

Eosinophilic myelocyte

Polychromatophilic erythroblast

Metamyelocyte

Normoblast

Polychromatophilic erythrocyte

Band

Erythrocyte

Basophil

Neutrophil

Eosinophil

Figure 9.10 Illustration of the morphologically recognizable stages of erythrocytic and granular leukocytic differentiation in myeloid tissue. Drawn are normal human bone marrow cells as they would typically appear in a smear. Romanovsky-type stain. (From Ham AW, Cormack DH: *Histology*, 8th ed. Philadelphia, JB Lippincott, 1979.)

or hepatic phase, still early in development, hemopoietic centers appear in the liver (and lymphatic tissues), and for a time, the liver is the major blood-forming organ in the fetus. The third phase of fetal hemopoiesis involves the bone marrow (and other lymphatic tissues). After birth, hemopoiesis occurs in the red bone marrow of the bones and in the other lymphatic tissues. Red and white blood cells develop in the bone marrow; lymphocytes also develop in the other lymphatic tissues.

For a long time, there was controversy among investigators as to whether all blood cells arise from a common stem cell, the *unitarian* or *monophyletic theory,* or each blood cell type arises from its own stem cell, the *dualistic* or *polyphyletic theory.* Recent experiments indicate that the mono-

phyletic theory is correct. The studies demonstrate that the blood cells are derived from *pluripotential* stem cells that are able to differentiate into different types of mature blood cells.[1] In essence, the experiments involve the exposure of an experi-

[1] Spangrude, Heimfeld, and Weissman (*Science* 241:58–62, 1988) recently reported on their success in isolating pure populations of bone barrow stem cells in the mouse. This work confirms the potential of stem cells to differentiate into precursors for various types of blood cells. Work is in progress to isolate human stem cells by similar methods and to determine if human stem cells have the same potential to generate all of the different blood cell types. The isolation of purified stem cells also will make possible the study of microbiological environments on the cell's final differentiated state. For example, injection of stem cells into the thymus results in differentiation of cells only into T-lymphocytes.

mental animal to a lethal dose of irradiation. The irradiation results in a critical depletion of hemato-poietic tissue. Death can be prevented by the injection of a suspension of marrow cells from a healthy nonirradiated animal. Some of the injected cells colonize the spleen of the irradiated animal forming nodules of hemopoietic tissue that are distinguished easily from the damaged host splenic tissue. The nodule contains developing forms of all blood cell types. Moreover, modifications of this type of experiment provide evidence that shows that the splenic nodules are a clone, that is, all cells within the nodule have derived from one parent cell, the stem cell.

The easiest way to begin the study of blood cell development is to refer to a diagram such as the one in Figure 9.10. The figure outlines those stages in blood cell development that can be recognized by an experienced individual in a section or smear of bone marrow.

Development of Erythrocytes (Erythropoiesis)

The recognizable cell that begins the process of erythropoiesis is called the *proerythroblast*. It is a relatively large cell, measuring about 15 μm in diameter. It contains a large spherical nucleus with one or two visible nucleoli. The cytoplasm shows mild basophilia due to the presence of free ribosomes. The next stage in development is represented by the *basophilic erythroblast*. It is somewhat smaller than the proerythroblast and has a smaller nucleus. The cytoplasm shows strong basophilia due to an increased number of free ribosomes (polyribosomes), which synthesize the intracellular protein hemoglobin. The accumulation of the intracellular protein in the cell changes the staining reaction of the cytoplasm because hemoglobin stains with eosin. At this stage, the cytoplasm displays both eosinophilia, due to the staining of hemoglobin, and basophilia, due to the staining of the ribosomes. Because of this double staining reaction, the cell is now called a *polychromatophilic erythroblast*. The nucleus of the polychromatophilic erythroblast is smaller than that of the basophilic erythroblast. The next named stage in erythropoiesis is the *normoblast*. This cell has a small, compact, intensely stained nucleus and eosinophilic cytoplasm due to its large amount of hemoglobin (Fig. 9.11). The normoblast then loses its nucleus by extruding it from the cell and it is ready to pass into a blood sinus of the red marrow. Some polyribosomes, still able to synthesize hemoglobin, are retained in the cell. These polyribosomes im-

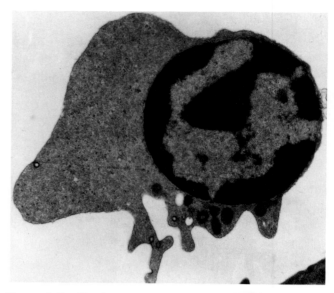

Figure 9.11. Electron micrograph of a normoblast just before extrusion of the nucleus. The cytoplasm reveals mitochondria, a few small vacuoles, a coated pit and some coated vesicles. The latter are recognizable by their dense outline, a reflection of the coat. The fine dense particles in the cytoplasm are polysomes. × 10,000. Courtesy of Dorothea Zucker-Franklin.

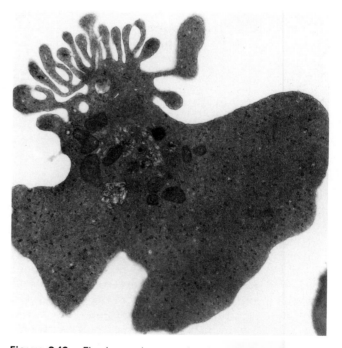

Figure 9.12. Electron micrograph of a reticulocyte. The nucleus is no longer present and the cytoplasm shows the characteristic fimbriated processes that occur just after nuclear extrusion. Mitochondria are still present, as are degradation vacuoles and polysomes. × 16,500. Courtesy of Dorothea Zucker-Franklin.

part a slight degree of basophilia to the otherwise eosinophilic cells and because of this, these new red blood cells are called *polychromatophilic erythrocytes* (Fig. 9.12). The polyribosomes of the new red blood cells can also be demonstrated with special stains that cause the polyribosomes to clump and form a reticular network. Because of this, the polychromatophilic erythrocytes are also, and more frequently, called *reticulocytes.* In normal blood, reticulocytes (new red blood cells) constitute about 1 to 2 percent of the red blood cells. However, if increased numbers of red blood cells enter the bloodstream (as during increased erythropoiesis to compensate for loss of blood) the number of reticulocytes increases. Red blood cell formation is under the influence of a kidney hormone called *erythropoietin.*

Red blood cells have a life-span of about 120 days in humans. At this time, they become fragile and subject to breakage. The macrophage system of the spleen, bone marrow, and liver plays a role in the phagocytosis of the red blood cells undergoing degradation. The iron is separated from the hemoglobin for reuse in hemoglobin synthesis. Other parts of the hemoglobin molecule are removed by the liver and excreted via the gallbladder as the bilirubin of the bile.

Development of Granulocytes (Granulopoiesis)

The recognizable cell that begins the process of granulopoiesis is the *promyelocyte.* The promyelocyte has a large spherical nucleus and the cytoplasm contains azurophilic granules; it gives rise to myelocytes. The *myelocyte* has a more or less spherical nucleus. Each of the specific cell lines (basophilic, neutrophilic, and eosinophilic) is distinguished by specific granules in the cytoplasm. The *metamyelocyte* (basophilic, neutrophilic, and eosinophilic) is an intermediate stage in which the specific granules increase in number and the nucleus becomes indented, thereby beginning the formation of a lobulated nucleus. The next stage is the mature basophil, the mature eosinophil, and an immature form of the neutrophil called a *band cell.* Band cells are sometimes seen in the circulation along with the mature granulocytes. Continued maturation of the band cell involves segmentation of the nucleus, thereby forming the three to five lobes typical of the adult.

Granulocytes remain in the circulating blood for an average of about 8 to 12 hours in the human. By means of labeling granulocytes with radioactive tags, it has been possible to study the ki-

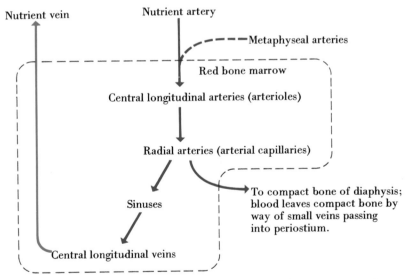

Figure 9.13 Schematic diagram of blood vessels in bone marrow of a young long bone. The **dashed line** surrounds vessels within the marrow cavity. A nutrient artery enters the cavity through a large nutrient foramen in the shaft of the bone. Other arteries typically enter the cavity near the ends of the bone. These are designated as metaphyseal arteries. At least one large nutrient vein leaves the marrow cavity through the nutrient foramen in company with the nutrient artery. Blood vessels also pass from the narrow cavity into the compact bone of the shaft. The vessels leaving the compact bone of the shaft exit as periosteal vessels.

netics of these cells. Such investigations show that the red bone marrow contains a ready reserve of mature granulocytes and metamyelocytes. These investigations also show that there are two pools of granulocytes in the blood vessels, namely, a *circulating pool* and a *marginating pool.* Marginating cells are in capillaries through which blood is not actively circulating. Such capillaries are temporarily excluded from the circulation and they contain granulocytes adhering to the endothelium.

BONE MARROW

The red bone marrow lies entirely within the spaces of bone, either in the medullary cavity of young long bones or in the spaces of spongy bone. It consists of blood vessels, specialized units of blood vessels called *sinuses,* and a sponge-like network of hemopoietic cells. In sections, the hemopoietic cells appear to lie in "cords" between sinuses or between sinuses and bone.

The sinus of red bone marrow is unique vascular unit. Its relationship to other blood vessels in the medullary cavity of a long bone is shown schematically in Figure 9.13. The sinus occupies the position normally occupied by a capillary, that is, it is interposed between arteries and veins. The sinus wall is described by Weiss (Fig. 9.14) as consisting of an endothelial lining, a basal lamina, and an outer *adventitial cell* layer. The endothelium con-

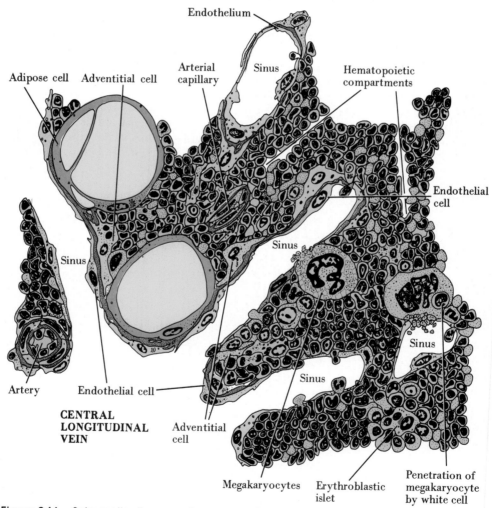

Figure 9.14. Schematic diagram of a cross-section through the marrow of a young long bone showing active hemopoiesis. To be noted are the erythroblastic islets engaged in the formation of red blood cells; megakaryocytes discharging platelets into the sinuses; endothelial cells adjacent to a basal lamina that is sparse in places and absent where blood cells are entering the sinuses; and adventitial, or reticular, cells extending from the basal lamina into the hemopoietic compartment. (L. Weiss, 1977.)

sists of simple squamous epithelium. It is not phagocytic. The adventitial cell, also called a *reticular cell,* sends sheet-like extensions into the substance of the hemopoietic cords and these thin cellular sheets provide some degree of support for the developing blood cells. In addition to providing support, the adventitial cell is able to produce reticular fibers. It may also play a role in stimulating the differentiation of stem cells into blood cells. When blood cell formation and passage of mature blood cells into the sinuses is active, the adventitial cell and the basal lamina become displaced by the mature blood cells as they approach the endothelium to enter the sinus. As a maturing blood cell or a megakaryocyte pushes against an endothelial cell, a transitory opening, called an *aperture,* is produced; that is, the migrating cell or the megakaryocyte process literally pierces the endothelial cell. Each blood cell must squeeze through such an aperture in order to enter the lumen of a sinus. Similarly, a megakaryocyte process must protrude through an aperture so that the platelets can be emptied into the sinus lumen. The aperture is lined by the plasma membrane, thus maintaining the integrity of the endothelial cell during the transcellular passage. As the blood cell completes its passage through the aperture or the megakar-

yocyte that has extruded its platelets withdraws its process, the endothelial cell repairs itself and the aperture disappears.

In active red bone marrow, the cords of hemopoietic cells contain chiefly developing blood cells and megakaryocytes. The cords also contain macrophages, mast cells, plasma cells, and some fat cells. Although the cords of hemopoietic tissue appear to be unorganized, specific types of blood cells develop in nests or clusters. Each nest in which red blood cells develop contains a macrophage. These nests are located near the sinus wall. Megakaryocytes are also adjacent to the sinus wall, and they discharge their platelets directly into the sinus through apertures in the endothelium. Granulocytes develop in cell nests farther from the sinus wall. When mature, the granulocyte migrates to the sinus and enters the bloodstream.

Marrow now active in blood cell formation chiefly contains fat cells, giving it the character of adipose tissue. It is called *yellow bone marrow.* It is the chief form of marrow in the medullary cavity of bones in the adult. However, the yellow marrow retains its hemopoietic potential, and when necessary, as after severe loss of blood, it can revert to red marrow, a sign that hemopoiesis is under way.

PLATE 25. Erythrocyes and Agranulocytes

In examining a blood smear, it is useful to survey the smear with a low-power objective in order to ascertain which parts of the preparation show an even distribution of blood cells. In general, the periphery of a blood smear should be avoided, the cells being either distorted, too close to each other (at the end where the drop of blood was placed, or too widely dispersed (at the opposite end, where the smear ended). Furthermore, the edges of a blood smear do not show a true percent distribution of white cells.

Figure 1 shows a low-power view of a smear with the blood cells well distributed. Most of the cells are erythrocytes. They are readily identified because of their number and lack of a nucleus. Scattered among the red cells are four white blood cells that can be distinguished from the erythrocytes without difficulty by their larger size and their staining characteristics. Interspersed among the cells are a number of small speck-like objects. These are blood platelets that have aggregated into small groups and, thus, can be readily observed even at this low magnification. They can be visualized better at higher magnification in **Figures 2, 3 and 4 (arrows).**

Erythrocytes have a biconcave shape. In the circulating blood, they measure about 8.0 μm, in diameter, in blood smears about 7.5 μm, and in sectioned material they range from 6 to 10 μm depending upon the method used for preserving the tissue. (A size of 7 μm for the erythrocyte in sectioned material is useful to remember because it enables one to ascertain the approximate size of other structures in a histological section by comparison without resorting to a micrometer.) Erythrocytes stain uniformly with eosin, a component of the usual dye mixture (for example, Wright's) used to stain blood smears. However, because of the biconcave form of the erythrocyte, its center is thinner and appears lighter than the periphery.

In order to distinguish the different kinds of leukocytes in a blood smear, it is advantageous to use the highest available magnification, usually an oil immersion lens. This enables one to use the morphological features of the cytoplasm in addition to nuclear morphology and cytoplasmic staining in identifying the cell type.

Lymphocytes and monocytes are classified as agranulocytes, that is, they are usually free of specific cytoplasmic granules. Moreover, their nuclei

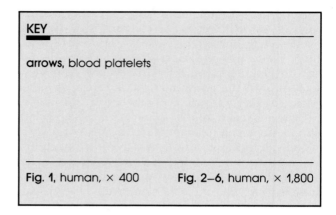

are nonlobed. Thus, they are distinguished from granulocytes, which possess specific cytoplasmic granules as well as a lobed or segmented nucleus.

Figures 2 to 4 illustrate characteristic features of lymphocytes. The nucleus stains intensely, generally has a rounded shape and, as illustrated in Figure 2, may possess a slight indentation. These cells measure about 8, 10, and 12 μm in diameter, respectively (circulating lymphocytes range from 6 to 12 μ). In a small lymphocyte **(Figure 2)** only a small amount of cytoplasm is evident and the nucleus seems to constitute most of the cellular volume. In large lymphocytes of circulating blood **(Figures 3 and 4),** there is a larger amount of cytoplasm. (Large lymphocytes of circulating blood are equivalent to the medium-sized lymphocytes of lymphatic tissue. The large lymphocytes of lymphatic tissue are not a characteristic feature of circulating blood except in certain abnormal conditions.) The cytoplasm of lymphocytes may stain a pale blue and sometimes a distinct, lightly stained Golgi area is evident. In addition, lymphocyte cytoplasm may contain azurophilic granules as shown in **Figures 3 and 4.**

Figures 5 and 6 show characteristic features of monocytes. These cells measure approximately 12 and 15 μm in diameter, respectively (monocytes range from 9 to 18 μm). The nucleus is indented, with the indentation facing the larger cytoplasmic area of the cell. The nucleus is somewhat less "compact" than the nucleus of lymphocytes. The cytoplasm, like that of lymphocytes, stains lightly, but tends to have a grayer or duller blue tint. Azurophilic granules are also present in the cytoplasm.

PLATE 25

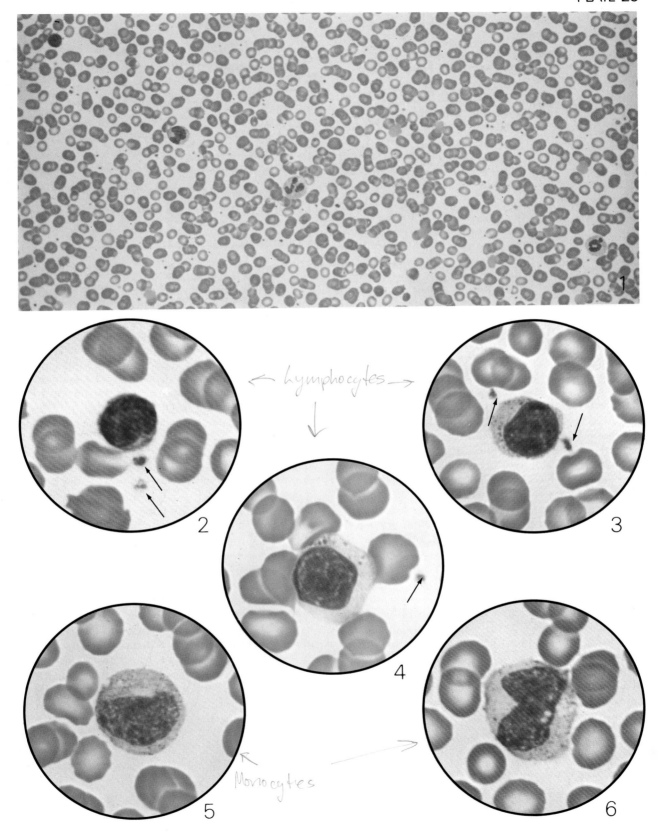

← lymphocytes →

2

3

4

Monocytes

5

6

PLATE 26. Granulocytes

Granulocytes are characterized by a lobed nucleus and specific granules within the cytoplasm. Three kinds of granuloctyes are present in a peripheral blood smear: *eosinophils,* about 2 to 5 percent of the white blood cell count; *neutrophils,* 55 to 60 percent of the white cells; and *basophils,* 1 percent or less of the white cells.

Eosinophils are shown in **Figures 1 and 2.** These cells measure about 13 μm in diameter (eosinophils range from 10 to 14 μm). The most conspicuous feature of eosinophils is the presence of numerous cytoplasmic granules that stain with eosin. The granules virtually fill the cytoplasm. The eosinophilic granules have specific morphological characteristics that can be used in the identification of the cells. They are relatively uniform in size within a particular cell; they are about 0.6 μm in diameter, significantly larger than granules of neutrophils; and they are typically closely packed. In going "through focus," eosinophilic granules often display a marked refractility. The nucleus of the eosinophil is usually bilobed as seen in **Figure 2.**

Neutrophils develop in the red bone marrow from cells that have a rounded nucleus. During their maturation the nucleus changes from a rounded to a segmented, or lobed, form. A fully developed neutrophil nucleus may have as many as five lobes. The configuration and number of lobes vary from one cell to another **(Figures 3 to 5)** and, on the basis of the variable nuclear morphology, these cells are sometimes called polymorphonuclear leukocytes. It should be understood, however, that each cell has only one nucleus, each lobe being joined to its neighbor by a strand of nuclear material.

Neutrophils usually measure from 9 to 14 μm in diameter. The cytoplasm of these cells contains granules that range from 0.1 to 0.4 μm in diameter and stain variably, either azure, light blue, or violet. Although neutrophils contain specific granules, the identification of these cells can usually be accomplished on the basis of the distinctive lobulation of the nucleus. Moreover, because these cells are the most numerous of the leukocytes in a smear of normal blood, their number is an aid in their identification.

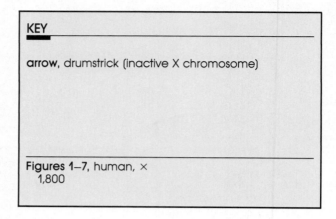

KEY

arrow, drumstrick (inactive X chromosome)

Figures 1–7, human, ×
1,800

The neutrophil in **Figure 5** shows a small projection from one of the nuclear lobes **(arrow).** This is referred to as a drumstick. It is the inactive female X chromosome. Its presence is sufficient to identify the blood as having come from a female assuming that the normal complement of chromosomes is present. Because the visualization of the drumstick requires a fortuitous orientation of the nuclear lobes, many cells usually need to be examined before a recognizable drumstick profile is found.

Basophils are shown in **Figures 6 and 7.** They measure about 8 and 14 μm in diameter, respectively (this represents the range in basophil size). These cells contain cytoplasmic granules of variable size that stain intensely with the methylene blue of the blood stain. The granules are randomly distributed throughout the cell, usually superimposed over the nucleus and obscuring it to such a degree that all its boundaries barely can be distinguished. Some of the granules shown in **Figure 7** are larger than the eosinophilic granules, others are smaller, and some are as small as those found in the neutrophils. The range in size of basophil granules (in contrast to the more uniform size of granules in eosinophils) is another characteristic that may aid in the identification of these cells. Because the basophil is so rare, it may be necessary to examine a significant part of the blood smear before one can be found.

PLATE 26

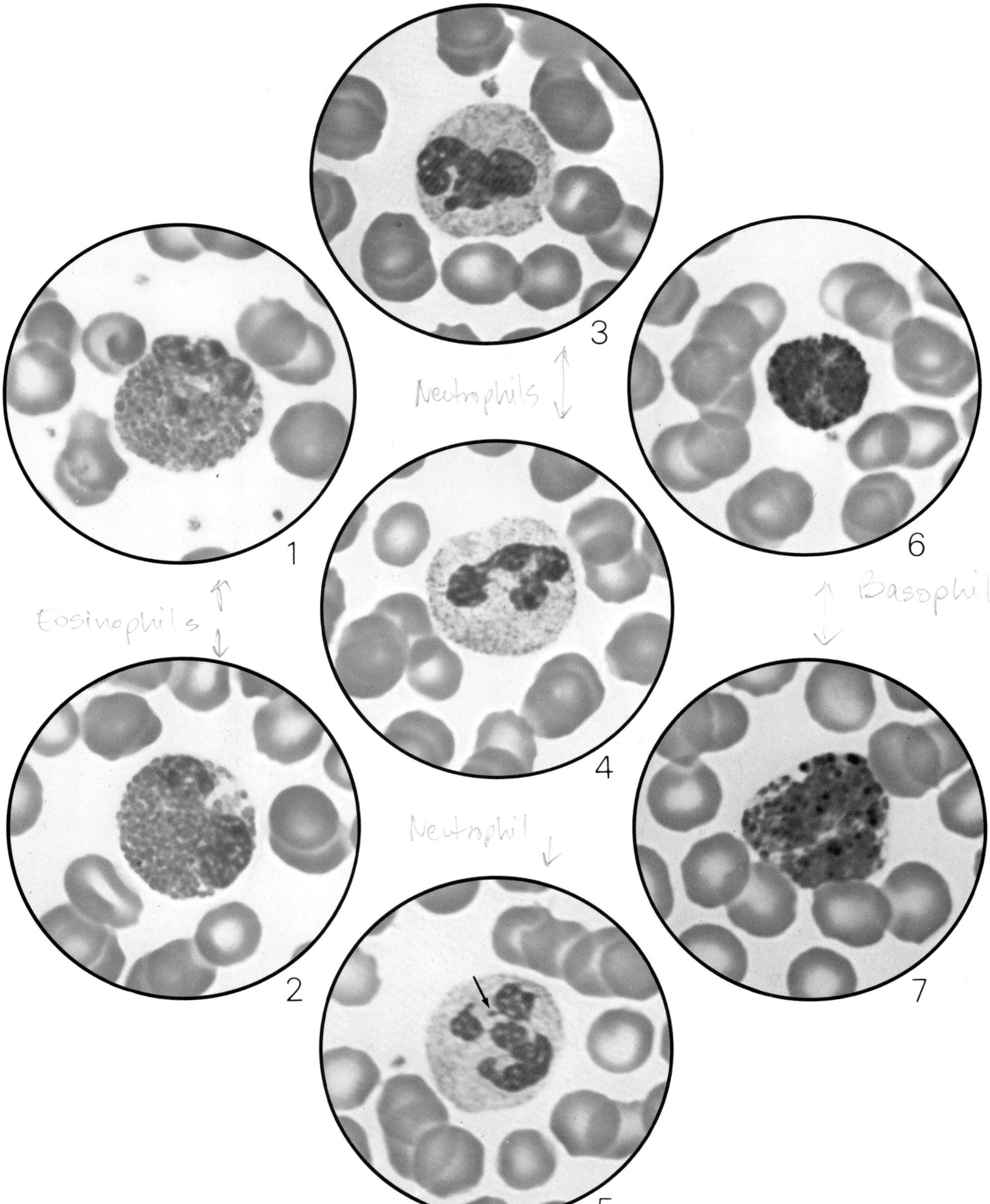
3
Neutrophils
1
6
Basophils
Eosinophils
4
2
Neutrophil
7
5

Muscular Tissue

Muscular tissue is characterized by aggregates of specialized cells whose primary role is contraction. The cells are elongate and arranged in parallel arrays, allowing them to work together effectively to produce movement. The principal components of the muscle cell related to contractibility are the myofilaments. There are two types of myofilaments, one comprised primarily of the protein actin, the other of the protein myosin. Myofilaments occupy the bulk of the muscle cell cytoplasm. Actin and myosin are also demonstrable in most other cell types, where they play a role in movement of the cell or part of the cell, for example, in the movement of microvilli, cytokinesis, exocytosis, and cell migration. However, compared to other cells, the muscle cell has an enormous number of coaligned contractile filaments that it utilizes for the singular purpose of producing mechanical work at the organ level of body structure.

CLASSIFICATION OF MUSCULAR TISSUE

Muscular tissue can be subclassified on the basis of the appearance and location of the contractile cells. Thus, we refer to striated muscle, which exhibits cross-striations at the light microscopic level, and nonstriated or smooth muscle, which does not. The striated muscle can be divided further into skeletal muscle and cardiac muscle on the basis of its location in the skeletal muscles or in the heart, respectively.[1] The arrangement of the myofilaments is the same in both of the striated muscle cell types; the chief differences between the two

are the size of the individual cells and their arrangement relative to one another. Smooth muscle cells do not exhibit cross-striations because the myofilaments do not achieve the same degree of order in their arrangement and the myosin-containing myofilaments are highly labile. Smooth muscle is largely restricted to the viscera and blood vessels.

SKELETAL MUSCLE

A skeletal muscle consists of parallel striated muscle cells, surrounded and held together by connective tissue (Fig. 10.1). The striated muscle cells are also called *fibers.* At its end, the muscle contains a tendon or some other arrangement of collagenous fibers whereby it attaches, usually, to bones. The muscle has a rich blood supply. A "capillary bed" is arranged so that the capillaries are, for the most part, parallel to the muscle fibers. The muscle cells are also richly innervated and they respond to impulses conducted by motor neurons of the spinal cord or brain stem. The contact made by the terminal branches of the axon with the muscle is called the *motor end plate.* Together, the neuron and the muscle cells it innervates are called a *motor unit,* or a *neuromotor unit.* A single motor neuron may contact from several to a hundred or more muscle fibers. Generally, muscles capable of the most delicate movements have fewer muscle cells per motor neuron in their motor units. For example, eye muscles have an innervation ratio of about one neuron to three muscle cells; in contrast, in muscles of the back, a single neuron may innervate hundreds of muscle cells. The nerve cell not only serves to instruct the muscle cells to contract but also exerts a trophic influence on the muscle cells, which is necessary in order for the muscle cells to maintain their structural integrity. If the nerve

---

[1] Striated muscle is also located in the tongue, pharynx, and upper part of the esophagus; this may be referred to as visceral striated muscle.

203

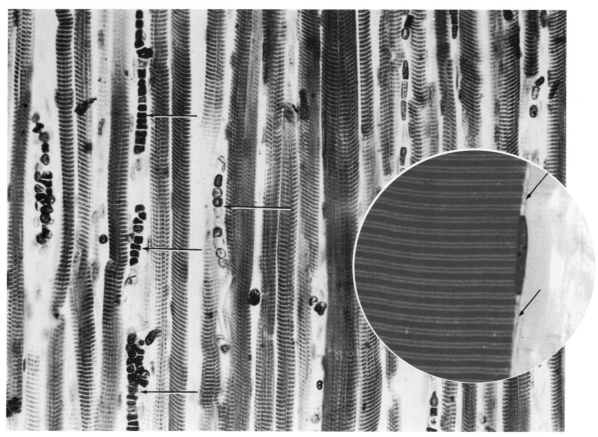

Figure 10.1. Photomicrograph of a longitudinally sectioned skeletal muscle. The muscle cells are arranged in parallel with the capillaries **(arrows)** between the fibers. The length of each fiber, or cell, extends far beyond the top and bottom limits of the micrograph. The cross-striations of the muscle fibers are readily apparent. The **inset** shows at higher magnification a portion of a single muscle cell. The sarcolemma and adherent substances **(arrows)** can be seen overlying a clear area of sarcoplasm. The visible striations include the Z line, the thin dark lines; the I band, the lighter-staining areas on each side of the Z line; and the A band, the wide darker-staining bands.

supply to the muscle is disrupted, the muscle cell undergoes regressive changes known as ***disuse atrophy.*** The most conspicuous indication of this atrophy is the thinning of the muscle and its cells. A skeletal muscle generally has two kinds of sensory receptors: the ***muscle spindle,*** within the substance of the muscle, and the ***Golgi tendon organ,*** within the tendon.

The connective tissue associated with skeletal muscle is designated by three names according to its arrangement with respect to the muscle fibers. ***Endomysium*** is the delicate, loose connective tissue immediately around each muscle fiber; it contains the capillaries. ***Perimysium*** surrounds bundles of muscle fibers or fascicles; it serves as the route for larger blood vessels. ***Epimysium*** is the relatively dense connective tissue surrounding the muscle.

The skeletal muscle cells are extremely long; they are multinucleated and, as already noted, display cross-striations. With the light microscope, it is usually possible to identify the cytoplasm, or ***sarcoplasm,*** and to distinguish the cytoplasmic boundary of the muscle cell, the ***sarcolemma.*** The nuclei are located immediately under this cytoplasmic boundary. It is now known that the boundary structure seen with the light microscope consists of the plasma membrane (also called the sarcolemma for muscle cells) and the basal or external lamina surrounding the muscle cell and possibly some reticular fibers.

Another feature of skeletal muscle is that some nuclei that appear to belong to the muscle cell are actually nuclei of small cells called ***satellite cells.*** These cells are interposed between the plasma membrane of the muscle cell and its basal lamina; they are dormant stem cells that may proliferate after minor injury to give rise to new myoblasts. As long as the basal lamina remains in-

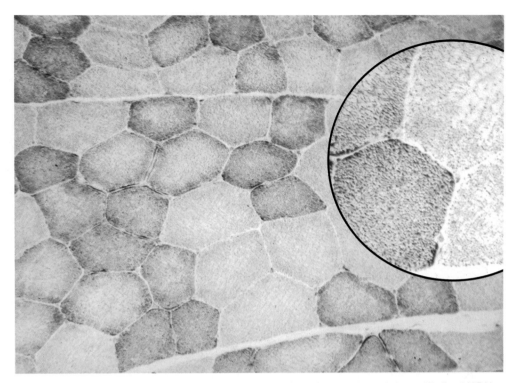

Figure 10.2. Cross-section of muscle fibers demonstrating two fibers types with the NADH-TR reaction. The deeply stained, smaller muscle fibers exhibit a strong reaction and correspond to the red muscle fibers. The lighter-staining larger fibers correspond to the white fibers. The **inset** shows portions of the two fiber types at higher magnification. The reaction enables one to visualize the mitochondria that contain the enzymes. The contractile components, the myofibrils, are unstained. (Original slide specimen courtesy of Dr. W. Ballinger.)

tact, the myoblasts fuse within the basal lamina to form myotubes, which then mature into a new fiber. In contrast, disruption of the basal lamina results in fibroblast repair of the injured site with scar tissue formation.

Red and White Fibers

It has been known from the early days of cytology that skeletal muscle cells differ in diameter and color. These differences are not conspicuous in hematoxylin and eosin (H&E) sections, but special cytological and histochemical reactions based on oxidative enzyme activity (Fig. 10.2) enable the microscopist to distinguish several types of fibers (cells), the most obvious of which are the red fibers and the white fibers. *Red fibers* are smaller in diameter, have relatively large numbers of mitochondria, and display a strong NADH-TR[2] or succinic dehydrogenase reaction (mitochondrial enzymes). Red fibers make up slow-twitch motor units, have a

_____
[2] Nicotinamide adenine dinucleotide-tetrazolium.

great resistance to fatigue, and generate relatively less muscle tension than white fibers. *White fibers* are larger, possess fewer mitochondria, and display a weak NADH-TR or succinic dehydrogenase reaction. White fibers make up fast-twitch motor units, fatigue rapidly, and generate a large peak muscle tension. They are innervated by neurons with axons of above average diameter that are capable of conducting impulses with above average velocity. Fibers with intermediate characteristics are called *intermediate fibers.* Although some muscles have predominantly one or the other of the two main types, generally both types of fibers are found in a single muscle.

Organization of Myofibrils and Myofilaments in a Skeletal Muscle Fiber

The organization of a skeletal muscle from the gross level to the molecular level is shown in Figure 10.3. The muscle fiber contains large numbers of myofibrils, which are just visible with the light mi-

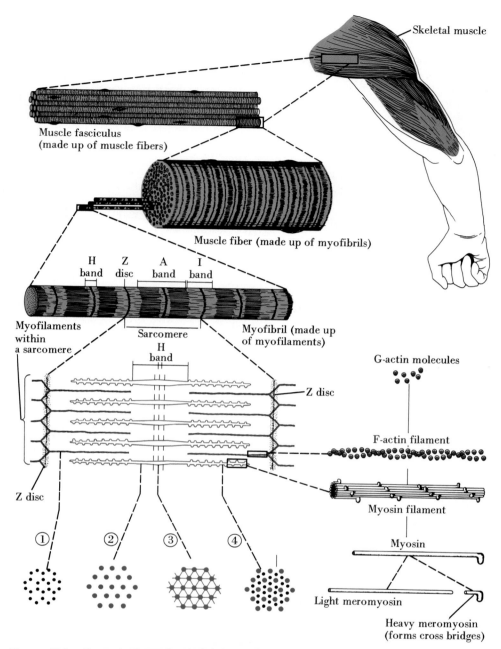

Figure 10.3. Organization of a skeletal muscle. A skeletal muscle consists of bundles of muscle fibers called fasciculi. In turn, each fasciculus consists of a bundle of elongate muscle fibers (cells). Within the muscle cell are longitudinal units, the myofibrils, which, in turn, are made up of myofilaments of two types: myosin (thick) filaments and actin (thin) filaments. The myofilaments are organized in a specific manner that impart to the myofibril and, in turn, to the fiber, a cross-striated appearance. The functionally significant repeating unit of the myofibril is the sarcomere; it extends from one Z disc to the next Z disc. The A band marks the extent of the myosin filaments. Actin filaments extend from the Z band into the region of the A band, where they interdigitate with the myosin filaments as shown in the illustration. Items 1 to 4 show cross-sections through different regions of the sarcomere: **(1)** through actin filaments of the I band; **(2)** through myosin filaments of the H band; **(3)** through the center of the A band where adjacent myofilaments are linked to form the M line; and **(4)** where actin and myosin filaments interdigitate in the A band, each myosin filament is within the center of a hexagonal array of actin filaments. Actin filaments can be broken down into globular actin molecules. Myosin filaments consist of myosin molecules; each one can be further broken down to a light and heavy meromyosin. (From Bloom W, Fawcett DW: *A Textbook of Histology,* 10th ed. Philadelphia, WB Saunders, 1975.)

croscope. In turn, the myofibrils are comprised largely of two populations of myofilaments, namely *myosin,* which appears in the electron microscope as *thick filaments,* and *actin,* which appears as *thin filaments.* It is the relationship and alignment of the thick and thin filaments that are responsible for the characteristic banding pattern of striated muscle. Since the myofibrils are aligned and in register, the banding patterns established within the individual myofibrils are seen as the striations across the muscle fiber.

The cross-striations of a muscle fiber, which are most readily seen in a stained section with the light microscope, are the *A band,* the *I band,* and the *Z line.* The A band stains more intensely than the I band. The Z line is actually a disc, which appears as a dark line bisecting the I band. It may be possible also to discern an H band bisecting the A band and an *M line* bisecting the *H band.* However, the H band and M line are demonstrated best in electron micrographs, such as that shown in the Atlas section, Plate 28. As already mentioned, the cross-banding pattern of striated muscle is due largely to the arrangement of the two kinds of myofilaments, and this arrangement now needs to be considered in more functional terms in order to understand the mechanism of contraction.

The Sarcomere. The functional unit of the myofibril is the sarcomere. This is the segment of the myofibril between two Z lines. The thick filaments are located within the sarcomere; they mark the extent of the A band: they are equidistant from the Z lines. The thin filaments are joined to the Z lines; they extend through the I band, where they are the only myofilaments present, and then partially into the A band, where they interdigitate with the thick filaments. Also to be noted is that in a longitudinal section of a sarcomere, the Z disc appears as a zigzag line with a matrix material, the Z matrix, bisecting the zigzag. The Z disc and its matrix material are construed to be skeletal or structural and the thin filaments are anchored to the angles of the zigzag. Cross-sections through different parts of the sarcomere provide additional information regarding the organization of myofilaments. Thus, a cross-section through the I band region shows only thin filaments (① in Fig. 10.3) and they are arranged in a hexagonal pattern. A section through the H portion of the A bands shows only thick filaments (② in Fig. 10.3). A cross-section through the M band shows a network presumably, binding the thick filaments together (③ in Fig. 10.3). The site where the thick and thin filaments interact in the sarcomere, namely the A band, reveals the spatial relationship between the two filaments (④ in Fig. 10.3). Note that here each

thick filament is surrounded by six thin filaments. This is one of the essential structural features of the sliding filament mechanism of contraction.

Sliding Filament Mechanism of Contraction

The basis for contraction resides in the interaction of thick and thin filaments so that the thin filaments are made to move past the thick filaments toward the center of the sarcomere. As they do so, the length of the sarcomere is shortened and each successive sarcomere is simultaneously shortened. The thin filaments are made up of *F-actin, tropomyosin,* and *troponin;* the thick filaments are made up of myosin molecules with a head at one end. When the myosin molecules are assembled into a filament, the heads project outward to form crossbridges that connect with and move the actin filaments during contraction. In the absence of calcium, the tropomyosin and troponin form a complex that prevents a linkage between the actin and myosin (Fig. 10.4, left panel). When calcium is present, a repositioning of the troponin-tropomyosin occurs, thereby allowing for contact between the myosin and actin, "bending" of the myosin head, and movement of the actin filament (Fig. 10.4, right panel). Since the action of one myosin head can account for movement of less than 10 nm, it is concluded that a series of repetitive interactions between myosin and actin occur to bring about the observed shortening of the sarcomere. The distance between the thin and thick myofilaments is increased during the contraction of the muscle and this accounts for the bulging of the contracting muscle (Fig. 10.5). The energy for the bending of the myosin molecule is provided by adenosine triphosphate (ATP). ATP is involved not only in the process of contraction, but also in relaxation. Without ATP, the actin and myosin filaments remain bound and the muscle cannot relax. It is the unavailability of ATP that accounts for the rigidity, called *rigor mortis,* after death.

Sarcoplasmic Reticulum and T Tubules

Calcium must be available for the reaction between actin and myosin, that is, it must be available for contraction to occur and, after contraction, the calcium must be removed. This rapid delivery and removal of calcium is accomplished by the combined work of the endoplasmic reticulum, also called the *sarcoplasmic reticulum* in muscle cells, and the plasma membrane. The sarcoplasmic reticulum is arranged in networks around or between a group of myofilaments (such a group of myofila-

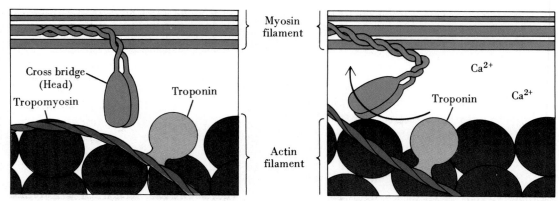

Figure 10.4. Diagram of the sliding filament mechanism of contraction. During relaxation (left), tropomyosin blocks the active site on actin (hatched area) and prevents interaction with the myosin crossbridge. During contraction (right panel) the configuration of the troponin is altered by calcium ions. This causes tropomyosin to move away from the active site on actin and allows the actin and myosin head to interact at the now exposed active site on actin. The movement of many cross-bridges (only one is shown) causes the actin filament to "slide" along the length of the myosin filaments. The ratcheting process is repeated many times during a single contraction, thereby causing a shortening of the individual sarcomeres. (From Ganong WF: *Review of Medical Physiology*, 9th ed. Los Altos, CA, Lange, 1979.)

ments is recognized as a myofibril with the light microscope). In the most highly developed arrangements, one network of sarcoplasmic reticulum surrounds the A band and another network surrounds the I band (Fig. 10.6). Where the two networks meet, at the junction between A and I

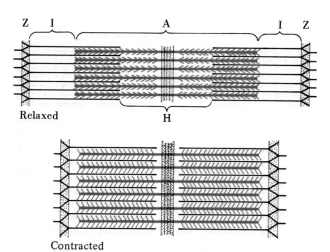

Figure 10.5. Relaxed and contracted sarcomere. In the relaxed state, interdigitation of actin and myosin filaments is not complete; the H band and I bands are relatively wide. During contraction, the interdigitation of the actin and myosin filaments is increased according to the degree of contraction. The length of the A band remains the same; the length of the H and I bands is diminished, again in proportion to the degree of contraction. (Based on Schultz E, Leblond CP: In Ham AW, Cormack DH (eds): *Histology*, 8th ed: Philadelphia, JB Lippincott, 1979.)

bands, the sarcoplasmic reticulum forms a slightly more regular ring-like channel around the filaments of the myofibril, called the **terminal sac.** Between the two facing terminal sacs an invagination of the plasma membrane forms an additional tubule, called the **transverse** or **tubule.** Together, the T tubule and the two contiguous terminal sacs constitute the **triads** seen with the transmission electron microscope. The T tubules provide for the rapid transmission of the surface membrane excitation to the terminal sacs throughout the thickness of the muscle fiber. In turn, the terminal sacs release and then reaccumulate calcium according to messages provided by the T tubules (see Fig. 10.9). Also located between the myofibrils are large numbers of mitochondria, which provide energy for the reactions involved in contraction. Glycogen granules, a reserve form of energy, are also located in the region between the myofibrils.

Motor End Plate

The junctional site that includes the axonal ending of a motor neuron and the receptor region of the striated muscle fiber that it innervates is referred to as the **motor end plate** (Fig. 10.7). The myelin cover of the axon terminates just before the axon reaches the motor end plate. The axon is, however, still covered by Schwann cells, here also referred to as **teloglia.** The axon terminal lies in a depression or groove in the muscle cell, called the **neuromuscular synaptic clefts** (Fig. 10.8). The axon terminal contains numerous synaptic vesicles and

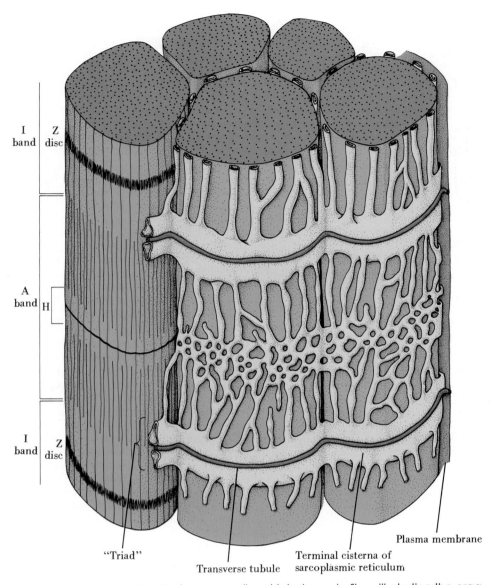

I band | Z disc

A band | H

I band | Z disc

"Triad"

Transverse tubule

Terminal cisterna of sarcoplasmic reticulum

Plasma membrane

Figure 10.6. Diagram of part of a mammalian striated muscle fiber, illustrating the organization of the sarcoplasmic reticulum and its relationship to the myofibrils. In the myofibril at the left, the A, I, and H bands and the Z lines are indicated. The sarcoplasmic reticulum is shown surrounding the myofibrils at the middle and right of the illustration. Note that in mammalian striated muscle fibers two transverse (T) tubules supply a sarcomere. Each T tubule is located at the A–I band junction, where it is associated with two terminal cisternae of the sarcoplasmic reticulum, one cisterna on either side of the T tubule. The triple structure as seen in cross-section, where the two terminal cisternae flank a transverse tubule at the A–I junction, is referred to as a triad. (Based on Leblond CP: In Ham AW, Cormack DH (eds): *Histology,* 8th ed. Philadelphia, JB Lippincott, 1979.)

mitochondria; the sarcoplasm in the receptor region of the muscle fiber also contains numerous mitochondria. In this same region, many narrow furrows, referred to as **subneural clefts,** are formed by folds of the sarcolemma. These junctional folds increase the receptor surface of the muscle. The basal lamina extends into the neuromuscular synaptic cleft and also into the subneural clefts. The synaptic vesicles release acetylcholine into the cleft; it reacts with specific acetylcholine receptors on the sarcolemma and initiates the processes leading to muscle contraction. Acetylcholinesterase quickly inactivates the acetylcholine to prevent continued stimulation.

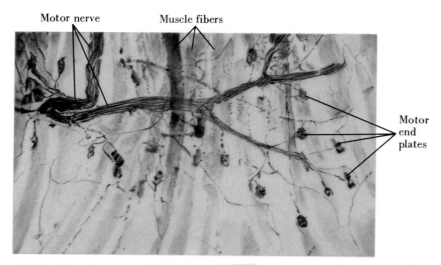

Figure 10.7. Drawing of a silver preparation showing a motor nerve and its final branchings which lead to the motor end plates. The skeletal muscle fibers are oriented vertically in the field. The motor nerve is vertically disposed where it enters the field in the upper left; it then turns and is horizontally disposed.

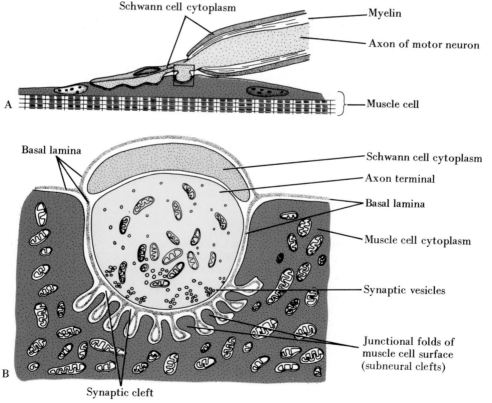

Figure 10.8. Diagram of neuromuscular junction. In **(A)** an axon is shown making contact with the muscle cell. An area similar to the one shown in the small rectangle is diagrammed at higher magnification in **(B)**. Note how the junctional folds of the muscle cell augment the surface area within the synaptic cleft. The basal lamina extends throughout the cleft area. The cytoplasm of the Schwann cell is shown covering the axon terminal. (Based on Couteaux R: In Ham AW, Cormack DH (eds): *Histology,* 8th ed. Philadelphia, JB Lippincott, 1979.)

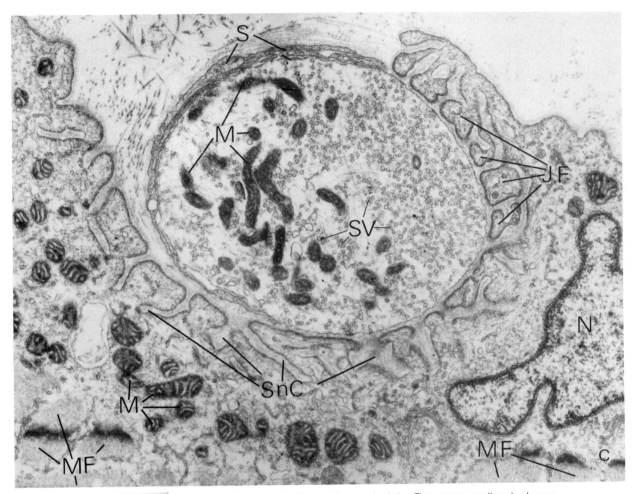

Figure 10.8. (C). Electron micrograph of a motor end plate. The axon ending is shown here within the synaptic cleft of a skeletal muscle fiber. It reveals an aggregation of mitochondria (M) and numerous synaptic vesicles (SV). The portion of the motor axon ending that is not in apposition with the muscle fiber is covered by Schwann cell cytoplasm (S), but no myelin is present. The muscle fiber shows the junctional folds (JF) and the subneural clefts (SnC) between them. The basal lamina of the muscle fiber is barely evident within the subneural clefts. Other structures present are the aggregated mitochondria of the muscle fiber (M) in the region of the end plate, a nucleus (N) of the muscle fiber, and some myofibrils (MF). Courtesy of George D. Pappas.

In *myasthenia gravis,* and autoimmune disease characterized by extreme muscular weakness, the acetylcholine receptors on the sarcolemma become blocked by antibodies. The number of functional receptor sites thus is reduced and the muscle fiber then can respond to the nerve stimulus in only a feeble manner.

Summary of Events Leading to Contraction of Skeletal Muscle

The event that leads to the contraction of a skeletal muscle fiber is the arrival of nerve impulses at the neuromuscular junction, that is, the motor end plate (Fig. 10.9. The numbers in parentheses below refer to the numbers in Fig. 10.9). The nerve cell conducting these impulses is called a motor neuron. The cell body of this neuron is within the spinal cord (or in the brain stem). It sends a long cytoplasmic process, called the axon or nerve fiber, to the skeletal muscle where the axon branches to innervate several muscle fibers (Fig. 10.7). The nerve impulses are measured as an action potential of the nerve fiber (1). The nerve impulses are transmitted to the muscle cell (2) and this results in a depolarization of the plasma membrane and in the generation of an action potential by the membrane of the muscle cell (3). The depo-

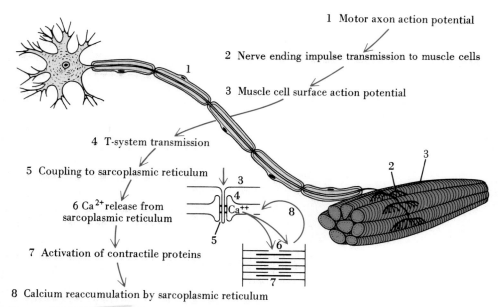

Figure 10.9. Diagram showing summary of events leading to contraction of skeletal muscle and the sites where these occur. See the text section for a description of the events indicated by the numerals. (Based on Peachey LD: In: *Bicore* XVIII. New York, McGraw-Hill, 1974.)

larization action potential spreads over the muscle cell and continues via the T tubules into the substance of the muscle cell (4). At the muscle cell triads, the T tubules are in close contact with enlargements of the sarcoplasmic reticulum and, at this point, the excited (depolarized) T tubule membrane (5) causes calcium to be released from the sarcoplasmic reticulum into the cytoplasmic matrix (6). The calcium then activates the contractile proteins (7) as outlined above and contraction ensues. The calcium is returned to the cisterns of the sarcoplasmic reticulum (8) at the end of these events.

Neuromuscular Spindle

The *neuromuscular spindle* is a receptor unit in a muscle consisting of special muscle fibers and neuron terminals surrounded by a capsule (Fig. 10.10). A large fluid-filled space separates the special muscle cells and the capsule. Two kinds of muscle cells are found within the spindle: *nuclear bag fibers* and *nuclear chain fibers.* A typical spindle may have four nuclear bag fibers and twice as many nuclear chain fibers. A nuclear bag fiber is expanded in the midregion to accommodate an aggregate of nuclei; a nuclear chain fiber contains nuclei in a chain. The nuclear bag fiber is contacted by neuron terminals (primary afferent endings) that spiral around it; the nuclear chain fiber receives primary afferent spiral nerve endings about its midregion and secondary afferent nerve

endings on each end of the fiber. Both nuclear bag and nuclear chain, fibers also receive an efferent innervation by nerve fibers designated as *gamma fibers.* Functionally, the muscle spindle responds to stretch, and it is the receptor for the two-neuron stretch reflex (e.g., the knee jerk reflex). The muscle spindle also functions in a more complex manner in the control of coordinated muscle contraction.

Tendon Organs

Tendon organs are encapsulated nerve endings in the tendon of the muscle and they respond to stretch. Unlike the muscle spindle, which contains both afferent and efferent endings, the tendon organ contains only afferent endings.

CARDIAC MUSCLE

It was long ago established with the light microscope that cardiac muscle consists of long fibers that, like skeletal muscle, are cross-striated. The cross-striations are due to the arrangement of thick and thin filaments attached to Z discs in a manner similar to that of skeletal muscle. The cardiac muscle also contains special cross-bands, the *intercalated discs,* which are not present in skeletal muscle (Fig. 10.11). With the electron microscope, the intercalated discs have been shown to be end-to-end junctions between individual cardiac muscle cells

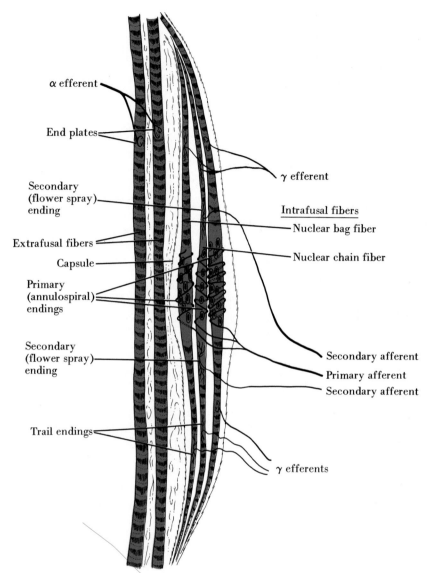

α efferent

End plates

Secondary (flower spray) ending

γ efferent

Intrafusal fibers

Nuclear bag fiber

Extrafusal fibers

Nuclear chain fiber

Capsule

Primary (annulospiral) endings

Secondary (flower spray) ending

Secondary afferent

Primary afferent

Secondary afferent

Trail endings

γ efferents

Figure 10.10. Schematic diagram of a muscle spindle illustrating the innervation of the nuclear bag fibers and nuclear chain fibers, as determined from muscles of the cat. There are up to 12 intrafusal fibers (up to 10 of these being of the nuclear chain type); only two nuclear bag fibers and one nuclear chain fiber are shown here for clarity. The afferent nerve fibers supplying the spindle are classified as primary afferents and secondary afferents. See text for further details. The β-innervation has been omitted and the diameter of the spindle was expanded in order to show details. (From Ham AW, Cormack DH: *Histology,* 8th ed. Philadelphia, JB Lippincott, 1979.)

(see Atlas Section, Plate 35). Thus, unlike skeletal muscle in which the muscle fiber is a single multinucleated protoplasmic unit, in cardiac muscle the muscle fiber consists of numerous mononucleated cells aligned end-to-end. Some cells in a fiber may join with two other cells (rather than a single cell); thus, creating a branching of the fiber.

The cardiac muscle cell contains numerous large mitochondria, frequently a full sarcomere in length. It also contains a well-developed sarcoplasmic reticulum. However, the sarcoplasmic reticulum does not display a well-organized association with the system of T tubules, and so triads similar to those of skeletal muscle are not common. The T

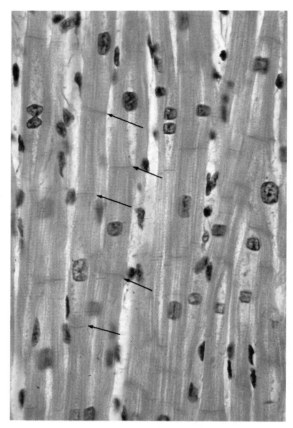

Figure 10.11. Photomicrograph of longitudinally sectioned cardiac muscle. The **arrows** point to the intercalated discs. The discs represent specialized end-to-end junctions of adjoining cells. Also note the apparent branching of the muscle fibers.

system (Fig. 10.12) also differs from that of skeletal muscle in that it is made up of tubules that have a large diameter and surround the myofibrils at the level of the Z bands. The basal (or external) lamina adheres to the invaginated sarcolemma of the T tubule as it penetrates into the substance of the muscle. T tubules are regularly found in the muscle cells of the ventricles, but they are sparse or absent in the cells of the atria.

Mitochondria and sarcoplasmic reticulum are located between the myofibrils, but they do not always totally surround the myofibrils. In many places, myofilaments of one myofibril are continuous with myofilaments of adjacent myofibrils.

Whereas nuclei of skeletal muscle cells are usually under the sarcolemma, at the periphery of the cell, those of cardiac muscle are situated more in the center of the cell; cardiac muscle cells may be binucleate. The myofilaments separate to bypass the nucleus and thereby outline a juxtanuclear region of sarcoplasm; this region is rich in mitochon-

dria and contains a Golgi apparatus, pigment granules (lipofuscin), and glycogen. In the atria, but not in the ventricles, the juxtanuclear region contains atrial granules (0.3 to 0.4 μm in diameter). Recent evidence indicates that they have an endocrine function regulating the renal excretion of sodium.

Mature cardiac muscle cells do not divide and thus destroyed cells are not replaced by new cells. An injury to cardiac muscle tissue is repaired by the formation of fibrous connective tissue.

The innervation of cardiac muscle and the special properties of the intrinsic conducting system are described in Chapter 12.

SMOOTH MUSCLE

Smooth muscle consists of fusiform cells that range in length from 20 μm in the walls of small blood vessels to as much as 200 μm in other locations. The cells, also called fibers, are thickest in their midregion and taper at each end (Fig. 10.13). As in striated muscle, the contractile elements are myofilaments, but they are not arranged in the ordered, paracrystalline manner of those in striated muscle; there are no sarcomeres. In a standard electron micrograph only one type of contractile filament, the thin (actin) filament, is evident (Fig. 10.14). However, in appropriately prepared specimens thick (myosin) filaments and also intermediate filaments can be displayed. Moreover, actin and myosin can be isolated chemically from smooth muscle cells and a sliding filament mechanism is evidently operational in the contraction of this muscle. The myofilaments of smooth muscle occupy large regions of the smooth muscle cell. Interspersed among the myofilaments and on the inner surface of the plasma membrane are irregular electron-dense areas. The dense areas, usually referred to as *cytoplasmic densities* or *dense bodies,* contain a protein, α-*actinin,* which is also found in the Z discs of striated muscle. Together, the intermediate filaments and dense bodies are thought to serve a skeletal function like that of the Z disc of striated muscle. In support of this concept is the finding that the dense bodies, when observed in the electron microscope, sometimes appear as linear structures. Moreover, in some fortuitous sections, they exhibit a branching configuration consistent with a three-dimensional anastomosing network that extends from the sarcolemma into the interior of the cell (Fig. 10.15).

Although the smooth muscle cells have no T system, they do have large numbers of pinocytotic vesicles associated with the sarcolemma and with the sarcoplasmic reticulum. The vesicles and the

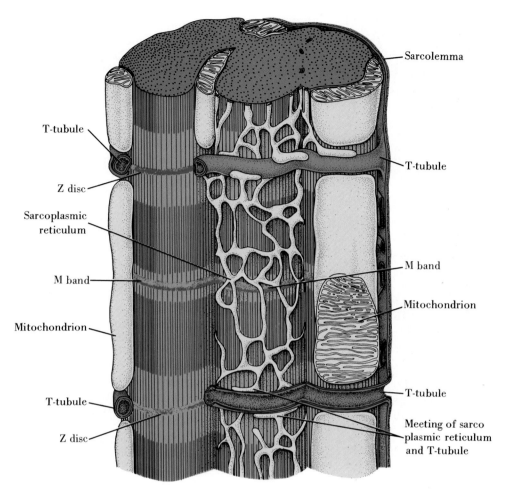

Figure 10.12. Organization of mammalian ventricular cardiac muscle fiber. The transverse tubules are much larger than the T tubules of skeletal muscle and carry an investment of basal lamina material into the cell. They also differ in that they are located at the level of the Z disc. The portion of the sarcoplasmic reticulum adjacent to the T tubule is not in the form of an expanded cisterna, but rather it is organized as an anastomosing network. (From Fawcett DW, McNutt S: *J Cell Biol* 42:1, 1969.)

sarcoplasmic reticulum have been shown to sequester calcium.

In the sarcoplasm adjacent to each nuclear pole, there are numerous mitochondria, some rough endoplasmic reticulum (rER), free ribosomes, glycogen, and a small Golgi apparatus. Smooth muscle cells make contact with neighboring cells by gap junctions. The gap junction between two smooth muscle cells was originally designated as a **nexus;** that term is still in use today.

Smooth muscle is innervated by postganglionic neurons of the autonomic nervous system. The nerve fibers pass among the smooth muscle cells, and enlargements in the passing nerve fiber occur adjacent to those muscle cells that are to be innervated. The enlargements contain synaptic vesicles with neuromuscular transmitters. The neuromuscular contact is not comparable to the motor end plate of striated muscle. Rather, a considerable distance, usually 10 to 20 μm, but in some locations up to 200 μ, may separate the nerve terminal and the smooth muscle. The neurotransmitter released by the nerve terminal needs to diffuse across this distance in order to reach the muscle.

The description of autonomic innervation according to the sympathetic and parasympathetic classification and their respective adrenergic and cholinergic transmitters may be more complex than traditionally thought. Viewed in the electron microscope, nerve terminals with empty-appearing synaptic vesicles are interpreted to be cholinergic,

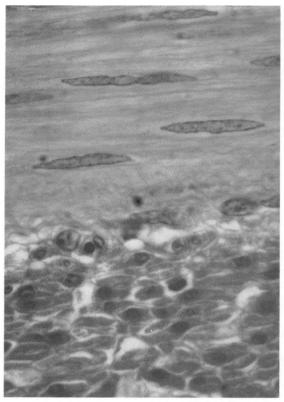

Figure 10.13. Photomicrograph of smooth muscle from the small intestine. The muscle is arranged in two layers. The upper portion of the micrograph shows the muscle cells cut in longitudinal section. Where the cells are cross-sectioned, some have the nucleus included in the plane of section, whereas others do not. This is a reflection of the much greater length of the cell compared to its width. Note, it is usually the smaller cross-section profiles that lack the nucleus. They represent the tapering ends of the muscle cells. Also note that the longitudinal smooth muscle cells are not easily delineated from one another. This is due to the way they lie over one another within the thickness of the section.

secreting the neurotransmitter acetylcholine; those nerve terminals with dense granular material in the synaptic vesicles are interpreted to be adrenergic, secreting the neurotransmitter norepinephrine. Other transmitters have also been identified, but they are not as well understood as the two mentioned. They have been collectively grouped under the heading of *purinergic,* and they are likely to consist of large vesicles with an opaque content. Nerve endings in smooth muscle tissue that contain primarily mitochondria and no vesicles are construed to be sensory. Both sympa-

thetic and parasympathetic fibers innervate smooth muscle and it is most difficult to distinguish between the fibers. Autonomic fibers are efferent. In some smooth muscle, the adrenergic transmitters stimulate and the cholinergic transmitters inhibit contraction; in other smooth muscle, the reverse is true.

The contractions of smooth muscle cells are much slower and generate much less tension than the contractions of striated muscle. In most organs, the smooth muscle cells appear to act as though they were made up of functionally connected sheets or bundles. Such functional groups are poorly innervated and not every cell is contacted by an efferent nerve ending. However, the gap junctions that join the cells are thought to connect the cells into functional groups. In other organs, such as the ductus deferens, even though there are gap junctions, each cell is contracted by an efferent nerve ending.

Smooth muscle cells are surrounded by a basal (or external) lamina except at the nexus. The smooth muscle cells produce the basal lamina. They also produce the collagen and elastic material that surrounds them in certain locations, such as in the walls of blood vessels. Smooth muscle cells in some locations are capable of division (for example, in the uterus), but generally the regenerative capacity of smooth muscle is limited. Large areas of destroyed smooth muscle are usually repaired by scar formation.

OTHER CONTRACTILE CELLS

In addition to the striated and smooth muscle cells that have been recognized traditionally as comprising muscular tissue, there are cells in other tissues that have contractile properties. These include myofibroblasts, myoepithelial cells, myoid cells of the testis, and cells of the perineurium. Each of these contain myofilaments as a notable feature of the cytoplasm, yet these cells are not classified as muscular tissue. Myofibroblasts are not surrounded by a basal lamina and, for this and other reasons, they can be considered to be cells of the connective tissue. Myoepithelial cells are found in sweat glands, mammary glands, salivary glands, and the iris; they are components of the epithelial tissue. The comparative anatomy of the myoid cells of the testis indicates that they have a special functional and structural relationship to the seminiferous tubules. The perineurium consists of cells with morphological and histochemical features that indicate that they function as contractile-transport-barrier cells.

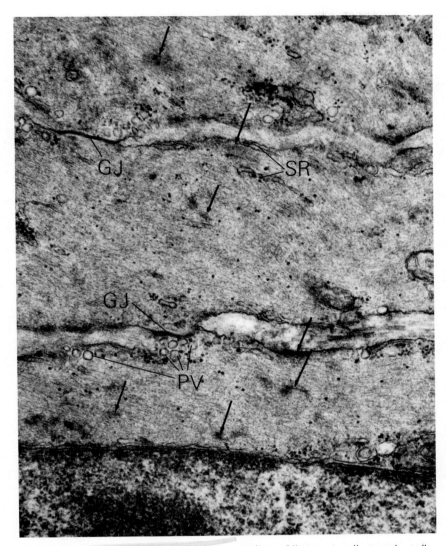

Figure 10.14. Electron micrograph of a portion of three smooth muscle cells. The nucleus of one cell is the lower part of the micrograph. The bulk of the cytoplasm is occupied by actin filaments, which are just recognizable at this magnification. The α-actinin-containing dense areas are indicated by the **arrows.** Elements of the sarcoplasmic reticulum (SR) and the pinocytotic vesicles (PV) are also indicated. The small dark particles are glycogen. Lastly, the presence of a gap junction (GJ), or nexus, between each of the cells can also be seen, $\times$ 30,000.

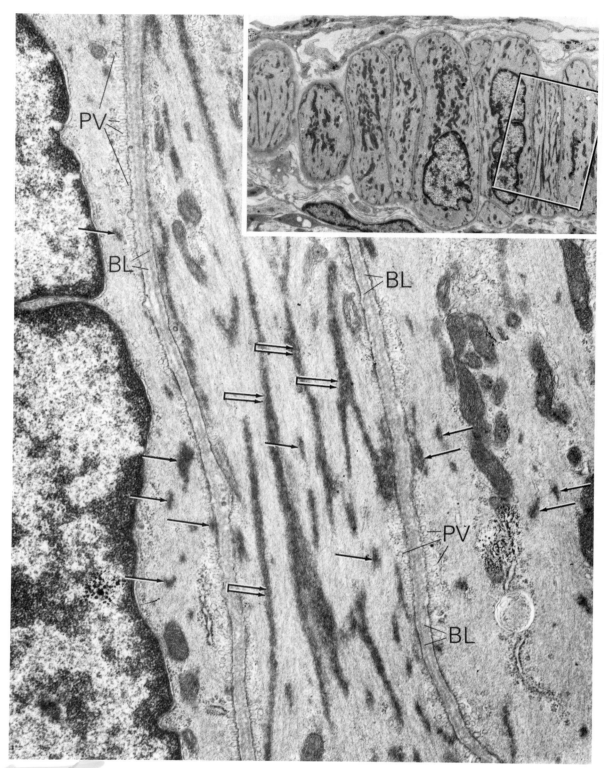

Figure 10.15. Electron showing the cytoplasmic densities in vascular smooth muscle cells. The plane of section includes only the smooth muscle cells in the wall of the vessel (see **inset**). The **rectangle** in the **inset** shows portions of three smooth muscle cells that appear at higher magnification in the large micrograph. The α-actinin containing cytoplasmic densities (**single arrows**) usually appear as irregular masses, some of which are in contact with and attached to the sarcolemma. The cell in the center of the micrograph has been cut in a plane closer to the cell surface and reveals these same densities as a branching structure (**double arrows**). A three-dimensional model of the cytoplasmic densities would reveal an anastomosing network. BL, basal (external) lamina; P, pinocytotic vesicles. ×30,000; **inset**, ×4000.

ATLAS PLATES

27–36

PLATE 27. Skeletal Muscle

Skeletal muscle cells, also called fibers, are long multinucleated protoplasmic units arranged in parallel with their neighbors. Their multiple nuclei are at the periphery of the cell, just under the plasma membrane (sarcolemma). The main volume of the cell is occupied by the contractile elements and these have a very orderly and specific relationship to each other. The organization of contractile filaments is particularly well-ordered and their specific arrangement accounts for the cross-striations seen in a longitudinal section of the skeletal muscle fibers and is also the basis for their familiar name, ***striated muscle.*** Skeletal muscle is richly supplied with blood and each fiber is usually in proximity to several capillaries.

A section of skeletal muscle fibers in longitudinal profile is shown in **Figure 1.** Note the parallel alignment of the fibers (**M**); they are vertically oriented in the illustration. The fibers appear to be of different thickness. This is largely a reflection of the cross-sectioned aspect of the muscle fibers. For example, note the polygonal shape of the fibers when cross-sectioned, as in **Figures 2 and 3.** By drawing a random imaginary line across either micrograph, as if the line were the plane of a longitudinal section, considerable variation would occur with respect to the width of each fiber included in the section. Some fibers might be sectioned along their broadest dimension, some at their narrowest dimension, and others at a variety of intermediate dimensions.

The cross-striations are the bands that appear at right angles to the long axis of the fibers. They are seen at higher magnification in the circular **inset.** Two major bands, the darker or more heavily stained A band and the lighter I band, have been labeled. In addition, the **inset** shows a thin line that bisects the I band; this is the Z line. The other bands, that is, the M and H bands, are not evident despite the relaxed state of the muscle fibers. (The relatively wide I band is an indicator of the relaxed state of the muscle.)

Examination of the cytoplasm about the nucleus in the **inset** reveals that the cross-striations do not extend into the cytoplasmic areas adjacent to the nuclear poles. This cytoplasm stains lightly (**asterisk**) and contains a concentration of organelles not directly involved in the contractile process.

Between the muscle fibers is a small amount of delicate connective tissue, the ***endomysium.*** Also to be noted in **Figure 1** are two capillaries (**C**) within the endomysium. While they do not display the structural features of the vessel walls, they can be identified by virtue of the red blood cells in the lumen. The nuclei directly associated with the capillary belong to endothelial cells. Note how they appear to bulge into the lumen (see **inset**).

A cross-section of striated muscle cells is shown in **Figure 2.** As already noted, the muscle fibers, (**M**) appears as polygonal profiles. They are partially outlined by numerous nuclei, however, at the relatively low magnification shown in **Figure 2** it is not easy to ascertain if these nuclei belong to the muscle cells, to the capillary endothelial cells, to the satellite cells, or to the fibroblasts in the endomysium, which surrounds the individual muscle cells. A larger amount of connective tissue (**CT**) separates bundles of muscle fibers; this connective tissue is called ***perimysium;*** it contains small arteries and veins (**BV**).

Several cross-sectioned muscle cells are shown at higher magnification in **Figure 3.** The nuclei (**N**) that bulge into the cytoplasm belong to the muscle cell. (However, it should be noted that some nuclei in this position may belong to satellite cells. These are undifferentiated cells on the muscle side of the basal lamina and they cannot be definitely identified in H&E sections.) This higher magnification also reveals numerous ring-like structures (**asterisks**) in the endomysium; these are "empty" capillaries. Other capillaries have been cut more obliquely or longitudinally; these contain red blood cells (**arrows**). During maximal muscular activity, the capillaries are all patent; in a less active state, only some of the capillaries are patent at a particular time.

The striated muscle cell contains longitudinal units called ***myofibrils*** (see Atlas section, Plate 29). The cut ends of the myofibrils (sarcostyles) account for the stippled appearance seen in the cross-sectioned muscle cells in **Figure 3.**

KEY

A, A band
BV, blood vessels (small artery and vein)
C, capillary
CT, connective tissue (perimysium surrounding muscle fascicles)
arrows, red blood cells in capillaries
asterisks, Fig. 1, myofibril free region of cytoplasm
asterisks, Fig. 3, empty capillaries

I, I band
M, muscle fiber
N, nuclei of muscle cells
Z, Z line

Fig. 1, × 400
Fig. 2, × 260

Fig. 3, × 640.

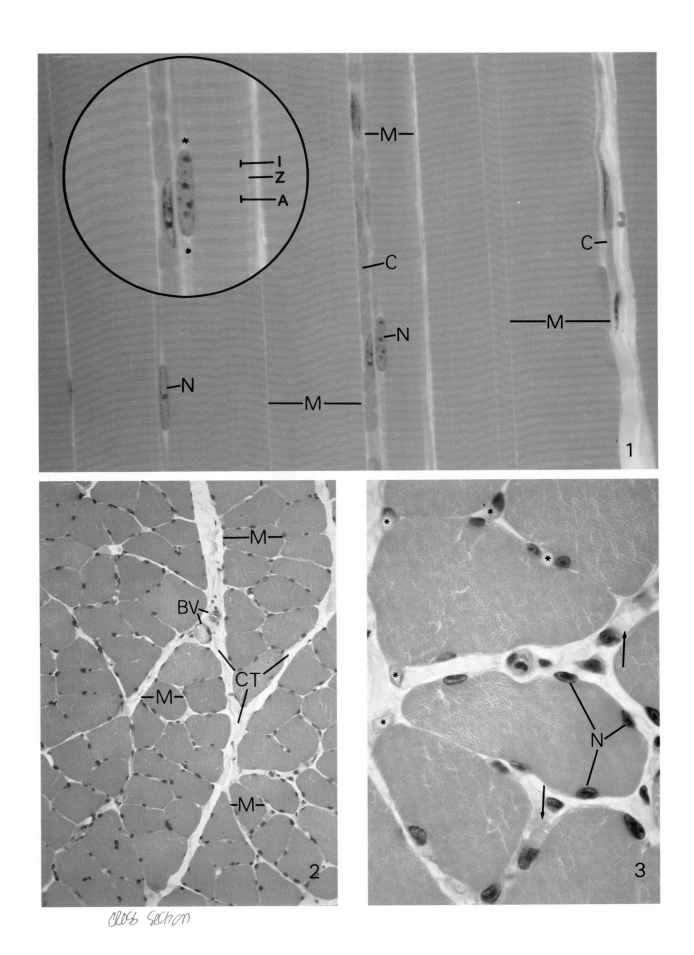

cross section

PLATE 28. Skeletal Muscle I, Electron Microscopy

The cytological organization and functional units of the skeletal muscle cell are revealed in this low power electron micrograph. For purposes of orientation it should be noted that only a small portion of two muscle cells (fibers) are included in the micrograph. Both are seen in longitudinal profile. One of the sectioned muscle cells occupies the upper two-thirds of the figure and reveals a nucleus (**N**) at its periphery. Below, and largely covered by the **inset,** is part of the second muscle cell. The connective tissue in the extracellular space between the two cells, that is, the collagen fibrils (**Col**) and fibroblast (**Fib**), constitutes the endomysium of the muscle.

The individual myofibrils (**Myf**), which were not perceptible in the light micrograph, are clearly seen here in longitudinal profile. The myofibrils, which are more or less cylindrical structures, extend across the micrograph. Each is separated from neighboring myofibrils by a thin sheath of surrounding sarcoplasm (**Sp**).

Each repeating part of Z lines (from the German *zwischenscheibe,* "intercalated line") in a striated muscle fiber represents a sarcomere. In the electron micrograph shown here two sarcomeres (**S**), one following the other but in adjacent myofibrils, have been marked. Each sarcomere extends from one Z line, the thin dark line, to the next Z line. The essential features of a sarcomere are shown at higher magnification in the **inset.** Here, the filamentous nature of the myofibrils is evident. For example, the I (isotropic) band, which is bisected by the Z line, is seen to consist of thin (5 nm) barely visible filaments. The thin filaments, which are composed of actin, are joined to the Z line and extend across the I band into the A (anisotropic) band. The thick filaments, composed of myosin, account for the full width of the A band. In the A band there are additional bands or lines. One of these, the M line (from the German *mitte,* "middle"), is seen at the middle of the A band. This line appears to be due to the presence of a substance which binds the thick filaments to one another. A

second subband within the A band is the H band (from the German *helle,* "light"). This band appears as the less dense segment within the A band and it consists of only myosin filaments. The lateral segments (**double-headed arrows**) of the A band are rather dense. This more dense-appearing area is a reflection of the extent to which the actin filaments have extended into the A band and interdigitated with the thick filaments. Because contraction involves the interdigitation of the thick and thin filaments, increasing degrees of contraction result in continued narrowing of the I and H bands. Inasmuch as the individual thick filaments do not change in length, the width of the A band is always the same.

The cross-banded pattern that characterizes the striated muscle fiber is a reflection of the arrangement, in register, of the individual myofibrils. Additionally, the cross-banded pattern of the myofibril is a reflection of the arrangement, in register, of the myofilaments (**inset**). The in-register arrangement of myofibrils is an important feature relating to impulse propagation within the cell; this is considered in Atlas section, Plate 29.

KEY

A, A band
I, I band
H, H band
M, M band
Z, Z line
CM, cell membrane (sarcolemma)
Col, collagen fibrils
Fib, fibroblast
Myf, myofibril

N, nucleus
S, sarcomere
Sp, sarcoplasm between adjacent myofibrils
arrowhead, glycogen
double-headed arrow, overleap in A band of thick and thin filaments

Fig., × 6,500 (inset, × 30,000)

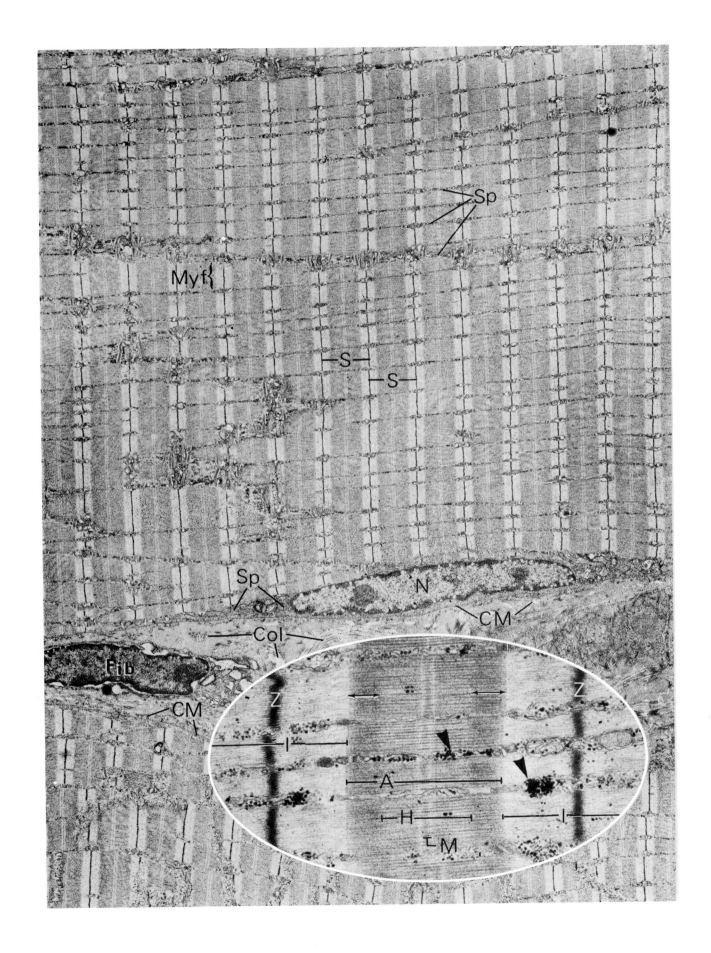

PLATE 29. Skeletal Muscle II, Electron Microscopy

The electron micrograph shown here illustrates the nature of the sarcoplasm, especially the membrane system that pervades it. It also again demonstrates the filamentous components that make up the myofibril.

The muscle fiber is longitudinally sectioned, but it has been turned so that the direction of the fiber has a vertical orientation. The various bands and lines of a single sarcomere are labeled in the myofibril on the left of the illustration. The thin actin filaments are especially well resolved in the I band in the lower left corner and easily can be compared with the thicker myosin filaments of the A band. The point of juncture or insertion of the actin filaments into the Z line is also readily apparent.

In contrast to the relatively nondescript character of the sarcoplasm as seen in the light microscope, the electron microscope reveals a well-developed membrane system called the sarcoplasmic reticulum **(SR).** The reticulum consists of segments of anastomosing tubules that form a network around each myofibril. The electron micrograph here fortuitously depicts a relatively wide area of sarcoplasm in a plane between two myofibrils. Prominent in this area are numerous glycogen particles **(G).** Somewhat less apparent but nevertheless evident are the anastomosing tubules of the sarcoplasmic reticulum **(SR).** Near the junction of the A and I bands the tubules of the reticulum become confluent, forming flattened sac-like structures, the terminal cisternae. These cisternae come in proximity to another membrane system, the T (transverse) system.

The *T system* consists of tubular structures **(T),** each tubule originating as an invagination of the sarcolemma. The tubules course transversely through the muscle fiber. Because of the uniform register of the myofibrils, each T tubule comes to surround the myofibrils in proximity to the juncture of the A and I bands. In effect, the T system is not simply a straight tubule, but rather it is a grid-like system that surrounds each myofibril at the level of the A-I junction. Thus, in a section passing tangentially to a myofibril, as is seen in the center of the micrograph and in the **upper inset,** the lumen of the T tubules may appear as elongate channels **(arrows)** bound by a pair of membranes. The

inner, facing pair of membranes belongs to the T tubule. The outer membranes, on either side, belong to the terminal cisternae of the sarcoplasmic reticulum. The communication between a terminal cisterna and the tubular portion of the sarcoplasmic reticulum is marked by an **arrowhead** in the **upper inset.** In contrast, a longitudinal section passing through two adjacent myofibrils (see **lower inset**) reveals the T tubule to be flattened with the terminal elements of the sarcoplasmic reticulum **(SR)** on either side. The combination of the T tubule and the adjoining dilated terminal cisternae of the sarcoplasmic reticulum on either side is referred to as a *triad.*

The nature and geometric configuration of the triad helps explain the rapid and uniform contraction of a muscle fiber. It is postulated that the depolarization of the sarcolemma continues along the membranes of the T tubules and thereby results in an inward spread of excitation to reach each myofribil at the A-I junction. This initiates the first stage in the contraction process, that of causing the release of calcium ions from the immediately adjacent terminal cisternae. Relaxation occurs through the recapture of calcium ions by the sarcoplasmic reticulum. In terms of energetics, it is also of interest that the mitochondria **(Mi)** occupy a preferential site in the sarcoplasm, being oriented in a circular fashion around the myofibrils in the region of the I band.

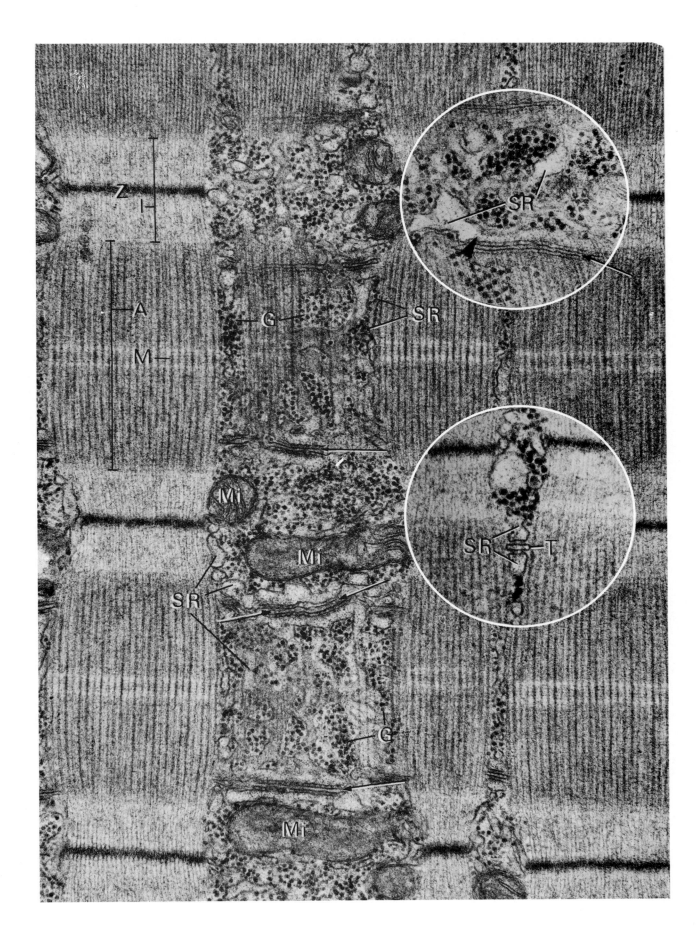

PLATE 30. Musculotendinous Junction & Neuromuscular Junction

Skeletal muscle fibers attach at their ends to collagen fibers. The latter may be part of a tendon, fibrous sheet (aponeurosis), periostium, or a raphe. In a musculotendinous junction as shown in **Figure 1,** the muscle fibers appear to terminate directly on the tendon. The muscle fibers (**M**) are in the left half of the figure. They stain more red than the tendon (**T**), which typically stains in a more pale manner. The skeletal muscle fibers have been cut obliquely and the boundaries between individual muscle cells are not distinct. However, in many places, there is a slight separation of the muscle fibers, and along with the orientation of the muscle cell nuclei, this separation tends to show their general direction. Cross-striations can be identified at right angles to the direction of the fibers. In contrast, the tendon gives no obvious indication of how the collagen fibers are arranged. This needs to be surmised by the direction of the fibroblast nuclei, which usually have their long axis parallel to the direction of the fibers. While the nuclei of the fibroblasts are readily identified, the cytoplasm of these cells is not distinguishable from the collagen of the tendon. At the actual junction between the muscle cell and tendon, the end of the cell becomes serrated and the cytoplasmic projections of the muscle cell interdigitate with the collagen fibrils of the tendon. This arrangement is, at best, only suggested in **Figure 1,** but it is clearly evident in an electron micrograph of the junction (**Fig. 2**).

The electron micrograph shows four finger-like projections of the muscle cell. The basal lamina (**BL**) is directly adjacent to the plasma membrane (**PM**) of the muscle cell and follows the finger-like projections. Actin filaments (**arrows**) of the terminal sarcomeres extend into the finger-like projections and insert into densities on the inner face of the plasma membrane (**arrowheads**). Note that the terminal sarcomeres possess only one Z disc (**ZD**). Also to be seen within the muscle cell cytoplasm are triads (Tr), glycogen granules (G),

and mitochondria (Mi). External to the cell are fibrils of the tendon (T).

A neuromuscular junction is shown in **Figure 3.** A special stain has been used to visualize the neural elements, and in this staining procedure, the skeletal muscle cells are not revealed to best advantage. They are horizontally disposed in the illustration, and in some muscle fibers, cross striations (**arrows**) are visible. The nerve (**N**) enters the field from the left; intitially it dips downward and then it turns in an upward direction. As it does, it can be seen to divide into smaller branches and finally as it nears the muscle cells, the nerve fiber branches to make contact with several muscle cells. At the terminal between nerve fiber and each muscle cell, the nerve fiber arborizes to form a disc-like structure, the motor end plate (**MEP**), on the surface of the muscle cell. The motor end plate is the physiological contact between nerve and muscle; it is in fact a neuromuscular synapse station at which the neurotransmitter acetylcholine is liberated. This transmitter initiates a sequence of muscle membrane events that lead to contraction of the muscle.

KEY	
BL, basal lamina	T, tendon
G, glycogen	Tr, triad
M, striated muscle	ZD, Z disc
MEP, motor end plate	**arrowheads,**
Mi, mitochondria	attachment of actin
N, nerve	filaments into plasma
PM, plasma membrane	membrane
(sarcolemma)	**arrows,** actin filaments
Fig. 1, × 350	Fig. 3, × 280
Fig. 2, × 24,600	

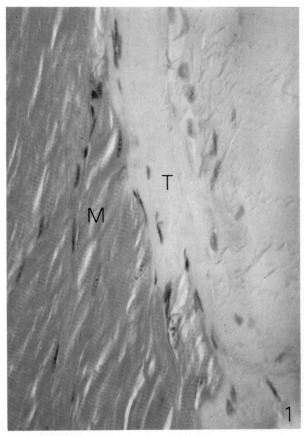

1

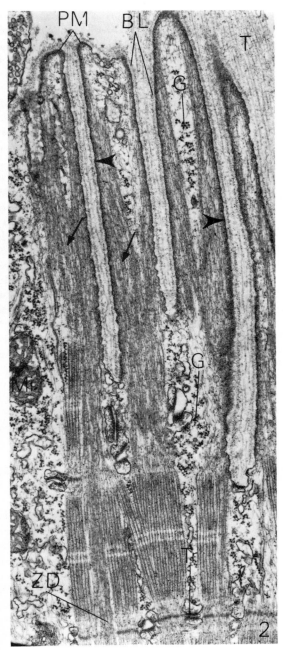

2

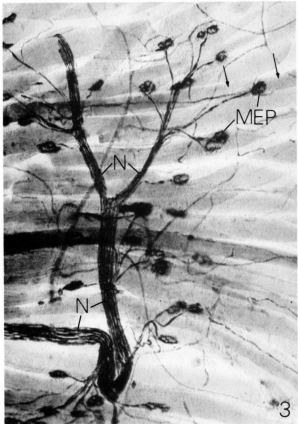

3

PLATE 31. Cardiac Muscle

Cardiac muscle consists of fibers, which possess the same cross-banding patterns that are present in striated skeletal muscle. Thus, it is also striated. However, cardiac muscle differs in many other respects from skeletal muscle. The histologically obvious differences are: The presence of intercalated discs, the location of the cardiac cell nuclei in the center of the fiber, and the branching nature of the muscle fiber. All of these are evident in a well-prepared longitudinal section of the muscle.

Figure 1 shows a longitudinal section of cardiac muscle. The muscle fibers are disposed horizontally in the illustration and they show cross-striations. However, in addition to the regular cross-striations (those of greater frequency), there is another group of very pronounced cross-bands, namely, the intercalated discs (**ID**). Intercalated discs most often appear as a straight band, but sometimes they are arranged in a stepwise manner (see also **Fig. 2** and Atlas section, Plate 32). These discs are not always displayed in routine H&E sections and so, one may not be able to depend on these structures for identifying cardiac muscle. Intercalated discs are opposing cell to cell contacts, thus, cardiac muscle fibers differ in a very fundamental respect from fibers of skeletal muscle. The cardiac muscle fiber consists of an end-to-end alignment of cells; in contrast, the skeletal muscle fiber is a single protoplasmic unit.

In examining a longitudinal section of cardiac muscle, it is useful to scan specific fibers along their long axis. By doing so, one can find places where the fibers obviously branch. Two such branchings are indicated by the **arrows** in **Figure 1**.

Like skeletal muscle, the cardiac muscle is comprised of linear contractile units, the *myofibrils.* These are evident in **Figure 2** as the longitudinally disposed linear structures that extend through the length of the cell. The myofibrils separate to bypass the nuclei and, in doing so, they delineate a perinuclear region of cytoplasm which is free of myofibrils and their cross-striations. These perinuclear cytoplasm areas (**asterisks**) contain the cytoplasmic organelles, which are not directly involved in the contractile process. Many cardiac muscle cells are binucleate; both nuclei typically occupy the myofibril-free region of cytoplasm as shown in the cell marked by the **asterisks.** The third nucleus in this region appears to belong to the connective tissue either above or below the "in focus" plane of section. Often, the staining of muscle cell nuclei in a specific specimen is very characteristic, especially when seen in face view as in **Figure 2.** Notice, in the nucleus between the **asterisks,** the well-stained nu-

cleolus and the delicate pattern of the remainder of the nucleus. Once such features have been characterized for a particular specimen, it becomes easy to identify nuclei having a similar staining character throughout the specimen. For example, see again **Figure 1** and survey the field for nuclei with similar features. Having done this, it is substantially easier to identify nuclei of connective tissue cells (**CT**), which display different staining properties and are not positioned in the same relationship to the muscle cells.

Figure 3 shows cross-sectioned cardiac muscle fibers. Many have rounded or smooth contoured polygonal profiles. However, some fibers are generally more irregular and elongate in profile. These probably reflect a profile of both a fiber and a branch of the fiber. The more lightly stained region in the center of many fibers represents the myofibril free region of the cell already referred to above and indicated by the **asterisks** in **Figure 2.** Delicate connective tissue surrounds the individual muscle fibers. This contains capillaries and sometimes larger vessels such as the venule (**V**) in the center of the bundle of muscle fibers. Larger amounts of connective tissue (**CT**) surround bundles of fibers and this contains larger blood vessels such as the arteriole (**A**) marked in the figure.

At higher magnification (**Fig. 4**) it is possible to see the cut ends of the myofibrils. These appear as the numerous red areas, which give the cut face of the muscle cell a stippled appearance. The nuclei (**N**) occupy a central position surrounded by myofibrils. (In contrast, nuclei of skeletal muscle fibers are located at the perimeter of the cell.) Note also that, as already mentioned, the nuclear free central area of the cell, devoid of myofibrils, shows areas of perinuclear cytoplasm similar to that marked in **Figure 2** with **asterisks.**

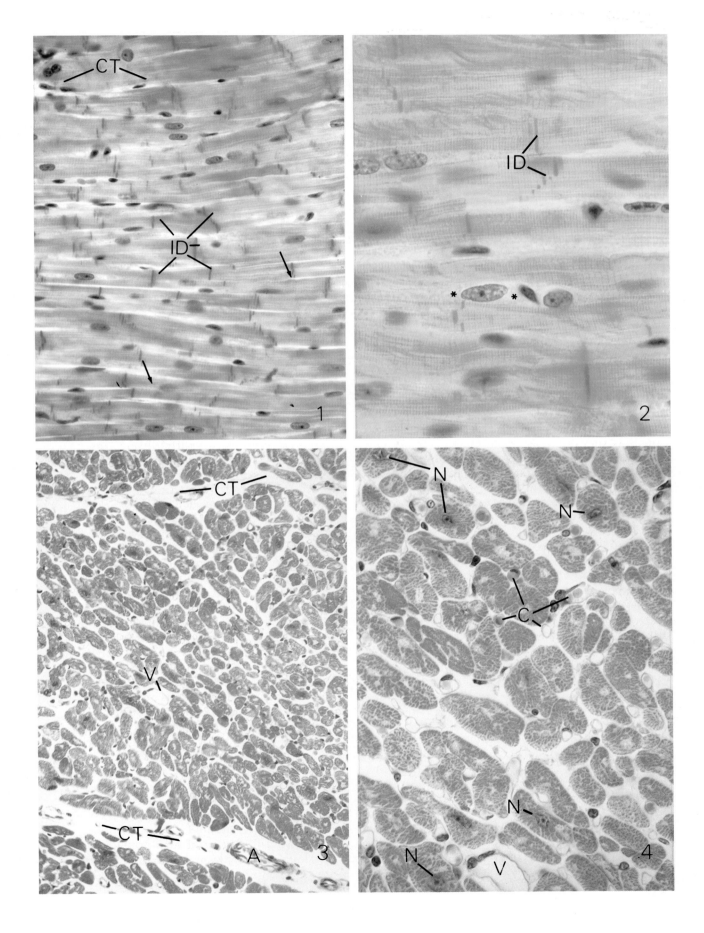

PLATE 32. Cardiac Muscle, Intercalated Disc, Electron Microscopy

This electron micrograph reveals portions of two cardiac muscle cells including the site where they join in end-to-end apposition. The apposition between the two cells can be followed in its entirety across the micrograph. It takes an irregular, step-like course making a number of near right angle turns so that part of the junction is disposed crosswise, part is disposed longitudinally, and part is disposed obliquely. In its course, different junctional specializations of the intercalated disc are evident. These include the macula adherens, fascia adherens, and gap junction. It is principally the fascia adherens and, to some extent, the macula adherens that correspond to the intercalated disc of light microscopy.

The macula adherens **(MA)** in the upper left of the illustration has been enlarged in **insert 1.** It displays the typical features seen in macula adherens in other tissues (referred to as desmosomes with the light microscope), namely, a thickening of the inner leaflet of the plasma membrane, a condensation of the adjacent cytoplasm, and an intermediate dense line seen in the middle of the intercellular space. Typically, intermediate filaments form loops in the adjacent cytoplasmic condenation and although the loops are not evident, the intermediate filaments **(arrow)** can be seen in the macula adherens **(MA),** which has been sectioned obliquely on the right side of the illustration. The macula adherens is a plaque-like site of contact between cells thought to provide for adhesion between the two cells.

The fascia adherens **(FA)** is more extensive than a macula, being disposed in a larger area of irregular outline. Thin sections showing the fascia adherens on edge **(inset 3)** reveal the plasma membranes of the neighboring cells to be separated by a space of 15 to 20 nm. In each cell the fascia adherens is typified by a condensation of the subplasmalemmal cytoplasm. The thin actin filaments of the myofibril are anchored in the cytoplasmic density. The fascia adherens of the intercalated

disc corresponds to the zonula adherens of other tissues (see Atlas section, Plate 5).

The gap junctions **(GJ)** are seen in those portions of the intercalated disc that are disposed longitudinally with respect to the direction of the myofilaments. (This orientation may not be significant because gap junctions also appear cross-wise in some electron micrographs.) In electron micrographs of routinely prepared tissues **(inset 2),** the gap junction appears as two dense lines, each representing a thickened inner layer of plasma membrane, and a barely discernible intermediate line. The intermediate line represents the outer layers of the plasma membranes of the two adjacent cells. Gap junctions are looked upon as sites where excitation spreads from one cell to another and where small molecules or ions pass readily from one cell to another.

Other features typical of striated muscle are also revealed in the illustration, namely, mitochondria **(Mi),** sarcoplasmic reticulum **(SR),** and components of the sarcomere, including Z lines **(Z),** M band **(M),** and myofilaments. This particular specimen is in a highly contracted state and consequently the I band is practically obscured.

KEY

FA, fascia adherens	**Z,** Z lines
GJ, gap junction	**arrow,** intermediate
M, M band	filaments
MA, macula adherens	**Inset 1,** macula
Mi, mitochondria	adherens
SR, sarcoplasmic	**Inset 2,** gap junction
reticulum	**Inset 3,** fascia adherens

Fig., × 30,000 (insets, × 62,000)

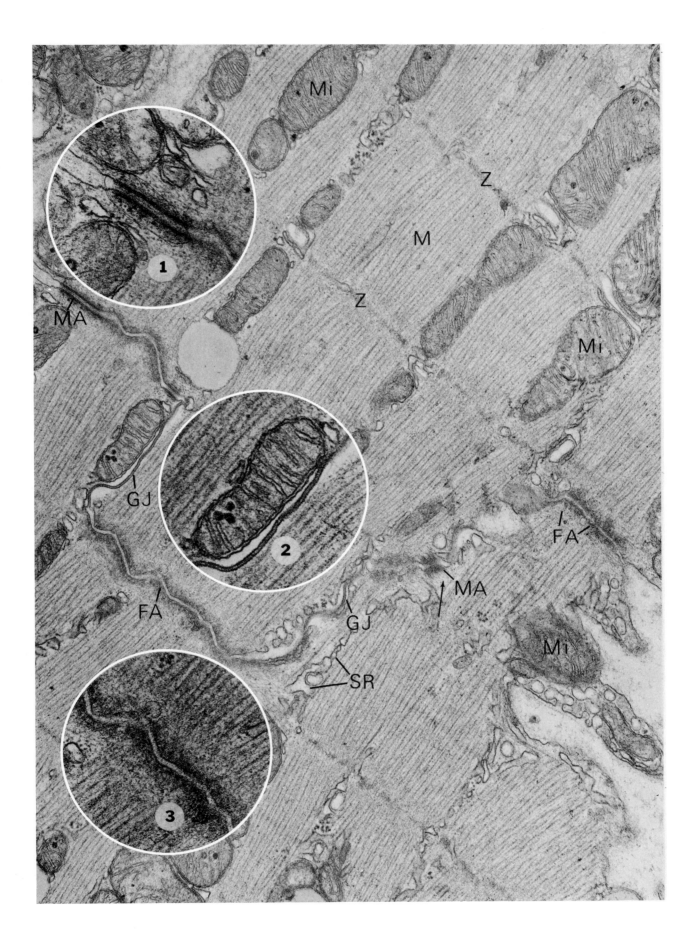

PLATE 33. Cardiac Muscle, Purkinje Fibers

Some of the muscle cells within the heart are specialized to conduct impulses from the AV node through the ventricular septum into the ventricles. Within the ventricular septum the cells are grouped into a bundle, the AV bundle. The bundle quickly branches into two main components, one going into each ventricle. These special conducting fibers are responsible for the final distribution of the electrical stimulus to the myocardium. As the bundles ramify in the ventricle, the specialized conducting cells are given the name *Purkinje fibers.*

A section of cardiac muscle and Purkinje fibers is shown in a relatively low-power view in **Figure 1.** The cardiac muscle fibers **(CM)** appear in the left of the figure; the Purkinje fibers **(PF)** occupy much of the remainder of the field. Connective tissue separates groups of Purkinje fibers from each other and from the cardiac muscle. Small blood vessels **(BV)** and nerves **(NF)** are also present within the connective tissue.

The nature of the Purkinje fibers and their architecture are seen more advantageously at higher magnification **(Fig. 2).** The fibers are individual cells of irregular shape that maintain extensive contact with one another. Intercalated discs are not observed, but desmosomes are present joining adjacent cells of the fiber.

The cytoplasm of a Purkinje cell contains a large amount of glycogen. The glycogen-rich areas **(G)** appear as homogeneous, pale-staining regions that usually occupy the center portion of the cell. The periphery of the cell contains the myofibrils

KEY	
BV, blood vessel	Mf, myofibrils
CM, cardiac muscle fibers	N, nucleus of Purkinje cell
CT, connective tissue	NF, nerve fibers
G, glycogen-rich area	PF, Purkinje fibers
GC, ganglion cell	
Fig. 1, sheep, × 160	**Fig. 2**, sheep, × 350

(Mf). The nucleus is round and much larger than the nucleus of the cardiac muscle cell. Because of the considerable size of the Purkinje cells, the nuclei are often not included in the section and one may get a misleading impression as to the disposition and number of cells that make up a fiber. On the other hand, since the myofibrils tend to be located at the periphery of the cell, they can be used to locate the cell boundaries and, thus, help delineate the individual cells of the bundle. The Purkinje fibers ultimately terminate by joining cardiac muscle fibers, thereby permitting direct passage of the impulse to the cardiac muscle fiber.

The connective tissue through which the Purkinje fibers course may also contain nerves **(NF)** and ganglion cells **(GC).** These neural elements belong to the autonomic nervous system, which regulates the activity of the Purkinje fibers and heart muscle.

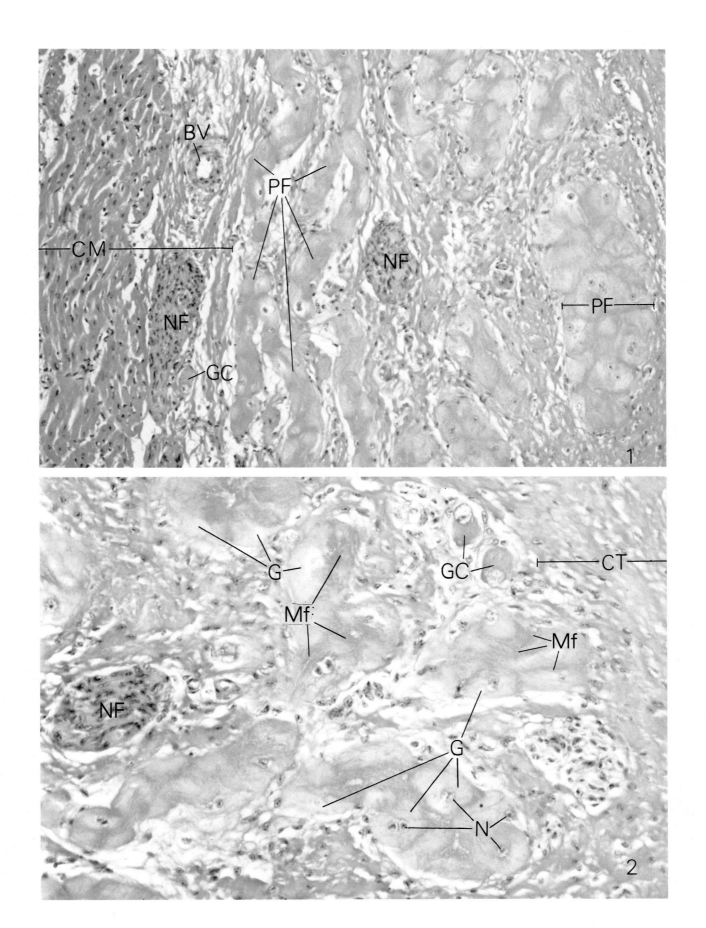

PLATE 34. Smooth Muscle

Smooth muscle tissue is comprised of cells that are typically fusiform or spindle-shaped and organized in parallel arrangements. In longitudinal section smooth muscle cells appear elongate (**Fig. 1**). Their nuclei (**N**) are also elongated and conform to the general shape of the cell. In this preparation the nuclei appear slightly twisted, like a corkscrew; this is a characteristic of contracted cells. In this specimen, the cells are sufficiently separated from one another to allow one to delineate the cell boundaries. However, the boundaries cannot always be seen in H&E sections (see **Fig. 4**).

A cross-section through smooth muscle cells from the same specimen is shown in **Figure 2.** The cells now appear as circular or polygonal profiles with variations in size. The nuclei (**N**) also appear as circular profiles and are included in some cells. However, in most of the cells, the nuclei have not been included in the section and only the eosinophilic cytoplasm appears. Because the cells are staggered, some are cut through the thick central portion, in which case the nuclei are included, while others are cut through the tapering ends, in which case only the cytoplasm is seen (**asterisks**). The differences in diameter between neighboring cells and the variable nuclear profiles are characteristic features of cross-sectioned smooth muscle. Typically, smooth muscle cells are grouped in ill-defined bundles. Note the connective tissue (**CT**) surrounding part of the bundle. Lesser amounts of extracellular connective tissue fibers and, occasionally, a fibroblast (**F**) are between the individual muscle cells within a bundle.

The smooth muscle cells (**SM**) of a blood vessel (arterial) wall are shown in **Figure 3.** These cells are arranged in a circular pattern forming part of the vessel wall. When the blood vessel is bisected longitudinally, as it is in the upper part of the figure, the smooth muscle cells are cut in cross-section and the nuclei appear rounded (**arrows**), as they are in **Figure 2.** In addition, most of the cells display cross-sectioned profiles of only cytoplasm for the reasons given above. In the bottom of the figure the blood vessel presents a different profile. It has turned and is leaving the plane of section. Here the blood vessel is cut in essentially a cross-section. The smooth muscle cells are now seen as longitudinal curved profiles as evidenced by the

---

KEY

BV, blood vessel
CT, connective tissue
F, nucleus of fibroblast
L, lumen of arteriole
N, nucleus of smooth
   muscle cells
SM, smooth muscle cell

arrow, nucleus of
   cross-sectioned
   smooth muscle cell
arrowhead, nucleus of
   longitudinally
   sectioned smooth
   muscle cell
asterisks, cytoplasm of
   smooth muscle cell
interrupted lines,
   boundaries of bundles
   of smooth muscle cell

Figs. 1–2, intestine,
  monkey, × 900

Fig. 3, human, × 425
Fig. 4, human, × 160.

---

elongate profiles of the nuclei (**arrowheads**). The vertically disposed nuclei between the two lumenal profiles (**L**) are nuclei of endothelial cells. Connective tissue (**CT**) is external to the smooth muscle cells.

Interlacing bundles of smooth muscle cells from the uterus are shown in **Figure 4.** These bundles are separated from each other by connective tissue. However, it is not always easy to distinguish between connective tissue and the smooth muscle. Three bundles of smooth muscle cells have been delineated by the interrupted lines. In each there are smooth muscle cells which are arranged in predominately one direction: longitudinally, obliquely, and in cross-section. Careful examination of these areas will reveal nuclei whose profile can be used to estimate the orientation of the cells. Having noted the orientation of the cells and the nuclei, it is now appropriate to note their number per given area of tissue. Comparing the smooth muscle with the connective tissue (**CT**), it should be noted that the connective tissue shows far fewer nuclear profiles per given area of tissue. The lumen in the upper part of the figure belongs to a blood vessel (**BV**) whose mural components blend imperceptibly with the surrounding connective tissue.

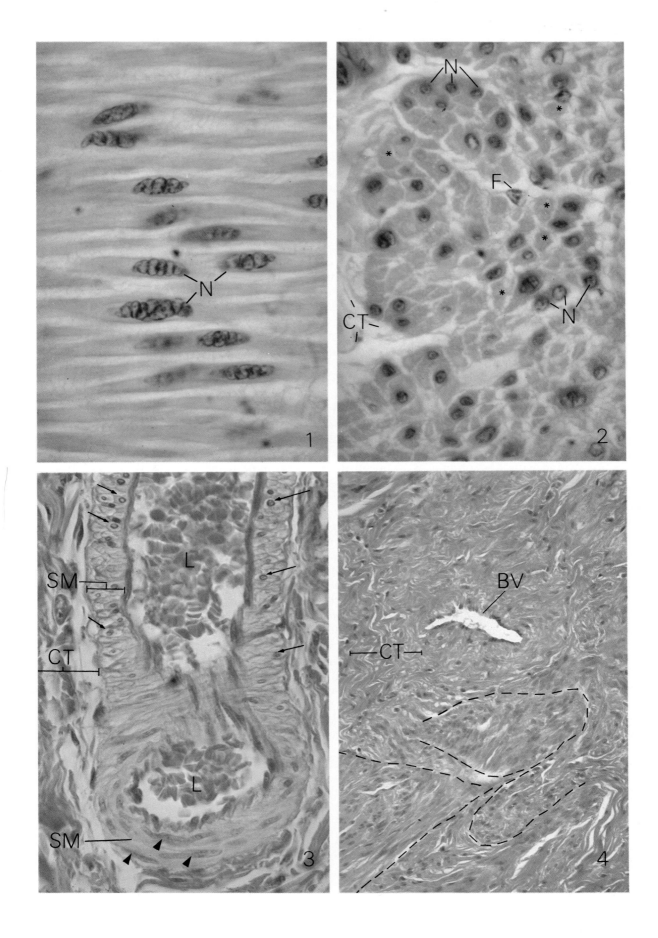

PLATE 35. Smooth Muscle, Longitudinal Section, Electron Microscopy

The electron micrograph illustrated here shows smooth muscle comparable to that shown in the light micrograph of **Figure 1** in the preceding plate. The muscle cells are longitudinally oriented and are seen in a relatively relaxed state as evidenced by the smooth contour of their nuclei. The intercellular space is occupied by abundant collagen fibrils (**C**) that course in varying planes between the cells.

At the low magnification utilized here much of the cytoplasmic mass of the muscle cells has a homogeneous appearance. This homogeneous appearance is due to the contractile components of the cell, namely, the thin (5-nm) actin filaments that are oriented in parallel array in the direction of the long axis of the cell. (The thicker myosin filaments of mammalian smooth muscle cells are extremely labile and tend to be lost during tissue preparation.) The nonhomogeneous-appearing portions of the cytoplasm contain mitochondria and other cell organelles. To illustrate these differences, the area within the small circle in the lower right of the micrograph is shown at higher magnification in the **inset** nearest the right hand margin of the micrograph. The particular site selected for the inset reveals a filamentous area (**F**) as well as a region containing mitochondria (**M**), a few profiles of rER (**arrows**), and numerous dense particles, most of which are glycogen. While the distinction between the filament-containing regions of cytoplasm and those areas containing the remaining organelles are clearly evident in the electron microscope, the routine H&E preparation of light microscopy reveals only a homogeneous eosinophilic cytoplasm.

Fibroblasts and other connective tissue cells, when present, are also readily discernible in electron micrographs among the smooth muscle cells of various organs. In this micrograph, several fibroblasts (**Fib**) are evident. In contrast to the smooth muscle cell, their cytoplasm exhibits numerous profiles of rER, as well as other organelles throughout all but the very attenuated cytoplasmic

---

KEY	
C, collagen fibrils	N, nucleus of smooth
F, filamentous area of	muscle cell
cytoplasm	**arrows**, endoplasmic
Fib, fibroblast	reticulum
M, mitochondria	

Fig., × 5500 (insets × 20,000)

---

processes. For purposes of comparison, the **small circled area** of the fibroblast on the left side of the micrograph is shown at higher power in the adjacent **inset.** Note the more numerous dilated profiles of endoplasmic reticulum (**arrows**) and the multitude of small particles (ribosomes), most of which are associated with the membranes of the reticulum. The ribosomes are slightly smaller and stain less intensely than the glycogen particles of the smooth muscle cells. The presence of rER in both the fibroblast and the smooth muscle cell is consistent with the finding that smooth muscle cells, in addition to their contractile role, have the ability to produce and maintain collagen and elastic fibers.

The tissue utilized in this micrograph is from a young animal and it contains fibroblasts in a relatively active state, hence, the well-developed endoplasmic reticulum and abundant cytoplasm. With the light microscope it is not likely that one would be able to distinguish readily between the fibroblasts shown here and the smooth muscle cells. However, less active fibroblasts, as in a more mature tissue or in an older individual, have less extensive cytoplasm and, accordingly, are more easily distinguished from the smooth muscle cells.

PLATE 35

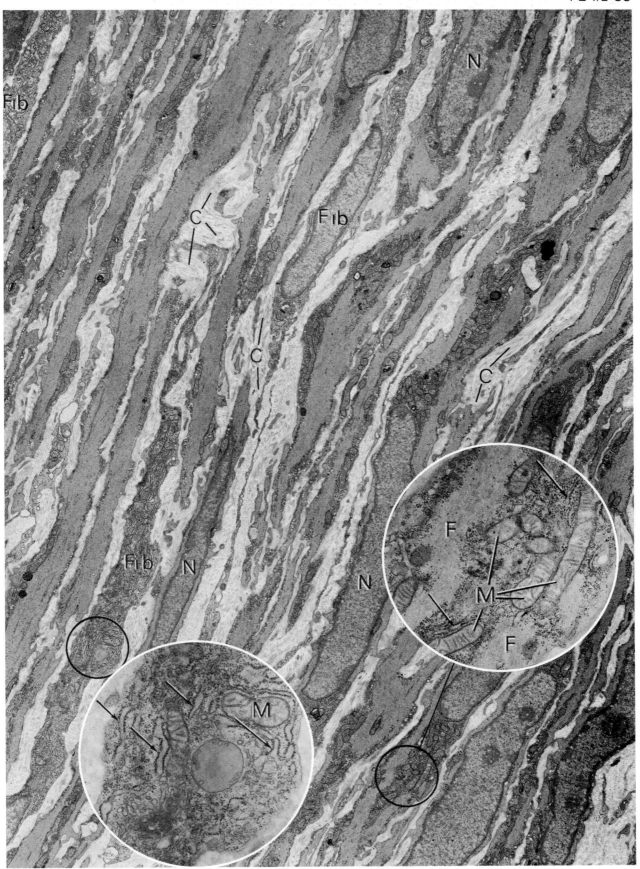

PLATE 36. Smooth Muscle, Cross-Section, Electron Microscopy

The specimen from which the micrograph was obtained is the same as that shown in the previous plate, namely, the oviduct. It is an electron micrograph of cross-sectioned smooth muscle cells and shows, at higher resolution, many of the features of smooth muscle cells seen already with the light microscope. For example, it can be seen that the muscle cells are arranged in bundles comparable to those seen with the light microscope in **Figures 2 and 4** of Atlas section, Plate 34. The bundle arrangement is not readily apparent, even in electron micrographs, when the muscle cells are longitudinally sectioned as in the proceding plate. The cross-sectioned profiles of the greatest diameter depict the midportion of the muscle cell and these show nuclei, whereas the profiles of lesser diameter depict the tapered ends of the cell and show cytoplasm only. The smooth muscle cells display cytoplasmic areas that appear homogeneous due to the presence of myofilaments. The homogeneous areas are evident, but the individual myofilaments are not. Also seen within the cytoplasm are mitochondria. Other cytoplasmic constituents are not resolved at this relatively low magnification.

Generally the cross-sectioned smooth muscle cells **(SM)** show an irregular contour when seen at the electron microscopic level. This is due, in part, to the better resolution obtained with the electron microscope, but, even more so, it is a reflection of the extreme thinness of the section. At this low magnification numerous sites are seen where a cell appears to contact its neighbor. Most of these sites do not reflect true cell-to-cell contacts. However, there are places where the smooth muscle cells do make contact by means of a nexus or gap junction **(inset).** These junctions are similar to gap junctions in other cells. They are considered to be the structural sites of easy ion movement from cell to cell and for the spread of excitation from one cell to another. Usually, special staining procedures are employed to demonstrate the nature of the junction. When seen in face view, the special stains reveal hexagonal patterns on the opposing plasma membranes. In routinely prepared electron micrographs of a gap junction **(arrow, inset),** it appears as though the adjacent plasma membranes make contact (see also Atlas section, Plate 32).

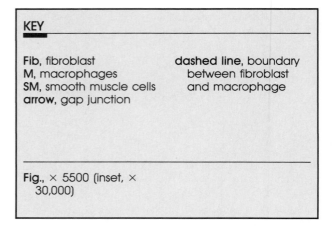

KEY

Fib, fibroblast
M, macrophages
SM, smooth muscle cells
arrow, gap junction

dashed line, boundary
between fibroblast
and macrophage

Fig., × 5500 (inset, × 30,000)

The electron micrograph shows connective tissue cells associated with the bundles of smooth muscle cells. Fibroblasts are the most numerous of the connective tissue cells. The processes of the fibroblasts tend to delineate and define the limits of the bundles. Note the very thin fibroblast processes **(Fib)** coursing along the periphery of the two muscle bundles (one bundle occupying the left half of the micrograph, the other occupying the right half). Although the nuclei of the fibroblasts would be evident with the light microscope, the cellular processes would not. In addition to fibroblasted, another cell type is also seen about or between the bundles of smooth muscle cells. These are the macrophages **(M),** readily identified with the electron microscope by the presence of lysosomal bodies within the cytoplasm. With the light microscope, these cells would be difficult to identify because the lysosomes are not evident without the use of special histochemical staining procedures. However, if the macrophages contain phagocytosed particles of large size or of distinctive coloration (e.g., hemosiderin), their identification with the light microscope becomes easier.

In the electron micrograph shown here the macrophages appear to have taken up a preferential position, lying in immediate apposition with the fibroblasts. The relationship is so close that, at this magnification, the intercellular space is difficult to discern. The **dashed line** indicates the boundary between the two cell types.

PLATE 36

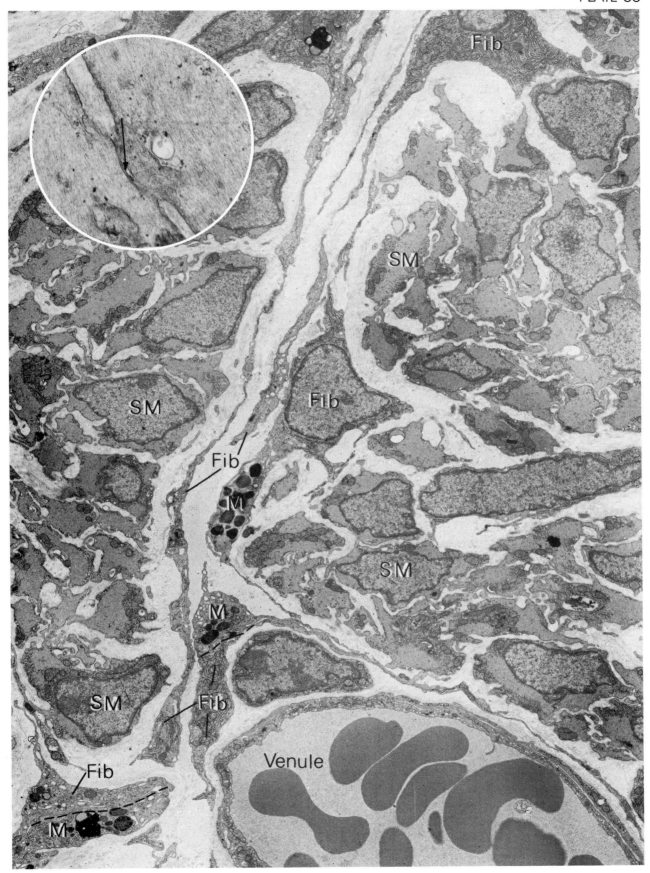

Nervous Tissue

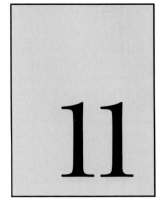

The nervous system consists of all the nervous tissue in the body. It can be divided into a **central nervous system** (CNS) and a **peripheral nervous system** (PNS). The CNS consists of the **brain** and the **spinal cord;** these are located within the cranial cavity and the spinal canal, respectively. All nervous tissue other than the brain and spinal cord is designated as the PNS; it consists of **nerves, ganglia,** and **receptors.**

NERVOUS TISSUE

Nervous tissue consists of two principal types of cells: the nerve cells and their supporting cells. The functional units of nervous tissue are the nerve cells, or **neurons.** These cells are specialized to receive information and conduct it, as impulses, to other parts of the nervous system. The nerve cells are arranged as an integrated communications network, and several neurons arranged in a chain-like fashion typically are involved in sending information from one part of the system to another. The specialized contacts between neurons that provide for the transmission of information from one neuron to the next in the chain are called **synapes.** Cells that play the supporting roles in nervous tissue are the **neuroglia,** or simply **glia,** in the CNS and the **Schwann cells** and the **satellite cells** of ganglia in the PNS.

In addition to the two components of nervous tissue, there are blood vessels in both the CNS and the PNS. The blood vessels are separated from the nervous tissue by the interposition of basal laminae and, for the larger vessels, a perivascular sheath of delicate connective tissue. However, in the CNS, the boundary between blood vessels and nervous tissue has long been recognized as special in that certain tracer substances that readily leave blood vessels to enter other tissues do not enter the nervous tissue successfully. Although the structural components of this barrier are not yet completely defined, the selective restriction of blood-borne substances in the CNS is designated as the **blood-brain barrier.**

The nervous system evolved from the simple neuroeffector system of lower animals, which allowed for the reception of stimuli from the external environment and primitive responses to these stimuli. In higher animals, the nervous system retains the capability of responding to stimuli from the external environment through the action of effector cells (such as skeletal muscles), but the neuronal responses are infinitely more varied. They range from simple reflexes requiring only the spinal cord to complex operations of the brain that bring to bear the memory of past experiences. In addition, the nervous system of higher animals has a second major function in regulating the activity of the organs of the body. The specific effectors in the organs that respond to the instructions of the neurons are smooth muscle, cardiac muscle, and glandular epithelium; the part of the PNS innervating these effectors is referred to as the **autonomic nervous system.** The regulation of the organs involves a close cooperation between the nervous system and the endocrine system and, in the area of interchange between the two systems, some nerve cells display functions designated as **neuroendocrine** (see hypothalamus and neurohypothesis).

NEURON

It is estimated that there are 10^{10} to 10^{11} neurons in the human nervous system. They are generally classified into three main categories: **sensory neurons,** which convey impulses from receptors to the CNS; *motor neurons,* which convey impulses from the CNS to effector cells; and a great intermediate network interposed between the sensory and the motor neurons called *interneurons, internuncial neurons, intercalated neurons,* or *central neurons.* It is estimated that about 99.98 percent of all neurons belong to the greater intermediate network.

Despite the great differences in size and shape, most neurons share certain structural features that make it possible to identify three functionally distinct regions of the cell: the *cell body,* the *dendrites,* and the *axon.* The cell body contains the nucleus and the main concentration of organelles of the cell. Dendrites and axons are processes of the cell body. Based on how many processes extend from the cell body, neurons are classified as *multipolar,*

one axon and two or more dendrites; *bipolar,* one axon and one dendrite; or *unipolar* (also called pseudounipolar), one axon which divides close to the cell body into two long branches (Fig. 11.1).

Motor neurons (Fig. 11.2) and interneurons are multipolar. In these cells (and it should be recalled that these cells constitute most of the neurons in the nervous system) the physiological direction of impulses is from dendrite to cell body to axon or from cell body to axon. Thus, from the functional point of view, the dendrites and cell body of multipolar neurons are the receptor portions of the cell and their plasma membranes are specially adapted for impulse generation. The axon is the conducting portion of the cell and its plasma membrane is specialized for impulse conduction. The terminal portions of the axons are

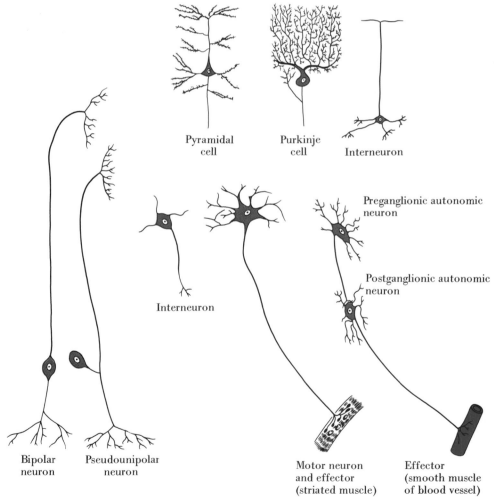

Figure 11.1. Diagram of different types of neurons. Bipolar, pseudounipolar (unipolar), and postganglionic autonomic neurons have their cell body in a ganglion outside of the CNS. (From Junqueira LC, Carneiro J: *Basic Histology,* 3rd ed. Los Altos, CA, Lange, 1980.)

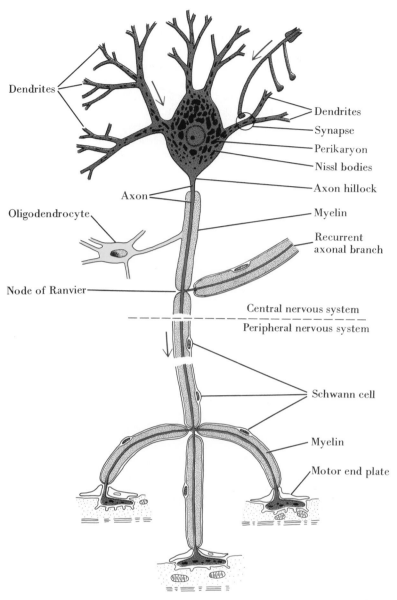

Dendrites

Dendrites
Synapse
Perikaryon
Nissl bodies
Axon hillock
Axon
Myelin
Oligodendrocyte
Recurrent axonal branch
Node of Ranvier
Central nervous system
Peripheral nervous system
Schwann cell
Myelin
Motor end plate

Figure 11.2. Diagram of a motor neuron. The perikaryon, dendrites, and initial part of the axon are within the CNS. The axon leaves the CNS and, while in the PNS, it is part of a nerve (not shown) as it courses to its effectors (striated muscle). While in the CNS, the myelin for the axon is produced by, and is actually part of, an oligodendrocyte; in the PNS, the myelin is produced by, and is actually part of, a Schwann cell. (From Junqueira LC, Carneiro J: *Basic Histology,* 3rd ed. Los Altos, CA, Lange, 1980.)

the transmitter or effector portion of the cell and they are terminal enlargements that contain transmitter substances for synaptic transmission.

Sensory neurons are unipolar. The cell body of a neuron is situated in a ganglion close to the CNS; one axonal branch extends to the periphery and one extends to the CNS. (The cell body of a sensory spinal neuron is located in a dorsal root ganglion.) Functionally, impulses are generated in the peripheral arborizations of the neuron and these arborizations are the receptor portion of the cell; the two axonal branches are the conducting units. Unipolar neurons are also sometimes called *pseudounipolar* because developmentally they originally exist as bipolar neurons that then become unipolar as they differentiate into their mature form.

Bipolar neurons are found in the retina and in the ganglia of the vestibulocochlear (VIII) nerve.

Neurons associated with the receptors for the special senses (taste, smell, hearing, sight, and equilibrium) often do not fit the generalizations made above. For example, the amacrine cells of the retina have no axons; the olfactory receptors resemble neurons of primitive neural systems in that they retain a surface location.

Cell Body

The cell body, or *perikaryon,* contains numerous mitochondria, rough endoplasmic reticulum (rER), free ribosomes, a large Golgi apparatus arranged as a network about the nucleus, lysosomes, microtubules, neurofilaments, vesicles, and inclusions (Fig. 11.3). Some cell bodies are large and filled with the organelles just listed, especially Golgi, rER, and ribosomes. Typically, with the light microscope, these large cell bodies are seen to contain a large, pale-staining round nucleus with a prominent nucleolus; much of the chromatin is in the extended configuration (euchromatin). In the

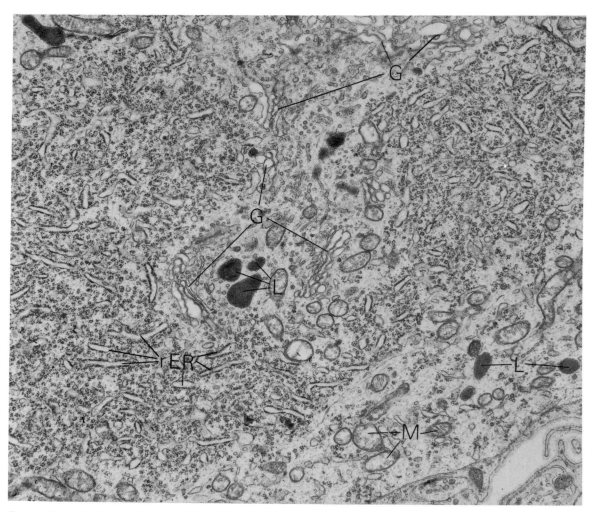

Figure 11.3. Electron micrograph showing a portion of a nerve cell body. The cytoplasm is occupied by masses of free ribosomes and profiles of rough endoplasmic reticulum (rER) that constitute the Nissl bodies of light microscopy. The Golgi apparatus (G) is arranged as a network but appears in a tissue section as isolated areas containing profiles of flattened sacs, vesicles, and anastomosing tubules. Other characteristic organelles include mitochondria (M) and lysosomes (L). The neurofilaments and neurotubules are difficult to discern at this relatively low magnification. × 15,000.

cytoplasm, large clusters of ribosomes and rER appear as areas of basophilia called *Nissl bodies.* All of these features speak of a cell that is metabolically very active. The significance of this metabolic activity, which by morphological criteria involves a substantial amount of protein synthesis, is related to the relative life-span of the cell and its components. Neurons do not divide; they must last for a lifetime. However, components within the neuron, such as enzymes and other complex molecules, have turnover times (molecular life-spans) that are measured in days and months, and these must be renewed. The renewal of these enzymes and complex molecules occurs in the cell body and the morphological features of the nucleus and cytoplasm are a reflection of this activity. It is also required that the newly synthesized molecules be transported to distant locations within the neuron; that is accomplished by a process referred to as *axonal transport.*

Dendrites and Axons

Generally speaking, dendrites are located in the vicinity of the cell body and they tend to branch, forming arborizations (Fig. 11.2). Many dendrites have short, spinous processes that serve as sites of synaptic contact. In multipolar neurons, the dendrites are extensions of the cell body and there is no sharp delineation between the cytoplasm of the dendrites and that of the cell body. Whereas Golgi network remains close to the nucleus, other organelles characteristic of the cell body proper, including ribosomes and rER, are found in the dendrites and especially in the base of the dendrites. In contrast to the multiple dendritic processes, there is only one axon for each neuron and this may be extremely long. In the case of the motor neurons the axon is always long, leaving the CNS to reach its effector cells. Although an axon may give rise to a recurrent branch near the cell body and other collateral branches, the branching of the axon is most extensive in the vicinity of its targets. The base of the axon, that is, the part of the axon that joins the cell body, is cone-shaped and it is called the *axon hillock.* This cone of cytoplasm is free of rER and is a discharge region of the cell body. Molecules synthesized in the cell body and destined to pass down the axon are sometimes delayed in this junctional region as though they were awaiting their turn for a position in the axonal transport system.

The plasma membrane of the axon is called the *axolemma;* the cytoplasm of the axon is called the *axoplasm.* The axoplasm contains numerous neurofilaments, microtubules, vesicles, and mitochondria. Typically, the axon in the CNS is insulated by a myelin sheath; in the PNS, the axon may or may not be myelinated. If it is not myelinated, it is surrounded by a Schwann cell (see below).

Synapse

Special histological staining methods show that the receptor portion of a typical multipolar neuron (e.g., the cell body and dendrites) receives numerous synaptic contacts from other neurons. The synaptic contacts appear as oval-shaped bodies on the surface of the receptor neuron (Fig. 11.4). A small segment of the incoming axon is also darkened giving the appearance of a tail. Typically, an axon from a particular neuron makes several synaptic contacts with the receptor portion of the neuron it contacts. Often, the axon travels along the surface of the neuron to be contacted and, at several places, thickenings of the axon, *boutons en passage,* make synaptic contacts. The axon

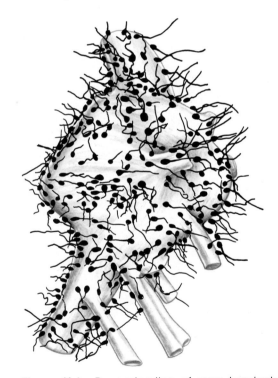

Figure 11.4. Reconstruction of axon terminals making contact on a neuron cell body and its dendrites. The axon terminals appear as the numerous ovoid bodies with a tail-like appendage. This tail is the terminal segment of the axon which is also stained by the special procedure. The remainder of the axon is unstained and, therefore, not visible. (Based on Hagger RA, Barr ML: *J Compar Neurol* 93:17, 1950.)

then continues to end finally as a terminal twig. The synaptic contact made by the terminal twig is called an **end bulb** or **terminal bouton.**

The synapse itself consists of three distinct parts: a **presynaptic knob,** that is, the terminal bouton (axonal ending) or the boutons en passage of one neuron; the **synaptic cleft,** a narrow extracellular space (about 20 nm) between the presynaptic neuron and the postsynaptic neuron; and the **postsynaptic membrane,** the receptor membrane of the second neuron (Fig. 11.5). The bouton contains synaptic transmitters stored in numerous **synaptic vesicles.** When an impulse reaches the bouton, calcium enters the bouton. The action of the calcium causes the vesicles to migrate to and fuse with the presynaptic membrane and then discharge the transmitter into the synaptic cleft by exocytosis. The transmitter diffuses across the synaptic cleft and binds to receptors in the postsynaptic membrane. The transmitter-receptor reaction causes channels to open in the membrane, which, in turn, allow ions to pass, depolarizing the membrane and thereby generating a nerve impulse. The firing of impulses in the postsynaptic neuron is due to the action of hundreds of synapses. While **excitatory** synapses depolarize the membrane of the postsynaptic neuron, **inhibitory synapses** hyperpolarize the membrane, and this tends to cancel out the effects of the excitatory synapses. Most synapses involve contact of an axon with the dendrites or cell body of the next neuron, but axon-to-axon synapes also occur (Fig. 11.6).

A number of transmitter chemicals have been identified by neurobiologists. These include acetylcholine (ACh), norepinephrine (NE), dopamine (DA), gamma aminobutyric acid (GABA), sertonin, glutamic acid, and glycine. ACh and NE act not only as transmitters between nerve cells, but also as transmitters between axon and effector in the autonomic nervous system. ACh is the transmitter between axon and striated (skeletal) muscle.

After a transmitter is released at the synapse, its action is rapidly terminated by enzymatic degradation or by rapid reincorporation into the bou-

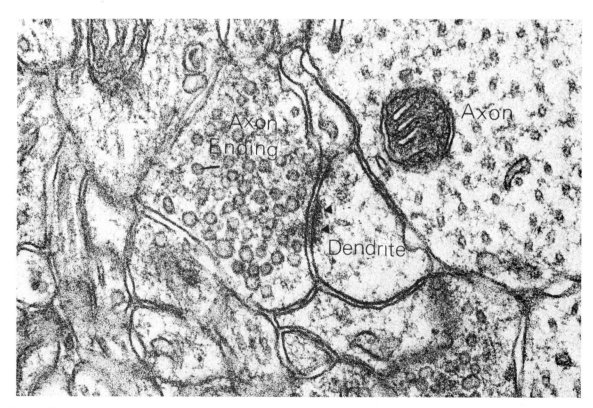

Figure 11.5. Electron micrograph of nerve processes in the cerebral cortex. A synapse can be seen in the center of the micrograph where an axon ending is in apposition with a dendrite. The ending of the axon exhibits numerous transmitter-containing vesicles, which appear as circular profiles. The postsynaptic membrane of the dendrite characteristically shows a dense material **(arrowheads).** A substance of similar density is also present in the synaptic cleft (intercellular space) at the synapse. × 76,000. (Courtesy of Dr. George P. Pappas and Virginia Kriho.)

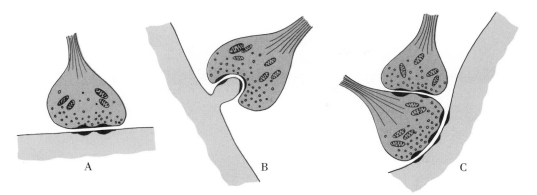

Figure 11.6. Schematic diagram of different types of synapses: **(A)** axodendritic or axosomatic; **(B)** axodendritic in which an axon terminal synapses with a dendritic spine; and **(C)** axoaxonic. (From Barr ML: *The Human Nervous System,* 4th ed. New York, Harper & Row, 1983.)

ton. The enzyme *acetylcholinesterase* (AChE) inactivates ACh; catechol-O-methyltransferase (COMT) inactivates NE.

In addition to the chemical synapses described above, there are also electrical synapses. These are similar to gap junctions in that they allow for the passage of ions between neurons and for their electrical coupling. Relatively little is known about how they participate in the specialized conducting functions of nerve tissue.

The function of synapses is not simply to transmit information in an unchanged manner from one neuron to another. Rather, synapses allow for the processing of information. Typically, the information passing from the presynaptic to the postsynaptic neuron is modified at the synaptic station by other neurons that, although not in the direct pathway, nevertheless have access to the synaptic station. These other neurons influence the membrane of the postsynaptic neuron and facilitate or inhibit the transmission of impulses.

Axonal Transport

It is now known that the axon serves not only for the transmission of the impulses, essentially a membrane phenomenon, but also for the transport of molecules between the cell body and the terminal bouton. The transport is a function of the axoplasm and it appears to involve microtubules and neurofilaments. Axonal transport is in two directions: *anterograde,* from the cell body to the terminal bouton, and *retrograde,* from the bouton to the cell body. Moreover, there appear to be two different systems: a *slow transport system* conveying substances from the cell body to the bouton at a speed of about 1 mm per day and a *fast transport system* going in both directions at a rate of about 10 to 20 cm per day. The slow transport appears to convey components needed for growth and regeneration of the axon, whereas the fast transport appears to convey components such as enzymes needed for the resynthesis of transmitters within the terminal bouton.

Dendritic transport also occurs, but it has not been studied as extensively as axonal transport. It evidently serves the same kind of functions for the dendrite as axonal transport does for the axon.

SUPPORTING CELLS OF NERVOUS TISSUE

Schwann Cells and the Myelin Sheath

With the light microscope, it was learned that many axons of the PNS are surrounded by a lipid-rich tubular cover called the *myelin sheath* and, external to this, a cellular sheath called the *sheath of Schwann* or the *neurilemma* (Fig. 11.7). Only the *initial segment* of the axon, that is, the tapered axon hillock, and the terminal ramifications are devoid of the myelin cover. Subsequent studies with the electron microscope showed that the myelin consists of plasma membrane of the Schwann cell. The Schwann cell is wrapped around the axon in a spiral fashion for a variable number of times and the cytoplasm between the membranes is extruded (Fig. 11.8). The thickness of the myelin depends on how many wrappings are made. Inner leaflets of the plasma membrane fuse to form the *major dense lines* observed in the myelin; fusion of the outer leaflets results in the *intraperiod lines* of myelin. It is the fused plasma membranes, i.e., the major dense lines and the intraperiod lines and the material between these lines that constitute the myelin. Each Schwann cell covers only a small seg-

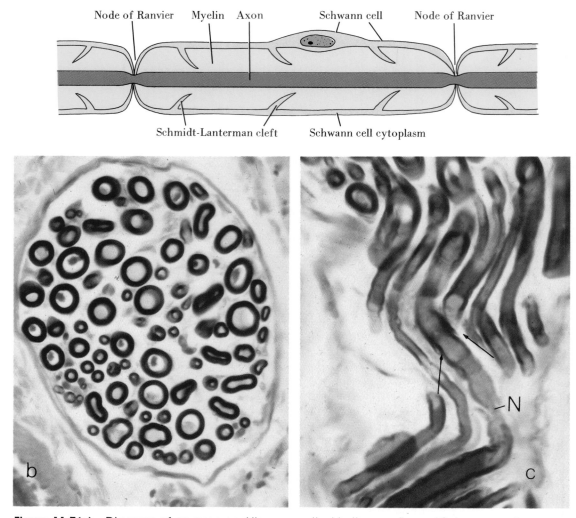

Node of Ranvier   Myelin   Axon   Schwann cell   Node of Ranvier

Schmidt-Lanterman cleft   Schwann cell cytoplasm

Figure 11.7(a). Diagram of an axon and its cover—that is, the myelin and Schwann cell—as seen with the light microscope. A single Schwann cell (also referred to as the sheath of Schwann or the neurilemma) surrounds the axon from one node of Ranvier to the next. The Schmidt-Lanterman cleft represents cytoplasm of the Schwann cell. (From Barr ML: *The Human Nervous System*, 4th ed. New York, Harper & Row, 1983.) **(b and c).** Photomicrographs of nerves fixed and stained with osmium. The nerve in the micrograph on the left **(b)** is seen in cross-section. On the right **(c)**, another nerve is seen in longitudinal section. The myelin appears as the **black rings** in the cross-sectioned profile. Note the variation in diameter of the fibers. A node of Ranvier (N) and a Schmidt-Lanterman cleft **(arrows)** can be seen in one of the fibers of the longitudinally sectioned nerve.

ment of the axon (0.08 to 0.1 mm) and the entire myelin sheath is made up of the membrane wrappings of successive Schwann cells. The junction where two adjacent Schwann cells meet and where a small length of axon is not covered by myelin is called the **node of Ranvier.**

The myelin is lipid-rich because as the Schwann cell winds around the axon, its cytoplasm, as just noted, is extruded from between the opposing layers of the plasma membranes. However, electron micrographs typically show small amounts

of cytoplasm in several locations (Fig. 11.9): the **inner collar of Schwann cell cytoplasm** between the axon and the myelin; the **Schmidt-Lanterman clefts,** small islands within successive lamellae of the myelin; **perinodal cytoplasm,** at the node of Ranvier; and the **outer collar of perinuclear cytoplasm** around the myelin (this is what light microscopists identified as the Schwann cell). If one conceptually unrolls the Schwann cell, as shown in Figure 11.10, its full extent can be appreciated and it can be seen that the inner collar of Schwann cell cytoplasm is

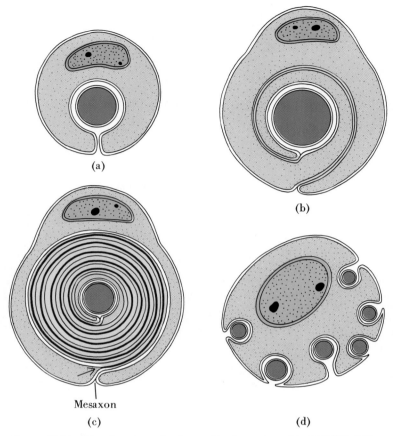

(a)

(b)

(c)

Mesaxon

(d)

Figure 11.8(a-d). A series of schematic diagrams showing the successive stages in the formation of myelin by a Schwann cell. **(a)** The axon is initially surrounded by a Schwann cell. **(b)** The Schwann cell then wraps around itself and the axon forming multiple layers. **(c)** During the process the cytoplasm is extruded from between the two apposing plasma membranes, which then fuse, inner leaflet to inner leaflet, to form the major dense line **(arrow)**. The outer opposing leaflets also fuse to form the less conspicuous intraperiod line. The outer mesaxon represents invaginated plasma membrane extending from the outer surface of the Schwann cell to the myelin. The inner mesaxon extends from the inner surface of the Schwann cell (the part facing the axon) to the myelin. **(d)** A Schwann cell and its unmyelinated axons. Each axon is invaginated in a recess of the Schwann cell, but no myelin is present. (From Barr ML: *The Human Nervous System,* 4th ed. New York, Harper & Row, 1983.)

continuous with the body of the Schwann cell through the Schmidt-Lanterman clefts and through the perinodal cytoplasm.

Axons that are unmyelinated are nevertheless enveloped by a Schwann cell, as illustrated in Figure 11.8d and f. The unmyelinated nerve fibers lie within invaginations of the Schwann cell. Either a single axon or a group of axons may be enveloped in the cytoplasmic invagination. In turn, a basal lamina surrounds the Schwann cell and its contained axons, as is also the case of Schwann cells of myelinated nerve fibers.

Neuroglia

Within the CNS, the supporting cells are referred to as neuroglia. Three types of cells are customarily classified as neuroglia: ***astrocytes, oligodendrocytes,*** and ***microglia.*** These cells have long been thought to be supporting cells of nerve tissue in the physical sense and, while this concept is at least partially correct, it is gradually being extended to emphasize the functional interdependence of neuroglial cells and nerve cells. The most obvious example of physical support occurs during

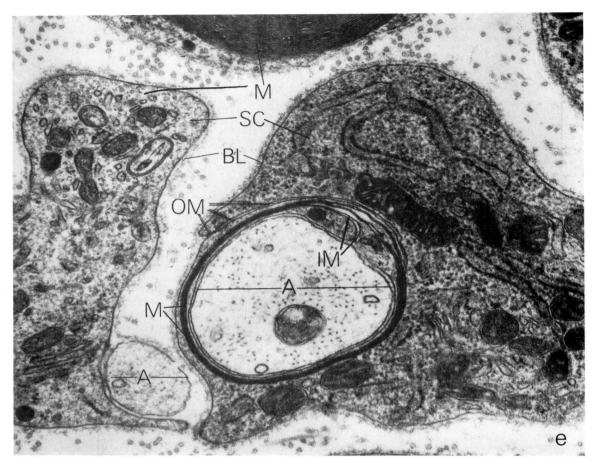

Figure 11.8(e) Electron micrograph of an axon (see A, center of field) in the process of being myelinated. At this stage of development, the myelin (M) consists of about six membrane layers. The inner mesaxon (IM) is represented by the apposition of the internal opposing processes of the Schwann cell (SC). Similarly, the outer mesaxon (OM) is represented by the outer fold, or lip, of the Schwann cell where it meets itself. Another axon (A) is present **(lower left)** that has not yet been enwrapped by the Schwann cell. Other features of note include the Schwann cell basal lamina (BL) and the considerable amount of Schwann cell cytoplasm associated with the myelinization process. The mature myelinated axon, part of which is shown at the top center of the micrograph, exhibits only a thin outer collar of Schwann cell cytoplasm. × 50,000. (Courtesy of Dr. Stephen G. Waxman.)

development. The brain and spinal cord develop from the embryonic neural tube. In the head region, the neural tube undergoes remarkable thickening and folding, leading ultimately to the final structure, which is the brain. During the early stages of the process, glial cells extend through the entire thickness of the neural tube in a radial manner. These radial glial cells serve as a physical substrate for the migration of neurons to their appropriate position in the brain.

Microglia. In considering adult neural tissue, it is useful to separate microglia from astrocytes and oligodendrocytes. Microglia are known to be macrophages of the CNS. There is evidence that they remove debris of cells that die during the normal development of the nervous system. They

are also implicated in phagocytosis in other situations. Microglia are small cells with relatively small nuclei. They contain lysosomes, inclusions, and vesicles characteristic of macrophages and only sparse rER and few microfilaments or microtubules.

Astrocytes. Astrocytes are the largest of the neuroglia. Two kinds of astrocytes have been identified, **protoplasmic** and **fibrous.** The protoplasmic astrocyte is more prevalent in gray matter; the fibrous astrocyte is more prevalent in white matter. Both types have numerous processes that extend to blood vessels and to neurons where they expand. The expanded processes, called **end feet,** cover a greater part of the vessel or neuron. Because the end feet cover so much of the blood ves-

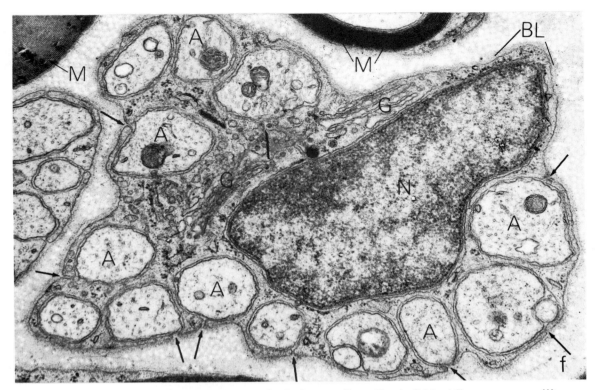

Figure 11.8(f). Electron micrograph of unmyelinated nerve fibers. The individual fibers, or axons (A), are embedded in the cytoplasm of the Schwann cell. The **arrows** indicate the site of the mesaxon. In effect, each axon is enclosed by the Schwann cell cytoplasm except for the intercellular space of the mesaxon. Other features evident in the Schwann cell are its nucleus (N), the Golgi apparatus (G), and the surrounding basal lamina (BL). In the upper part of the micrograph, myelin of two myelinated nerves is also evident. × 27,000.

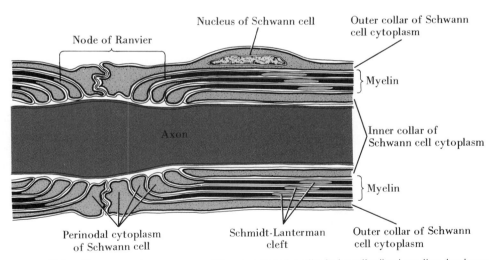

Figure 11.9. Diagram of an axon and its covering sheaths in longitudinal section to show the relationship between the axon, the myelin, and the cytoplasm of the Schwann cell and the node of Ranvier. Schwann cell cytoplasm is present at four locations. These are **(1)** the inner and **(2)** outer cytoplasmic collars of the Schwann cell, **(3)** the perinodal location, and **(4)** the Schmidt-Lanterman clefts. It should be noted that the cytoplasm throughout the Schwann cell is continuous, and it is not a series of cytoplasmic islands as it appears in the digram (see Fig. 11.10). The node of Ranvier is the location where successive Schwann cells meet. The adjacent plasma membranes of the Schwann cells are not tightly apposed at the node, and extracellular fluid has free access to the neuronal plasma membrane. Also, the node is where depolarization of the neuronal plasma membrane occurs during the transmission of the nerve impulse. (Based on Leblond CP: In Ham AW, Cormack DH (eds): *Histology*, 8th ed. Philadelphia, JB Lippincott, 1979.)

251

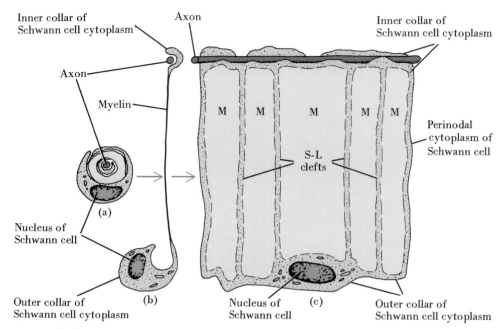

Figure 11.10(a-c). Diagrams to aid in conceptualizing the relationship of myelin and cytoplasm of a Schwann cell. **(a)** A cross-section of a myelinated axon. **(b)** A hypothetically uncoiled Schwann cell viewed on edge. **(c)** The same uncoiled Schwann cell in face view. Note how the cytoplasm of the Schwann cell is continuous. S-L clefts = Schmidt Lanterman clefts; M = myelin. (Modified from Webster H deF: *J Cell Biol* 48:348, 1971.)

sels, it is thought that they have a role in the regulated movement of blood-borne materials to the neurons. While the tight junctions of the capillaries and venules of the CNS seem to be the structure responsible for the blood-brain barrier, recent evidence strongly indicates that the astrocytes induce the formation of the tight junctions.

Oligodendrocytes. Oligodendrocytes are known to produce the myelin of myelinated axons in the CNS, and thus, they are CNS counterparts of the Schwann cells. They differ from Schwann cells in that the oligodendrocytes typically myelinate several axons, as shown in Figure 11.11.

Ependyma

The cells that constitute the ependyma are sometimes classified as neuroglia. The ependyma consists of cuboidal to columnar cells (Fig. 11.12) that form a lining of the ventricles and spinal canal (fluid-filled cavities in the brain and spinal cord, respectively). In several locations, the ependymal lining of the cavities in the brain is modified to produce cerebrospinal fluid from the adjacent capillary loops. The modified ependymal cells and associated capillary loops are called the ***choroid plexus.***

Impulse Conduction, Myelin, and the Node of Ranvier

The nerve impulse can be measured as a rapid sweep of an ***action potential*** along an axon, much as a flame travels along the fuse of a firecracker. The action potential is due to changes in permeability of the axolemma, an influx of sodium ions into the axoplasm, and a consequent voltage reversal (depolarization) of the membrane.[1] Initially, the charge internal to the resting membrane is negative (-70 mV); after the influx of the sodium ions it is positive ($+30$ mV) and this voltage reversal constitutes the action potential. Return to the original polarity is associated with an efflux of potassium ions. As a consequence of these ion movements, more sodium is inside the cell and more potassium is outside the cell than usual. This alteration due to the passage of the impulse is quickly remedied as the sodium and potassium ions are returned to their original resting locations and

---

[1] Traditionally, the term depolarization has been used to describe the voltage change in the membrane that accounts for the action potential. However, the change is actually a voltage reversal. Thus, the expression *voltage reversal* is more accurate than *depolarization*.

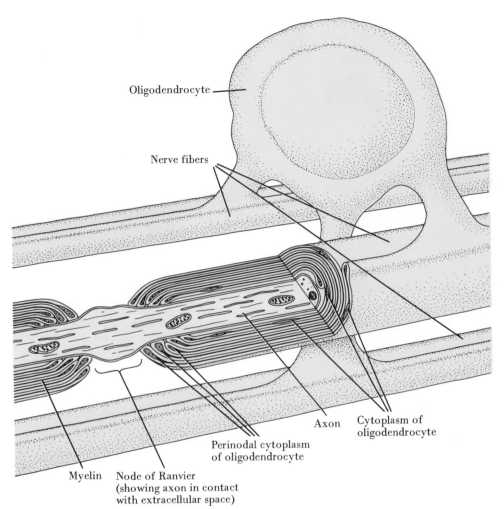

Oligodendrocyte

Nerve fibers

Axon

Cytoplasm of
oligodendrocyte

Perinodal cytoplasm
of oligodendrocyte

Myelin   Node of Ranvier
(showing axon in contact
with extracellular space)

Figure 11.11. A three-dimensional view of an oligodendrocyte as it relates to three axons. Cytoplasmic processes from the oligodendrocyte cell body form flattened cytoplasmic sheaths that wrap around each of the axons. The relationship of cytoplasm and myelin is essentially the same as that found in Schwann cells. (Based on Bunge et al: *J Biophys Biochem Cytol* 10:67, 1961.)

concentrations by the work of ion pumps in the axolemma. These ion pumps move sodium out of the axoplasm in exchange for potassium.

In unmyelinated axons, the impulse is conducted as a continuous wave of voltage reversal to the end of the axon. In myelinated axons, the voltage reversal is not a continuous wave. It occurs at the nodes of Ranvier where the axolemma is exposed to the extracellular fluids, but not in the internodal segments of the axon that are covered by myelin. Because of the insulating effect of the myelin, the electrical alteration (and, thus, the impulse) jumps as "current flow" from one node of Ranvier to the next. This process is designated as *saltatory conduction;* it is more rapid than a contin-

uous wave of voltage reversal. The speed of saltatory conduction is related not only to the thickness of the myelin, but also to the thickness of the axon, it being more rapid in the axons of greater diameter.

ORIGIN OF CELLS OF NERVOUS TISSUE

In the CNS, neurons derive from postmitotic cells in the neural tube. After they have migrated to their predestined location and have differentiated into mature neurons, they no longer divide. Astrocytes and oligodendrocytes also derive from postmitotic cells of the neural tube. Studies with

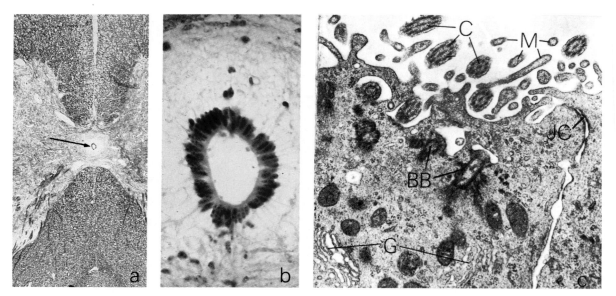

Figure 11.12(a-c). **(a)** Light micrograph of center region of spinal cord with an **arrow** pointing to the central canal. **(b)** At higher magnification the ependyma, which lines the canal, can be seen to consist of columnar cells. **(c)** TEM showing a portion of the apical region of two columnar ependymal cells. They are joined by a junctional complex (JC), which separates the lumen of the canal from the lateral intercellular space. The surface of the ependymal cells contain cilia (C) and microvilli (M). Basal bodies (BB) and a Golgi (G) within the apical cytoplasm are also marked. (Light micrographs, courtesy of G. Pappas; TEM, courtesy of Dr. P. Reier.)

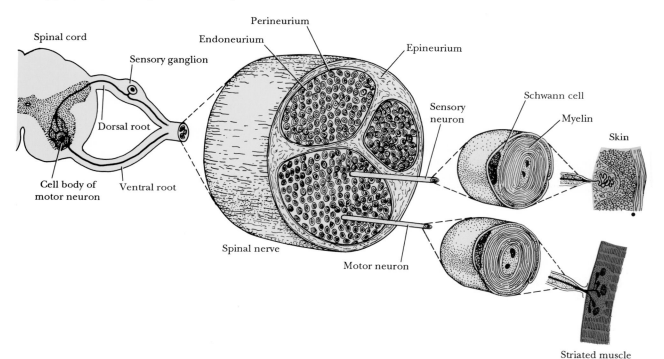

Figure 11.13. Schematic diagram showing arrangement of motor and sensory neurons. The motor neuron has its cell body in the ventral gray matter of the spinal cord. The axon covered with myelin leaves the cord via the ventral root and becomes part of the spinal nerve, which continues to its destination to a striated (skeletal) muscle. The sensory neuron originates in the skin and continues as a component of the spinal nerve, entering the spinal cord via the dorsal root. Note the location of the cell body in the sensory ganglion of the dorsal root. A segment of the spinal nerve is enlarged to show the relationship of the nerve fibers to the endoneurium and the location of perineurium and epineurium. In addition, segments of the sensory and motor neurons have been enlarged to show the relationship of the axons to the Schwann cells and myelin. (Autonomic nerve fibers are not shown in the diagram.) (Based on Ham AW: *Histology,* 6th ed. Philadelphia, JB Lippincott, 1969.)

tritiated thymidine indicate that these two types of neuroglial cells may undergo a slow turnover. Microglia are now believed to derive from the mononuclear cells of blood along with other macrophages of the body. However, there is some question as to whether they are still able to divide after they have reached the nerve tissue.

The development of ganglion cells involves the migration of postmitotic cells from the neural crest to their future ganglionic site, a second wave of mitosis at the site, and then the development of processes that reach the cells' target tissues (smooth muscle cells to be innervated or sensory territory). In the second mitotic wave, more cells are produced than are needed. Evidently, those that do not make functional contact with a target tissue undergo cell death.

Schwann cells also originally arise from the neural crest, but they undergo mitoses in the developing nerve. Most Schwann cells are formed by mitosis of parent Schwann cells in the peripheral nerves rather than by the migration of postmitotic cells from the neural crest.

ARRANGEMENT OF NERVE CELLS IN THE PERIPHERAL NERVOUS SYSTEM

As a general statement, a **nerve** is a bundle of nerve fibers, myelinated and unmyelinated, held together by connective tissue in a specific **manner.**[2] **Ganglia** contain not only nerve fibers, but also clusters of neuronal cell bodies. These cell bodies may belong to sensory neurons and their distribution is restricted to specific locations (Table 11.1 and Fig. 11.13), or they may belong to postsynaptic "motor" neurons of the autonomic nervous system (see Table 11.1 and Fig. 11.16).

The nerve cells in the peripheral system connect the periphery of the body with the brain and spinal cord. In considering the arrangement of nerve cells in the PNS, it is necessary also to consider certain parts of the CNS. The reason for this is that all motor neurons going to skeletal muscles originate in the CNS (spinal cord or brain stem); in addition, certain autonomic neurons (preganglionic) also originate in the CNS. Sensory neurons enter the CNS (again, spinal cord or brain stem). Sensory neurons have their cell body in ganglia outside of but close to the CNS. For our purpose,

the spinal cord will be used to illustrate these points. The spinal cord is a cylindrical structure; it is directly continuous with the brain. It is divided into 31 segments (8 cervical, 12 thoracic, 5 lumbar, 5 sacral, and 1 coccygeal) and each segment is connected to a pair of spinal nerves. Each spinal nerve is joined to its segment of the cord by a number of roots, or rootlets, grouped as **posterior (dorsal) roots** or as **anterior (ventral) roots** (see Fig. 11.19). A cross-section through the spinal cord reveals that within the inner substance of the cord there is tissue that has a general profile of an H. This is the gray matter of the spinal cord (Fig. 11.13). It is the part of the spinal cord where cell bodies and their dendrites are to be found along with other components of nerve tissue (axons and neuroglia). The gray matter is surrounded by white matter, which

TABLE 11.1. Peripheral Ganglia

I. Ganglia that contain cell bodies of sensory neurons (not synaptic stations)
  1. Dorsal root ganglia of all spinal nerves
  2. Sensory ganglia of cranial nerves
    a. Trigeminal (semilunar, Gasserian) ganglion of trigeminal (V) nerve
    b. Geniculate ganglion of facial (VII) nerve
    c. Spiral ganglion (contains bipolar neurons) of vestibulocochlear (VIII) nerve
    d. Vestibular ganglion (contains bipolar neurons) of vestibulocochlear (VIII) nerve
    e. Superior and inferior ganglia of glossopharyngeal (IX) nerve
    f. Superior and inferior ganglia of vagus (X) nerve
II. Ganglia that contain cell bodies of autonomic (postsynaptic) neurons (synaptic stations)
  A. Sympathetic ganglia
    1. Sympathetic trunk (paravertebral or vertebral chain) ganglia (the highest of these is the superior cervical ganglion)
    2. Prevertebral ganglia (adjacent to origins of large branches of abdominal aorta); includes celiac, superior mesenteric, inferior mesenteric, and aorticorenal ganglia
  B. Parasympathetic ganglia
    1. Head ganglia
      a. Ciliary ganglion of oculomotor (III) nerve
      b. Geniculate ganglion of facial (VII) nerve
      c. Submandibular ganglion of facial (VII) nerve
      d. Pterygopalatine (sphenopalatine) of facial (VII) nerve
      e. Otic ganglion of glossopharyngeal (IX) nerve
    2. Terminal ganglia (near or in wall of organs); includes ganglia of Meissner's and Auerbach's plexuses and isolated ganglion cells in a variety of organs

Practical Note: Neuron cell bodies seen in tissue sections such as tongue, pancreas, alimentary canal, urinary bladder, and heart are invariably terminal ganglia or "ganglion cells" of the parasympathetic nervous system.

---

[2] The term *nerve fiber* is used in different ways. It can be used to mean the axon with all of its covers (myelin and Schwann cell) or the axon alone. It is also used to refer to any process of a nerve cell, either dendrite or axon, especially if sufficient information is not available to identify the process as either an axon or dendrite.

contains only axons traveling to and from other segments of the spinal cord and to and from the brain. Thus, only in the gray matter can synapses occur.

Motor neurons destined to innervate striated muscle have their cell body and dendrites in the anterior prong of the H. This portion of the spinal cord is called the **anterior horn,** and, accordingly, one of the names given to the motor neuron is **anterior horn cell.** The axon of the motor neuron leaves the spinal cord, passes through the anterior root, becomes a component of the spinal nerve, and, as such, is conveyed to the muscle. The axon is myelinated except at its origin and termination. Near the muscle cell the axon divides into numerous terminal branches that form neuromuscular synapses with the muscle cell. Because the motor neuron conducts impulses away from the CNS, it is called an **efferent neuron.**

The sensory neuron has its cell body in a ganglion on the posterior root of the spinal nerve. It is a unipolar neuron. Its single axon divides into a peripheral segment "coming from" the periphery and a central segment that enters the spinal cord. Impulses are generated in the terminal receptor arborization of the peripheral segment. They are then conducted along the peripheral segment of the myelinated axon toward the cell body and then along the central segment of the axon to the spinal cord. Because the sensory neuron conducts impulses to the CNS, it is called an **afferent neuron.** It should be noted that with respect to the neurons considered thus far, one neuron with its cell body in the spinal cord conducts the impulse all the way

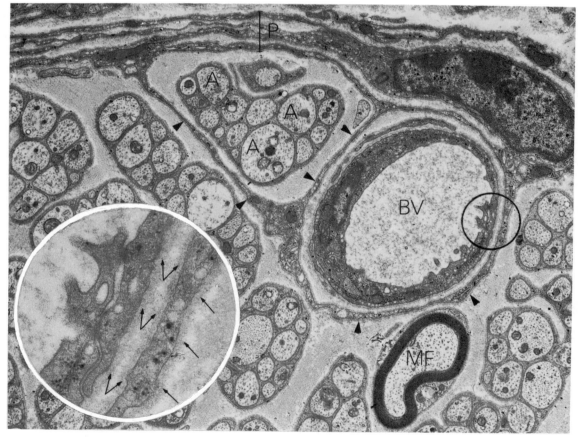

Figure 11.14(a). Electron micrograph of unmyelinated nerve fibers and a single myelinated fiber (MF). The perineurium (P), consisting of several cell layers, is seen in the upper portion of the micrograph. Perineurial cell processes **(arrowheads)** have also extended into the nerve to surround a group of axons (A) and their Schwann cell, as well as a small blood vessel (BV). The enclosure of this group of axons represents the root of a small nerve branch that has joined the larger fascicle. The area within the circle encompassing the endothelium of the vessel and the adjacent perineurial cytoplasm is shown in the inset at higher magnification. Note the basal laminae of the vessel and the perineurial cell **(arrows)**. The junction between endothelial cells of the blood vessel is also apparent. × 10,000; **inset,** × 46,000.

from the spinal cord to the skeletal muscle, and one neuron with its cell body in the dorsal root ganglion conducts the impulse all the way from the periphery to the spinal cord.

The nerve also has axons of sensory neurons coming from other locations such as the skeletal muscles, blood vessels, and other organs. Regardless of their origin, every sensory neuron (except some of those serving the special senses) has its cell body in a ganglion that is outside of the CNS; the ganglia are either dorsal root ganglia of the spinal nerves or sensory ganglia of certain cranial nerves.

Finally, nerves contain axons of motor neurons going to smooth muscle and glands, and these are typically unmyelinated. The arrangement of these neurons is slightly different; they belong to the autonomic nervous system and they have their cell body in a peripheral (autonomic) ganglion.

Structural Organization of a Nerve

The bulk of a peripheral nerve consists of nerve fibers and their supporting Schwann cells. The nerve fibers and their associated Schwann cells are surrounded by connective tissue, referred to as **endoneurium,** which is comprised of delicate collagen fibers and a relatively sparse population of fibroblasts. Other kinds of connective tissue cells usually associated with loose connective tissue, with the exception of mast cells, are not present under normal conditions. (It may be noteworthy that the mast cell is prevalent in nerves of certain laboratory animals.)

Surrounding the nerve bundle is a cellular sheath, the **perineurium,** which serves as a semipermeable barrier. It may be one or more cell layers thick, depending upon the nerve diameter. The cells that comprise this layer are squamous in shape and exhibit a basal lamina (Fig. 11.14). They are contractile cells and contain an appreciable amount of the microfilaments characteristic of smooth muscle cells. Moreover, in those instances where there are two or more perineurial cell layers (as many as five or six layers may be present in larger nerves), collagen fibrils are present between the perineurial cell layers, but typical fibroblasts are absent. In effect, the arrangement of these cells to form a barrier, and the presence of basal lamina material, likens them to an epithelioid tissue. On the other hand, their contractile nature and the apparent ability to produce collagen fibrils also likens them to smooth muscle cells as well as to

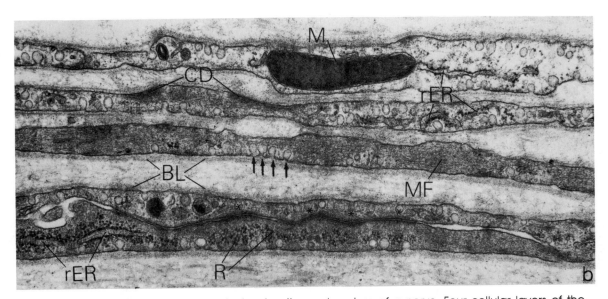

Figure 11.14(b). Electron micrograph showing the perineurium of a nerve. Four cellular layers of the perineurium are present. Each layer has associated with it on both surfaces a basal lamina (BL). Other features associated with the perineurial cell include an extensive population of microfilaments (MF) known to consist of actin, pinocytotic vesicles **(arrows)**, and cytoplasmic densities (CD). These features are characteristic of smooth muscle cells. The cytoplasm of the peripheral cell layer is less electron-dense due to a paucity of microfilaments. However, the presence of a basal lamina in association with this cell indicates that it is a perineurial cell. The innermost perineurial cell layer exhibits a junctional specialization **(asterisks)** where one cell is overlapping a second cell in forming the sheath. Such junctions (fascia adherens) are associated with strong adhesion between neighboring cells. Other features seen in the cytoplasm are mitochondria (M), rough endoplasmic reticulum (rER), and free ribosomes (R). × 27,000.

fibroblasts. These features are considered further in the Atlas Section, Plate 41. However, for our purposes here, it should simply be pointed out that the absence of connective tissue cells other than fibroblasts and mast cells within the endoneurium is undoubtedly a reflection of a protective role that the perineurium plays and that it excludes the need for the presence of cells (other than the mast cell) belonging to the immune system.

The last component associated with the structural organization of a nerve is the *epineurium.* This is simply a connective tissue covering that may surround one or more perineurial bundles, binding them together and forming the outermost tissue of the nerve. It is a dense connective tissue that also carries the blood vessels serving the larger nerves. Branches of these vessels penetrate the perineurium, initially carrying with them a perineurial sheath, and then travel within the nerve to provide for its blood supply (see Fig. 11.14).

AUTONOMIC NERVOUS SYSTEM

Traditionally, the autonomic nervous system has been defined as being that portion of the PNS that conducts impulses to smooth muscle, cardiac muscle, and glandular epithelium. These effectors are the functional units in the organs that respond to regulation by nervous tissue. The term *visceral* is sometimes used in referring to the autonomic nervous system or its neurons. It is known that sensory neurons also leave the organs to convey impulses to the CNS, but these visceral afferent neurons have the same arrangement as other sensory neurons, that is, their cell body is in sensory ganglia and they possess long peripheral and central axons, as already described.

The main organizational difference between the efferent flow of impulses to skeletal muscle (the somatic effector) and the efferent flow to smooth muscle, cardiac muscle, and glandular epithelium is that one neuron conveys the impulses from the CNS to the somatic effector (Fig. 11.15a), whereas a chain of two neurons conveys the impulses from the CNS to the autonomic effectors (Fig. 11.15b). Thus, there is one synaptic station in a ganglion outside of the CNS where a preganglionic, or presynaptic, neuron makes contact with postganglionic, or postsynaptic, neurons. Each presynaptic neuron synapses with several postsynaptic neurons.

The autonomic nervous system is divided into two parts, *sympathetic* and *parasympathetic.* The presynaptic neurons of the sympathetic system leave the CNS from the thoracic and upper lumbar

segments of the spinal cord. These neurons synapse in ganglia of the vertebral chain and in prevertebral ganglia (Figs. 11.15b and c). The presynaptic neurons of the parasympathetic nervous system leave the CNS from the brain as components of cranial nerves III, VII, IX, and X and from the sacral region of the spinal cord (Fig. 11.16). These presynaptic neurons synapse in terminal ganglia (ganglia in the walls of organs or close to the organs) and in head ganglia (ciliary, sphenopalatine, sublingual, and otic) (see Table 11.1). Both parts of the autonomic nervous system sometimes supply the same organs. In these cases, the actions of the two are often antagonistic. An obvious example of this is that sympathetic stimulation brings on increased activity of cardiac muscle, whereas parasympathetic stimulation inhibits activity.

Many functions of the sympathetic nervous system are similar to those of the adrenal medulla, an endocrine gland. This is partly explained by the fact that the cells of the adrenal medulla are related to postganglionic sympathetic neurons. They both derive from the same neural crest origin; they are both innervated by preganglionic sympathetic neurons; and they produce closely related physiologically active agents, epinephrine and NE. The difference is that the sympathetic neurons deliver the agent directly to the effector, whereas the cells of the adrenal medulla deliver the agent indirectly through the bloodstream. It should be noted that the innervation of the adrenal medulla constitutes an exception to the rule that autonomic innervation consists of a two-neuron chain from CNS to an effector; for the adrenal medulla, it is only one neuron.

SUMMARY OF AUTONOMIC DISTRIBUTION (see Fig. 11.16)

1. *Extremities and body wall.* The extremities and body wall have numerous effectors that receive an autonomic innervation. Anatomically, the innervation is only sympathetic and it conforms to the scheme shown in Figure 11.15b, that is, each spinal nerve contains postganglionic sympathetic fibers of neurons whose cell bodies are in the vertebral chain of ganglia. These fibers are unmyelinated and are designated visceral efferent. Anatomically, the extremities and body wall do not receive an outflow from the parasympathetic system; nevertheless, the parasympathetic influence might be represented functionally, at least with respect to the innervation of sweat glands, since the neurotransmitter

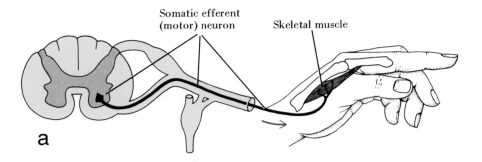

Somatic efferent
(motor) neuron

Skeletal muscle

a

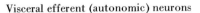

Visceral efferent (autonomic) neurons

Preganglionic   Postganglionic

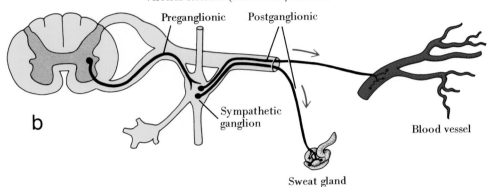

Sympathetic
ganglion

Blood vessel

b

Sweat gland

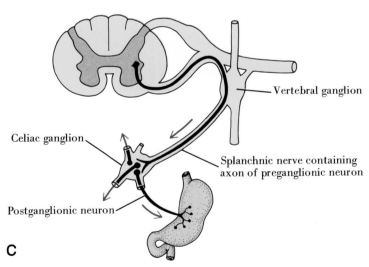

Vertebral ganglion

Celiac ganglion

Splanchnic nerve containing
axon of preganglionic neuron

Postganglionic neuron

c

Figure 11.15(a-c). Comparison between arrangement of **(a)** efferent neurons of the somatic system supplying skeletal muscle and **(b)** efferent neurons of the autonomic (sympathetic) nervous system supplying smooth muscle (as in a blood vessel) or glandular epithelium (as in a sweat gland). In the somatic system **(a)**, one neuron conducts the impulses from CNS to the effector (skeletal msucle); in the autonomic system **(b)**, the impulses are conducted by a chain of two neurons. Moreover, each preganglionic neuron makes synaptic contact with more than one postganglionic neuron. Neurons of the autonomic (sympathetic) nervous system supplying organs of the abdomen reach the abdominal organs by way of the splanchnic nerves **(c)**. In the case shown, the splanchnic nerve joins with the celiac ganglion where most of the synpases of the two-neuron chain occur. Note that the one preganglionic neuron makes contact with several postganglionic neurons. (From Reith EJ, Breidenbach, Lorenc, et al: *Textbook of Anatomy and Physiology,* 2nd ed. New York, McGraw Hill, 1978.)

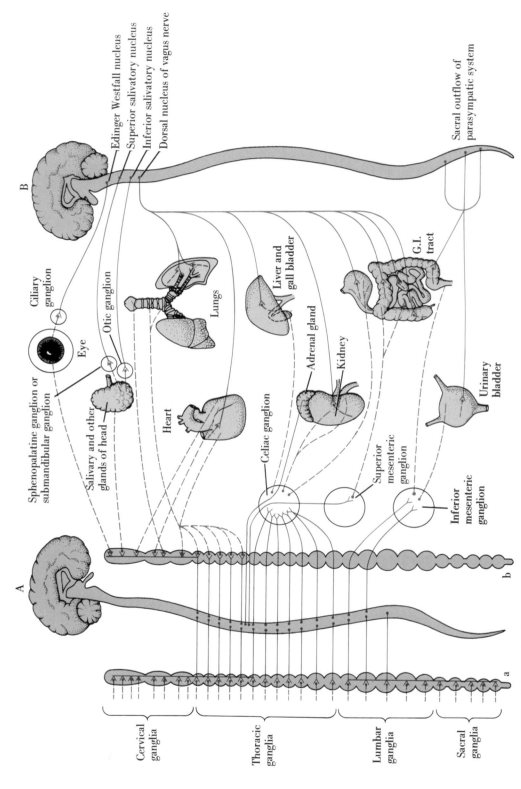

Figure 11.16. Schematic diagram showing general arrangement of sympathetic and parasympathetic neurons of the autonomic nervous system. The sympathetic outflow is shown in **A**. There are two chains of vertebral ganglia: **(a)** and **(b)**. Both contain the same neuronal components, but **(a)** shows only the outflow destined for the smooth muscle and glands in somatic territories (for example, smooth muscle in blood vessels of the limbs), whereas **(b)** shows the outflow to the viscera of the body. The sympathetic outflow leaves the CNS from the thoracic and upper lumbar segments of the spinal cord. The parasympathetic outflow **(B)** leaves the CNS from the brain stem and sacral spinal cord segments and is distributed to the viscera. The viscera, thus, contain both a sympathetic and parasympathetic innervation. Note that a two-neuron chain carries impulses to all effectors except the adrenal medulla. (From Reith EJ, et al: *Textbook of Anatomy and Physiolgy.* 2nd ed. New York, McGraw Hill, 1978.)

delivered to these glands by the "sympathetic" neurons is ACh instead of the usual NE.

2. **Head.** The parasympathetic preganglionic outflow to the head leaves the brain with the cranial nerves as indicated in Figure 11.16, but the routes are quite complex. For the histology student, it is important to know that cell bodies might also be found in structures that are clearly not the head ganglia listed in Table 11.1 and Figure 11.16. For example, cell bodies might be found in the tongue. These are "terminal" ganglion cells of the parasympathetic system.

The sympathetic preganglionic outflow to the head comes from the thoracic region of the spinal cord. The postganglionic neurons have their cell bodies in the superior cervical ganglion and the axons leave the ganglion in a nerve network that hugs the wall of the internal carotid artery. The nerve is called the **internal carotid nerve** or the **internal carotid plexus.** Some postganglionic fibers also reach the head by a much smaller **external carotid nerve** and plexus.

3. **Thorax.** Parasympathetic preganglionic outflow to the thoracic viscera is via the vagus (X) nerve. The postganglionic neurons have their cell bodies in the walls or in the substance of the organs of the thorax. Sympathetic postganglionic neurons for the heart are mostly in the cervical ganglia. The axon of these neurons make up nerves called **cardiac nerves.** Postganglionic sympathetic neurons for the other thoracic viscera are in ganglia of the thoracic part of the sympathetic chain. The axons are in small **splanchnic nerves,** which travel from the sympathetic chain to the organs.

4. **Abdomen and pelvis.** Parasympathetic preganglionic outflow to the abdominal viscera is via the vagus (X) and pelvic nerves. Postganglionic neurons of the parasympathetic system to abdominopelvic organs are in terminal ganglia that, for the most part, are in the walls of the organs themselves. Examples of these ganglia are the ganglionic portion of Meissner's plexus and Auerbach's plexus.

The sympathetic preganglionic outflow to the abdominopelvic organs is from the thoracic and upper lumbar segments of the spinal cord. Postganglionic neurons have their cell bodies mostly in the prevertebral ganglia (see Fig. 11.15c). However, some of the sympathetic synapses occur in the vertebral chain itself as the sympathetic pathway passes through the chain to enter the splanchnic nerves.

HISTOLOGICAL FEATURES OF THE CENTRAL NERVOUS SYSTEM

Examination of a cut surface of any part of the CNS reveals that it consists of gray matter and white matter. These have specific locations within different parts of the CNS. In the spinal cord, the gray matter occurs in the core of the organ, presenting the general form of an H on the cut surface (see Fig. 11.13). Surrounding the gray matter of the spinal cord is white matter. The cerebrum and cerebellum have a reverse arrangement. For these two parts of the brain there is an outer cover of gray matter, designated as the **cortex,** and an inner core of white matter.

The white matter contains only axons of nerve cells plus the associated neuroglial cells and blood vessels. These axons travel from one part of the nervous system to another. Whereas many of the fibers (axons) going to or coming from a specific location are grouped into bundles called **tracts,** the tracts themselves do not stand out as delineated bundles of fibers. The demonstration of a tract in white matter of the CNS requires some special procedure such as the destruction of cell bodies, which contributes fibers to the tract. The damaged fibers can be displayed by the use of appropriate methods and then traced. Even in the spinal cord, where the grouping of tracts is most pronounced, there are no sharp boundaries between adjacent tracts.

In contrast the white matter, the nerve tissue of gray matter contains cell bodies, fibers (both axons and dendrites), and the associated neurological cells. The gray matter is the site for synapses.

In addition to the gray matter of the cortex, the deeper substance of the cerebrum and cerebellum contains islands of gray matter called **nuclei.** In this context, the term nucleus means a cluster or group of neuronal cell bodies plus fibers and neuroglia.

The kinds of cell bodies found in the gray matter vary according to which part of the brain or spinal cord is being examined. Each functional region of the gray matter has a characteristic variety of cell bodies associated with a meshwork of axonal dendritic and glial processes. The organization of this meshwork of processes, called the **neuropil,** is not demonstrable in hematoxylin and eosin-stained (H&E) sections.

It is left for methods other than H&E histology to decipher the cytoarchitecture of the gray matter. Although general histology programs do not generally deal with the actual arrangements of the nerve cell in the CNS, it is believed that certain examples will add to the appreciation of the H&E

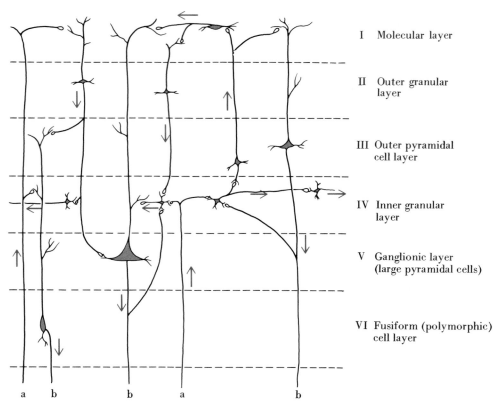

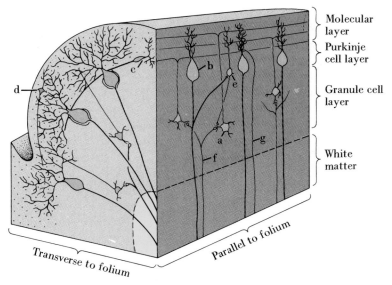

Figure 11.17. Simple scheme of intracortical circuits: **(a)** cortical afferent fibers; **(b)** cortical efferent fibers. The interneurons are unlabeled. The **arrows** show direction of impulses. The numbers and labels on the right correspond to the layers of the cerebral cortex in the Atlas section, Plate 42. (Based on Barr ML: *The Human Nervous System,* 4th ed. New York, Harper & Row, 1983.)

Figure 11.18. Cytoarchitecture of the cerebellar cortex: **(a)** granule cell; **(b)** Purkinje cell; **(c)** basket cell; **(d)** stellate cell; **(e)** Golgi cell; **(f)** mossy fiber; **(g)** climbing fiber. (Based on Barr ML: *The Human Nervous System,* 4th ed. New York, Harper & Row, 1983.)

specimen. The two examples are a region of the cerebral cortex (Fig. 11.17) and the cerebellar cortex (Fig. 11.18). These figures refer to neuron types illustrated in the Atlas section, Plates 42 and 43. The figures should be correlated with the description of those plates.

The midbrain, pons, and medulla are collectively referred to as the brain stem. Their organization is closely, but not entirely, associated with the cranial nerves. Histologically, the brain stem contains numerous islands of gray matter surrounded by white matter. Some of this white matter is comprised of more or less distinct tracts. In other cases, the definition between white matter and gray matter, as in the *reticular substance,* is not very clear. Many of the nuclei in the brain stem contain cell bodies of motor neurons of the cranial nerves. These motor nuclei are counterparts of the anterior horns of the spinal cord.

CONNECTIVE TISSUE OF THE CENTRAL NERVOUS SYSTEM

The brain and spinal cord are covered by connective tissue membranes called the **meninges.** The three meninges are the ***dura mater,*** the ***arachnoid,*** and the ***pia mater.***

The dura mater is a tough, relatively thick sheet made up of dense connective tissue. In the cranial cavity, the outer surface of the dura is directly connected to the bone and, in fact, constitutes the periosteum of the bone. Separations in the dura mater, called the ***venous sinuses,*** serve as channels for venous blood. Sheet-like extensions of the dura mater form incomplete partitions between certain parts of the brain. In the spinal canal, the dura mater constitutes a tube separated from the vertebrae (Fig. 11.19).

The arachnoid is a delicate sheet of connective tissue joined to the inner surface of the dura mater. It sends delicate trabeculae to the pia mater. Between the arachnoid and the pia mater is the ***subarachnoid space.*** This space contains cerebrospinal fluid (Fig. 11.20).

The pia mater consists of delicate connective tissue directly on the surface of the brain and spinal cord. The connective tissue of the pia mater is continuous with the perivascular connective tissue sheath of blood vessels in the brain and spinal cord.

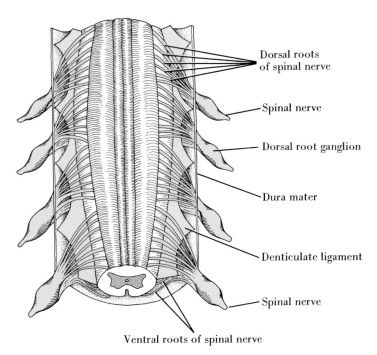

Dorsal roots of spinal nerve

Spinal nerve

Dorsal root ganglion

Dura mater

Denticulate ligament

Spinal nerve

Ventral roots of spinal nerve

Figure 11.19. Dorsal view of exposed spinal cord showing that each spinal nerve joins the cord by a number of dorsal and ventral roots. Also shown are the dura mater and the denticulate ligaments. The former is the outer layer of the meninges covering the cord; the latter is a delicate connective tissue sheet which aids in anchoring the cord. (Based on Barr ML: *The Human Nervous System,* 4th ed. New York, Harper & Row, 1983.)

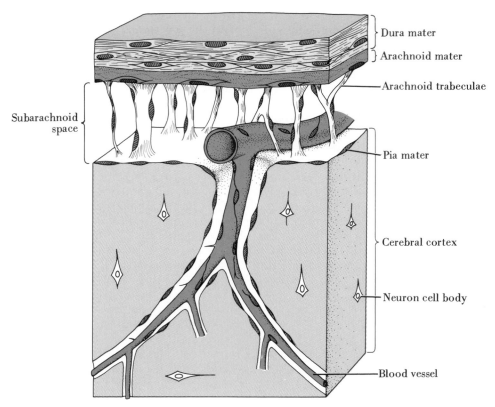

Figure 11.20. A schematic diagram of the cerebral meninges. The outer layer, the dura mater, is joined to adjacent bone of the cranial cavity (not shown). The inner layer, the pia mater, rests directly on the neural tissue. The intervening layer, the arachnoid mater, is attached to the dura mater and sends delicate trabeculae to the pia mater. Between the arachnoid and the pia mater is the subarachnoid space; it contains cerebrospinal fluid. The space also contains the larger blood vessels that send branches into the substance of the brain. A sheath of cells, which is continuous with the pia mater and surrounds the branches of the blood vessels supplying the brain, is indicated by the nuclei of the cells located on the external surface of the vessels. (Based on Weed, 1934. In Junqueira LC, Carneiro J: *Basic Histology,* 3rd ed. Los Altos, CA, Lange, 1980.)

REGENERATION OF NERVOUS TISSUE

Although neurons cannot divide to replace those that were destroyed, there is some measure of regeneration of nerve fibers. The regeneration of fibers in peripheral nerves has been studied extensively and it is illustrated in Figure 11.21. When the fiber is cut, the segment of the fiber separated from the cell body undergoes degeneration; this is called *Wallerian degeneration.* Some degeneration of the fiber occurs in a retrograde direction, but only for an internodal segment or two. Changes also occur in the cell body, the most conspicuous being the disorganization of the Nissl bodies, a process called *chromotolysis,* and a migration of the nucleus to a more peripheral location in the cell body. The amount of axoplasm separated from the cell body by the injury has a direct effect on how

severely the cell body reacts to the injury. If the axon is cut far from the cell body, separating only a relatively small amount of axoplasm, the changes in the cell body are not so severe. In some instances, there are only minimal reactions in the cell body even though a substantial amount of axoplasm appears to have been lost due to injury; in these cases it has been postulated that axoplasm of collateral branches sustain the cell body. Extensive loss of axoplasm, as when the injury is close to the cell body, may result in death of the cell. When the fiber is cut, the muscle innervated by the neuron undergoes atrophy.

The peak of the chromatolysis reaction is manifest about 2 weeks after the injury. During this time, macrophages enter the Schwann cell sheath and remove fragments of axon and myelin. At the same time, the Schwann cells multiply and

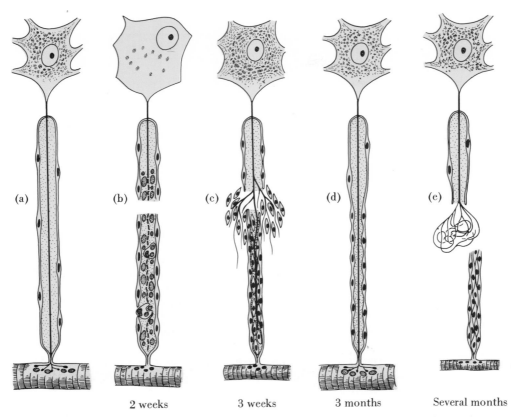

(a)   (b)   (c)   (d)   (e)

2 weeks   3 weeks   3 months   Several months

Figure 11.21(a-e). Main changes that take place in an injured nerve fiber. **(a)** Normal nerve fiber, with its perikaryon and the effector cell (striated skeletal muscle). Note the position of the neuron nucleus and the amount and distribution of Nissl bodies. **(b)** When the fiber is injured, the neuronal nucleus moves to the cell periphery and Nissl bodies become greatly reduced in number. The nerve fiber distal to the injury degenerates along with its myelin sheath. Debris is phagocytosed by macrophages. **(c)** The muscle fiber shows a pronounced disuse atrophy. Schwann cells proliferate, forming a compact cord penetrated by the growing axon. The axon grows at a rate of 0.5–3 mm per day. **(d)** In this example, the nerve fiber regeneration was successful. Note that the muscle fiber was also regenerated after receiving nerve stimuli. **(e)** When the axon does not penetrate the cord of Schwann cells, its growth is not organized. (Based on Willis RA, Willis AT: *The Principles of Pathology and Bacteriology,* 3rd ed. Woburn, MA, Butterworth, 1972 and from Junquera LC, Caneiro J: *Basic Histology,* 3rd ed. Los Altos, CA, Lange, 1980.)

form a cord of cells along the route of the damaged fiber and axonal sprouts begin to grow from the cut end of the proximal stump. A successful sprout manages to follow the route to the effector that was reestablished by the cord of Schwann cells. Other nerve sprouts without appropriate guidance from the Schwann cells regress. The successful sprout grows at a rate of about 3 mm per day and ulti-mately reestablishes contact with the muscle. After functional contact is reestablished by the nerve the muscle returns to its healthy state. By this time the Nissl bodies of the cell body and the position of the nucleus have returned to their original conditions. If the axonal sprout does not re-establish contact with the cord of Schwann cells, it grows in a disor-ganized manner and the muscle stays atrophic.

PLATE 37. Sympathetic and Dorsal Root Ganglia

Sympathetic ganglia constitute a major sub-class of autonomic ganglia (parasympathetic ganglia constitute the other subclass). Autonomic ganglia are peripheral motor ganglia containing cell bodies of postsynaptic neurons. These neurons conduct nerve impulses to smooth muscle, cardiac muscle, and glands. Synapses between presynaptic neurons (all of which have their cell body in the CNS) and postsynaptic neurons occur in autonomic ganglia.

A sympathetic ganglion stained with silver and counter stained is illustrated in **Figure 1.** Shown to advantage in the preparation are several discrete bundles of nerve fibers **(NF)** and numerous large circular structures, namely, the cell bodies **(CB)** of the postsynaptic neurons. In addition to the organized nerve fibers, more random patterns of nerve fibers are also seen. Moreover, careful examination of the cell bodies shows that some display several processes joined to the cell bodies. Thus, these are multipolar neurons, one of which is contained within the **rectangle** and is shown at higher magnification in **Figure 2.** Generally, the connective tissue is not conspicuous in a silver preparation, although it can be identified by virtue of its location about the larger blood vessels **(BV),** particularly in the upper part of **Figure 1.**

The cell bodies of the sympathetic ganglion are typically large, and the one labeled in **Figure 2** shows several processes **(P).** In addition, the cell body contains a large, pale-staining spherical nucleus **(N),** and this in turn contains a spherical intensely staining nucleolus **(NI).** [These features, namely, a large pale-staining nucleus (indicative of much extended chromatin) and a large nucleolus, reflect a cell that is metabolically active in protein synthesis.] Also shown in the cell body are accumulations of pigment; this is lipofuscin **(L),** a yellow pigment that is darkened by the silver. Because of the large size of the cell body, sometimes the nucleus is not included in the section, in which case the cell body appears as a rounded cytoplasmic mass. Whereas the silver preparation displays the multipolar cell bodies and nerve fibers to great advantage, other methods need to be used to display satellite cells and myelin better.

Dorsal root ganglia differ from autonomic ganglia in a number of ways. Whereas the latter contain multipolar neurons and have synaptic con-

nections, dorsal root ganglia contain unipolar sensory neurons and have no synaptic connections.

Part of a dorsal root ganglion stained with H&E is shown in **Figure 3.** The specimen includes the edge of the ganglion, and here it is covered with connective tissue **(CT).** The dorsal root ganglion contains large cell bodies **(CB)** that are typically arranged as closely packed clusters. Also, between and around the cell clusters, there are bundles of nerve fibers **(NF).** Most of the fiber bundles indicated by the label have been sectioned longitudinally. At higher magnification of the same ganglion, as seen in **Figure 4,** the constituents of the nerve fiber show their characteristic relationship, namely, a centrally located axon **(A)** surrounded by a myelin space (not labeled), which, in turn, is bounded on its outer border by the thin cytoplasmic strand of the neurilemma **(arrowheads).**

The cell bodies of the sensory neurons display large, pale-staining spherical nuclei **(N)** and intensely staining nucleoli **(NI)** with the same functional implications as mentioned above. Also seen in this H&E preparation are the nuclei of satellite cells **(SatC)** that completely surround the cell body. Note how much smaller these cells are than the neurons. In effect, the satellite cells form a sheath around the nerve cell body. They are continuous with the Schwann cells that invest the axon. Clusters of cells **(asterisks)** within the ganglion, which have an epithelioid appearance, are face views of satellite cells where the section tangentially included the satellite cells but barely grazed the adjacent cell body.

KEY	
A, axon	N, nucleus of nerve cell
BV, blood vessels	NI, nucleolus
CB, cell body of neuron	NF, nerve fibers
CT, connective tissue	P, processes of nerve
L, lipofuscin	cell body
arrowheads, Fig. 3.	Sat C, satellite cells
neurilemma	

Fig. 1, human, × 150	**Fig. 3,** cat, × 150
Fig. 2, human, × 500	**Fig. 4,** cat, × 350

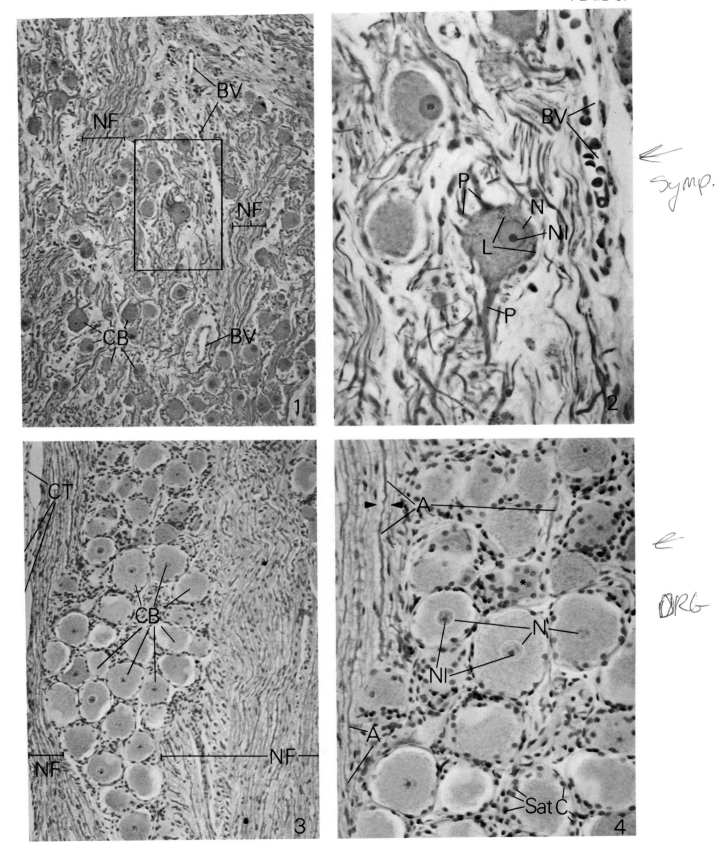

PLATE 37

PLATE 38. Sympathetic Ganglion I, Electron Microscopy

The specimen in the accompanying electron micrograph depicts a sympathetic ganglion similar to that seen in the light micrographs of the preceding plate. At the magnification utilized here, the neuron cell bodies (**CB**) along with a myriad of nerve fibers (**NF**) can be identified readily. Two of the cell bodies were sectioned in a plane that includes the nucleus (**N**) and one also reveals the nucleolus (**Nu**). The neuron cell body and one of its processes (within the rectangle) is shown at higher magnification in the Atlas section, Plate 39. Other cells within the ganglion, but somewhat less easy to identify at this magnification, include fibroblasts (**F**), Schwann cells, and satellite cells. Surrounding the ganglion is a specialized connective tissue, the perineurium (**P**), part of which can be seen in the **upper left corner** of the micrograph. It is continuous with the connective tissue covering of the nerve bundles that enter the ganglion. Perineurium is considered in some detail with respect to nerve in the Atlas section, Plate 40 and at the electron microscopic level in the Atlas section, Plate 41. Also seen in the ganglion is a small blood vessel (**BV**). The intercellular matrix consists largely of collagen that, together with the fibroblasts, comprises the endoneurium of the ganglion.

A feature not appreciated with the light microscope, but evident in electron micrographs is the relationship of the satellite cells to the neuron cell bodies. Each cell body is surrounded by a thin sheath of satellite cell cytoplasm that covers not only the cell body, but may extend for a short distance onto its processes. The attenuated satellite cell cytoplasm (**Sat**) is just barely recognizable at this low magnification. It can be seen best around the two cell bodies in the lower part of the micrograph. The cytoplasm of the satellite cell has slightly greater electron density than the neuron and, thus, gives the appearance of a thin rim around the neuron cell body. In the thin sections employed in electron microscopy, the nuclear region of the satellite cell is infrequently included in the plane of section; in the preparation shown here, only one satellite cell nucleus (**SatN**) is present.

Typically, both myelinated and unmyelinated fibers are present in sympathetic ganglia. How-

---

KEY

BV, blood vessel
CB, neuron cell body
F, fibroblast (endoneurial cell)
My, myelin
N, nucleus
NF, nerve fibers
Nu, nucleolus

P, perineurium
Sat, satellite cell cytoplasm
SatN, satellite cell nucleus
SCN, Schwann cell nucleus

Fig., human, × 4200

---

ever, only one of the many fibers included in the portion of the ganglion seen here is myelinated; it is just to the left of the blood vessel. The myelin sheath (**My**) surrounding the nerve fiber appears as the ovoid black ring. External to the myelin, one can identify the nucleus of the associated Schwann cell (**SCN**). All of the unmyelinated nerve fibers are also enclosed by Schwann cell cytoplasm. However, instead of a single axon being surrounded by Schwann cell cytoplasm as in the case of the myelinated fibers, the Schwann cells related to the unmyelinated nerve fibers will usually ensheath more than a single fiber. Generally, a number of sectioned fibers can be seen included within a Schwann cell. In effect, the Schwann cell has the same relationship to the nerve fiber as the satellite cell has to the cell body. Both are disposed as an intimate cellular sheath around the neural element. Although Schwann and satellite cells are designated by different names, they probably have the same function and may differ only in terms of location. Both satellite cells and Schwann cells can be looked upon as peripheral neurologia.

Connective tissue occupies the interstices of the neural elements within the ganglion. In this illustration, several fibroblasts (**F**) are evident. Some fibroblasts are located in close apposition to the neuron cell bodies. With the light microscope, it would be most difficult, if not impossible, to distinguish such a fibroblast nucleus from that of a satellite cell.

PLATE 38

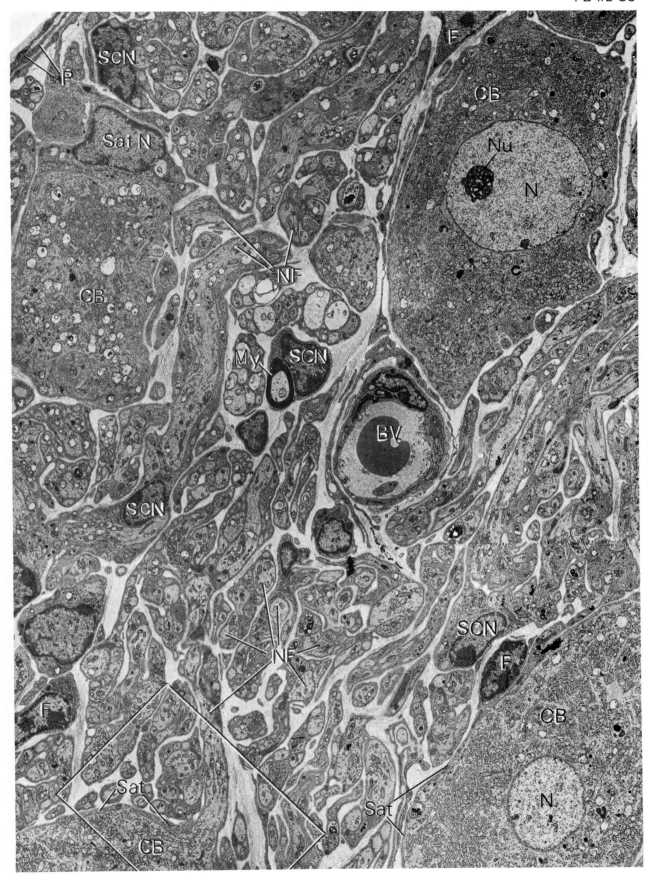

PLATE 39. Sympathetic Ganglion II, Electron Microscopy

The electron micrograph shown here reveals at higher magnification the **rectangular area** from the previous plate. The cytoplasm of the neuron cell body exhibits numerous mitochondria **(M),** clusters of polyribosomes **(R),** and profiles of rough-surfaced endoplasmic reticulum **(RER).** The ribosomes and elements of the endoplasmic reticulum tend to aggregate in recognizable masses. The limits of these ribosome-rich areas are not sharply defined. However, one such concentration is shown enscribed by the **broken line.** These localized regions of ribosome-rich cytoplasm may be visualized in the light microscope, after staining with a basic dye such as toluidine blue. The staining reaction results in the appearance of small colored bodies, referred to as Nissl bodies (see Fig. 3, Atlas section, Plate 44). Between the ribosome-rich areas, microtubules, neurofilaments, and mitochondria predominate, as they do throughout the cell process.

The satellite cell **(SatC)** can be distinguished from the neuron cell body simply by differences in cytoplasmic density; it appears conspicuously more electron dense than the neuron. The satellite cell provides a complete covering sheath about the cell body. In some areas, it may be extremely attenuated **(arrowheads).** Similarly, the nerve process emanating from the cell body is ensheathed by cytoplasm, identical in appearance to that covering the cell body. The neuronal process is covered by cytoplasm of the Schwann cell **(SC).** (The site at which the satellite cell terminates and the Schwann cell investment begins is not evident in the example shown here.)

The unmyelinated nerve fibers **(NF)** are sectioned in various planes. Each nerve fiber is surrounded by Schwann cell cytoplasm **(SC)** that displays the same electron opacity as the cytoplasm of the satellite cells. A few of these nerve fibers appear as singular profiles covered by Schwann cell cytoplasm **(asterisks).** Most of the nerve fibers, however, are embedded in groups within the confines of the Schwann cell. Both the satellite cell and Schwann cell are surfaced by basal lamina **(BL)** (see **inset).** Thus, the neuron, by means of its associated cell cover, is isolated from the collagen matrix **(C).**

KEY

A, axon terminal
BL, basal lamina
C, collagen
D, dendrite
L, lysosome
M, mitochondria
NF, nerve fiber
R, ribosome clusters
RER, rough-surfaced
  endoplasmic
  reticulum

SatC, satellite cell
SC, Schwann cell
arrow, synaptic cleft
arrowhead, attenuated
  satellite cell sheath
asterisk, nerve fiber
  covered by Schwann
  cell cytoplasm

Fig., human × 22,000
  (inset, × 45,000)

With respect to the individual fibers, it is not always possible to distinguish an axon from a dendrite. However, a general rule is that if the fiber displays synaptic vesicles (the small round profiles), it is identified as an axon terminal **(A);** if it displays profiles of granular endoplasmic reticulum, it is identified as a dendrite **(D).** Fibers that do not exhibit these specific characteristics are best referred to simply as nerve fibers. The axon **(A)** that has entered the satellite sheath of the neuron cell body contains numerous synaptic vesicles. Presumably it will make synaptic contact with the cell body in this vicinity (an axosomatic synapse).

The small **circle** encloses an axondendritic synapse which is shown at higher magnification in the inset. The axon **(A)** of this synapse reveals numerous synaptic vesicles most of which appear empty, but they contain the neurotransmitter acetylcholine. The vesicle with granules, several of which are seen in the inset, contain catecholamines. The space **(arrow)** between the axon and dendrite **(D)** is the synaptic cleft. It is across this space that the neurotransmitter substance passes to stimulate the membrane of the postsynaptic cell. The presence of ribosomes in the postsynaptic cytoplasm indicate a dendrite; thus, the synapse is an axondendritic synapse.

PLATE 39

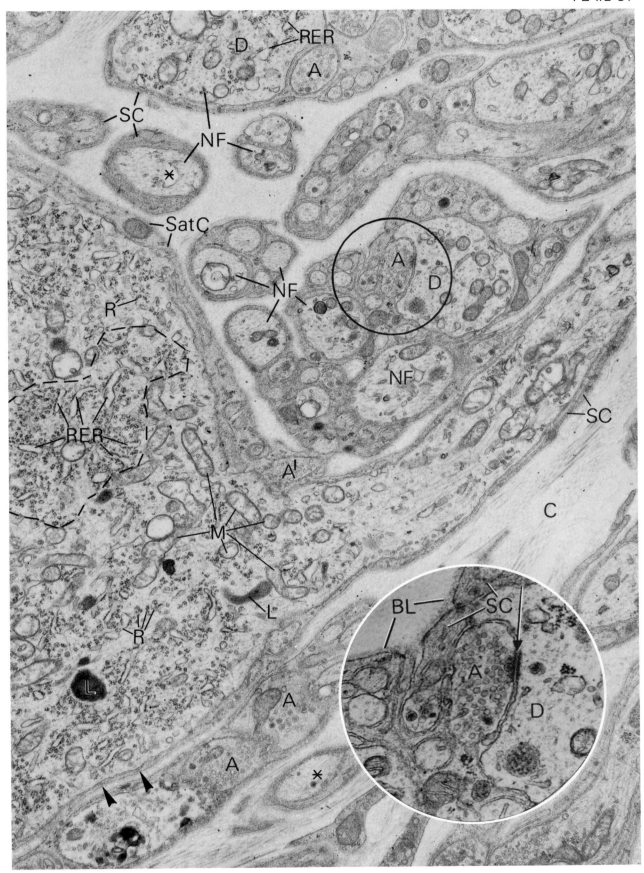

PLATE **40**. Peripheral Nerve

Nerves are comprised of bundles of nerve fibers held together by perineurium and connective tissue. Each nerve fiber[3] consists of an axon that is surrounded by a cellular investment called the neurilemma or the sheath of Schwann. In addition, the fiber may be myelinated or unmyelinated. The myelin, if present, is immediately around the axon and is, in turn, surrounded by the neurilemma.

A cross-section through a femoral nerve stained with H&E (**Fig. 1**) shows several bundles of nerve fibers (**BNF).** The external cover for the entire nerve is the epineurium (**Epn),** the layer of dense connective tissue that one touches when a nerve has been exposed during a dissection. The epineurium also serves as the outermost cover of the individual bundles. The epineurium contains blood vessels (**BV)** and it may contain some fat cells. Typically, adipose tissue (**AT)** is found about the nerve.

Figure 2 shows an area from the upper left of **Figure 1** at higher magnification. The illustration has been rotated, and the septum (marked in **Fig. 1** with **arrows)** is now vertically disposed (**arrows).**

The layer under the epineurium that directly surrounds the bundle of nerve fibers is the perineurium (**Pn).** As seen in the cross-section through the nerve, the nuclei of the perineurial cells appear flat and elongate; they are actually being viewed on edge and they belong to flat cells, which are also being viewed on edge. Again, as noted by the distribution of nuclei, it can be ascertained that the perineurium is only a few cells in thickness. The perineurium is a specialized layer of cells and extracellular material whose arrangement is not evident in H&E sections. They are shown in the following electron micrograph (Atlas section, Plate 41). The perineurium (**Pn)** and epineurium (**Epn)** are readily distinguished in the triangular area formed by the diverging perineurium of the two adjacent nerve bundles.

The nerve fibers included in **Figure 2** are mostly myelinated and, because the nerve is cross-sectioned, the nerve fibers are also. They have a characteristic appearance when seen in cross-section. Each nerve fiber shows a centrally placed axon (**A);** this is surrounded by a myelin space (**M)** in which some radially disposed precipitate may be retained as in this specimen; and external to the myelin space is a thin cytoplasmic rim representing the neurilemma (**NI).** On occasion, a Schwann cell

---
[3] See footnote on page 255.

nucleus (**SS)** appears to be perched on the neurilemma. As noted in the illustration, the upper edge of the nuclear crescent appears to occupy the same plane as that occupied by the neurilemma. These features enable one to identify the nucleus as belonging to a Schwann (neurilemma) cell. Other nuclei (**N)** are not related to the neurilemma but, rather, appear to be between the nerve fibers. Such nuclei belong to fibroblasts of the endoneurium. The latter is the delicate connective tissue between the individual nerve fibers; it is extremely sparse and contains the capillaries (**C)** of the nerve bundle.

The edge of the longitudinally sectioned nerve bundle is shown in **Figure 3.** The boundary between the epineurium (**Epn)** and perineurium is ill defined. Within the nerve bundle, the nerve fibers show a characteristic wavy pattern. Included among the wavy nerve fibers are nuclei belonging to Schwann cells and to cells within the endoneurium. Higher magnification (**Fig. 4)** allows one to identify certain specific components of the nerve. Note that the nerve fibers (**NF)** are now shown in longitudinal profile. Moreover, each myelinated nerve fiber shows a centrally positioned axon (**A),** surrounded by a myelin space (**M),** which, in turn, is bordered on its outer edge by the thin cytoplasmic band of the neurilemmal cell (**NI).** Another diagnostic feature of myelinated nerve fibers is also seen in longitudinal section, namely, the node of Ranvier (**NR).** This is where the ends of the two Schwann cells meet. Histologically, the node appears as a constriction of the neurilemma and sometimes the constriction is marked by a cross-band as in **Figure 4.** It is difficult to determine if the nuclei (**N)** shown in **Figure 4** belong to Schwann cells or to endoneurial fibroblasts.

PLATE 40

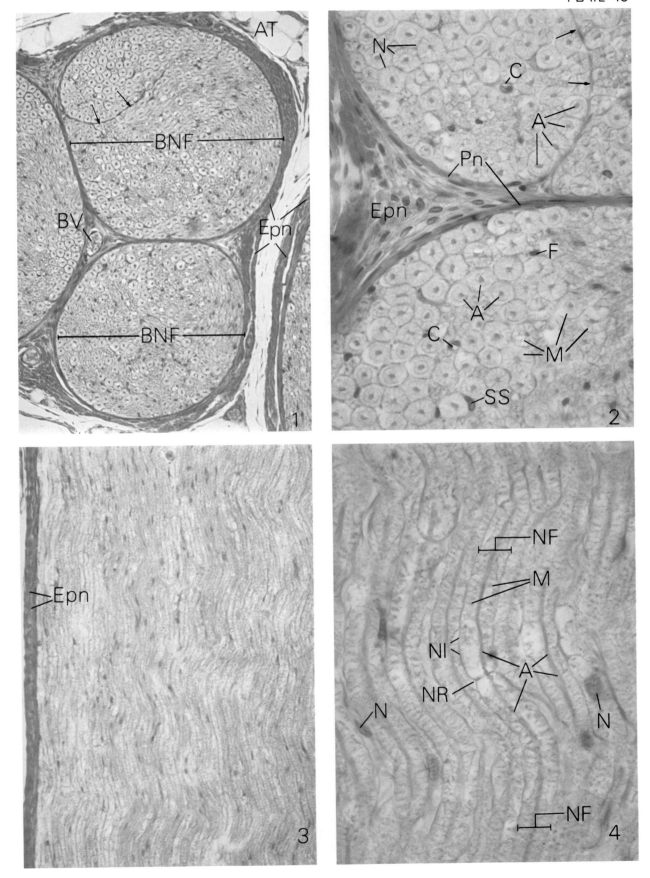

PLATE 41. Perineurium, Electron Microscopy

Perineurium has special characteristics that distinguish it from the connective tissue that comprises epineurium and endoneurium. Unlike epineurial and endoneurial cells, which are typical fibroblasts, perineurial cells exhibit epithelioid as well as myoid features.

The electron micrograph reveals the outer portion of a small nerve that has been longitudinally sectioned; an axon (A) that has been obliquely cut and its covering myelin sheath (M) is present in the upper right corner. The perineurium (Per) is to the left of the axon and appears as an orderly series of cellular layers. To the left of the perineurium is the epineurium, which contains a moderate amount of collagen (C), epineurial fibroblast processes (Epi F), and elastic material (E). The epineurium, unlike the perineurium, is less well defined. It tends to blend with the connective tissue more removed from the nerve. Thus, there is no discrete boundary between the epineurium and the surrounding connective tissue.

In examining the perineurium at this low magnification, the most notable feature is the relative uniformity of the individual cellular layers or lamellae. The cells that constitute each layer, in effect, are contiguous with one another. Typically, the edge of one cell meets in apposition with its neighbors, thus forming a series of uninterrupted concentric cellular sheaths, each of which completely surrounds the nerve bundle.

In contrast to the perineurial cells, a portion of another cell can be seen along the inner aspect of the perineurium. Although closely applied to the perineurium, this cell exhibits characteristics of a typical fibroblast and, as such, represents an endoneurial fibroblast (End F). Note that it does not form a continuous sheath-like structure, but rather exhibits a lateral margin (arrowhead) that does not meet on edge with another cell to provide continuity. This endoneurial cell is morphologically identical to the epineurial cell (Epi F); both are typical fibroblasts.

The cytological distinction between the fibroblasts of the epi- and endoneurium and the specialized perineurial cell can be appreciated better at

higher magnification (insets). The upper inset reveals a small portion of the perineurial cell; the lower inset, an epineurial cell. The specific site from which each is taken is indicated by the small ovals. In comparing the two cells, note that the perineural cell exhibits basal lamina (BL) on both surfaces; the fibroblast typically lacks this covering material. Both cell types reveal pinocytotic vesicles as well as mitochondria (Mi). However, the remainder of the cytoplasm in these two micrographs shows an important difference. The perineurial cell reveals numerous fine filaments, thought to represent myofilaments, and cytoplasmic densities (CD). Both are features characteristic of the smooth muscle cell. Again, the fibroblasts lack these elements. Although not evident here, the perineural cells also exhibit profiles of rER, but in lesser amount than that seen in the fibroblast (RER). The presence of rER in the perineurial cell suggests that it, like the fibroblast, produces collagen and, thus, could account for the deposition of collagen (C) between the cellular laminae. The myoid nature of the perineurial cells, as evidenced by the myofilaments and cytoplasmic densities, explains the shortening of a nerve when accidentally or surgically cut. Finally, the epithelial-like arrangement of the perineurial cells is regarded as a selective permeability barrier.

KEY

A, axon
BL, basal lamina
C, collagen fibrils
CD, cytoplasmic density
E, elastic fibers
End F, endoneurial fibroblast
Epi F, epineurial fibroblast

M, myelin
Mi, mitochondria
Per, perineurium
RER, rough endoplasmic reticulum
S, Schwann cell
arrowhead, margin of fibroblast

Fig., human, × 7,000
(insets, × 26,000)

PLATE 41

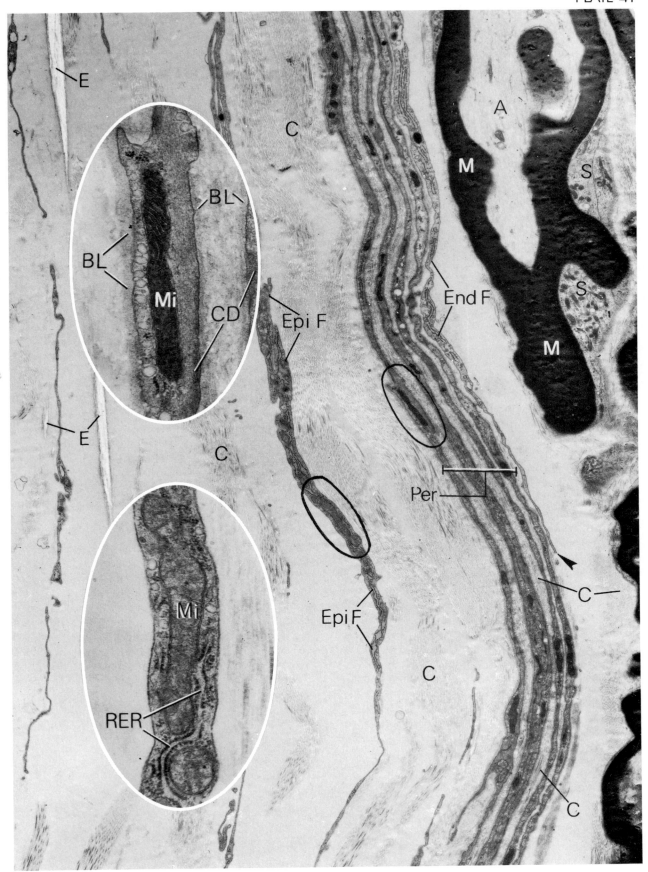

PLATE 42. Cerebrum

The cerebral cortex is described as containing six distinguishable layers. No sharp boundaries separate these layers; rather, they are distinguished on the basis of predominant cell type and fiber (axons and dendrites) arrangement. Although the various layers can be recognized in H&E preparations, these preparations do not provide information regarding the fiber arrangement.

Figure 1 is a low-power view of the cerebral cortex and includes a small amount of white matter below the lowest **broken line.** It is possible to recognize the two areas at a glance, inasmuch as the white matter contains many more nuclei than the cortex and, in addition, they are all of approximately the same size. These are nuclei of neuroglial cells (**NN**) and are shown at higher magnification in **Figure 5. Figure 5** also shows that the cytoplasm of the neuroglial cells is not distinguishable and, consequently, the cells appear as naked nuclei in a "no man's land," referred to as the neurophil (**Np**). Small blood vessels (**BV**) are also evident in the white matter.

The six layers of the cortex are marked in **Figure 1** and are best seen on the right side of the figure. None of these layers is sharply delineated; the **horizontal lines** represent only rough approximations. From the surface, the layers are: (**I**) The plexiform or molecular layer consists largely of fibers, most of which travel parallel to the surface, and relatively few cells. (**II**) The layer of small pyramidal cells (or outer granular layer) consists mainly of small cells, many of which have a pyramidal shape. (**III**) The layer of medium pyramidal cells (or layer of outer pyramidal cells) is not sharply marked from **layer II.** However, the cells are somewhat larger and possess a typical pyramidal shape. (**IV**) The granular layer (or inner granular layer) is characterized by the presence of many small stellate cells (granule cells). (**V**) The layer of large pyramidal cells (or inner layer of pyramidal cells) contains pyramidal cells that, in many parts of the cerebrum, are smaller than the pyramidal cells of **layer III,** but in the motor area are extremely large and are called Betz cells. (**VI**) The layer of polymorphic cells contains cells with diverse shapes, many of which have a spindle or

fusiform shape. These cells are called fusiform cells.

Three cell types have been referred to above: pyramidal cells, stellate cells (or granule cells), and fusiform cells. Two other cell types are also present in the cerebral cortex, but are not illustrated. They are the horizontal cells of Cajal, which are present only in **layer I** and send their processes laterally, and cells of Martinotti, which send their axons toward the surface (opposite to that of pyramidal cells).

Layer I is illustrated at higher magnification in **Figure 2** and reveals a blood capillary (**Cap**) and several nuclei. Most of these nuclei belong to neuroglial cells (**NN**). This conclusion is based on the fact that the cytoplasm belonging to these nuclei cannot be distinguished. One nucleus, however, is surrounded by cytoplasm (**arrow**) and, thus, is identified as part of a neuron cell body.

The **rectangle** in **Figure 1** is examined at higher magnification in **Figure 3.** The pyramidal cells (**PC**) contain an oval nucleus in which a small, intensely staining, round nucleolus is located. The cytoplasmic limits of the cell body appear roughly triangular. The base of the cell faces the white matter and sends a single axon in that direction. This process, however, is not evident. The apex of each cell body shows a large dendritic process, the apical dendrite, that extends toward the surface of the gray matter.

Figure 4 shows the small polymorphic cell bodies (**Pol C**) of **layer VI** and, again, neuroglial nuclei (**NN**).

PLATE 42

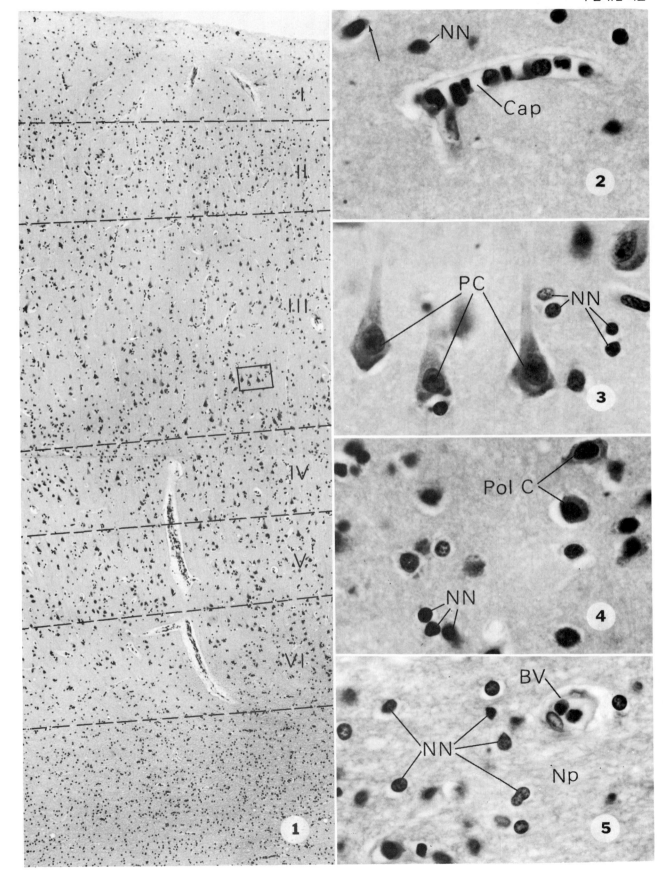

PLATE 43. Cerebellum

The cerebellar cortex is more or less the same in appearance regardless of which region is examined. **Figure 1** is a low-power view of the cerebellum stained by H&E. The outermost layer, the molecular layer (**Mol**), is lightly stained with eosin. Under this is the granular layer (**Gr**), which stains intensely with hematoxylin. Together, these two layers constitute the cortex of the cerebellum. Deep in the granular layer is another region that stains lightly with H&E and, except for location, shows no distinctive histological features. This is the white matter (**WM**). As in the cerebrum, it contains nerve fibers, supporting neuroglial cells and small blood vessels, but no neuronal cell bodies. The fibrous cover on the cerebellar surface is the pia mater (**Pia**). Cerebellar blood vessels (**BV**) can be seen in this layer. (Shrinkage artefact has separated the pia mater and blood vessels from the cerebellar surface).

The **rectangular area** in **Figure 1** is shown at higher magnification in **Figure 2**. At the junction between the molecular and granular layers are the extremely large flask-shaped cell bodies of the Purkinje cells (**Pkj**). These cells are characteristic of the cerebellum. They each possess numerous dendrites (**D**) that arborize in the molecular layer. The Purkinje cell has a single axon not usually evident in H&E sections. It should be noted that this nerve fiber represents the beginning of the outflow from the cerebellum.

Further reference to **Figure 2** explains the differences in H&E staining between the two cortical layers. The illustration shows relatively few neuron cell bodies, the basket cells (**BC**), in the molecular layer; they are widely removed from each other and, at best, show only a small amount of cytoplasm surrounding the nucleus. In contrast, the granular layer presents an overall spotted blue appearance due to the staining of numerous small nuclei (**Fig. 2**) with hematoxylin. These nuclei belong mostly to small neurons called granule cells. These cells receive incoming impulses from other parts of the CNS and they send axons into the molecular layer where they branch in the form of a T, so that the axons contact the dendrites of several Purkinje cells and basket cells. Incoming (mossy) fibers contact granule cells in the lightly stained areas called glomeruli (**arrows**). If one carefully examines the granular layer where it meets the molecular layer, there will be found a group of nuclei (**G**) that are larger than the nuclei of granule cells. These belong to Golgi type II cells.

KEY

BC, basket cells
BV, blood vessels
D, dendrites
F, fibers
G, Golgi type II cells
arrows, Fig. 2, glomeruli
arrow, Fig. 4, T
   branching of axon in
   molecular layer
rectangular area, Figs. 1
   and 3, areas shown at
   higher magnification
   in Figs. 2 and 4,
   respectively

Gr, granular layer
Mol, molecular layer
Pia, pia mater
Pkj, Purkinje cells
WM, white matter

Fig. 1, human, × 40
Fig. 2, human, × 40
Fig. 3, human, × 160

Fig. 4, human, × 400
Fig. 5, cat, × 160

The specimen in **Figure 3** has been stained with a silver procedure. Such procedures do not always color the specimen evenly as do H&E and it is easy to note that the part of the molecular layer on the right is much darker than that on the left. A **rectangular area** marked on the left has been selected for later examination at higher magnification. Even at the relatively low magnification shown in **Figure 3,** the Purkinje cells can be recognized in the silver preparation because of their large size, characteristic shape, and location between an outer molecular layer (**Mol**) and an inner layer (**Gr**). The main advantage of this silver preparation is that the white matter (**WM**) can be recognized as being comprised of fibers; they have been blackened by the silver staining procedure. The pia mater (**Pia**) and cerebellar blood vessels are also evident in the preparation.

At higher magnification (**Fig. 4**), the Purkinje cell bodies (**Pkj**) stand out as the most distinctive and conspicuous neuronal cell type of the cerebellum and numerous dendritic branches (**D**) can be seen. Note also the blackened fibers within the granular layer (**Gr**), about the Purkinje cell bodies, and in the molecular layer (**Mol**) disposed in a horizontal direction (relative to the cerebellar surface). The **arrow** indicates a T turn characteristic of the turn made by axons of granule cells. As these axonal branches travel horizontally, they make synaptic contact with numerous Purkinje cells.

278

PLATE 43

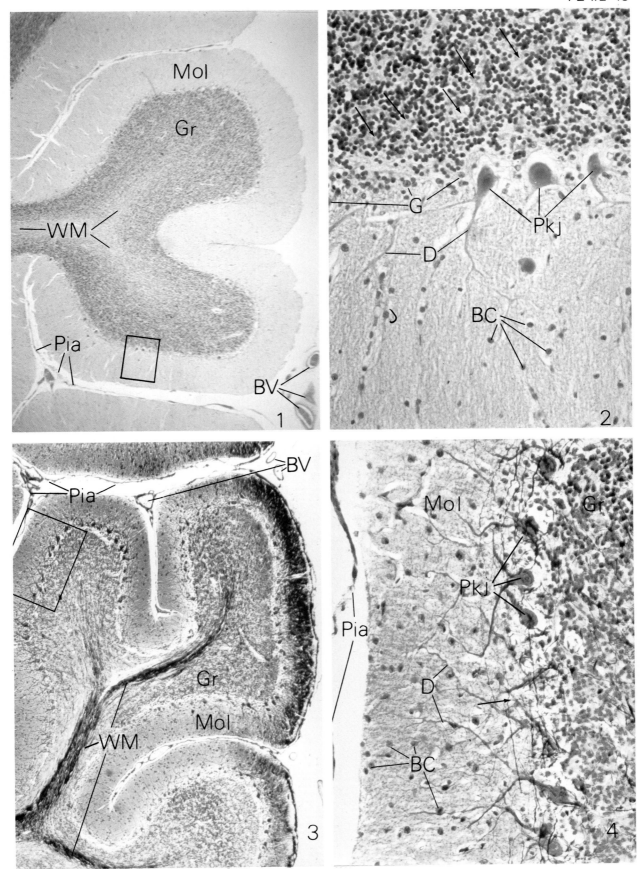

PLATE 44. Spinal Cord

The spinal cord is organized into two discrete parts. The outer part contains ascending and descending nerve fibers. This constitutes the white matter of the cord. The inner part contains cell bodies of neurons and nerve fibers. This is the gray matter of the spinal cord. Neuroglial cells are in both the white matter and the gray matter.

A cross-section through the cervical region of the spinal cord (human) is shown in **Figure 1.** The preparation is designed to stain the myelin that surrounds the ascending and descending fibers. Although the fibers that have common origins and destinations in the physiological sense are arranged in tracts, these tracts cannot be distinguished unless they have been marked by special techniques, such as causing injury to the cell bodies from which they arise.

The gray matter of the spinal cord appears roughly in the form of an H. The anterior and posterior prongs are referred to as anterior horns **(AH)** and posterior horns **(PH),** respectively. The connecting bar is called the gray commissure **(GC).** The neuron cell bodies that are within the anterior horns (anterior horn cells) are so large that they can be seen even at extremely low magnification **(arrows).** The pale-staining fibrous material that surrounds the spinal cord is the pia mater **(Pia).** It follows the surface of the spinal cord intimately and dips into the large ventral fissure **(VF)** and into the shallower sulci. Blood vessels are present in the pia mater. Some ventral **(VR)** and dorsal **(DR)** roots of the spinal nerves are included in the section.

An H&E preparation showing a region of an anterior horn is illustrated in **Figure 2.** The nucleus **(N)** of the anterior horn cell appears as the large, spherical, pale-staining structure within the

---

KEY

AH, anterior (ventral) horn
DR, drosal root
GC, gray commissure
N, nucleus of anterior horn cell
NB, Nissl bodies
NN, nucleus of neuroglial cell

Np, neuropil
PH, posterior (dorsal) horn
Pia, pia matter
VF, ventral fissure
VR, ventral root
arrows, Fig. 1, cell body of anterior (ventral) horn cell

Fig. 1, human, × 16
Fig. 2, human, × 640

Fig. 3, human, × 640

---

cell body. It contains a spherical, intensely staining nucleolus. The anterior horn cell contains many processes, two of which are seen in **Figure 2.** The illustration also shows a number of other nuclei that belong to neuroglial cells **(NN).** The cytoplasm of these cells is not evident. The remainder of the field consists of nerve fibers and neuroglial cell cytoplasm whose organization is hard to interpret. This is called the neurophil **(Np).** A capillary crosses through the field below the cell body.

A toluidine blue preparation of the spinal cord (a comparable area to that of **Fig. 2)** is shown in **Figure 3.** The toluidine blue reveals the Nissl bodies **(NB)** that appear as the large, dark-staining bodies in the cytoplasm. Nissl bodies do not extend into the axon hillock. (The axon leaves the cell body at the axon hillock.) The nuclei of neuroglial cells, **(NN)** are evident; the cytoplasm is not. The neurophil stains very faintly.

PLATE 44

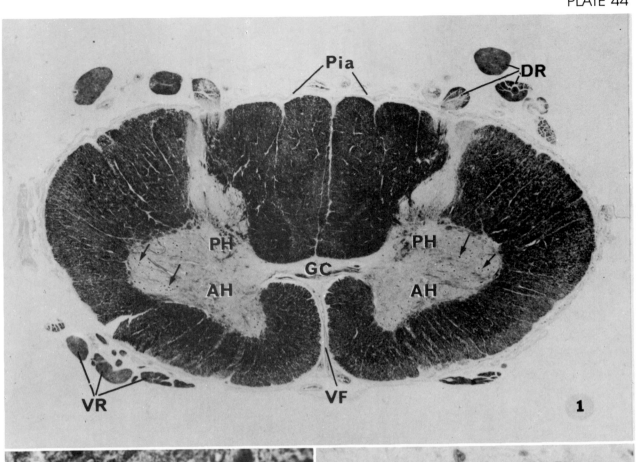

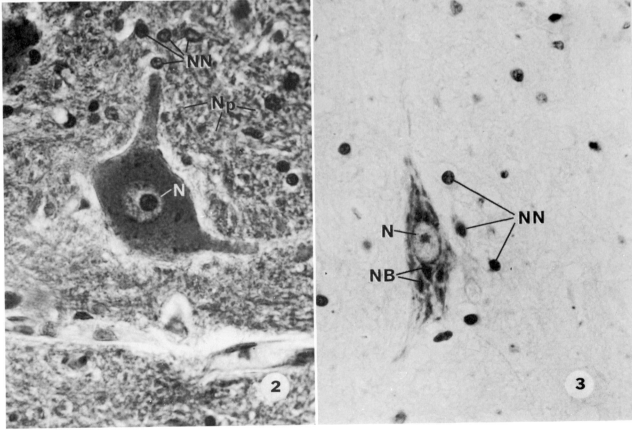

The Cardiovascular System

12

The cardiovascular system consists of blood vessels, which circulate blood to and from all parts of the body; the heart, which keeps the blood in motion; and the lymphatic vessels, an ancillary set of vessels, which circulate lymph. The different kinds of blood vessels are arranged so that the blood delivered from the heart quickly reaches a network of small, thin-walled vessels within or in proximity to the tissues in every part of the body. It is through the wall of these thin-walled vessels, the blood *capillaries*, that a two-directional exchange occurs between the blood and the tissues. Exchange also occurs through vessels called *postcapillary venules;* they are especially important as vessels that allow for the passage of certain blood cells into the tissues. This is particularly significant, for example, in the inflammatory reaction, during which large numbers of neutrophils can emigrate from these venules.

The blood vessels that deliver blood to the capillaries are the *arteries.* The smallest arteries, called *arterioles,* are functionally associated with the particular network of capillaries to which they deliver blood; they regulate the amount of blood going to the capillary network. Together, the arterioles, capillary network, and postcapillary venules are referred to as the *microcirculatory,* or *microvascular, bed* of that tissue (Fig. 12.1). Just as arteries deliver blood to the microvascular bed, veins collect blood from the microvascular bed and carry it away.

There are actually two circulations formed by the blood vessels and the heart; these are the *systemic circulation,* from the heart to the tissues of the body and back, and the *pulmonary circulation,* from the heart to the lungs and back (Fig. 12.2). The structure of arteries, capillaries, and veins in both circulations is basically the same. Although the general arrangement of blood vessels in both is from arteries to capillaries to veins, in some parts of the systemic circulation it is modified so that a vein is interposed between two capillary networks; this is called a *venous portal system.* Such an arrangement occurs in vessels carrying blood to the liver, namely, the *hepatic portal system,* and in vessels leading to the pituitary, the *hypothalamic-hypophyseal portal system.* Another modification is found in the *arterial portal system* of the kidneys where an arteriole is interposed between two capillary networks.

ARTERIES

Arteries are traditionally divided into three types: large or elastic arteries; medium or muscular arteries; and small arteries and arterioles. In all, the wall is divided into three major components: a *tunica intima,* a *tunica media,* and a *tunica adventitia.* Histologically, the types are distinguished from each other on the basis of thickness and differences in the composition of the various layers, especially the tunica media.

Elastic Arteries

The artery leaving the heart to supply the systemic circulation is the *aorta.* It has the largest diameter of any artery and it is an elastic artery (Fig. 12.3); the larger branches of the aorta are also elastic. From a functional point of view, the elastic arteries serve as conduction tubes, but they also facilitate the movement of blood along the tube. This occurs as follows: The ventricles of the heart pump blood into the elastic arteries during the contraction (systolic) period of the cardiac cycle. The pressure generated in the elastic arteries by the ventri-

283

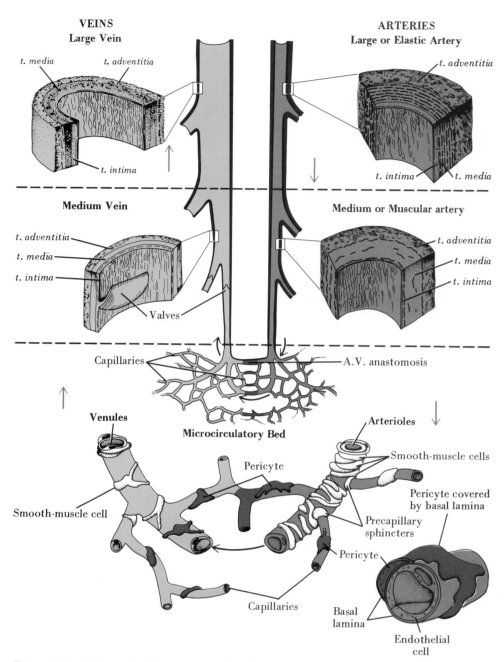

Figure 12.1. Schematic diagram of major structural features of blood vessels. The layers, or tunics, of the blood vessel walls are marked in the upper two frames. The arrangement of the microcirculatory bed in certain parts of the body is shown in the lowest panel. Note that the microcirculation shows an arteriovenous (AV) anastomosis and a thoroughfare channel (arteriovenous shunt). (Based on Rhodin JG: *Handbook of Physiology.* New York, Oxford University Press, 1963.)

cles moves the blood along the arterial tree; the pressure also causes the wall of the arteries, because of its elastic nature, to distend. The distension is limited by the network of collagenous fibers in the tunica media and tunica adventitia. Then, during the relaxation (diastolic) period of the car-

diac cycle, when no pressure is generated by the heart, the elastic recoil of the distended arterial wall serves to maintain arterial pressure and the resultant flow of blood within the vessel.

Tunica intima. The tunica intima of elastic arteries is relatively thick. It consists of a lining

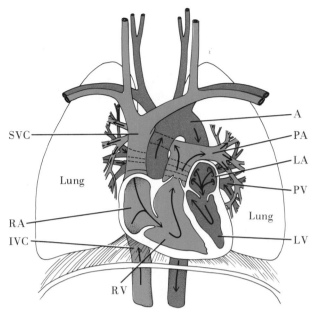

Figure 12.2. Diagram depicting circulations of blood through the heart. Blood returns from the tissues of the body via the superior vena cava (SVC) and inferior vena cava (IVC). These two major venous vessels return the blood to the right atrium (RA). Blood then passes into the right ventricle (RV), and from this chamber the blood is pumped into the pulmonary arteries (PA) that convey the blood to the lungs. The blood is aerated in the lungs and is then returned to the left atrium (LA) via the pulmonary veins (PV). Blood then passes to the left ventricle (LV), and from here it is pumped into the aorta (A), which conveys the blood to the tissues of the body. From the heart to the lungs and back to the heart constitutes the pulmonary circulation; from the heart to the tissues and back to the heart constitutes the systemic circulation.

endothelium with its basal lamina, a subendothelial layer of connective tissue, and a layer of elastic material, the ***internal elastic membrane.*** In elastic arteries, the internal elastic membrane is not conspicuous because it is one of many elastic layers in the wall of the vessel. Its identification is based on the fact that it is the innermost of the many elastic layers present in the arterial wall.

The endothelium is a simple squamous epithelium. The cells are typically flat, but they are elongate and oriented with their long axis parallel to the direction of the artery (Fig. 12.4). The cytoplasm is, in most respect, unremarkable. However, it does display several significant features. In forming the epithelial sheet, the cells are joined by tight junctions (zonulae occludentes) and gap junctions

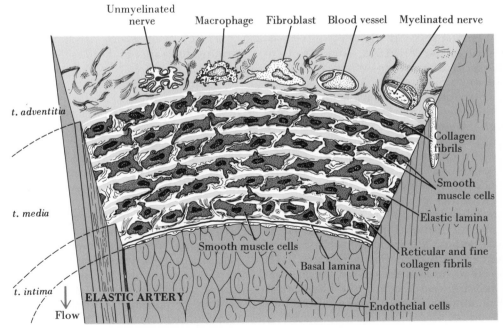

Figure 12.3. Schematic diagram of elastic artery showing the cellular and extracellular components. (Based on Rhodin JG: *Handbook of Physiology.* New York, Oxford University Press, 1963.)

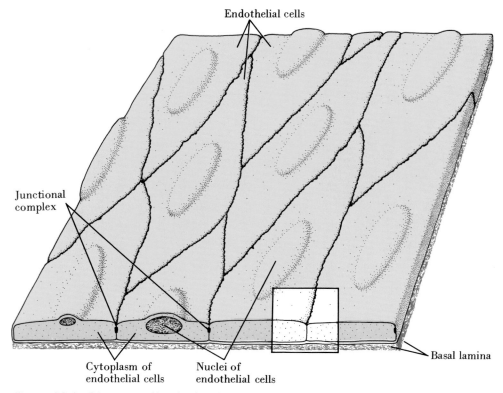

Endothelial cells

Junctional
complex

Cytoplasm of
endothelial cells

Nuclei of
endothelial cells

Basal lamina

Figure 12.4. Diagram of luminal surface and cut edge of endothelium. The cells are elongate; their long axis is parallel to the direction of blood flow. Nuclei of endothelial cells are also elongate in the direction of blood flow. The area marked by the **rectangle** is shown in Figure 12.5. (Based on Rhodin JG: *Handbook of Physiology.* New York, Oxford University Press, 1963.)

(Fig. 12.5). The endothelium, its tight junctions, and the basal lamina serve as a barrier to the passage of substances. Nevertheless, some transendothelial transport does occur. Whereas the full range of transport mechanisms has not yet been elucidated, pinocytotic vesicles have been shown to transport experimental markers, such as peroxidase, through the endothelium. The vesicles move these substances from the vascular lumen to the basal surface of the endothelial cell and to the lateral surface of the cell. This is illustrated by the series of pinocytotic vesicles marked with arrows in Figure 12.5. Another cytoplasmic feature associated with arterial endothelium, worthy of mention, is the presence of rod-like inclusions known as Weibel-Palade bodies. These electron-dense structures contain a coagulating factor (Factor VIII) that is believed to be synthesized by the arterial endothelial cell and secreted into the blood, thus giving the cell, among other activities, a secretory function.

In the larger elastic arteries, the subendothelial layer consists of connective tissue with both collagenous and elastic fibers. The main cell type of

this layer is the smooth muscle cell; it is not only contractile, but it also produces the extracellular ground substance and fibers. Macrophages are also present.

Tunica media. The tunica media of elastic arteries is the thickest of the three layers. It consists of sheets, or lamellae, of elastic material with intervening layers comprised of smooth muscle cells, collagenous fibers, and ground substance. The elastic lamellae are arranged as concentric fenestrated sheets. The fenestrations are said to facilitate the diffusion of substances through the arterial wall.

The smooth muscle cells appear to be circularly arranged, but they are actually arranged in a low-pitched spiral. The smooth muscle cells display gap junctions between neighboring cells. It is important to point out that fibroblasts are not present in the tunica media and that the smooth muscle cells are responsible for the production of the collagenous and elastic components of this layer.

Tunica adventitia. The tunica adventitia is a connective tissue layer. In elastic arteries it is relatively thin, usually less than half the thickness of

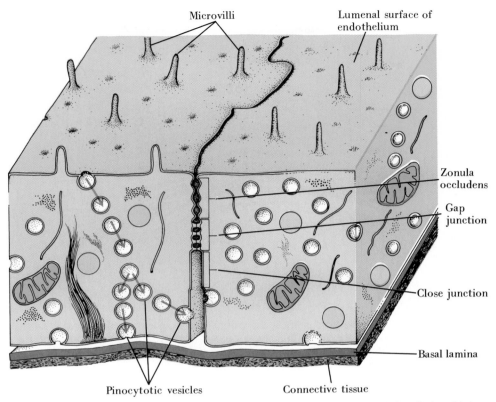

Microvilli

Lumenal surface of
endothelium

Zonula
occludens

Gap
junction

Close junction

Basal lamina

Pinocytotic vesicles

Connective tissue

Figure 12.5. Diagram depicting segments of two adjacent endothelial cells in which a junctional complex joins the cells. Pinocytotic vesicles in cell on the left have been positioned to suggest the pathway of vesicles from the lumen of the blood vessel to the base of the cell or to the basal-lateral intercellular space. A variety of markers have been traced through pinocytotic vesicles across the endothelial cell as suggested by the **arrows.** (Based on Rhodin JG: *Handbook of Physiology.* New York, Oxford University Press, 1963.)

the tunica media, but this varies. The main extracellular component of the tunica adventitia in elastic arteries is collagenous fibers. These aid in preventing the expansion of the arterial wall beyond physiological limits during the systolic period of the cardiac cycle. There is also a loose network of elastic fibers in the tunica adventitia. Cells of the tunica adventitia are fibroblasts and macrophages.

The tunica adventitia contains blood vessels (***vasa vasorum***) and nerves (***nervi vascularis***). Branches of each enter the tunica media to supply the blood vessel wall. The blood vessels supply only the outer portion of the arterial wall. The inner part is supplied from the lumen of the vessel.

Muscular Arteries

There is no sharp dividing line between elastic and muscular arteries (Fig. 12.6). Arteries are often intermediate between the two types and difficult to classify. Generally, in the region of transition, the amount of elastic material decreases and

smooth muscle cells become the predominant constituent of the tunica media. One of the features that distinguishes muscular arteries from elastic arteries is the presence of a prominent internal elastic membrane and an ***external elastic membrane.***

Tunica intima. The tunica intima of muscular arteries contains a lining of endothelial cells and a basal lamina similar to those in elastic arteries. The subendothelial connective tissue is sparse. In some muscular arteries it is so scant that the basal lamina of the endothelium makes contact with the internal elastic membrane. In histological sections, the internal elastic membrane usually appears as a well-defined undulating or wavy structure due to contraction of the smooth muscle in the tunica media.

Tunica media. The tunica media of muscular arteries contains smooth muscle cells, collagenous fibers, and relatively little elastic material. The smooth muscle cells are arranged in a spiral fashion in the arterial wall. Their contraction assists in maintaining the blood pressure in the ves-

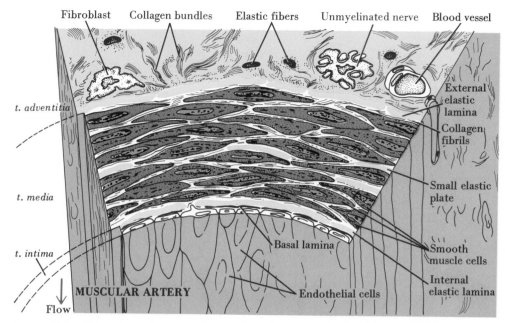

Figure 12.6. Schematic diagram of muscular artery. In certain locations, muscle cells are shown to be in contact to represent the presence of a gap junction (nexus) between the cells. (Based on Rhodin JG: *Handbook of Physiology.* New York, Oxford University Press, 1963.)

sels. As in the elastic arteries, the smooth muscle cells produce the extracellular collagenous and elastic fibers and there are no fibroblasts in this middle vascular layer. The smooth muscle cells are joined by gap junctions; they are invested by a basal lamina except where the gap junctions occur.

Tunica adventitia. The tunica adventitia of muscular arteries, like that of other arteries, is connective tissue. It is about as thick as the tunica media and, thus, is relatively thicker than the tunica adventitia of elastic arteries. Collagenous fibers are the principal extracellular component of the tunica adventitia. However, there is a concentration of elastic material adjacent to the tunica media. This is called the external elastic lamina or membrane.

Small Arteries and Arterioles

Small arteries and arterioles are arbitrarily distinguished from one another by the number of smooth muscle cells in the tunica media, although there are other differences as well. By definition, the arteriole has one or two layers of smooth muscle in the tunica media (see Atlas section, Plate 48), whereas the small artery may have up to about eight layers. The smooth muscle cells are arranged in a spiral pattern. Typically, the tunica intima of the small artery has an internal elastic membrane, whereas this layer may or may not be present in the arteriole. The endothelium in both is essentially similar to endothelium in other arteries except that there are junctions between endothelial cells and the smooth muscle cells of the tunica media; their function has not yet been clarified. The tunica adventitia is a thin, ill-defined sheath of connective tissue.

Arterioles serve as the stopcocks to the capillary networks. Contraction of the smooth muscle in the wall of these vessels can shut off the blood going to the capillaries.

VEINS

Veins are traditionally classified as large, medium, and small. The small veins, referred to as *venules,* are further subclassified as *postcapillary* and *muscular.* Large- and medium-sized veins usually travel with large- and medium-sized arteries; arterioles and muscular venules also sometimes travel together. While large and medium veins have three layers designated the tunica intima, tunica media, and tunica adventitia, these layers are not as well defined as they are in arteries. Moreover, veins have thinner walls than their accompanying arteries, and the lumen of the vein is usually larger than that of the arterial lumen. Many veins, especially those of the limbs, contain valves that allow blood to flow in one direction only. The valves are semilunar flaps consisting of a thin connective tissue core with an endothelial surface exposed to the blood.

Large Veins

The tunica intima of large veins (Fig. 12.7) consists of endothelium, its basal lamina, and a small amount of subendothelial connective tissue with smooth muscle cells. The boundary between the tunica intima and tunica media is not clear in that it is not always easy to decide if the smooth muscle cells close to the intimal endothelium should be classified as belonging to the tunica intima or to the tunica media. The tunica media is relatively thin; it contains smooth muscle cells, collagenous fibers, and some fibroblasts. On the other hand, the tunica adventitia is relatively thick and in the wall of large veins, such as the vena cava, it contains bundles of longitudinally disposed smooth muscle cells, some fibroblasts, collagenous fibers, and some elastic fibers. Near their entry to the heart, the walls of large veins contain cardiac muscle.

Medium Veins

The three layers of the venous wall are most evident in medium-sized veins (Fig. 12.8). In addition to the endothelium and its basal lamina, the tunica intima may have a small amount of subendothelial connective tissue with some smooth muscle cells and there may be a thin internal elastic membrane. The tunica media is much thinner than in medium-sized arteries. It contains circularly arranged smooth muscle cells and collagenous fibers. The tunica adventitia is usually thicker than the tunica media. It is made up of connective tissue with many longitudinally disposed bundles of smooth muscle cells, collagenous fibers, and networks of elastic fibers.

Venules

Postcapillary venules receive blood from capillaries. They possess a lining of endothelium, a basal lamina, and **pericytes.** Pericytes are cells that, while contractile, appear to be otherwise unspecialized. They are enclosed by basal lamina material that is continuous with that of the endothelium. The endothelium of postcapillary venules is sensitive to vasocative agents, such as histamine and serotonin. The response to such agents results in the extravasation of fluid and emigration of white blood cells from the vessel during inflammation and allergic reactions. Postcapillary venules of lymph nodes also participate in the transmural migration of lymphocytes from the vascular lumen into the lymphatic tissue.

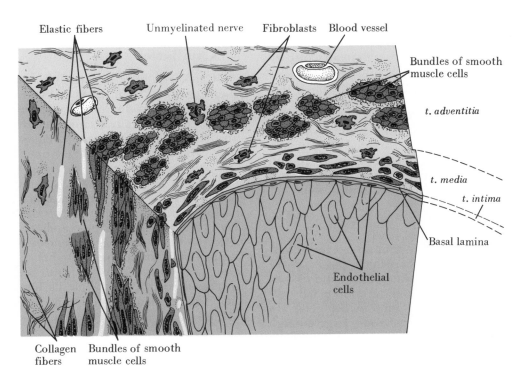

Figure 12.7.   Schematic diagram of large vein. (Based on Rhodin JG: *Handbook of Physiology.* New York, Oxford University Press, 1963.)

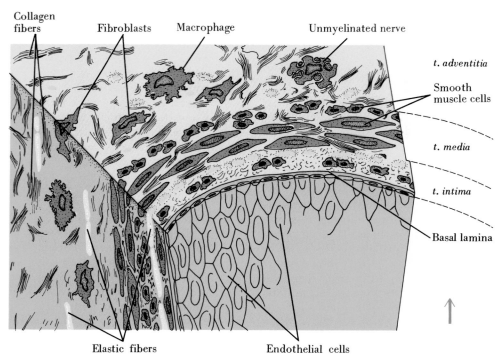

Collagen fibers | Fibroblasts | Macrophage | Unmyelinated nerve

t. adventitia

Smooth muscle cells

t. media

t. intima

Basal lamina

Elastic fibers | Endothelial cells

Figure 12.8.   Schematic diagram of medium-sized vein. (Based on Rhodin JG: *Handbook of Physiology.* New York, Oxford University Press, 1963.)

The next venules in the returning venous network are the ***muscular venules.*** Whereas postcapillary venules have no true tunica media, the muscular venules have one or two layers of smooth muscle and these constitute a tunica media. Muscular venules also possess an adventitia of connective tissue that forms a sheath around the tunica media.

The venous channels in the cranial cavity, called ***venous sinuses*** or the ***dural sinuses,*** have a special structure. They are essential endothelial-lined spaces in the dura mater. Veins in certain other locations (for example, retina, placenta, trabeculae of the spleen) also have atypical walls.

CAPILLARIES

The capillaries are the thin-walled blood vessels, arranged in a network, which allow for the exchange of substances between blood and tissues. They consist of a single layer of endothelial cells and a basal lamina. The endothelial cells are curved so that they form a tube just large enough to allow the passage of red blood cells one at a time. In cross-sections, the tube may be seen to be formed by only one cell or by portions of two and even three cells. The margins of the endothelial cells are joined by tight junctions (zonulae occludentes).

Continuous and Fenestrated Capillaries

Capillaries may be classified as ***continuous*** or ***fenestrated*** (Fig. 12.9). The main feature of continuous capillaries is the presence of pinocytotic vesicles that function in transepithelial transport. Fenestrated capillaries contain circular ***fenestrae*** or ***pores,*** whose diameters range from 80 to 100 nm. The pore is spanned by a diaphragm with a central thickening. The diaphragm is thinner than the plasma membrane. In certain capillaries, pericytes may be found in association with the endothelium (Fig. 12.9). As in the postcapillary venules, the pericyte, when present, is enclosed by a basal lamina that is continuous with that of the endothelium. The pericyte displays features of a relatively unspecialized cell, and while its function has not yet been clarified, it is thought to be capable of differentiating into other cell types.

Sinusoids

In addition to the two main types of capillaries, there is a category of specialized vessels found

CAPILLARIES

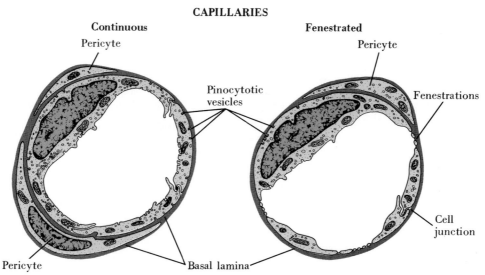

Figure 12.9. Schematic diagrams of continuous and fenestrated capillaries. Both may be surrounded partially by pericytes. The pericytes are enclosed by the same basal lamina which surrounds the capillary endothelium. (Based on Fawcett DW: In Orbison JL, Smith D (eds): *Peripheral Blood Vessels*. Baltimore, Williams & Wilkins, 1962.)

in the liver, spleen, and bone marrow, called *sinusoids* or *sinusoidal capillaries*. Sinusoids are generally larger in diameter than continuous and fenestrated capillaries. They are characterized by the presence of special lining cells and an incomplete basal lamina. The lining cells are specifically adapted to the function of the tissue. For example, in the liver the sinusoids contain phagocytic Kupffer cells; in the spleen, the sinusoidal lining cells have a unique rod-like shape that allows for passage of blood cells through the wall.

ARTERIOVENOUS SHUNTS

The general arrangement for a microvascular bed of a tissue is that arteries convey blood to the capillaries and veins convey blood away from the capillaries. However, all the blood does not necessarily pass from arteries to capillaries and thence to veins. In many tissues, there are more or less direct routes between the arteries and veins which divert blood from the capillaries. These routes are called *arteriovenous (AV) anastamoses* (see Fig. 12.1).

In addition, preferential thoroughfares, the proximal segment of which is called a *metarteriole* (Fig. 12.10), also exist that allow some blood to pass more directly from artery to vein. Capillaries originate from both the arteriole and from the metarteriole. While capillaries themselves have no smooth muscle in their wall, there is a sphincter of smooth muscle, called the *precapillary sphincter,* at their

origin from either the arteriole or the metarteriole. These sphincters control the amount of blood passing through the capillary.

HEART

The heart contains four chambers (two atria and two ventricles) *through* which the blood is pumped (Figs. 12.2 and 12.11). Valves guard the exits of the chambers, preventing backflow of blood. The wall of the heart includes the cardiac muscle, a fibrous "skeleton" for attachment of the valves, and a specialized internal conducting system involved in the regulation of heart rate.

The fibrous skeleton, comprised of dense connective tissue, is situated around the openings of the two arteries leaving the heart and around the openings between the atria and the ventricles (Fig. 12.12). Each annular arrangement of fibrous tissue serves for the attachment of valves that allows blood to flow in only one direction through the openings. The fibrous skeleton also includes an extension into the interventricular septum. This small part of the interventricular septum (the membranous portion) is devoid of cardiac muscle; it contains the short length of unbranched AV bundle. Elsewhere, the heart wall contains cardiac muscle.

The wall of the heart contains three layers: the *epicardium,* the *myocardium,* and the *endocardium* (see Atlas section, Plate 45). The layers are essen-

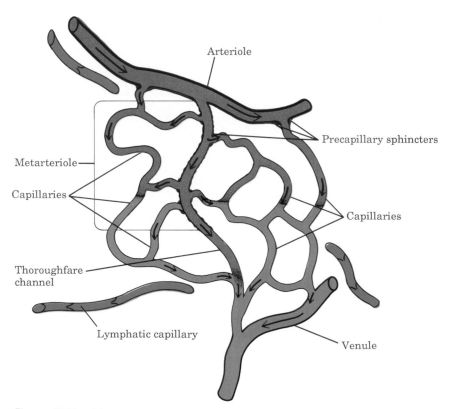

Figure 12.10. Diagram of microcirculation showing a metarteriole (initial segment of a thoroughfare channel) giving rise to capillaries. The precapillary sphincters of the arteriole and metarteriole control the entry of blood into the capillaries. The distal segment of the thoroughfare channel receives capillaries from the microcirculatory bed, but no sphincters are present where the afferent capillaries enter the thoroughfare channels. Blind ending lymphatic vessels are shown in association with capillary bed. (Courtesy of B. Zweifach.)

Figure 12.11. Chambers of the heart and the impulse-conducting system. The heart has been cut open in the coronal plane to expose its interior and the main parts of its impulse-conducting system (indicated in red). Impulses are generated in the sinoatrial (S-A) node; they are transmitted through the atrial wall to the atrioventricular (A-V) node and then along the atrioventricular (A-V) bundle to the Purkinje fibers. The valve guarding the entrance to the aorta is a semilunar valve. (Based on Shepard RS: *Human Physiology*. Philadelphia, JB Lippincott, 1971, p. 584.)

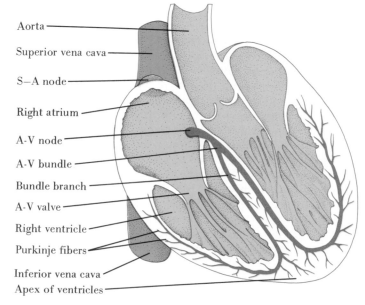

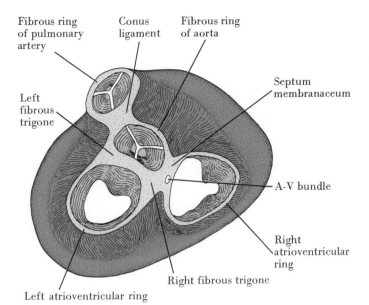

Fibrous ring
of pulmonary
artery

Conus
ligament

Fibrous ring
of aorta

Left
fibrous
trigone

Septum
membranaceum

A-V bundle

Right
atrioventricular
ring

Right fibrous trigone

Left atrioventricular ring

Figure 12.12. Fibrous skeleton of the heart as seen with the two atria removed. This fibrous network serves for the attachment of the cardiac muscle; it also serves for the attachment of the cuspid valves between the atria and ventricles, and for the semilunar valves of the aorta and the pulmonary artery. The atrioventricular bundle passes the right atrium to the ventricular septum via the membranous septum of the fibrous skeleton. (Based on Tandler J: *Lehrbuch der Systematiaschen Anatomie,* Vol. 3. Leipzig, Vogel, 1926.)

tially the same in the atria and the ventricles. The epicardium consists of a lining of mesothelial cells and an underlying layer of connective tissue. Blood vessels and nerves supplying the heart lie within the epicardium, often surrounded by adipose tissue. The myocardium consists of cardiac muscle (described in Chapter 10). The myocardium of the ventricles is substantially thicker than that of the atria due to the large amount of cardiac muscle in the pumping chambers. The endocardium can be divided into three layers: an inner layer of endothelium and subendothelial connective tissue; a middle layer comprised of connective tissue and smooth muscle cells; and an outer layer, also called the subendocardial layer, which is continuous with the connective tissue of the myocardium.

The *interventricular septum* serves as the wall between the right and left ventricles. It contains cardiac muscle except in the membranous portion. Endocardium lines each surface of the interventricular septum. The *interatrial septum* is much thinner than the interventricular septum. Except for certain small areas that contain fibrous tissue, it has a center layer of cardiac muscle with a lining of endocardium facing each chamber. The valves of

the heart have a center sheet of fibrous tissue and on all surfaces exposed to blood they are covered by endothelium. Fibrous thread-like cords, called the *chordae tendineae,* extend from the free edge of the atrioventricular valves to muscular projections from the wall of the ventricles called *papillary muscles.*

Regulation of Heart Rate

Cardiac muscle is capable of contracting in a rhythmic manner without any direct stimulus from the nervous system. The pace of this beating action is initiated at the *sinotrial (SA) node,* a group of specialized cardiac muscle cells located near the junction of the superior vena cava and the right atrium (see Fig. 12.11). Because of this function, the SA node is referred to as the *pacemaker.* The SA node initiates an impulse which spreads over the cardiac muscle of the atria and through or along internodal tracts composed of modified cardiac muscle fibers. The impulse is then picked up at the *atrioventricular (AV) node* and conducted across the fibrous skeleton to the ventricles by the *bundle of His (atrioventricular bundle).* The bundle divides into smaller *right* and *left bundle branches* and then into **Purkinje fibers.** The bundle of His, the bundle branches, and the Purkinje fibers are modified cardiac muscle cells that are specialized to conduct impulses (see the Atlas section, Plate 33). The components of the conducting system convey the impulse at a rate approximately four times faster than the cardiac muscle fibers. The conducting elements are the only elements that can convey impulses across the fibrous skeleton and serves to coordinate the contracts of the atrias and ventricles. The contraction is initiated in the atria forcing blood into the ventricles than a wave of contraction begins at the apex forcing blood from the heart through the aorta and pulmonary trunk.

The heart is innervated by both divisions of the autonomic nervous system. The nerve supply does not initiate contractions of the cardiac muscle, but rather regulates the heart rate according to the body's immediate needs. The parasympathetic fibers terminate chiefly about the SA and AV nodes; the sympathetic fibers are found chiefly in the epicardium about the blood vessels that supply the heart. The autonomic fibers regulate the rate of impulses eminating from the SA node. Under the influence of the sympathetic component of the autonomic nervous system the rate of contractions increases; the parasympathetic component, causes a decrease in the rate of contraction.

RECEPTORS

Receptors for physiological reflexes are located in the walls of large blood vessels near the heart. The receptors are located at the bifurcation of the carotid arteries and in the aortic arch and are called the **carotid** and **aortic bodies,** respectively. The carotid body consists of cords and irregular groups of epithelioid cells. Associated with these cells is a rich supply of nerve fibers. The neural elements are both afferent and efferent. The structure of the aortic bodies is essentially similar to that of the carotid bodies. Carotid and aortic body receptors serve to detect alterations in carbon dioxide and oxygen tensions and in pH. Special neuroreceptors in the arteries serve neural reflexes that adjust cardiac output and respiratory rate.

LYMPHATIC VESSELS

In addition to blood vessels, there is a set of vessels that circulates fluid, called lymph, through certain parts of the body. These **lymphatic vessels** are an adjunct to the blood vessels. Unlike the blood vessels, which convey blood to and from tissues, the lymphatic vessels are unidirectional, conveying fluid only from tissues. The smallest lymphatic vessels are called **lymphatic capillaries.** They are especially numerous in the loose connective tissues under the epithelium of the skin and mucous membranes. The lymphatic capillaries begin as "blind ending" tubes in the microcapillary beds (Fig. 12.10). Lymphatic capillaries converge into increasingly larger vessels called **lymphatics,** which ultimately unite to form two main channels that empty into the blood vascular system by draining into the large veins in the base of the neck. They enter the vascular system at the junctions of the internal jugular and subclavian veins. The largest lymphatic vessel, draining most of the body and emptying into the veins on the left side, is the **thoracic duct.** The other main channel is the **right lymphatic duct.**

Lymphatic capillaries are more permeable than blood capillaries and they are more effective than blood capillaries in removing protein-rich fluid from the intercellular spaces. Lymphatic vessels also serve as a preferential conveyance for lipid absorbed from the small intestines. Before lymph is returned to the blood, it passes through **lymph nodes** where it is exposed to the cells of the immune system. Thus, the lymphatic vessels serve not only as an adjunct to the blood vascular system, but they are also an integral component of the immune system.

Lymphatic capillaries are essentially tubes of endothelium that, unlike the typical blood capillary, lack a basal lamina. The lack of a basal lamina can be correlated with their extreme permeability. As lymphatic vessels become larger, the wall becomes thicker. The increasing thickness is due to connective tissue and bundles of smooth muscle. Lymphatic vessels possess valves that channel the lymph toward the large veins in the neck.

ATLAS PLATES

45–49

PLATE 45. Heart

A section through the wall of the atrium is shown in **Figure 1.** The outermost part is the epicardium **(Epi),** the thick middle portion is the myocardium **(Myo),** and the inner part is the endocardium **(End).** The mycocardium is by far the thickest component. It consists of bundles of cardiac muscle. These do not all travel in the same direction; therefore, in most sections cardiac muscle fibers may be cut longitudinally, in cross-section, or obliquely. Connective tissue **(CT)** separates the bundles of cardiac muscle. A large amount of connective tissue is in the vicinity of the blood vessel **(BV)** that is in the periphery of the myocardium.

The epicardium **(Epi)** is shown at higher magnification in **Figure 2.** It is surfaced by mesothelium. Under the mesothelium is the supporting connective tissue **(CT),** the fibrous elements of which are loosely arranged. Elastic fibers are present in the connective tissue; however, they are not evident in routine hematoxylin and eosin-stained (H&E) preparations. A small nerve **(N),** which has probably just entered the myocardium, is present in the connective tissue between the muscle bundles. The nerve appears as a bundle of thin wavy fibers that are significantly thinner than the muscle fibers.

The endocardium **(End)** is shown at higher magnification in **Figure 3.** It can be divided into three layers: **(1)** an inner layer, which is comprised of endothelial cells that rest on a subendothelial layer of delicate collagenous fibers; **(2)** a middle layer, which is somewhat thicker and contains not only collagenous fibers, but also smooth muscle cells **(SM)** and elastic fibers (not evident); and **(3)** an outer layer, which consists of loose connective tissue and is called the subendocardial layer. The subendocardial layer is continuous with the con-

KEY	
BV, blood vessel	**1,** endothelium and
CT, connective tissue	subendothelial
End, endocardium	connective tissue
Epi, epicardium	**2,** middle layer of
Myso, myocardium	endocardium
N, nerve	**3,** subendocardial layer
SM, smooth muscle	

Fig. 1. human. × 44   **Fig. 2–3.** human. × 160

nective tissue of the myocardium. The subendocardial layer contains blood vessels **(BV),** collagenous and elastic fibers, but no smooth muscle.

The ventricles have essentially the same structure as the atria except that the myocardium is much thicker. In addition, the subendocardial layer of the ventricles contains special muscle fibers that belong to the intrinsic conducting system of the heart (Purkinje fibers).

The epicardium can be distinguished from endocardium in several ways. The larger blood vessels and nerves that supply the heart wall are in the epicardium; blood vessels in the endocardium are considerably smaller. The endocardium is layered and contains smooth muscle cells; the epicardium is not layered and contains large amounts of adipose tissue, particularly in the vicinity of the large vessels. Finally, Purkinje fibers, when included in the section, are found in or near the subendocardial layer of the endocardium (see Atlas section, Plate 33).

PLATE 45

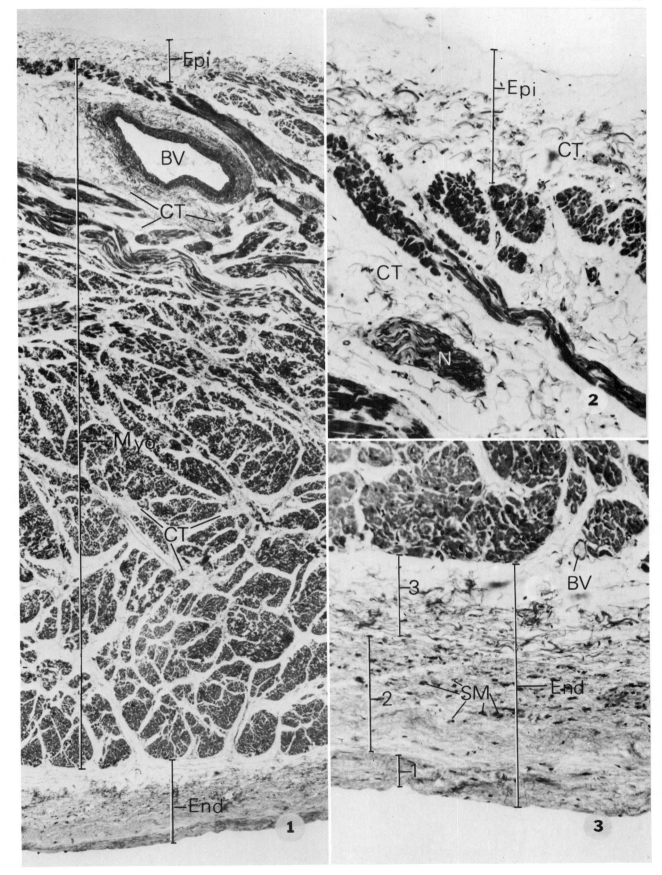

PLATE 46. Aorta

The aorta is the artery that carries blood away from the left ventricle. Because of the large amount of elastic material it contains, it is referred to as an *elastic artery*. The elastic material, however, is not readily evident without special stains.

The layers that make up the wall of the aorta are shown in **Figure 1.** This is a longitudinal section through the entire thickness of the arterial wall. Three layers can usually be recognized: the tunica intima (TI), tunica media (TM), and tunica adventitia (TA). The adventitia is the outermost part. It consists mainly of connective tissue, and contains the blood vessel (vasa vasorum) and nerves (nervi vascularis) that supply the arterial wall.

The tunica intima is shown at higher magnification in **Figure 2.** The boundary between it and the tissue below, the tunica media, is not sharply defined. However, largely because of staining characteristics and degree of cellularity, the two tunics are more easily distinguished at low magnification (**Fig. 1**). The tunica intima consists of a lining of endothelial cells that rest on a layer of connective tissue. However, the endothelium is difficult to preserve in these vessels and frequently is lost. Both collagenous fibers and elastic lamellae are in the connective tissue. Smooth muscle cells are also present in the intima of the aorta (*arrows*).

The tunica media contains an abundance of smooth muscle; however, the more distinctive feature is its large amount of elastic material. The elastic material is present not in the form of fibers, but rather as fenestrated membranes. **Figure 3** and the higher magnification of **Figure 5** are from a specimen stained to demonstrate elastic material. **Figure 3** reveals elastic laminae present in the media (TM) as well as the deep portion of the intima (TI). The adventitia (TA), however, essentially lacks these elastic laminae. Careful examination of the higher power of **Figure 5** reveals what appears to be interruptions of some of the laminae. These are actually the fenestrations or openings in the elastic membranes. **Figure 4** shows a higher power of the tunica media in the H&E preparation. Here,

the elastic laminae are unstained as is usually the case. (In some instances, the elastic material will stain lightly with eosin). The **arrowheads** reveal the site of some of the lamellae. Their presence is recognized by the apparent absence of structure, which, in turn, is due to the absence of staining of the elastic fibers. The smooth muscle cells of the media are arranged in a closely wound spiral between the elastic membranes. However, this arrangement is difficult to recognize in sectioned material.

The outermost layer of the aorta, the tunica adventitia, is shown in **Figure 6.** The tunica adventitia consists mostly of collagenous fibers that course in longitudinal spirals. (Their course, like the smooth muscle fibers, however, is unrecognizable in tissue sections.) There are no elastic laminae in the adventitia, but elastic fibers are present, though relatively few in number. The cells of the adventitia, represented by the nuclei seen in the adventitia in **Figure 6,** are fibroblasts. Occasionally, ganglion cells are present as well as some scattered smooth muscle cells. The ganglion cells, when present, are quite conspicuous, whereas the smooth muscle may be overlooked.

Other elastic arteries are the brachioephalic, the subclavian, the beginning of the common carotid, and the pulmonary arteries. The elastic arteries are also called conducting arteries.

PLATE 46

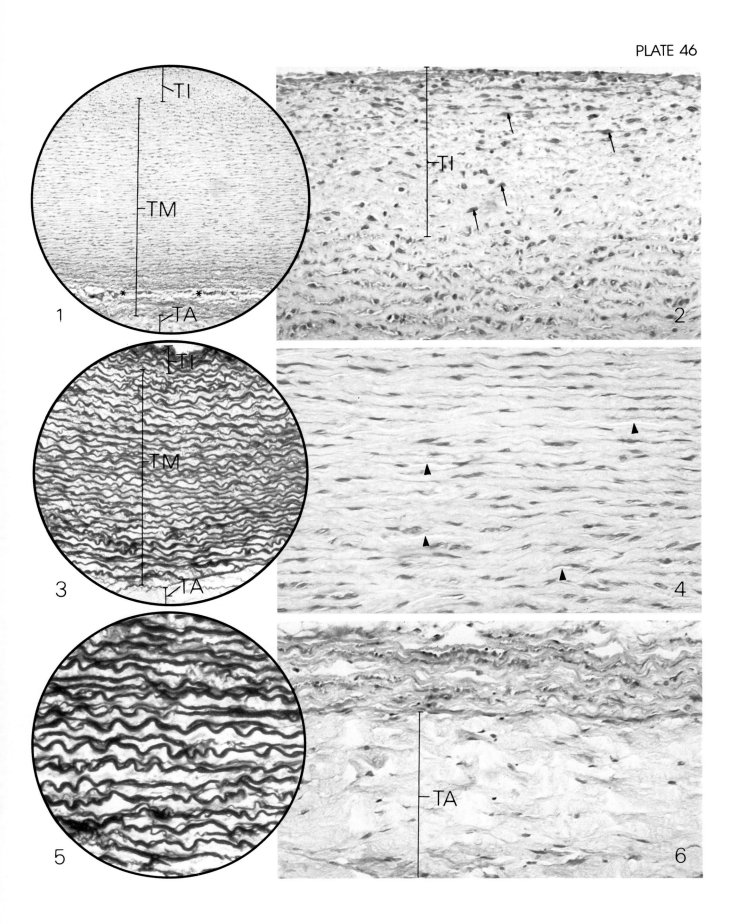

PLATE 47. Muscular Arteries and Veins

As the arterial tree is traced further from the heart, the elastic tissue is considerably reduced in amount, and smooth muscle becomes the predominant component in the tunica media. The arteries are then called muscular arteries, or arteries of medium caliber.

A cross-section through a muscular artery is shown in **Figure 1.** Some blood cells are in the lumen. The wall of the artery is divided into three layers: tunica intima **(TI),** tunica media **(TM),** and tunica adventitia **(TA).**

Figure 2 is a higher magnification of the area included in the **rectangle** in **Figure 1.** The tunica intima is comprised of an endothelial lining, its basal lamina (not evident), an extremely small amount of connective tissue, and the internal elastic membrane **(IEM).** The internal elastic membrane has a scalloped appearance and is highly refractile. The connective tissue is extremely scant and the endothelial cells appear to rest directly on the internal elastic membrane. The agonal contraction of the artery causes the internal elastic membrane to assume its scalloped formation and this contracts the endothelial cells so that the endothelial nuclei **[E(N)]** appear rounded and perched on the internal elastic membrane.

The tunica media consists mainly of circularly arranged smooth muscle cells. The nuclei of the smooth muscle cells **[SM(N)]** are elongated and oriented in the same direction. Their twisted appearance indicates that the smooth muscle cells are in a contracted state. The material between the nuclei is mainly cytoplasm of the muscle cells; however, the cytoplasmic boundaries are not evident. The refractile undulating material in the tunica media is elastic material **(EM).** Reticular fibers are also present, but they are not visualized in H&E preparations.

The tunica adventitia **(TA)** consists of connective tissue. The refractile scalloped sheet at the junction of the tunicae mediae and adventitia is the external elastic membrane **(EEM).** The nuclei

---

KEY

AT, adipose tissue
BV, small blood vessels in surrounding connective tissue
E, endothelium
EEM, external elastic membrane
EM, elastic material
E(N), endothelial nuclei

F(N), fibroblast nuclei
IEM, internal elastic membrane
SM(N), smooth muscle nuclei
TA, tunica adventitia
TI, tunica intima
TM, tunica media

Fig. 1, monkey, × 160
Fig. 2, monkey, × 640

Fig. 3, monkey, × 65
(inset, monkey, × 640

[F(N)] of some fibroblasts can be seen; the cytoplasm of these cells cannot be distinguished from the extracellular material.

The walls of veins that accompany muscular arteries can be divided into tunica intima, tunica media, and tunica adventitia. Although there is elastic material in the wall, it is significantly less in amount than in the artery. **Figure 3** enables one to compare a muscular artery with its accompanying vein. The lumen of the vein is larger than that of the artery, but the wall is thinner and the vessel frequently appears collapsed or flattened. The tunica intima **(TI)** is extremely thin **(inset)** and consists of a endothelial lining **(E)** that rests on a small amount of connective tissue. The tunica media **(TM)** is much thinner than that of the artery; the tunica adventitia **(TA)** is thicker. The tunica media consists largely of smooth muscle. The nuclei of the smooth muscle cells [SM(N)] are elongated and readily identified, but the cytoplasmic boundaries cannot be discerned.

The question of distinguishing between an artery and its accompanying vein or veins is simplified by their proximity, which enables one to compare histological features as in **Figure 3.**

PLATE 47

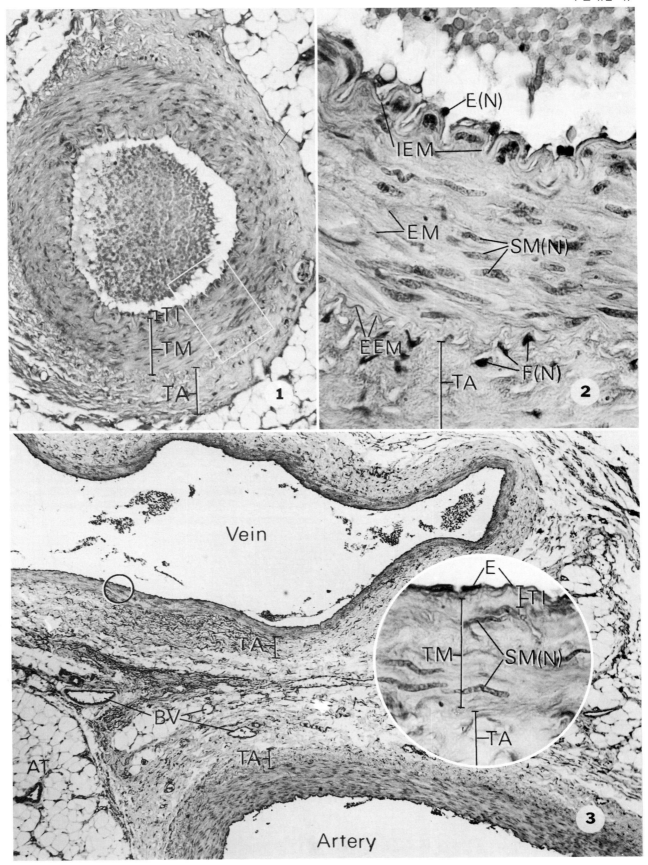

PLATE 48. Arterioles and Lymphatic Vessels

Arterioles. The terminal components of the arterial tree, just before the capillary bed or the arteriovenous shunt, are the arterioles. Arterioles contain an endothelial lining and smooth muscle in the wall. The muscle component is limited in thickness to one or two cells. There may or may not be an internal elastic membrane, according to the size of the vessel.

A longitudinal section through an arteriole is shown in **Figure 1.** It branches on the right. The elongated nuclei that line the lumen belong to endothelial cells (**arrows**). An elastic membrane cannot be seen. The round nuclei located in the wall of this vessel belong to smooth muscle cells [**SM(N)**] cut in cross-section. They should not be confused with cuboidal cells. The **rectangle** in **Figure 1** marks an area comparable to that seen in the electron micrograph in the following plate. **Figures 2 and 3** show how, by changing the focus of the optical system, one can obtain information relevant to this point. In **Figure 2,** one sees the elongated nuclei of the endothelial cells (**arrows**) as in **Figure 1.** Round nuclei are aligned in rows in the wall of the vessel. Four nuclei (**A**) are indicated on the left and seven (**B**) on the right. Notice the "shadows" related to the four nuclei on the left. By changing the focus (**Fig. 3**) one comes to realize that the round-appearing nuclei are really elongated nuclei that are wrapped around the vessel wall in a circular fashion. Note how the length of the four nuclei in **Figure 3** corresponds to the four nuclear "shadows" that are illustrated in **Figure 2.**

Lymphatic vessels have extremely thin walls. A lymphatic vessel from the mucosa of the pharynx is

shown in **Figure 4.** It has been cut longitudinally and two valves (**V**) are included in the section. One of the valves is shown at high magnification in **Figure 5.** The wall of the lymphatic vessel consists of almost nothing but an endothelial lining. The nuclei (**arrows**) of the endothelial cells appear to be exposed to the lumen. This is because the cytoplasm is so attenuated. At the nuclear poles, the cytoplasm continues as a thin thread. It is not possible to determine where one endothelial cell ends and the next begins. Connective tissue (**CT**) surrounds the lymphatic vessel. Some lymphocytes and precipitated lymph are within the lumen of the vessel. As a general statement, lymphatic vessels possess lumens of very large caliber in comparison to the thickness of the wall (see Atlas section, Plate 88, last paragraph).

KEY

A, smooth muscle cell nuclei at different focus levels
B, smooth muscle cell nuclei at different focus levels
CT, connective tissue
SM(C), smooth muscle cell cytoplasm
SM(N), smooth muscle cell nuclei
V, valves of lymphatic vessel
arrows, endothelial cell nuclei

Fig. 1–3, monkey, × 640
Fig. 4, human, × 160
Fig. 5, human, × 640

PLATE 48

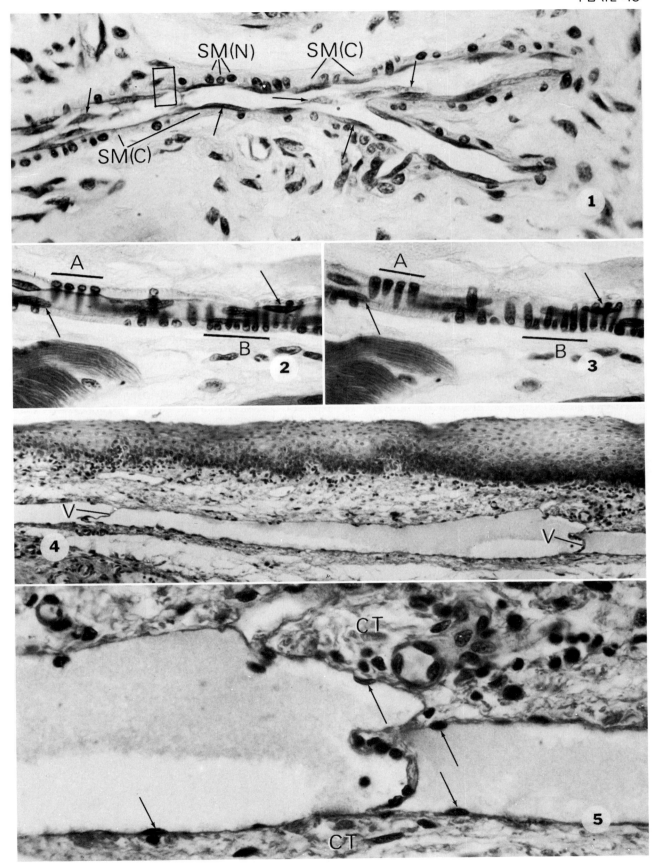

PLATE 49. Arteriole, Electron Microscopy

The electron micrograph shown here reveals a portion of the wall of a longitudinally sectioned arteriole. The vessel is comparable in size and general structural organization to the arteriole shown in Figure 1 of the preceding plate. For purposes of orientation, the portion of the vessel wall seen in the electron micrograph would correspond to the area indicated by the small **rectangle** in Figure 1.

In comparing the light and electron micrographs, note that with the light microscope the endothelial boundaries are not delineated, only the nuclei are clearly evident. Also, the cytoplasm of the individual smooth muscle cells blend together, only their nuclei when present in the section are readily discernible. In contrast, the electron micrograph reveals the individual smooth muscle cells **(SM)** of the vessel wall; each cell is separated from its neighbor by a definable intercellular space. Evident in the micrograph are portions of two endothelial cells **(End),** one of which includes part of its nucleus. At the site of apposition, the two endothelial cells are separated by a narrow (~20 nm) intercellular space **(arrows).**

Between the endothelium and the smooth muscle cells is an internal elastic membrane **(IEM).** This is typically lacking in the smallest arterioles. The elastic membrane in this vessel is a continuous sheath which is permeated by irregularly shaped openings **(arrowheads).** Together with the endothelium, it forms the tunica intima **(TI).** In sectioned material, the openings give the appearance of a discontinuous membrane, rather than a true sheath that simply contains fenestrations. The basal lamina **(BL)** of the endothelial and smooth muscle cells are closely applied to the elastic membrane; consequently, other than the elastic material, little extracellular matrix is present in the tunica intima of this vessel.

The tunica media is represented by the single layer of smooth muscle cells. The muscle cells are circumferentially disposed and appear here in cross-section; none includes a nucleus. Each muscle cell is surrounded by basal lamina **(BL).** However, there may be focal sites where neighboring smooth muscle cells come into more intimate apposition to form a nexus or gap junction. At these sites of close membrane apposition, the basal

---

KEY

BL, basal lamina
C, collegen fibrils
CD, cytoplasmic densities
E, elastic material
End, endothelial cell
F, fibroblast
IEM, internal elastic membrane
PV, pinocytotic vesicles

RBC, red blood cell
SM, smooth muscle cell
TA, tunica adventitia
TI, tunica intima
arrows, endothelial cell intercellular space
arrowheads, openings in internal elastic membrane

Fig., × 12,000 (**inset,** × 25,000)

---

lamina is absent. The cytoplasm of the muscle cell displays aggregates of mitochondria along with occasional profiles of rER. These organelles tend to be localized along the central axis of the cell at both ends of the nucleus. In addition, numerous cytoplasmic densities **(CD)** are present. They are adherent to the plasma membrane and extend into the interior of the cell to form a branching network. The cytoplasmic densities are regarded as attachment devices for the contractile filaments, analogous to the Z lines in striated muscle.

The tunica adventitia **(TA)** is comprised of elastic material **(E),** numerous collagen fibrils **(C),** and fibroblasts **(F).** The elastic material is somewhat more abundant nearest the smooth muscle. If the vessel shown here could be traced back in the direction of the heart, the elastic material would quantitatively increase, ultimately forming a more continuous sheath-like structure, namely, an external elastic membrane. The bulk of the adventitia consists of collagen fibrils, arranged in small bundles, separated by fibroblast processes.

The **inset** shows the area within the circle at higher magnification. It reveals with somewhat greater clarity the cytoplasmic densities **(CD)** of the smooth muscle cells, the basal lamina **(BL),** and the collagen fibrils **(C)** and elastic material of the adventitia. A series of pinocytotic vesicles **(PV)** along the plasma membrane are also evident.

PLATE 49

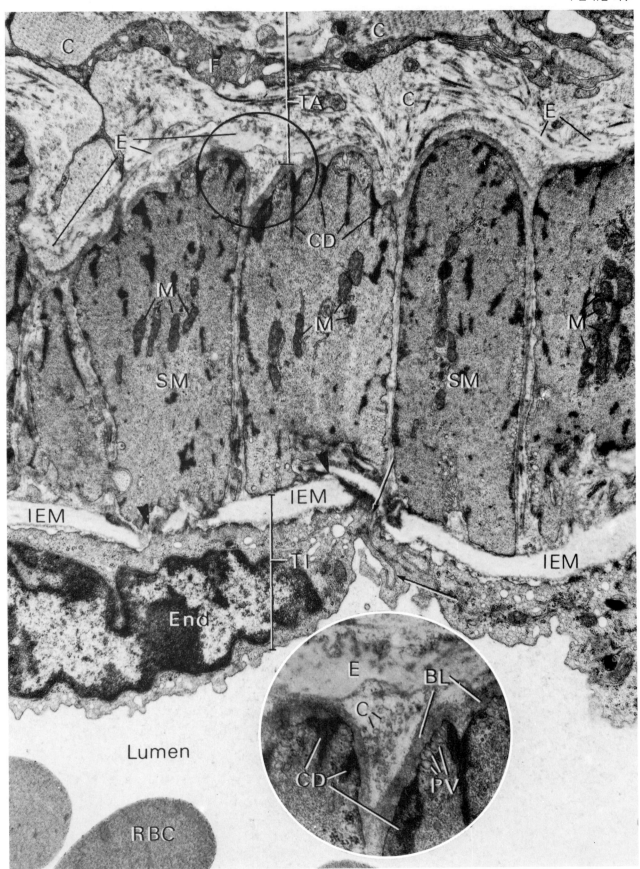

Lymphatic Tissue, Lymphatic Organs, and the Immune System

13

The terms *lymphatic* and *lymphoid* are used to identify or define the tissues or organs of the body in which lymphocytes represent a chief cellular constituent. The lymphatic tissues and organs include the *thymus, bone marrow, lymphatic nodules (lymphoid follicles), lymph nodes,* and *spleen* (Fig. 13.1). Although these forms of lymphatic tissue are often collectively referred to as the *immune system,* it is important to recognize that lymphocytes and other cells that are involved in the immune response are distributed throughout the connective and epithelial tissues of the body and are especially numerous in the lamina propria (the connective tissue underlying the epithelium) of the alimentary, genitourinary, and respiratory tracts. The term *lymphatic system* is sometimes used to describe the immune system, however, it is also used as a gross anatomical term to identify the portion of the circulatory system that collects and drains lymph from various tissue of the body.

Certain cells of the immune system, called *immunocompotent cells,* have the ability to distinguish between "self" (molecules normally present within an organism) and "nonself" (foreign molecules or those not normally present) and to provide for the inactivation or destruction of the foreign substances. This protective response of the lymphatic system is known as (acquired) *immunity*.

The lymphatic system is responsible for acquired immunity, that is, the body's acquired ability to resist the effects of disease-producing organisms or their toxins. For over 2000 years it has been known that people who recover from a disease are resistant to reinfection with the same disease. For example, children who recover from diseases like chickenpox, measles, or mumps are immune to reinfection. Another long-standing observation is that immunity is specific, that is, an immunity to

chickenpox will not prevent infection with measles. Unfortunately, the process by which the immune system protects the body can be turned against it in allergies and autoimmune diseases.

LYMPHATIC TISSUE, LYMPHOCYTES, AND THE IMMUNE RESPONSE

Lymphatic tissue is a specialized form of connective tissue containing large numbers of lymphocytes. Macrophages, while not conspicuous in histological sections, are present in lymphatic tissue as an essential functional component. The supporting framework of lymphatic tissue is a meshwork made up of *reticular cells* and *reticular fibers*. (The thymus is an exception to this in that its supporting framework consists of stellate epithelial cells, referred to as epithelioreticular cells.) The function of lymphatic tissue is surveillance and defense. Lymphocytes, with the cooperation of other cells (macrophages), protect the body from foreign cells, from microbes such as viruses and bacteria, and from cancer cells.

Lymphocytes are the main functional cells of the *lymphatic* or *immune system.* The cells, tissues, and organs of the immune system protect our bodies from exogenous (or foreign) macromolecules that contact or enter the body as free substances or attached to the surface of invading viruses, microorganisms, or cells. The immune system also has a surveillance function to watch constantly for the appearance of abnormal endogenous constituents of the body (for example, the transformation of normal cells into cells that are capable of producing tumors). In the tissues associated with the immune system, three groups of lymphocytes can be identified according to size: small, medium, and large, ranging in size from 6 to 18

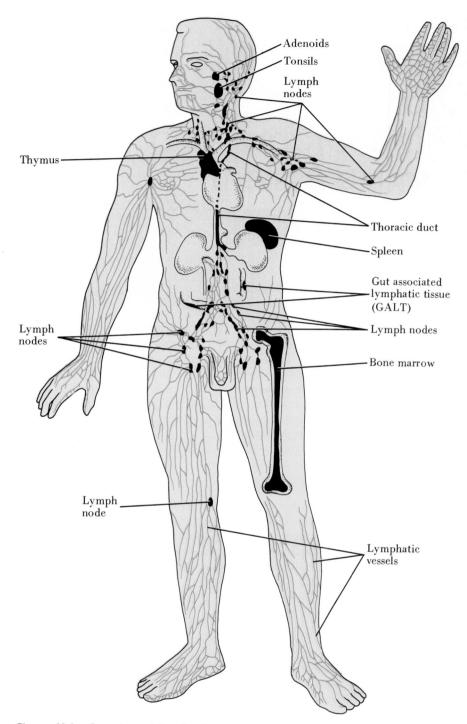

Figure 13.1. Overview of the structures constituting the lymphatic system. Since lymphatic tissue is the main component of some organs, they are regarded as organs of the lymphatic system (spleen, thymus, lymph nodes). Lymphatic tissue is present as part of other organs, namely, red marrow of bones; as lymphatic nodules of the alimentary canal (tonsils, Peyer's patches) and respiratory system (adenoids); and, not shown in the illustration, as diffuse lymphatic tissue of mucous membranes. The lymph nodes are interspersed in the path of lymphatic vessels, and ultimatlely, the lymphatic vessels empty into the bloodstream by joining the large veins in the root of the neck. The thoracic duct is the largest of the lymphatic vessels. (Based on Jerne NK: *Sci Am* 229:52, 1973.)

um. In contrast, in the bloodstream, only small and medium lymphocytes are present; the vast majority being small lymphocytes. In understanding the function of the lymphocytes, it is important to realize that the majority of the lymphocytes found in blood or lymph represent *recirculating immunocompetent cells.* These are cells that have developed the capacity to recognize and respond to foreign antigen and are in transit from one site of lymphatic tissue to another.

The study of the differentiation and function of lymphocytes has established the existence of two classes or categories of cells: (1) *T-lymphocytes* or *T-cells* and (2) *B-lymphocytes* or *B-cells.* Precursors of the two classes of lymphocytes originate in the bone marrow in late fetal life. The precursor cells continue to proliferate during postnatal life. The undifferentiated cells migrate to the bone marrow or thymus where they undergo differentiation and the production of unique membrane proteins that are essential to the functional activities of the cells. The *T-lymphocytes,* which have a long life-span and are involved in cell-mediated immunity, differentiate into immunocompetent cells in the thymus. The *B-lymphocytes,* which have variable life-spans and are involved in the production of antibodies, differentiate into immunocompetent cells in the bone marrow.

In the early 1960s, investigators using chickens embryos demonstrated that the *bursa of Fabricius,* a mass of lymphoid tissue associated with the cloaca of birds, was one of the anatomic sites of lymphocyte differentiation. The studies showed that when this tissue was destroyed in the chicken embryos (by removing it surgically or by administering high doses of testosterone) the adult chickens lack the ability to produce antibodies (*humoral immunity* was impaired). The chickens also demonstrated a marked reduction in the number of lymphocytes found in specific (*bursa dependent areas*) regions of the spleen and lymph nodes. The affected lymphocytes were identified as *B-lymphocytes* or *B-cells.* The bursa equivalent in mammals (including humans) is believed to be in special microenvironments in the bone marrow, where the B-lymphocytes differentiate into immunocompetent cells.

Investigators studying newborn mice found that removal of the *thymus* resulted in profound deficiencies in the *cell-mediated immune responses* (immune responses requiring the presence of cells of the immune system, in contrast to humoral responses involving circulating antibodies or immunoglobulins). The rejection of transplanted skin from a heterologous donor is an example of cellular immune response. Thymectomized mice

demonstrated a marked reduction in the number of lymphocytes found in specific regions (*thymus-dependent areas*) of the spleen and the lymph nodes. The ares of depletion were different from those identified after removal of the bursa Fabricius in the chicken. The affected lymphocytes were identified as *T-lymphocytes* or *T-cells.*

The bone marrow (or bursa of Fabricius in birds) and thymus are identified as *primary* or *central lymphoid organs.* Lymphocytes undergo their initial differentiation into immunocompetent cells in these organs and then migrate to *secondary* or *peripheral* areas of the body where the lymphatic tissue is found in diffuse, encapsulated, or organ form.

At this point let us summarize:

(1) The response of the immune system to antigen progresses along two distinctive pathways: (a) the *cell-mediated response,* leading to *cell-mediated immunity,* and (b) the *humoral response,* leading to *antibody-mediated immunity.* The humoral response is mediated by *B-lymphocytes,* which produce antibodies that act on an invading agent directly. In some diseases, for example, tetanus, a nonimmune person can be rendered immune by receiving an injection of antibody from an immune person or animal. The effectiveness of this passive transfer proves that it is the antibody that is responsible for the protection. With other diseases, for example, smallpox, the passive transfer of antibody is of no value. In these instances, in order to obtain protection, it is necessary to transfer lymphocytes, or more specifically *T-lymphocytes.*

(2) *T-* and *B-lymphocytes* both derive originally from stem lymphocytes in the bone marrow (Fig. 13.2), but they mature by different routes. Lymphocytes engaged in the cell-mediated response derive their immunologic competency in the thymus. For this reason, the response is also called the *thymus-dependent* response and the effector lymphocytes are designated as T-lymphocytes. The site of maturation from original stem cells for B-lymphocytes is not as well understood. In birds, the lymphocytes are processed in the bursa of Fabricius, a gut-associated lymphoid organ. In mammals, it appears that B-lymphocytes derive their immunologic competence in the bone marrow but some evidence suggests that this may occur in gut-associated lymphoid tissue, therefore, the *B* can be considered to refer the bursa of birds or to the bursa equivalent of mammals.

B-lymphocytes

When activated by contact with antigen, B-lymphocytes transform into *immunoblasts* (plas-

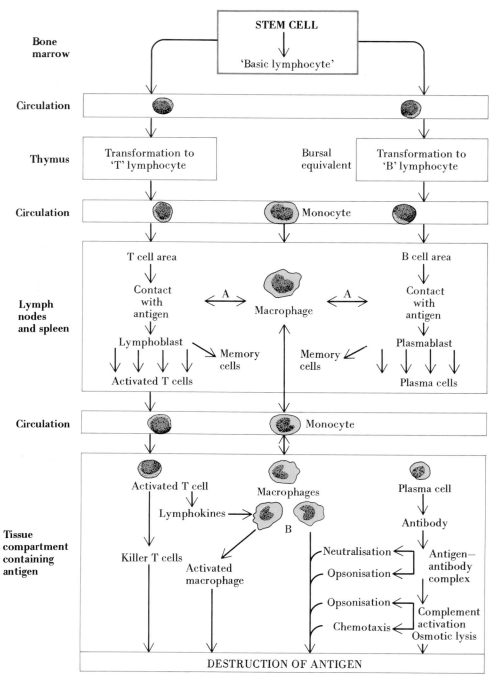

Figure 13.2. Outline of lymphocyte interactions. Mature lymphocytes are designated as either T- or B-lymphocytes according to whether they are transformed within the thymus or the bursal equivalent in mammals. T- and B-lymphocytes from the thymus and bursal equivalent populate the spleen, lymph nodes, and lymphatic nodules. Upon exposure of the lymphatic tissue to antigen, new lymphocytes are generated in these lymphatic organs. The new lymphocytes are activated so that they can react with the specific antigen responsible for their generation. The activated T-cells and plasma cells react with the antigen by mechanisms that result in the destruction and removal of the antigen. Reactions involving chiefly the T-lymphocytes are referred to as constituting the cellular response; reactions involving chiefly B-lymphocytes are referred to as constituting the humoral response. In both, macrophages participate with the lymphocytes at two differ-

mablasts) that proliferate and then differentiate into *plasma cells* or into *memory cells.* The plasma cells synthesize and secrete antibody. The antibodies bind to the foreign substance (antigen) and imitate a variety of reactions which eliminate the antigen (Fig. 13.2). For example, the antibodies may activate *complement,* a group of blood or serum constituents that attack invading microorganism or foreign cells by binding to them and causing them to lyse. In all of these reactions, the antigen-antibody complexes are finally eliminated by phagocytosis, by macrophages (and in some cases by eosinophils), or by lysis. Bacteria or toxins produced by bacteria are examples of antigenic agents eliminated by antibodies produced by B-lymphocytes.

The memory cells do not participate in the initial or *primary response* to a specific antigen. Rather, they are programmed to be ready to respond to the same antigen should it appear again. This second response to the same antigen upon a subsequent exposure is called the *secondary response.* It is more rapid and intense than the primary response because of the presence of a population of specific B-memory lymphocytes already programmed to respond to that antigen.[1]

Table 13.1 summarizes the characteristics of human immunoglobulins (Ig) and Figure 13.3 presents the structure of an antibody molecule in schematic form. Antibodies are produced by B-cells and by plasma cells, one of the cell types derived from the B-cell.

---

[1] When an individual has been immunologically sensitized by an exposure to an antigen, a subsequent exposure may lead not just to a boosting of the immune response (secondary response), but to tissue-damaging reactions designated as *hypersensitivity reactions.* Such reactions are observed in sensitized human subjects following insect bites or injections of penicillin. One type of hypersensitivity reaction familiar to many is the allergic reaction. Certain aspects of a hypersensitivity reaction are brought about by the antibody-induced discharge of mast cell granules. These granules contain mediators such as histamine which account for the distressing features of hypersensitivity reactions. Eosinophils are attracted to the site of mast cell degranulation and neutralize the effects of the released mediators. Thus, eosinophils are frequently seen in allergic or other hypersensitivity reaction sites.

T-lymphocytes

As was described previously, three fundamentally different types of T-lymphocytes have been identified:

1. *Cytotoxic lymphocytes (CTL) or killer T-cells* that serve as the primary effector cells in cell-mediated immunity. The CTLs recognize other cells that have foreign antigens on their surfaces and kill the cells by causing them to lyse. A classic target of a CTL is a virus infected cell which displays viral glycoproteins on its surface.

2. *Helper T-lymphocytes (TH cells)* that assist B-cells as well as other T-cells in their response to antigens. The interaction between most antigens and the antibodies on the surface of B-cells is insufficient to stimulate B-cell growth, differentiation, and secretion of soluble antibody. Only multivalent antigen molecules, those with more than one antigenic site, can stimulate the B-cells by themselves. A major function of the TH cell is to recognize foreign antigens and then secrete factors (such as lymphokines[2]) that stimulate B-cells, or other cells that participate in immune reactions, such as CTLs or macrophages.

3. *Suppressor T-lymphocytes or (TS cells)* that suppress the activity of B-cells. They appear to dampen the response to foreign antigens and may play a role in suppressing the immune response to self molecules. The T-cells may also function in the regulation of erythroid cell maturation in the bone marrow. The activities of the various types of T-lymphocytes are mediated by molecules located on their surface. By employing immunolabeling technique, it has been possible to identify specific types of T-cells and study their function. Some T-lymphocytes also form memory cells.

---

[2] Lymphokines are soluble substances, released by sensitized lymphocytes, upon contact with a specific antigen. These substances stimulate the activity of monocytes and macrophages in the cell-mediated immune response. Included among these substances are chemotactic, mitogenic, and migration inhibitory factors, interferon, and lymphotoxin.

---

ent levels of the chain. They may participate in the initial presentation of antigen to the lymphocyte **(A)**, or they may be involved in the final destruction and disposal of the antigen **(B)**. Memory cells do not participate in the initial response to antigen; they remain in the body, programmed to react at a later time with the same specific antigen in what is designated as the secondary response. The outline depicts those reactions of lymphocytes that are beneficial to the host and which result in the development of immunity. (Modified from Wheater PR, et al: *Functional Histology.* New York, Churchill Livingstone, 1969, p. 146.)

TABLE 13.1. Characteristics of Human Immunoglobulins

ISOTOPE	MOLECULAR WEIGHT	AVERAGE ADULT SERUM LEVEL (mg/ml)	CELLS TO WHICH BOUND VIA Fc REGION	BIOLOGICAL PROPERTIES
IgG	150,000	12	Macrophages, neutrophils, eosinophils, and large granular lymphocytes	Activates complement (a group of serum constituents having the capacity to lyse cells and bacteria); crosses placenta providing the newborn with passive immunity; principal Ig produced during secondary antibody response
IgM	190,000 (950,000)*	1	Lymphocytes	Fixes complement; activates macrophages; rheumatoid factor; Ig produced during primary antibody response
IgA	160,000 (385,000)†	2	Lymphocytes	Antibody present in body secretions including tears, colostrum, saliva, and vaginal fluid, and in the secretions of the nasal cavity, bronchi, intestine, and prostate (IgA provides protection against the proliferation of microorganisms in these fluids and aids in the defense against microbes and foreign molecules penetrating the body via the cells lining these cavities)
IgD	175,000	0.03	None	Found mainly on surface of lymphocytes (only traces in serum) and is involved in the differentiation of lymphocytes
IgE	190,000	0.0003	Mast cells and basophils	Stimulates mast cells to release histamine, heparin, leukotrienes (slow-reacting substance of anaphylaxis), and eosinophils chemotactic factor of anaphylaxis, (mediates anaphylaxis, allergy)

* IgM found in serum as a pentameric molecule
† IgA found in serum as a dimeric molecules

Large Lymphocytes

Large lymphocytes, also called *"null cells,"* account for 5 to 10 percent of the lymphocytes in peripheral blood (see Atlas Section, Plate 25, Figs. 3 and 4). These cells contain large azurophilic cytoplasmic granules and are nonadherent and nonphagocytic. In contrast to T-killer cells whose activity is dependent upon activation by antigen, a subset of large lymphocytes have *natural killer (NK) cell* activity and do not depend upon antigen activation. These cells, lacking the surface molecules associated with the activities of T- or B-lymphocytes, can also effect lysis of target cells. The killing of target cells, usually malignant cell types, is a nonimmune, nonantibody-mediated process. This population of large lymphocytes may play an important role in immune surveillance and the destruction of cells which undergo spontaneous transformation into malignant cells. Another subset of the large lymphocytes mediates *antibody-dependent cellular cytotoxicity (ADCC).* ADCC involves binding of an antibody-coated (opsonized) target cell to an Fc receptor-bearing effector cell.

The binding, through the Fc region of the antibody, results in the lysis of the target cell.

Antigen-Presenting Cells

In order for the effector cells of the immune system to function effectively, antigens are processed and presented to them by *antigen-presenting cells.* Although the molecular events involved in this process have not been defined, it is clear that several cell types are involved, including some macrophages (such as the Kupffer cells of the liver), Langerhans cells in the epidermis, and *follicular dendritic cells* found in the germinal center of lymphoid nodules. The follicular dendritic cells, considered to be a subclass of the lymphoid dendritic cells, are pale-staining, nonphagocytic cells with long motile cytoplasmic processes. These cells, as well as other antigen presenting cells, do not phagocytize foreign antigens, but retain them on their surfaces for long periods of time as complexed antigens bound to membrane proteins.

Table 13.2 presents a brief summary of the characteristics of the effector cells of the immune

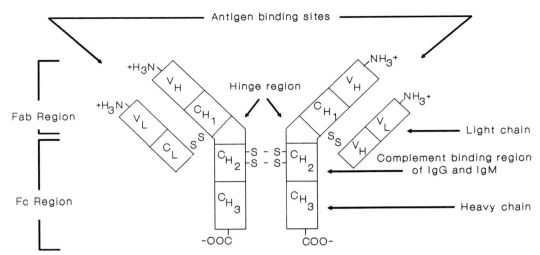

Figure 13.3. Schematic representation of an antibody molecule. The Y-shaped molecule binds antigens at the two sites indicated where the heavy and light chains are associated with each other. The immunoglobulin isotypes (see Table 13.1) are determined by the type of heavy and light chains present. The four chains (two heavy and two light) making up the molecule are covalently linked by disulfite bonds. Each polypeptide chain is composed domains of amino acids, which are constant (C) or variable (V) in the sequence. The subscripts, H and L, refer to the heavy and light chains. Two regions, Fab and Fc, having unique functions are also indicated. Enzymes can be used to cleave the molecule into two fragments which bind to antigens (Fab) and one fragment which is composed of constant regions of the heavy chains and in some isotypes binds complement (Fc). The constant regions of the heavy chain are involved in biological functions of the immunoglobulin molecules. The isotypes demonstrate specific amino acid domains in the three CH regions of the molecule indicated as C_H, C_{H2}, and C_{H3}. The C_H region at the carboxy terminus functions in the binding of the molecule to Fc receptors of macrophages, lymphocytes, mast cells, basophils, eosinophils, neutrophils, and large granular lymphocytes (see Table 13.1).

system and the functions associated with their unique cell surface membrane proteins.

Typically, in a response to a foreign substance, both cellular and humoral immune systems are involved, also though one system generally predominates in favor of the other according to the stimulus.

Macrophages are closely associated with lymphocytes in the two types of immune responses. At an early stage, the macrophage may concentrate antigen and present it to the lymphocytes (A in Fig. 13.2) or the macrophage may be the instrument for final destruction or disposal of antigen (B in Fig. 13.2).

While antigens are generally foreign substances, on occasion, body constituents may be identified as foreign by the immune system and elicit an immune response. This is the basis for the body's defense against cancerous cells, but it is also the basis for autoimmune diseases.

Although the components of the immune system discriminate between self and nonself, not all foreign substances can induce an immune response. A familiar example is carbon in the form of coal dust that is disposed of by phagocytosis independent of the immune system.

LYMPHATIC VESSELS AND THE CIRCULATION OF LYMPHOCYTES

Lymphatic vessels begin as networks of "blind" capillaries in the loose connective tissues of the body. Lymphatic capillaries are most numerous under the epithelium of skin and mucous membranes. These vessels remove substances and fluid from the extracellular spaces of the connective tissues. Because the walls of the lymphatic capillaries are more permeable than the walls of blood capillaries, large molecules and cells, including foreign substances, gain entry more readily into the lymphatic capillaries than into blood capillaries. In circulating through the lymphatic vessels, the lymph passes through lymph nodes. Here any foreign substances (antigens) being conveyed by the lymph are concentrated and exposed to the lymphocytes, and this leads to the cascade of steps which constitute the immune response. Lymphatic vessels ultimately drain the lymph into the bloodstream by

TABLE 13.2. Characteristics of the Effector Cells of the Immune System*

CELL TYPE	FUNCTIONAL SURFACE MOLECULE	CELLULAR FUNCTIONS MEDIATED BY THE SURFACE MOLECULES
T-lymphocyte	T3/T-cell antigen receptor complex (involving T3 receptors and other surface molecules)	Antigen recognition; T-cell activation
	T11	T-cell activation
	T4	Molecule present on helper and some cytotoxic T cells; T4 molecules facilitate antigen recognition. The AIDS (HTLV) infects the subset of T cells carrying this surface molecule
	T8	Molecule present on suppressor and cytotoxic T-cells that facilitates recognition of antigens via the major histocompatibility complex (MHC) molecules.
	Interleukin 2 (IL-2) receptor	Binds IL-2 to T-cells
B-lymphocyte	Surface immunoglobulins (sIg)†	Antigen recognition; cell activation
	IgG Fc receptors	Bind immune complexes
	C3 (complement) receptors	
Large granular lymphocyte	IgG receptors	Bind immune complexes
Monocyte-macrophage	IgG Fc receptors	Bind and phagocytose immune complexes
	C3 (complement) receptors	
	Major histocompatibility complex (MHC) class II antigens	Presentation of antigen to T- and B-cells
	Chemotactic receptors	Chemotaxis and polarization of cells
Neutrophils	IgG Fc receptors	Bind and phagocytose immune complexes
	C3 (complement) receptors	
	Chemotactic receptors	Chemotaxis and polarization of cells
Eosinophil	IgG Fc receptors	Bind and phagocytose immune complexes
	C3 (complement) receptors	
Basophil-mast cell	IgE Fc receptors	After binding of antigen (allergen)-IgE complexes to receptors, release of granules containing histamine, slow reacting substance of anaphylaxis, eosinophil chemotactic factor of anaphylaxis, platelet activation factor, neutrophil chemotactic factor, leukotactic activity, heparin, and basophil kallikrein of anaphylaxis
	C3 (complement) receptors	

* Modified from Haynes BF, Faver AS: 1987. Introduction to clinical immunology. In: *Harrison's Principals of Internal Medicine,* 11th Edition. McGraw-Hill, New York, pages 328–337.)
† Precursor B cells contain immunoglobulin M in their cytoplasm (cIgM). As they mature in the bone marrow they express IgM on their surface (sIgM) and they no longer express cIgM. With continued maturation, prior to exposure to specific antigens (i.e. antigen independent maturation), the production of immunoglobulins switches so that IgD molecules are express on the cell surface along with either IgM, IgG, IgA, or IgE. Each B-cell expresses Ig molecules of only one heavy and light chain variable and thus are specific for a specific antigen. On contact with that antigen, mature B cells terminally differentiate into antibody secreting plasma cells or proliferate to produce long-lived memory cells.

joining the veins at the junction of the internal jugular and subclavian veins in the neck.

Lymphocytes are migratory cells and they circulate through the lymphatic vessels and through the bloodstream. The circulation of lymphocytes enables them to move from one part of the lymphatic system to another at different stages in their development and also to reach sites within the body where they are needed. An outline of lymphocyte circulation showing a lymph node as a starting point is depicted in Figure 13.4. It shows lymphocytes conveyed in the lymph entering the node via afferent lymphatic vessels and lymphocytes conveyed in the blood entering the node

through the wall of postcapillary venule. Some of these lymphocytes pass to B- and T-territories of the node, others pass through the substances of the node to leave via the efferent lymphatic vessels. The latter lead ultimately to the right lymphatic duct or as shown in the illustration to the thoracic duct. In turn, both of these channels empty into the blood circulating by draining into the large veins in the root of the neck. The lymphocytes are conveyed to and from the various lymphatic tissues via the blood vessels. (The venous component of the blood vascular circulation has not been included in the scheme.) The scheme actually depicts a recirculation of lymphocytes and it should be

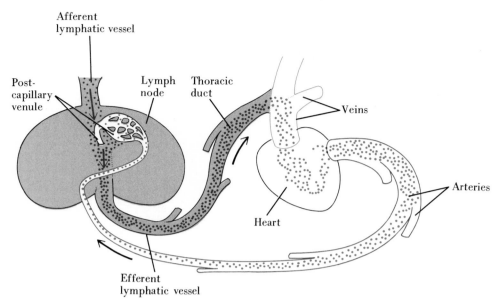

Figure 13.4. Diagram depicting circulation of lymphocytes beginning at a lymph node. Lymphocytes enter lymph nodes by two routes: (1) afferent lymphatic vessels (only one is shown) and (2) through the wall of the postcapillary venules. Some lymphocytes move to the T and B domains of the lymph node; others pass through the substance of the node and leave via an efferent lymphatic vessel. Ultimately, the lymphocytes enter a major lymphatic vessel, in the illustration the thoracic duct, which opens into the large veins in the root of the neck, whereupon the lymphocytes become components of the blood. The lymphocytes continue to the arterial side of the circulation and via the arteries to the lymphatic tissues of the body or to tissues where they participate in immune reactions. From the lymphatic tissues, lymphocytes again return to the lymph nodes to gain entry via the postcapillary venules. The above scheme describes a recirculation of lymphocytes that involves all lymphatic tissue except the thymus. (Based on Gowans JE: *Hosp Pract* 3:34, 1968.)

noted that all lymphatic tissue except the thymus appear to be in the recirculation route. While these migratory lymphocytes look alike when viewed with the light microscope, they reflect different levels of development, immunological competence, activation, and commitment.

The story of the lymphocyte biology is a major part of the subject matter of immunology and beyond the scope of a concise histology book. The introductory comments presented here are intended to alert the reader to the realization that the lymphatic system is a dynamic system in which the lymphocyte population of lymphatic tissues is constantly changing; that lymphocytes, as they are studied in histology, are actually a heterogeneous group of cells; that the lymphatic organs and tissues are interdependent; and that the lymphocytes and the antibodies may need to function in parts of the body which are beyond the boundaries of the lymphatic system as depicted in Figure 13.1. It is also useful in the study of the following sections to bear in mind the overall functions of the lymphatic system, namely:

1. to concentrate antigens in certain lymphoid organs,
2. to circulate lymphocytes through these organs so that they can come into contact with antigens,
3. to convey the products of the immune response (effector T-lymphocytes, humoral antibodies) to tissues where they are needed, and
4. to eliminate antigen from the body.

DIFFUSE LYMPHATIC TISSUE AND LYMPHATIC NODULES

The alimentary canal, respiratory passages, and genitourinary tract are guarded by accumulations of lymphatic tissue that are not enclosed by a capsule. The lymphocytes are disposed in an apparently random manner in the lamina propria (subepithelial tissue) of these tracts and this lymphatic tissue is called *diffuse lymphatic tissue* (Fig. 13.5). The cells of diffuse lymphatic tissue are not static; rather, they are strategically situated to intercept and react with antigen. The regular presence of large numbers of plasma cells, especially in

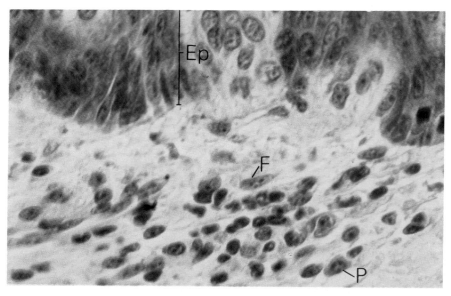

Figure 13.5. Light micrograph of diffuse lymphatic tissue in the tongue. The connective tissue underlying the epithelium (Ep) is very cellular. Included in this cell population are some fibroblasts (F); the bulk of the cells, however, are lymphocytes and, to a lesser extent, plasma cells (P).

the lamina propria of the gastrointestinal tract, is a morphological indication of antibody formation, and similarly, the presence of large numbers of eosinophils (frequently observed in the mucosa of the respiratory and intestinal passages) is an indication of hypersensitivity reactions.

In addition to the diffuse lymphatic tissue, there are localized concentrations of lymphocytes in the walls of the alimentary canal, respiratory passages, and genitourinary tract. These concentrations show a structural organization and are called **nodules** or **follicles** (Fig. 13.6). Generally, the

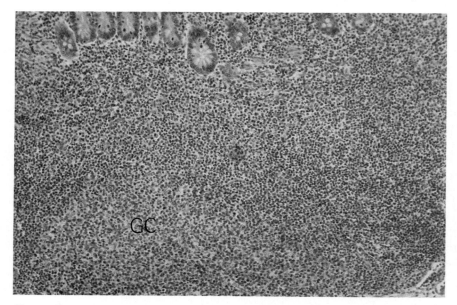

Figure 13.6. Light micrograph of a lymphatic nodule in the small intestine. The basal part of some of the intestinal glands are present in the upper portion of the micrograph. The remainder of the figure is occupied by the nodule, a compact mass of cells, comprised mostly of lymphocytes. In the lower left of the nodule, a germinal center (GC) is evident. The lymphocytes here are larger; they have more cytoplasm and, collectively, their nuclei appear as a less compact mass.

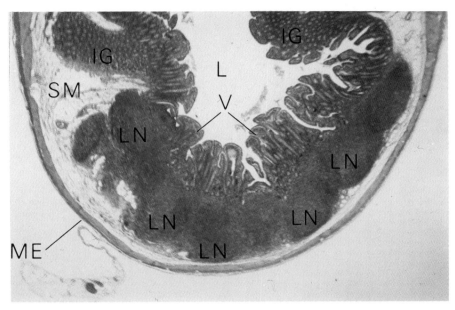

Figure 13.7. Light micrograph showing an aggregation of lymph nodules (LN) in the wall of the ileum. Such an aggregation is called a Peyer's patch. The lymph nodules are located partly in the mucosa, and they extend into the submucosa (SM). L, lumen of ileum; ME, muscularis externa; V, villi.

nodules are disposed singly in a random manner. However, in the alimentary canal some aggregations of nodules are found in specific locations, as in the appendix and where the oral cavity meets the pharynx. At the latter junction, aggregations of nodules are the *pharyngeal tonsils* or *adenoids,* located in the roof of the pharynx; the *palatine tonsils* or simply the tonsils, on either side between the faucial pillars; and the *lingual tonsils* in the base of the tongue. The small intestine also contains, in addition to isolated nodules, aggregations of nodules which are most numerous in the ileum; these are called *Peyer's patches* (Fig. 13.7). The diffuse lymphatic tissue and the nodules of the alimentary canal together are referred to as the *G*ut *A*ssociated *L*ymphatic *T*issue (GALT). All of these nodules are reactive lymphatic tissue and they become enlarged during encounters with antigen.

A lymphatic nodule is an oval concentration of lymphocytes contained in a meshwork of reticular cells. If the nodule consists chiefly of small lymphocytes, it is called a *primary nodule.* However, many, if not most, nodules display a central region that in histological sections, appears to stain less intensely than the outer ring of small lymphocytes. This central, lighter staining region is called a *germinal center* (see Fig. 13.6). It is a reaction center that develops when a primary nodule is exposed to antigen. The lighter staining is due to the fact that the germinal center contains large lymphocytes *(lymphoblasts and plasmablasts)* that have large amounts of the more dispersed euchromatin in their nuclei rather than the dense heterochromatin of the small lymphocytes. The germinal center is a morphological indication of lymphatic tissue response to antigen. The germinal center depicts a cascade of events, which include proliferation of lymphocytes, differentiation of plasma cells, and antibody production. Frequently, mitotic figures are observed in the germinal center, a reflection of the proliferation of new lymphocytes at this site.

LYMPH NODES

Lymph nodes are small, oval, encapsulated lymphatic organs. They range in size from about a millimeter (barely visible with the naked eye) to about 1 to 2 cm in their longest dimension. Lymph nodes are interposed in the pathway of lymphatic vessels (Fig. 13.8) and they serve as filters through which lymph percolates on its way to the blood. The lymphatic vessels entering the node are designated *afferent lymphatic vessels* and they enter the node at various point on the convex surface of the capsule. *Efferent lymphatic vessels* leave the node at a hilus which also serves for the entry and exit of blood vessels and nerves.

The supporting elements of the lymph node are the *capsule,* comprised of dense connective tissue, which surrounds the node; the *trabeculae,* also

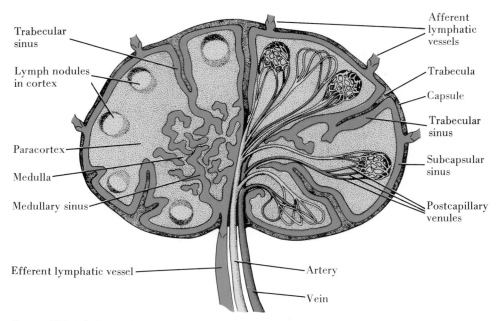

Figure 13.8. Schematic diagram of a lymph node. The left side of the figure depicts the general features of a lymph node as seen in a section. The substance of the lymph node is divided into a cortex, including a paracortical region, and a medulla. The cortex is the outermost portion; it contains spherical or oval aggregates of lymphocytes called lymph nodules. In an active lymph node, these contain a lighter center called the germinal center. The medulla is the innermost region of the lymph node and extends as far as the hilus of the node. It consists of regions of lymphatic tissue, appearing as irregular cords in section, separated by lymph sinuses, which because of their location in the medulla are referred to as medullary sinuses. The dense population of lymphocytes between the cortex and the medulla constitutes the paracortex. This is the region of the node which contains the postcapillary venules. Surrounding the lymph node is a capsule of dense connective tissue from which trabeculae extend into the substance of the node. Under the capsule and adjacent to the trabeculae are lymph sinuses designated as subcapsular or cortical, and trabecular, respectively. Afferent lymphatic vessels penetrate the capsule and empty into the subcapsular sinus. The subcapsular sinus and trabecular sinuses communicate with the medullary sinuses. The right side of the lymph node also shows an artery and vein and the location of the postcapillary venules of the lymph node. (Based on Bloom W, Fawcett DW: *A Textbook of Histology,* 10th ed. Philadelphia, WB Saunders, 1975.)

comprised of dense connective tissue, which extend from the capsule into the substance of the node forming a framework; and ***reticular tissue*** comprised of reticular cells and reticular fibers that form a fine supporting meshwork throughout the remainder of the organ (Fig. 13.9). The reticular cells produce and surround the reticular fibers so that the fibers are essentially separated from the microcompartment occupied by the lymphocytes (Fig. 13.10).

The parenchyma of the lymph node is divided into cortex and medulla (Fig. 13.11). The cortex forms the outer portion of the node except at the hilus. It consists of a dense mass of lymphatic tissue (reticular framework, lymphocytes, macrophages, and plasma cells) and lymph sinuses. The lympho-

cytes in the outer part of the cortex are organized into nodules. As elsewhere, these are designated as primary nodules if they consist chiefly of small lymphocytes and as secondary nodules if they possess a germinal center. [The structural and functional properties of germinal centers of lymph nodes are the same as those described for germinal centers in lymphatic nodules (see Fig. 13.6)]. The portion of the cortex adjacent to the medulla is free of nodules; it is called the ***deep cortex.*** Other names applied to the deep cortex are the juxtamedullary cortex, the paracortical zone, and the tertiary cortex. Nodules are the territory of B-lymphocytes; the deep cortex is the territory of the T-lymphocytes. Both B- and T-lymphocytes are present where the deep and nodular cortex meet.

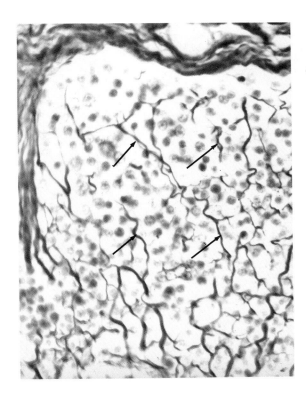

Figure 13.9. Photomicrograph of a lymph node, silver preparation, showing the connective tissue capsule at the top and trabeculum extending from it at the left. The reticular fibers **(arrows)** form an irregular anastomosing network.

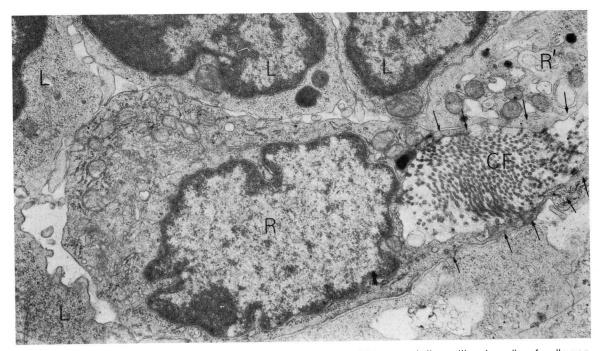

Figure 13.10. An electron micrograph showing a reticular cell (R) in association with a bundle of collagen fibrils (CF). With the light microscope and special staining procedures, the bundle of collagen fibrils would be recognized as a reticular fiber. Also present in the micrograph are parts of four lymphocytes (L) and the cytoplasm of another reticular cell (R'). The collagen fibrils are surrounded by the body and by the processes **(arrows)** of the reticular cells. Thus, the collagen fibrils are not exposed to the lymphocytes.

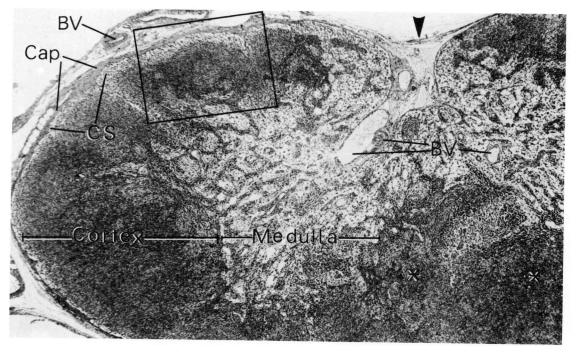

Figure 13.11. Light micrograph of a lymph node. The outermost portion of the lymph node, except at the hilus **(arrowhead)**, is the cortex. It contains dense aggregations of lymphocytes, many organized as lymph nodules. The rectangle shows a lymph nodule with a more lightly stained germinal center. The deep part of the cortex, usually nodule-free **(asterisks)**, is referred to as the paracortex or deep cortex. The innermost portion of the lymph node is the medulla. It extends to the surface of the node at the hilus where blood vessels (BV) enter or leave and where efferent lymphatic vessels leave the node. The medulla contains cords of lymphatic tissue and medullary sinuses. Surrounding the lymph node is the capsule (Cap) and immediately under this is the cortical sinus. Afferent lymphatic vessels enter the lymph node through the capsule and drain into the cortical sinus.

The lymph sinuses in the cortex are arranged in a special manner. Just under the capsule there is a lymph sinus interposed between the capsule and the cortical lymphocytes. This is called the **cortical** or **subcapsular sinus.** Afferent lymphatic vessels drain lymph into this sinus. Other lymph sinuses extend through the cortex as **trabecular, or peritrabecular, sinuses** and drain into the medullary sinuses. The region of the cortex adjacent to the medullar is called the **paracortical, or deep cortical, area.** As was stated above, this area is of functional significance because it is populated by T-lymphocytes. Lymphocytes and macrophages, or their processes, readily pass between lymph sinuses and parenchyma of the lymph node. The sinuses have a lining of endothelium that is continuous where it is directly adjacent to the connective tissue of the capsule or trabeculae, but is discontinuous where it faces the lymphatic parenchyma. Even though a macrophage may be in the lymphatic parenchyma, it often sends pseudopods (long cytoplasmic processes) into the sinus through the endothelial discontinuities (see Atlas section, Plate 53). These

pseudopods monitor the lymph as it percolates through the sinus.

The medulla is the inner part of the node. It consists of cords of lymphatic tissue separated by lymph sinuses, called **medullary sinuses.** As already mentioned, a network of reticular cells and fibers traverses the medullary cords and medullary sinuses and serves as the framework of the parenchyma. In addition to reticular cells, the medullary cords contains lymphocytes, macrophages, and plasma cells. The medullary sinuses converge toward the region of the hilus where they drain into efferent lymphatic vessels.

Not only lymph, but also lymphocytes constantly circulate through the lymph nodes. Although some lymphocytes enter nodes through afferent lymphatic vessels as components of lymph, more enter the node through the wall of postcapillary venules, located in the deep cortex (see Fig. 13.8 and Atlas section, Plate 51, Fig. 2). The postcapillary venules are lined by high cuboidal cells which play a role in the passage of lymphocytes from the blood to the substance of the lymph node.

Lymph Node Functions

Lymph nodes serve as filters of the lymph. The phagocytosis of particulate material by phagocytic cells within the lymph nodes can be considered a basic aspect of filtration. The physical obstruction of a lymph node by microorganism and particulate substances conveyed in the lymph and the phagocytosis of the particulate material may lead to concentration of an antigen, thus enhancing its presentation to lymphocytes. As antigens conveyed in the lymph, percolate through the sinuses and penetrate the lymph nodules, some of them are trapped on the surface of specialized cells known as *follicular dendritic cells.* Exposed in this way the antigens are presented to immunocompetent memory B-cells. Recognition of an antigen by a B-cell may necessitate the involvement of T-cells to facilitate activation of the B-cells. Activated B-cells migrate to germinal centers and undergo as series of mitotic divisions giving rise to immature immunoblasts. These cells proliferate and give rise to plasma cells and memory B-cells. The plasma cells migrate to the medullary cords where they synthesize and release specific antibodies into the lymph flowing through the sinuses. The memory cells may leave the lymph nodes and circulate to various regions through the body. If antigen is encountered the cells proliferate in the manner just described. The presence of memory cells, scattered in various sites throughout the body, results in a more rapid response to an antigen when it is next encountered (i.e., the secondary or amnestic immune response). Lymph nodes in which lymphocytes demonstrate response to an antigenic or infective agents undergo enlargement reflecting formation of germinal centers and proliferation of lymphocytes. Plasma cells account for 1 to 3 percent of the cells in resting lymph nodules. Their number increases dramatically during an immune response, thereby increasing the amount of circulating immunoglobulins.

THYMUS

The thymus is a bilobed structure that develops bilaterally from the third and sometimes also the fourth branchial (oropharyngeal) pouch. During development, the thymic rudiment grows caudally as a tubular prolongation of endodermal epithelium into the mediastinum of the chest. The advancing tip proliferates and ultimately becomes disconnected from the branchial epithelium. Lymphocytes invade the epithelial rudiment and occupy the spaces between the epithelial cells so that the thymus develops into a lymphoepithelial organ. Although many lymphocytes come to lie between the epithelial cells, the cells remain joined to one another by desmosomes at the end of long cytoplasmic processes. As a consequence, these epithelial cells assume a stellate shape. They form a cytoplasmic reticulum within the parenchyma of the thymus and they are designated as *epithelioreticular cells.* The epithelioreticular cells serve as a framework for the thymic lymphocytes, and, thus, they correspond structurally to the reticular cells and their associated reticular fibers in the other lymphoid tissues and organs.

The essential features of thymic structure are illustrated in Figure 13.12. Externally, there is a connective tissue capsule from which trabeculae extend into the substance of the organ. In addition to collagenous fibers and fibroblasts, this connective tissue contains variable numbers of plasma cells, granulocyte, lymphyocytes, mast cells, fat cells, and macrophages. The capsule and trabeculae also contain blood vessels, efferent lymphatic vessels (but not afferent lymphatic vessels), and nerves.

The outer portion, or cortex, of the thymic parenchyma contains a higher concentration of lymphocytes than the inner portion, or medulla. Because the lymphocytes in the cortex are small, are closely packed, and possess densely-staining nuclei (mostly heterochromatin), the cortex appears extremely basophilic. In contrast, the medulla stains less intensely because it contains, like germinal centers of nodules, large lymphocytes with paler-staining nuclei and quantitatively more cytoplasm as well as proportionally more epithelioreticular cells. In addition to the numerous lymphocytes and epithelioreticular cells, the thymic cortex contains many macrophages engaged in the phagocytosis of degenerating lymphocytes. Macrophages that are heavily laden with lysosome can be displayed with the PAS reaction, and these macrophages have been designated as *PAS cells.* The thymic medulla seen in a histological section is more heavily infiltrated with lymphocyte than is shown in the schematic diagram depicted in Figure 13.12.

The medulla also contains an unusual structure, the *thymic,* or *Hassall's, corpuscles* (Fig. 13.13). These are isolated masses of closely packed, concentrically arranged epithelioreticular cells. The center of a thymic corpuscle may display evidence of keratinization, a not surprising feature since the cells are of epithelial character.

The characteristic features of thymic structure persist until about the time of puberty. At this time, although it continues to function, it involutes and comes to contain large numbers of fat cells.

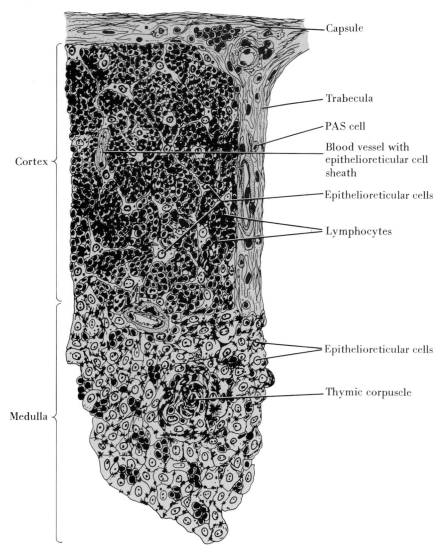

Capsule

Trabecula

PAS cell

Blood vessel with
epithelioreticular cell
sheath

Epithelioreticular cells

Lymphocytes

Cortex

Epithelioreticular cells

Thymic corpuscle

Medulla

Figure 13.12. Diagram illustrating a portion of a thymic lobule with cortex, medulla, capsule, and trabecula. The cortex contains numerous lymphocytes that are distributed in an apparently random manner between the epithelioreticular cells. The epithelioreticular cells remain joined to each other by means of desmosomes at the ends of long processes. As a consequence, the epithelioreticular cells assume a stellate shape. Fewer lymphocytes are present between the epithelioreticular cells of the medulla. Nevertheless, in the actual thymic section there are more lymphocytes than are depicted in the diagram. Blood vessels within the substance of the thymus are surrounded by epithelioreticular cells or their processes. The concentrically arranged epithelioreticular cells in the medulla constitute a thymic (Hassall's) corpuscle. The capsule and trabecula consist of dense connective tissue. (L. Weiss, 1972.)

Blood-Thymic Barrier

Blood vessels enter the substance of the thymus from the trabeculae. Typically, the blood vessels enter the medulla from the deeper parts of the trabeculae and carry a sheath of connective tissue along with them. The perivascular connective tissue sheath varies in thickness, being thicker around larger vessels and becoming increasingly thinner around smaller vessels. Where it is thicker, it contains reticular fibers, fibroblasts, macrophages, plasma cells, and other cells found in loose connective tissue; where it is thinnest, it may contain only reticular fibers and occasional fibroblasts.

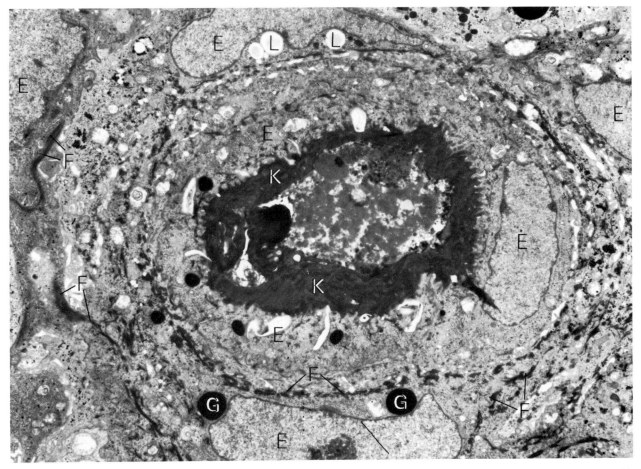

Figure 13.13. Lower power electron micrograph of a Hassall's corpuscle. Note the presence of nuclei of concentrically arranged epithelioreticular cells (E); keratohyalin granules (G); bundles of cytoplasmic filaments (tonofilaments) (F); lipid droplets (L); fully keratinized epithelioreticular cell (K). (J. G. Rhodin, 1974.)

A unique feature of the perivascular connective tissue sheath is that it is itself ensheathed by expansions of the epithelial reticular cells. Typically, a basal lamina is interposed between the expansions of the epithelial reticular cells and the perivascular connective tissue. Together these various layers constitute a ***blood-thymic barrier*** between the thymic lymphocyte and the lumen of the smallest blood vessels. In essence, the components of the barrier are:

1. the capillary endothelium,
2. its basal lamina,
3. a thin perivascular sheath of connective tissue,
4. the epithelioreticular cell sheath, and
5. its basal lamina.

The epithelioreticular cell layer surrounding the vasculature and endothelium of the capillaries in the cortex are the key function elements of the blood-thymic barrier. The endothelium has been shown to be highly impermeable to macromolecules and is considered to be the major structural component of the barrier.

Thymic Function

During fetal life, the thymus is populated by stem lymphocytes from the liver. When blood cell formation moves from the liver to the bone marrow, the marrow becomes the source of stem lymphocytes. Within the thymus there is large-scale proliferation of lymphocytes and large-scale cell death, so that most of the newly formed lymphocytes die within a few days. Nevertheless, the thymus releases large numbers of lymphocytes that are carried by the blood to the lymph nodes, spleen, and other lymphatic tissue where they colonize specific parts of these organs and tissues. The lymphocytes released by the thymus are the T-lymphocytes. Under the proper stimulus, T-lymphocytes proliferate and participate in the cell-mediated immune response. The T-lymphocytes survive for long periods and recirculate through lymphatic tissues.

The transformation of primitive or stem lymphocytes into T-lymphocytes is promoted by a thymic humoral factor called *thymosin*. There is evidence that the thymic epithelioreticular cells produce this factor.

When the thymus of the newborn mouse is removed, lymph nodes and spleen do not develop normally due to a depletion of T-lymphocytes and, as previously noted, there is an impairment in the cell-mediated immune response. Thus, in newborn thymectomized mice, tissue grafts from other mice may persist indefinitely, whereas the same type of graft would be rejected by thymus-intact animals. In adult animals, nonthymic lymphatic organs are well-stocked with T-lymphocytes and, therefore, graft rejection occurs even in thymectomized animals.

SPLEEN

The spleen is a large lymphatic organ in the upper left quadrant of the abdominal cavity. In addition to large numbers of lymphocytes, it contains specialized vascular spaces, a meshwork of reticular cells and reticular fibers, and a rich supply of macrophages. These contents allow the spleen to monitor the blood immunologically, much as the macrophages of the lymph nodes monitor the lymph.

The spleen is surrounded by a capsule of dense connective tissue from which trabeculae extend into the substance of the organ (Fig. 13.14). The connective tissue of the capsule and trabeculae contains myofibroblasts. These cells are not only contractile, but they also produce the extracellular connective tissue fibers. The spleen has the ability to hold large volumes of red blood cells in reserve. The contraction of the myofibroblasts in the capsule and trabeculae help discharge cells into the blood vessels thereby producing an immediate augmentation of vascular red blood cells. A hilus on the medial surface provides for the passage of the splenic artery and vein, for nerves, and for lymphatic vessels. The lymphatic vessels originate in the white pulp near the trabeculae and constitute a route for lymphocytes leaving the spleen.

White Pulp

The substance of the spleen, other than the capsule and trabeculae, consists of splenic pulp.

This, in turn, is divided into *white pulp* and *red pulp*. In a fresh section of the spleen the white pulp is seen as circular or elongated gray areas surrounded by the red pulp. The white pulp consists of lymphatic tissue, mostly lymphocytes; in hematoxylin-stained sections, the white pulp appears as basophilic areas due to the presence of dense heterochromatin in nucleus of the numerous lymphocytes.

Branches of the splenic artery course through the capsule and trabeculae of the spleen and then enter the white pulp. Within the white pulp, the vessel is called the *central artery*. The aggregated population of lymphocytes around the central artery are designated as the *periarterial lymphatic sheath (PALS)*. The PALS has a roughly cylindrical configuration which conforms to the course of the central artery. In cross-sections, the sheath of lymphocytes appears circular and it may have the appearance of a nodule. However, the presence of the central artery distinguishes the PALS from the nodule. True lymphatic nodules do occur in the periarterial sheath. They appear as localized expansions of the PALS and they tend to displace the central artery so that it occupies an eccentric rather than a central position (see Plate 55, Fig. 3). Nodules are the territory of B-lymphocytes; other lymphocytes of the PALS are chiefly T-lymphocytes. The nodules usually contain germinal centers and, as in other lymphatic tissue, the germinal center is a reaction center that forms in response to antigen. In the human, the germinal centers may become extremely large and visible with the naked eye. The enlarged nodules are called *splenic nodules* or *Malpighian corpuscles*.

Red Pulp

The red pulp has a red appearance in the fresh state as well as in histological sections because it contains large numbers of red blood cells. Essentially, the red pulp consists of splenic sinuses separated by the splenic cords, or cords of Billroth. The splenic cords consist of a meshwork of reticular cells and reticular fibers containing large numbers of erythrocytes, macrophages, lymphocytes, plasma cells, and granulocytes. Many of the macrophages are engaged in the phagocytosis of damaged red blood cells. The iron from degenerating red blood cells is reutilized in the formation of new red blood cells and the macrophages begin the process of hemoglobin breakdown and iron reclamation. Megakaryocytes are also present in certain species (such as rodents and the cat, but not in humans except during fetal life).

The splenic, or venous, sinuses are special si-

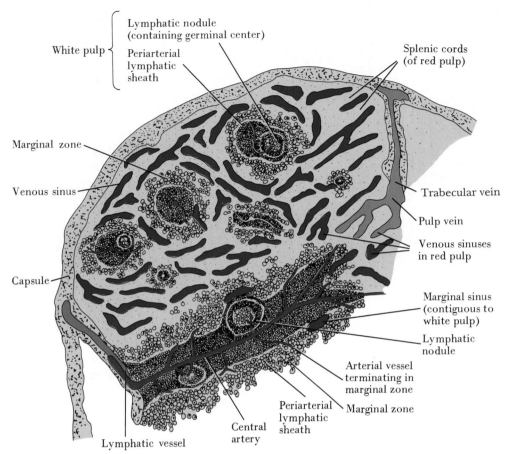

White pulp {
Lymphatic nodule (containing germinal center)
Periarterial lymphatic sheath
}

Splenic cords (of red pulp)

Marginal zone

Venous sinus

Capsule

Trabecular vein

Pulp vein

Venous sinuses in red pulp

Marginal sinus (contiguous to white pulp)

Lymphatic nodule

Arterial vessel terminating in marginal zone

Marginal zone

Periarterial lymphatic sheath

Central artery

Lymphatic vessel

Figure 13.14. This diagram outlines schematically those features of splenic structure that are evident in a histological section. The substance of the spleen is divided into white pulp and red pulp. White pulp consists of a cylindrical mass of lymphocytes arranged about a central artery. This mass of lymphocytes constitutes the periarterial lymphatic sheath. Lymphatic nodules occur along the length of the periarterial sheath, and when observed in cross-section through part of the sheath that contains a nodule (upper part of figure), the central artery appears excentrically located with respect to the lymphatic mass. The periarterial lymphatic sheath is surrounded by less densely packed lymphocytes that constitute the marginal zone. The red pulp consists of venous sinuses surrounded by splenic tissue called splenic cords or cords of Billroth. Surrounding the spleen is a capsule. Trabeculae project from the capsule into the substance of the spleen. Both capsule and trabeculae give the appearance of dense connective tissue. The cells in the capsule and trabeculae are myofibroblasts. Blood vessels traverse the capsule and trabeculae before and after passage within the substance of the spleen. Lymphatic vessels begin in the white pulp near the trabeculae. (Based on Weiss L, Tavossoli M: *S&M Hematol* 7:372, 1970.)

nusoidal vessels that are lined by unusually shaped endothelial cells (Fig. 13.15). These cells are extremely long with their longitudinal axis parallel to the direction of the vessel. Instead of a continuous basal lamina, the splenic sinuses are surrounded by thick, ring-like formations of basal lamina material. This may contain scattered single reticular fibrils, but they are few in number. It is chiefly the basal lamina material that is displayed with silver-containing reagents or when stained with the PAS reaction. The endothelial cells are evidently not tightly adherent to their neighbors and they allow blood cells to pass into and out of the sinuses quite readily. Also, the process of macrophages extend between the endothelial cells and into the lumen of the sinuses to monitor the passing blood.

Splenic Circulation

Branches of the splenic artery enter the white pulp from the trabeculae (Fig. 13.16). In the white pulp, the central artery sends branches to the white pulp itself and to the sinuses at the perimeter of the white pulp called *marginal sinuses* (see Fig. 13.14). The central artery continues into the red pulp where it branches into several relatively straight arteries called *penicilli.* The penicilli then continue as arterial capillaries; they may be surrounded by concentrically arranged macrophages. Arteries containing such arrangements of macrophages are called *sheathed arteries.*

The exact route whereby blood moves from the arterial capillaries into the splenic sinuses is not yet clear. Two routes have been proposed and both may in fact be operational. In one, called the open route, the arterial capillaries open and discharge blood into the splenic cords; blood cells would then enter the sinuses by passing between the endothelial cells that constitute the wall of the sinus. In the proposed route, the closed route, arterial capillaries open directly into the splenic sinuses and then drain into branches of the splenic vein. These branches enter the trabeculae, ultimately converge into larger veins, and leave the spleen as the splenic vein.

Splenic Functions

Splenic functions related to the immune system are lymphocyte production and antibody production. The spleen also plays a major role in the destruction of damaged and aged red blood cells, in phagocytosis of particulate matter in the blood, in blood cell formation during early fetal development, and in storage of blood. Despite this variety of functions the spleen is not essential to life and can be surgically removed if necessary.

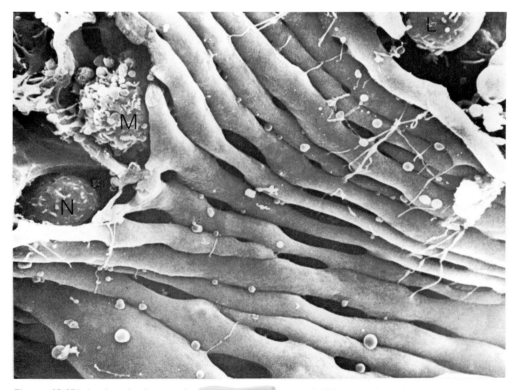

Figure 13.15(a). Luminal aspect of splenic sinus (human). This scanning electron micrograph shows the architecture of the sinus wall as seen from the luminal side. Rod cells run in parallel and are intermittently connected with each other by side processes. A nuclear swelling is shown on the bottom left. The tapered ends of a few of the rod cells are seen. The rod cells are provided with a few thread-like microprojections whose significance is unknown. The macrophage (M), neutrophil (N), and lymphocyte (L) are outside of the sinus. × 5,300. (From Fujita T, et al: *S&M Atlas of Cells and Tissues,* 1981.)

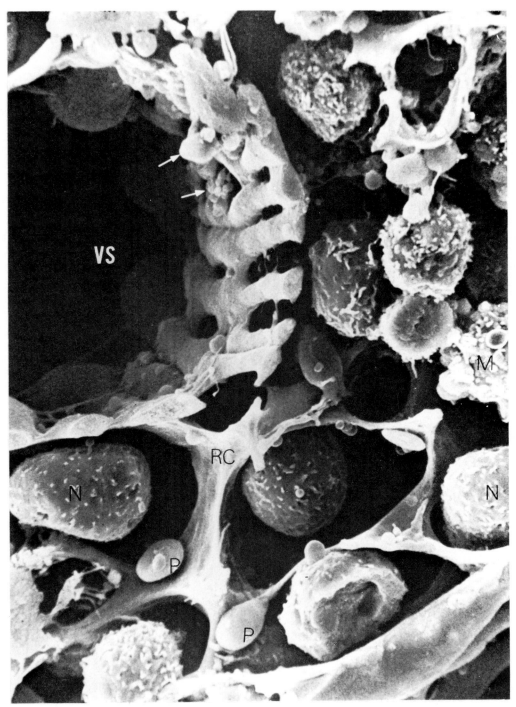

Figure 13.15(b).   Cross-section of splenic sinus and cord of Billroth (human). This scanning electron micrograph shows a cross-section view of a venous sinus (VS) on the left, revealing the lattice structure of its wall. Rod cells are connected with each other by their side processes. Through the apertures between the rod cells, processes of macrophages **(arrows)** may be inserted into the sinus lumen. The cord of Billroth is supported by the wing-like processes of reticular cells (RC) whose surface is characteristically smooth. The spaces of the reticular cell framework contain neutrophils (N), macrophages (M), and blood platelets (P). Red blood cells and many other free cells, which must have filled the spaces in the living state, have been washed away during perfusion. × 4,400. (From Fujita T, et al: *S&M Atlas of Cells and Tisuses*, 1981.)

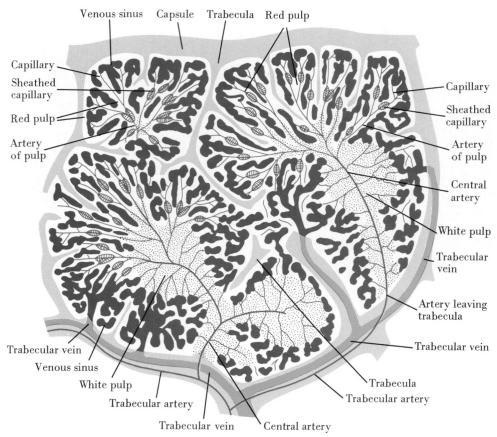

Figure 13.16. Diagram of splenic circulation according to the "closed circulation" theory. In the closed circulation theory, the central arteries give rise to arterial branches, which, in turn, lead to capillaries that open into the venous sinuses. Although not shown in the upper part of the diagram, it should be noted that all of the venous sinuses ultimately drain into trabecular veins as shown on the right and lower left side of the illustration. (Based on Bloom W, Fawcett DW: *A Textbook of Histology,* 10th ed. Philadelphia, WB Saunders, 1975.)

ATLAS PLATES

50–57

PLATE 50. Tonsil

The palatine tonsils (faucial tonsils)[3] are paired, ovoid structures that consist of dense accumulations of lymphatic tissue located in the mucous membrane of the fauces (the junction of oropharynx and oral cavity). The adjacent low-power survey micrograph shows the general structural features of part of the tonsil. The epithelium that forms the surface of the tonsil dips into the underlying connective tissue in numerous places, forming crypts, known as the tonsillar crypts. One of these crypts is seen in the adjacent survey micrograph (arrows). Numerous lymphatic nodules are readily evident in the walls of the crypts.

Figure 1 shows, at a higher magnification, part of this same crypt as well as the adjacent epithelium (EP) and one of the lymphatic nodules (LN). The crypt contains some cellular debris, a frequent occurrence. The lymphatic nodule exhibits a germinal center, the lighter central region of the nodule. The darker-staining peripheral portion of the nodule contains numerous closely packed small lymphocytes that are intimately related to the epithelium; they have actually become incorporated in the epithelium. Portions of the germinal center have also become incorporated into the epithelium.

The rectangular area in Figure 1 is shown at higher power in Figure 2. The stratified squamous epithelium (Ep) is just barely recognized due to the heavy infiltration of lymphocytes. However, the deeper portion of the epithelium is even more obscured. Epithelial cells are present, though difficult to identify, in the germinal center as well as in the periphery of the nodule (small arrows). The oval inscribed area is seen at higher magnification in the adjoining inset and shows the epithelial cells (arrows) more clearly. In effect, this nodule has literally grown into the epithelium, distorting it with the resulting disappearance of the well-defined epithelial-connective tissue boundary.

[3] In addition to the palatine tonsils, similar aggregations of lymphatic tissue are present beneath the epithelium of the tongue (called lingual tonsils), under the epithelium of the roof of the nasopharynx (called pharyngeal tonsils), and in smaller accumulations around the openings of the eustachian tubes.

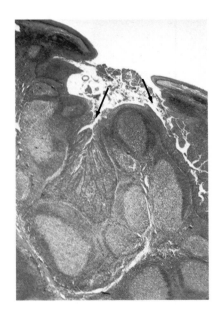

KEY

Ep, epithelium
LN, lymph nodule
LP, lamina propria
arrows, survey micrograph (above), crypt
large arrow, Fig. 1, crypt

small arrows, Fig. 2, strands of epithelial cells in nodule
rectangular area, Fig. 1, shown at higher magnification in Fig. 2

Survey micrograph, human, × 30
Fig. 1, human, × 180

Fig. 2, human, × 400 (inset, × 800)

PLATE 50

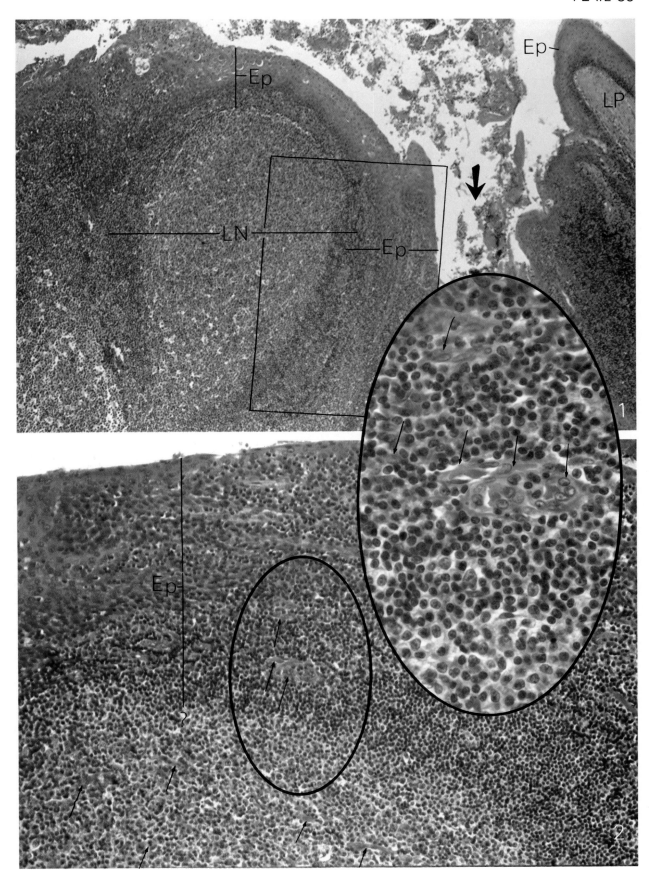

PLATE 51. Lymph Node I

Lymph nodes are small lymphatic organs that are located in the path of lymph vessels. A survey section through a lymph node is illustrated immediately to the right for orientation. The node is comprised of a mass of lymphoid tissue, arranged as a cortex **(C)** that surrounds a less dense area, the medulla **(M).** The cortex is interrupted at the hilus of the organ **(H),** where there is a recognizable concavity. It is at this site that blood vessels enter and leave the lymph node; the efferent lymphatic vessels also leave the node at this site.

An area from the cortex is shown in **Figure 1** at higher magnification. The capsule **(Cap)** is comprised of dense connective tissue from which trabeculae **(T)** penetrate into the organ to provide support. Immediately below the capsule is a sinus, the cortical or subcapsular sinus **(CS),** which receives the lymph from the afferent lymphatic vessels after they penetrate the capsule. The subcapsular sinus is continuous with the trabecular sinuses **(TS)** that course along the trabeculae.

The cortex contains the cortical or lymphatic nodules **(LN)** and a deeper component which lacks the nodules, known as the deep cortex. Whereas the lymph nodules and their lighter-staining germinal centers characterize the outer cortex, the more dense mass of lymphocytes, which impart a distinct basophilia, characterize the deep cortex. In contrast to these areas, the medulla is characterized by narrow strands of anastomosing lymphatic tissue containing numerous lymphocytes, the medullary cords **(MC),** separated by light-appearing areas, the medullary sinus **(MS).** The medullary sinuses receive lymph fluid from the trabecular sinuses as well as lymph that has filtered through the cortical tissue.

Figure 2, a higher magnification of a lymph nodule from **Figure 1,** contrasts the germinal center **(GC)** with its population of medium and large lymphocytes and the frequently observed dividing lymphocytes. (Germinal centers also contain a number of plasma cells.) The latter are shown at slightly higher magnification in the inset **(arrows),** which corresponds to the area in the **circle** in **Figure 2.** The **inset** also reveals nuclei of the reticular cells **(RC)** that form the connective tissue stroma throughout the organ. The reticular cell has a large pale-staining nucleus and is usually ovoid in shape. The cytoplasm forms long processes that surround the reticular fibers. In hematoxylin and eosin (H&E) preparations, the reticular fibers and the surrounding reticular cell cytoplasm are difficult to identify. However, the reticular cells are best seen in the sinuses where they extend across

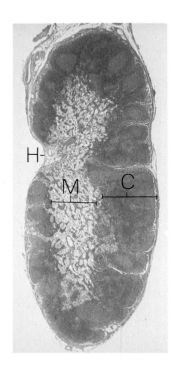

KEY	
C, cortex	MS, medullary sinus
Cap, capsule	PCV, postcapillary
CS, cortical or	venule
subcapsular sinus	RC, reticular cells
GC, germinal center	T, trabecula
H, hilus	TS, trabecular sinus
LN, lymph nodule	arrows, dividing
M, medulla	lymphocytes
MC, medullary cords	

Survey micrograph, × 14	Fig. 2, × 400 (inset, × 640)
Fig. 1, × 120	

the lymphatic space and are relatively unobscured by other cells.

A unique vessel, the postcapillary venule **(PCV),** is found in relation to the lymphatic nodules and particularly in the deep cortex. These vessels have an endothelium comprised of tall cells between which lymphocytes migrate from the vessel lumen into the parenchyma. The walls of the postcapillary venules are often infiltrated with migrating lymphocytes, sometimes making it difficult to recognize the vessel in some preparations.

PLATE 51

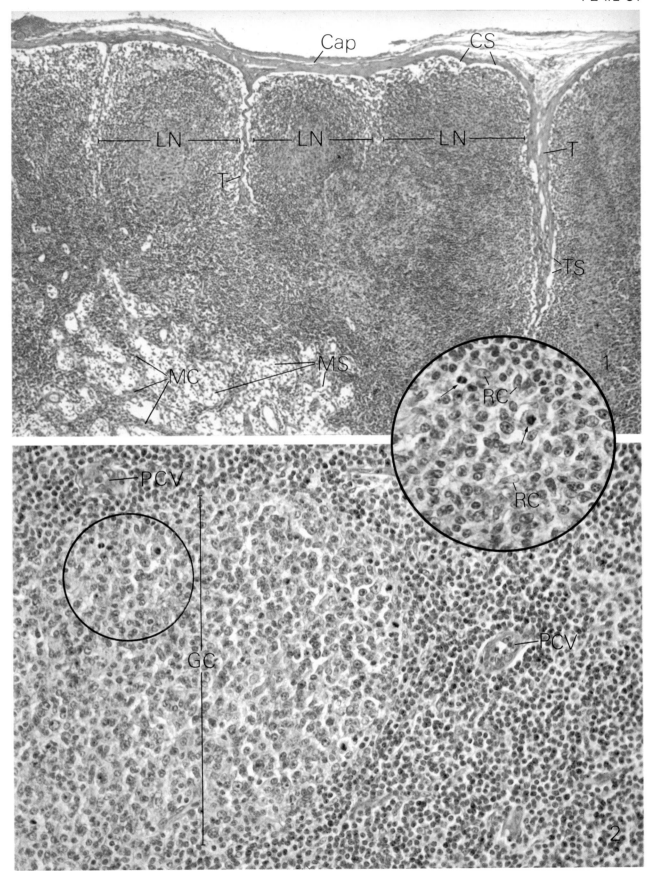

PLATE 52. Lymph Node II

The nature of the subcapsular (cortical) sinus is revealed at relatively high power in **Figure 1.** The capsule **(Cap)** is on the left, and a trabecula **(Tr)** extending into the substance of the node is seen at the bottom of the micrograph. The cortical sinus **(CS)** is bounded by endothelium that lines the undersurface of the capsule on the one side and by endothelium that covers the lymphatic parenchyma on the opposite side of the sinus. However, neither endothelial surface is clearly evident in the light microscope, particularly the endothelial layer adjoining the parenchyma. Extending across the lymphatic sinus are reticular cells **(RC)** and reticular fibers. The reticular cells and their associated fibers, though present throughout the node, are readily identified in the sinuses since here they are not obscured by large numbers of lymphocytes. The nuclei of the reticular cells are usually ovoid and pale staining. The cytoplasm extends into elongate processes that join with those of other reticular cells. The area within the **circle** is shown at high magnification in the **inset** and reveals the reticular cells with their characteristic processes **(asterisk).** Note how the cytoplasm of one cell appears to merge with its neighbor, forming a reticular configuration.

Figure 2, a silver preparation, reveals the distribution of the reticular fibers. They exhibit a blue-black color. Some are present in the capsule **(Cap)** and trabeculae **(Tr),** mixed with collagen fibers, but the majority of the reticular fibers **(RF)** can be seen, forming a network extending across the capsular sinus and into the substance of the lymphatic tissue. Associated with these fibers are the reticular cells that form a cytoplasmic sheath around the fibers. This relationship cannot be visualized in the light microscope but is readily apparent by electron microscopy (see Atlas section, Plate 54).

The sinuses of the node ultimately converge near the hilus of the node and empty into lym-

KEY	
A, artery	**Tr,** trabecula
Cap, capsule	**V,** valve
CS, cortical, or	**arrows,** openings in
subcapsular, sinus	which medullary
H, hilus	sinuses empty their
L, lymphocyte	contents into the
LN, lymph nodule	lymphatic vessel
Ly, lymphatic vessels	**asterisks,** reticular cells
M, macrophage	with their
RC, retulcar cell	characteristic
RF, reticular fiber	processes
Fig. 1, × 640 (inset, × 1,300)	**Fig. 3,** × 80
Fig. 2, silver preparation, × 500)	**Fig. 4,** × 360 (all monkey)

phatic vessels. **Figure 3** shows at low magnification the hilus **(H)** from which connective tissue penetrates into the node as an extension of the capsule. Within this connective tissue are lymphatic vessels **(Ly)** as wll as blood vessels. The lymphatic vessels leave the node at the hilus along with a vein. The artery enters the node at the same site; however, due to the nature of the section the vessels are not seen at the point where they enter and leave the hilus. **Figure 4** shows the area in the **rectangle of Figure 3** at higher magnification. Two of the vessels here represent the efferent lymphatics; both contain a valve **(V).** The upper lymphatic vessel exhibits what appears to be an incomplete wall. The openings **(arrows)** are sites in which the medullary sinuses (see area in **rectangle of Figure 3**) are emptying their contents into the lymphatic vessel. Also present are a small artery **(A)** and, at the top of the micrograph (unlabeled), a vein.

PLATE 52

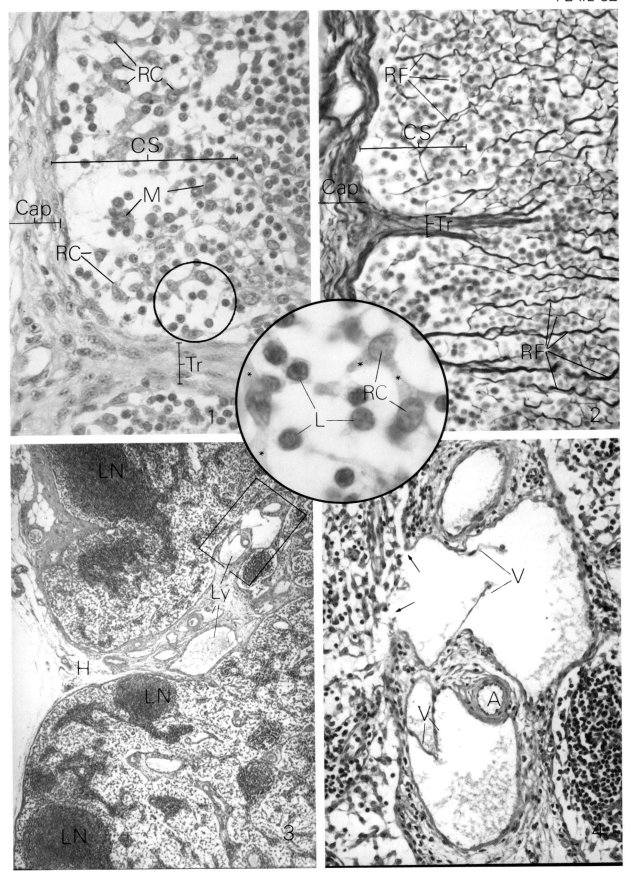

PLATE 53. Lymph Node III, Electron Miscroscopy

Some of the more significant aspects relating to the structural organization of the lymph node and its cells are evident in the accompanying electron micrograph. The region of the node shown here corresponds to the light microscopic picture in Atlas section, Plate 52, **Figure 1.**

The capsule of the lymph node is on the left side of the micrograph. It consists largely of collagen bundles **(C)** and some fibroblasts. The cortical sinus **(CS),** which lies just below the capsule, can be recognized at the electron microscopic level as a lymphatic channel. It is lined by endothelial cells **(En)** that, in effect, represent a continuation of the lining of the afferent lymphatic vessels that enter the node. The **inset** shows at higher magnification portions of two contiguous endothelial cells **(En)** immediately beneath the capsule **(Cap)** that are joined by an intercellular junction **(arrow).** The connective tissue of the capsule **(Cap)** is to the left of the endothelium and a portion of a lympocyte **(L)** within the sinus is seen on the right.

In contrast to the continuous nature of the endothelium that faces the capsule, the portion of the endothelium facing the deep surface of the sinus frequently shows discontinuities. Macrophages **(M)** located within the parenchyma of the node may abut on the sinus wall, or actually project into the sinus through these discontinuities **(curved arrows).** Here the endothelium **(En)** shows a gap and an extension of macrophage reaches the sinus in the vicinity of the gap. When interposed in this way, the macrophages can be regarded as a component of the sinus wall. However, it is not clear if these macrophages are actually fixed components of the wall or if they are more transient elements. In either case, the macrophage is in a position to monitor and phagoctytize substances within the sinus.

A second type of endothelial discontinuity is seen in the lower right of the micrograph **(arrowheads).** Here a lymphocyte is in the process of leaving the sinus and entering the parenchyma of the lymph node. The lack of contiguity of the endothelium in this instance is clearly transitory, since the endothelium is parted only during the interval that the lymphocyte is moving across the sinus wall.

In addition to the macrophages and the lymphocytes that constitute the bulk of the paren-

KEY	
C, collagen bundles	arrow, endothelial cell
Cap, capsule	junction
CS, cortical sinus	arrowheads, endothelial
En, endothelial cells	discontinuity
L, lymphocyte	curved arrow,
M, macrophage	macrophage
RC, reticular cell	extending into sinus
RF, reticular fiber	

Fig., × 4,300 (inset, × 16,000)

chyma of the node, reticular cells **(RC)** are also a conspicuous cell component when viewed at the electron microscopic level. In identifying these various cell types, the lymphocyte **(L)** is readily recognized by virtue of the dense chromatin (heterochromatin) of its nucleus and relative paucity of cytoplasm. On the other hand, the nuclei of both the macrophage and reticular cell display mostly diffuse chromatin and only a small amount of chromatin is in the condensed form. It is this feature that accounts for the relatively pale staining of reticular cells and macrophage nuclei as seen in the light microscope. In the electron micrograph, the reticular cell is distinguished from the macrophage by its relative lack of lysosomal granules. With the light microscope, it is difficult to distinguish macrophages from reticular cells of the parenchyma. However, the macrophages can be identified if their cytoplasm contains recognizable phagocytosed substances. An additional feature serves to aid in the identification of these cells in the light microscope, namely, macrophages are rarely seen in the cortical sinus. Thus, those cells in the sinus that exhibit lightly stained nuclei can be regarded as reticular cells, particularly if they also exhibit recognizable cytoplasmic processes.

The area within the **rectangle** in the upper right of the macrograph is shown in the next plate at higher magnification.

PLATE 53

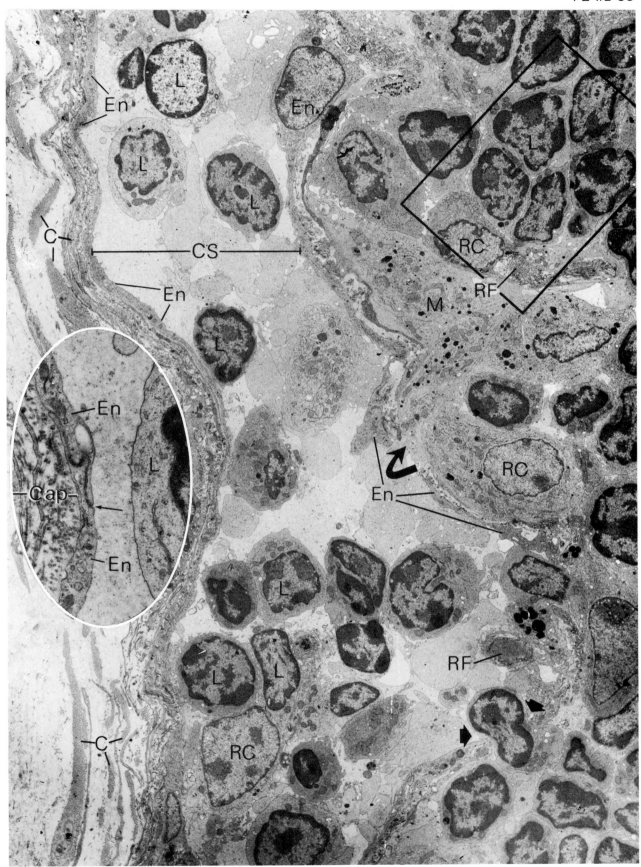

PLATE 54. Lymph Node IV, Electron Microscopy

The electron micrograph shown here illustrates the character of lymphocytes and reticular cells, and their relationship to the reticular fibers.

Lymphocytes **(L)** possess large numbers of ribosomes distributed throughout the cytoplasmic matrix that give the cytoplasm a stippled appearance. The Golgi area **(GA)** is relatively small and consequently inconspicuous. Mitochondria **(M),** though not numerous in terms of absolute numbers, occupy a relatively substantial portion of the available cytoplasmic volume. Profiles of rough-surfaced endoplasmic reticulum are rare; also, occasional granules are present. In paraffin sections prepared for the light microscope, the cytoplasm of the lymphocyte is inconspicuous, often appearing as nothing more than a light halo around a deeply stained nucleus. However, in blood smears where the cell is flattened, the cytoplasm is more evident. In such preparations, the cytoplasm is stained pale blue due to the ribosomes.

As already mentioned, the reticular cell can be distinguished from the lymphocyte by the relatively small amount of condensed chromatin in the nucleus. Thus, it is less deeply stained than the lymphocyte nucleus. The cytoplasm of the reticular cell **(RC)** resembles that of the fibroblast in that it contains moderate numbers of mitochondria **(M),** a relatively extensive Golgi apparatus **(GA),** and profiles of rough-surfaced endoplasmic reticulum. The most distinctive and unique feature of the reticular cell is its relationship to the reticular fibers. Unlike the fibroblast, the reticular cell virtu-

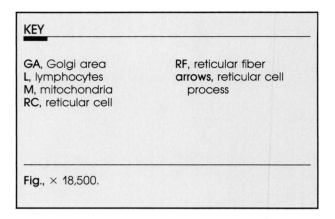

KEY

GA, Golgi area
L, lymphocytes
M, mitochondria
RC, reticular cell

RF, reticular fiber
arrows, reticular cell
process

Fig., × 18,500.

ally ensheaths the fiber. Cross-sections of the reticular fibers **(RF)** show that it is surrounded by cytoplasmic extensions **(arrows)** of the reticular cell. By virtue of this ensheathing, the reticular cell cytoplasm is interposed between the reticular fiber and the lymphocytes. It should be noted that the lymphocytes are tightly packed with little intercellular space separating the cells. As seen in the illustration, collagen fibrils are conspicuously absent from the space between the lymphocytes.

The reticular fiber of the lymph node consists of a bundle of collagen fibrils imbedded in and surrounded by a variable amount of matrix. The matrix contains specific polysaccharides that accounts for the special silver staining reactions that distinguishes reticular fibers from collagen fibers.

PLATE 54

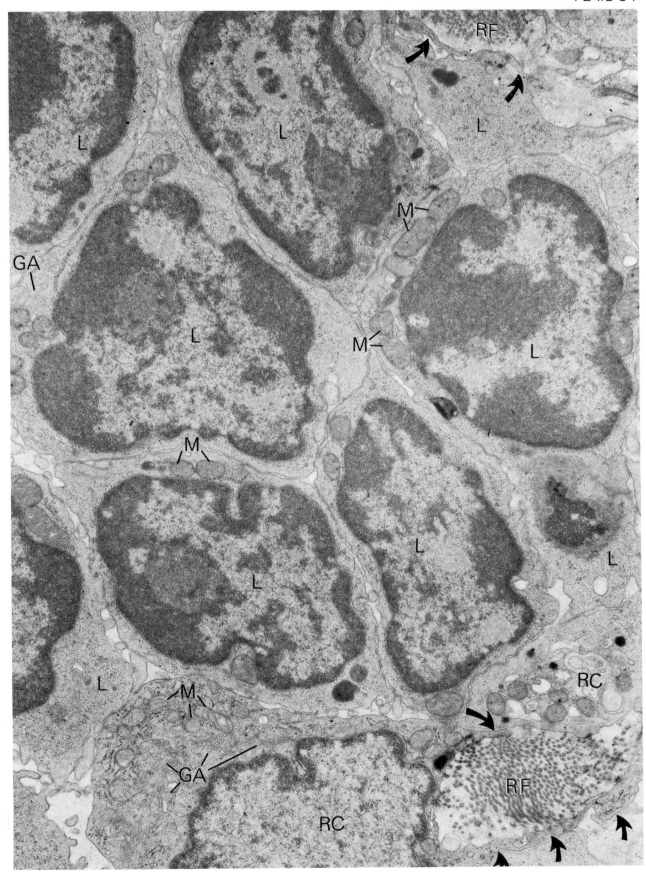

PLATE 55. Spleen I

The spleen is a lymphoid organ surrounded by a capsule and located in the path of the bloodstream (splenic artery and vein). A low-power micrograph of the spleen revealing its two major components, the red pulp (**RP**) and white pulp (**WP**), is shown in **Figure 1.** Also evident is a portion of the capsule (**Cap**) in the upper right of the figure, and in the center there is a *trabecula* containing a blood vessel, a trabecular vein (**TV**) through which blood leaves the organ. The red pulp constitutes the greater bulk of the splenic tissue. In life, the red pulp has pulp-like texture and is red due to the natural coloration of the numerous red blood cells present; hence its name, red pulp. The white pulp, on the other hand, is so named because its content of lymphocytes appears in life as whitish areas. In tissue sections, however, the nuclei of the closely packed lymphocytes impart an overall blue staining response. The lymphatic tissue that comprises the white pulp (**WP**) differs from nodules seen elsewhere in that it follows and ensheaths a blood vessel, the central artery. The lymphatic tissue surrounding the artery exhibits periodic expansions, thus forming the nodules. When this occurs, the central artery (**CA**) is displaced peripherally within the nodule (**Fig. 1**). In those regions where the lymphatic tissue is not in nodular form, it is present as a thin cuff around the central artery and is referred to as the periarterial lymphatic sheath (**PALS**). If the plane of section does not include the artery, the sheath may appear as a localized and irregular aggregation of lymphocytes (**asterisks**).

Figure 2 reveals at a higher magnification the red pulp and a portion of the trabecular vein from the area enclosed in the uppermost rectangle in **Figure 1.** The red pulp is comprised of two elements: venous sinuses (**VS**) and the splenic cords of Billroth, the tissue which lies between the sinuses. In this specimen, the venous sinuses can be seen to advantage because the red blood cells in the sinuses have lysed and appear as unstained "ghosts"; only the nuclei of the white cells are readily apparent. (This is seen better in Atlas section, Plate 56.) The paler unstained areas thus represent the sinus lumens.

Near the top of the micrograph, two venous sinuses empty into the trabecular vein (**arrows**),

thus, showing the continuity between venous sinuses and the trabecular veins. The wall of the vein is thin, but the trabeculum (**T**) containing the vessel gives the appearance of being part of the vessel wall. In man, as well as other mammals, the capsule and the trabeculae that extend from the capsule contain myofibroblasts. Under conditions of increasing physical stress, contraction of these cells will occur and cause rapid expulsion of blood from the venous sinuses into the trabecular veins and thus into the general circulation.

Figure 3 reveals at higher magnification the splenic nodule in the rectangle in the left portion of **Figure 1.** Present is a germinal center (**GC**) and a cross-section through the thick-walled central artery. As already noted, the central artery is eccentrically placed in the nodule. The marginal zone (**MZ**) is the area that separates white and red pulp. Small arterial vessels and capillaries, branches of the central artery, supply the white pulp and some pass into the reticular network of the marginal zone terminating there in a funnel-shaped orifice. Venous sinuses are also found in the marginal zone and, occasionally, arterial vessels may open into the sinuses. The details of the vascular supply are, at best, difficult to resolve in typical H&E preparations. The penicillar arteries, the terminal branches of the central artery, supply the red pulp, but likewise are difficult to resolve.

PLATE 55

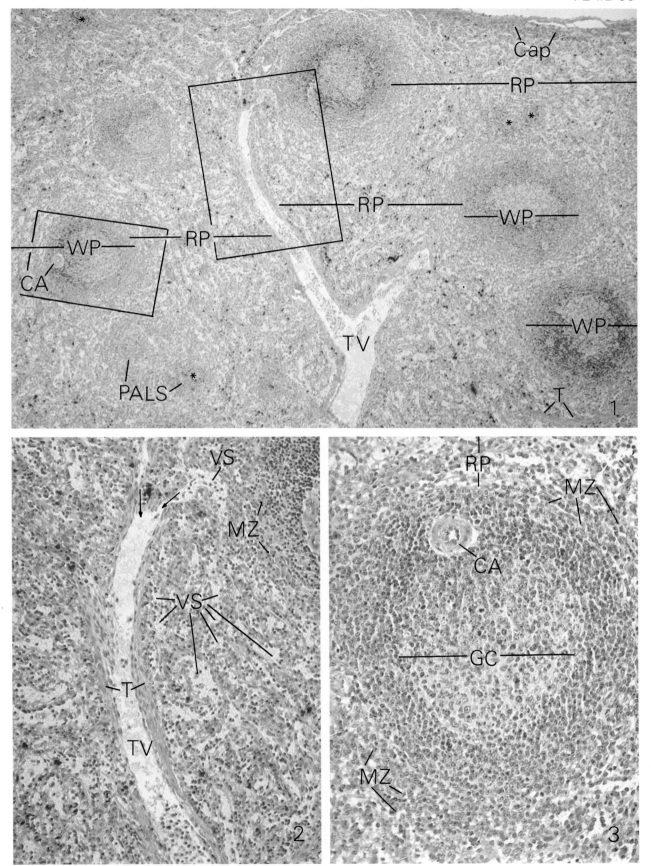

PLATE 56. Spleen II

The red pulp, as noted and described in the previous plate, is comprised of two components; venous sinuses, and the splenic cords of Billroth (**Fig. 1**). The venous sinuses (**VS**) can be recognized by their circumscribing endothelial wall. The red cells within the lumen of the vessels are apparent only by virtue of the their outline, the contents of the cells having been lost during preparation of the tissue, leaving only a ghost image. The cords are filled with a variety of cell types, among which are numerous lysed red blood cells. These red cells have left the vascular channels—that is, they are extravascular. Macrophages can be identified in this specimen by the pigment that they have sequestered (**arrows**), the breakdown product of old red blood cells.

Figure 2 reveals at higher magnification one of the venous sinuses and the surrounding Billroth's cord (**BC**) from the preceding figure. The wall of the sinus consists of elongated rod-like endothelial cells which are oriented parallel to each other in the long axis of the sinus. A narrow but clearly visible intercellular space is usually present between adjacent cells. (The space seen in light microscopic preparations is an exaggeration due to shrinkage during routine preparation.) When a venous sinus is cut in cross-section, as in **Figure 1**, the rod-shaped endotheilia lining cells are also cut in cross-section, and the cut edges of the adjoining cells are seen in the form of a ring. The narrow intercellular spaces then appear as slits between the cross-sectioned cells. Occasionally, the wall of a sinus is tangentially sectioned and the cytoplasm of the endothelial cells appears as a series of narrow stripes, as can be seen in the lower left of **Figure 1** (**asterisks**). Each linear component here is a single endothelial cell.

The endothelial cell nuclei (**En**) are located within the cell in a manner that they project into the sinus lumen. In effect, the nuclei form a bleb-like structure that then appears to sit within the lumen of the vessel. Unless carefully examined, they may give the impression that they are nuclei of white blood cells. This is especially true if the white bloods cells (**WBC**) within the lumen of the sinus are numerous.

The framework of the spleen consists of a capsule, trabeculae that extend from the capsule into the substance of the spleen, and a reticular stroma. The reticular stroma is illustrated in **Figure 3**, a silver preparation. In the white pulp, the germinal centers (**GC**) can be recognized by the circular ar-

rangement and, to some degree, the paucity of the blackened reticular fibers. The central arteries (**CA**) are surrounded by a relative abundance of reticular fibers—hence, the dense outline of these vessels. The arrangement of the fibers in the red pulp are more variable in appearance. A special arrangement of blackened fibers is seen in relation to the venous sinus (**VS**) of the red pulp. These fibers often appear as an organized lattice that circumscribe the vessel. The inset in **Figure 3** is a higher magnification of the area immediately above the inset. One of the vessels seen in the inset has been sectioned tangentially along its wall and the circumscribing fibers can be seen lying parallel to one another like the rungs of a ladder (**arrows**). The vessel above and in very close proximity (with the label **VS** in its lumen) has also been longitudinally sectioned, but the section passes deeper into the vessel; thus, the cut ends of the fibers are seen in cross-sectional profile (**arrowheads**) and give the appearance of a series of dots outlining the wall of the vessel. These fibers are actually comprised of basal lamina material. The basal lamina is thus not a thin sheath in this instance, but rather it forms a cord-like structure that facilates the passage of cells across the endothelium. The true reticular fibers (comprised of collagen fibrils) are darker staining and thicker. They can be seen between the closely apposed vessels.

KEY

BC, Billroth's cord (splenic cord)
CA, central artery
En, endothelial cell nucleus
arrows, Fig. 1, pigment (contained in macrophages)
arrows, Fig. 3 (inset), silver positive fibers (basal lamina material) circumscribing the venous sinus endothelium

GC, germinal center
VS, venous sinus
WBC, white blood cells

arrowheads, Fig. 3 (inset), above type fibers as seen in cross-sectional profile
asterisks, Fig. 1, wall of venous sinus seen in tangential section

---

Fig. 1, human, × 360
Fig. 2, human, × 1200

Fig. 3, human, × 120
(inset, human, × 300)

PLATE 56

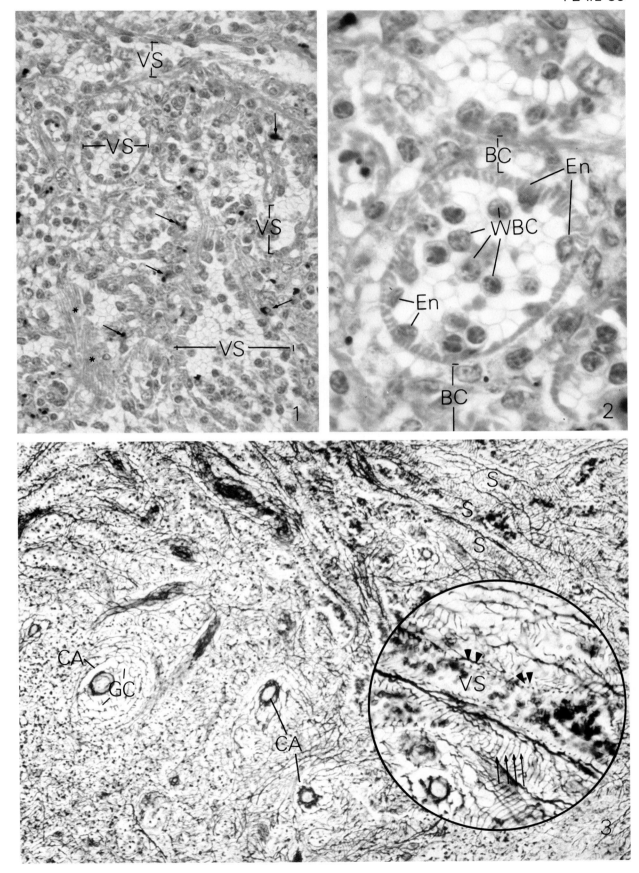

PLATE 57. Thymus

The thymus is a lymphoid organ that exhibits certain unique structural features. The supporting reticular stroma of the thymus arises from entodermal epithelium and produces a cellular reticulum. There are no reticular fibers associated with these cells; instead the cells, designated epithelioreticular cells, serve as the stroma. Lymphocytes come to lie within the interstices of the cellular reticulum, and these two cellular elements, the lymphocytes and the epithelial reticular cells, comprise the bulk of the organ. The lymphocytes migrate into the entodermal rudiment during embryonic development from the yolk sac and later from the red bone marrow. Upon entering the thymus, the lymphocytes proliferate. Some of these new lymphocytes migrate to other tissues; many of them also die in the thymus.

A connective tissue capsule (Cap) surrounds each lobe of the thymus (there are two lobes) and sends trabeculae (T) into the substance of the gland to form lobules. The lobules (L) are not completely separate units, but, rather, they interconnect owing to the discontinuous nature of the trabeculae.

Examination of the thymus at low magnification, as in **Figure 1,** reveals the lobules to be comprised of a dark-staining basophilic cortex (C) and a lighter-staining and relatively eosinophilic medulla (M). The cortex contains numerous densely packed lymphocytes, whereas the medulla contains fewer lymphocytes and is consequently less densely packed. It is the relative difference in the lymphocyte population (per unit area), and particularly the staining of their nuclei with hematoxylin, that creates the difference in appearance between cortex and medulla (Fig. 2). Note that some of the medullary areas bear a resemblance to germinal centers of other lymphoid organs because of the medulla appearing as isolated circular areas (upper left of Fig. 1). The medullary component, however, is actually a continuous branching mass surrounded by cortical tissue. Thus the "isolated" medullary profiles are in reality united with one another, though not within the plane of section. A suggestion of such continuity can be seen on the **right** in **Figure 1,** where the medulla appears to extend across several lobules.

The main cellular constituents of the thymus are (1) lymphocytes (thymocytes), with characteris-

tic small, round, dark-staining nuclei and (2) epithelial reticular supporting cells, with large, pale-staining nuclei. Both of the cell types can be distinguished in **Figure 3,** which provides a high-power view of the medulla. Because of the lesser number of lymphocytes in the medulla, it is the area of choice to examine the epithelial reticular cells. The thymus also contains macrophages, however, they are difficult to distinguish from the epithelial reticular cells.

The medulla usually possess varying numbers of circular bodies called Hassall's or thymic corpuscles (HC in Fig. 3). The corpuscles are large concentric layers of flattened epithelial reticular cells. They stain readily with eosin and can be distinguished easily with low power, as in **Figures 1 and 2 (arrows).** The center of the corpuscle, particularly the large ones, may show evidence of keratininzation, and appear somewhat amorphous.

The thymus gland remains as a large structure until the time of puberty. At this time, regressive changes occur that result in a significant reduction in the amount of thymic tissue. The young thymus is highly cellular and contains a minimum of adipose tissue (AT). On the other hand, in the older thymus much adipose tissue is present between the lobules, and with continued involution, adipose cells are found even within the thymic tissue itself. Also, occasional plasma cells may be present in the periphery of the thymic cortex of the involuting thymus gland.

PLATE 57

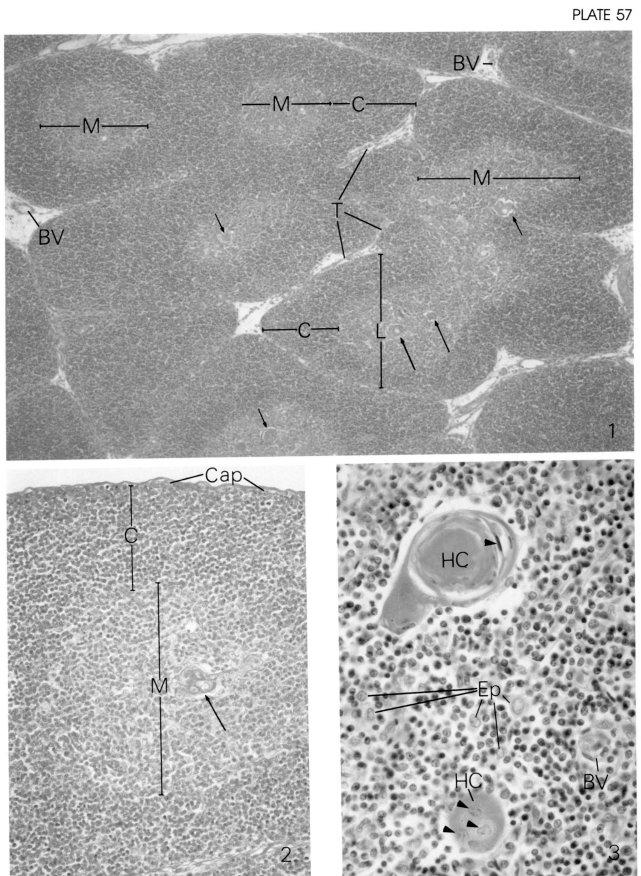

The Integumentary System

14

The **skin (integument, cutis)** and its derivatives constitute the integumentary system. The skin forms the external covering of the body. It consists of two main layers: the **epidermis,** composed of stratified squamous epithelium, and the **dermis,** composed of connective tissue. Under the dermis there is another layer of connective tissue, looser than that of the dermis, called the **hypodermis** (or, using a gross anatomical term, **superficial fascia**). It contains a variable amount of adipose tissue and, in the well-nourished individual, the thickness of the adipose tissue may be considerable. Associated with the skin are **epidermal derivatives** or **appendages,** namely, the **sudoriferous (sweat) glands, hairs, sebaceous glands,** and **nails.**

The integumentary system performs a number of functions related to its location on the surface of the body. It provides protection against physical, chemical, and biological injury; it prevents water loss; it serves as a large receptor for general sensation (pain, pressure, touch, temperature); it protects against ultraviolet radiation; it converts precursor molecules into vitamin D; it functions in heat regulation; and it excretes certain substances through the sweat glands. In addition, certain lipid-soluble substances are absorbed through the skin. This property, while not necessarily a "function" in the sense of having biological purpose, is taken advantage of in the administration of certain lipid-soluble therapeutic agents to the skin.

STRUCTURE OF THICK AND THIN SKIN

The character of the skin differs over most of the body surface. Although these differences are simply a question of degree, there are two locations where the skin is obviously different at both the gross and histological level. These are on the palms of the hands and soles of the feet. Here, there are no hairs. In addition, the epidermis in these two locations is much thicker than elsewhere and, consequently, this hairless skin is also called **thick skin.** Elsewhere, the epidermis is thinner and this skin is called **thin skin;** it contains hairs except in certain locations. One should recognize that the terms thin and thick skin as used in histology are, in part, misnomers. They refer only to the epidermis. Anatomically, the thickest skin in the body is found in the back, particularly the upper portion. This is due principally to the very thick dermis that is thought to have a protective function. The thickness of the epidermis of the back is, however, not remarkable and is comparable to that of thin skin found elsewhere in the body.

Epidermis

The epidermis is a layer of stratified squamous epithelium (Figs. 14.1 and 14.2). In thick skin, five layers can be discerned in the epidermis. Beginning with the deepest part of the epidermis and moving toward the surface, these are the **stratum basale,** the **stratum spinosum,** the **stratum granulosum,** the **stratum lucidum,** and the **stratum corneum.** The stratum lucidum is not present in thin skin.

The stratum basale is adjacent to the basal lamina. It is also called the **stratum germinativum** because it contains dividing cells. The newly produced cells move toward the surface to replace those that have sloughed off.

The stratum spinosum is several cells deep. Cells in this layer have spinous processes on their surfaces that meet similar spinous processes of neighboring cells. At the apices of the adjoining spines, the cells make contact by means of desmosomes. With the light microscope, the desmosome

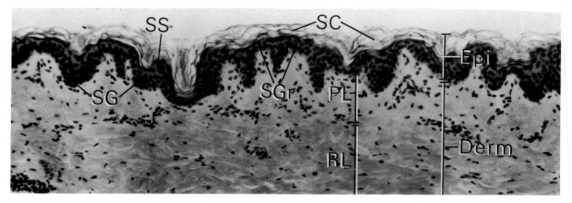

Figure 14.1. Light micrograph showing the layers of thin human skin, the two chief layers of which are epidermis (Epi) and dermis (Derm). The epidermis forms the surface; it consists of stratified squamous epithelium that is keratinized. The layers of the epidermis are identified on the basis of location as well as histological properties. Thus, the deepest layer of cells, adjacent to the dermis, is the stratum germinativum (SG), also called the stratum basale. Adjacent to this is a layer, several cells thick, designated as the stratum spinosum (SS). The most superficial layer of nucleated cells is the stratum granulosum (SGr), so designated because of its content of conspicuous cytoplasmic granules, keratohyaline granules, which stain with hematoxylin and give this layer a darker appearance than other layers of the epidermis. The superficial layer of the epidermis is the stratum corneum (SC). It consists of very flat keratinized cells that no longer possess a nucleus. The dermis consists of two layers: the papillary layer (PL), adjacent to the epidermis, and the reticular layer (RL), more deeply positioned. The boundary between these two layers is not conspicuous; however, it should be noted that the papillary layer is more cellular than the reticular layer. In addition, the collagen fibers of the reticular layer are thick; those of the papillary layer are thin. × 120.

appears as a slight thickening called a ***node of Bizzozzaro.*** In the early days of histology, it was thought that the two facing spinous processes actually formed an intercellular bridge and that the node of Bizzozzaro was simply a widened region of the bridge. The electron microscope has shown this to be an incorrect interpretation. They are not intercellular bridges, but rather, desmosomes.

The continuous production of new cells in the stratum basale pushes the overlying cells in the stratum spinosum toward the stratum granulosum. During this movement, the cells become flattened in a plane parallel to the surface of the skin.

The stratum granulosum is distinguished because the cells in this layer contain numerous granules, called ***keratohyaline granules,*** which stain with hematoxylin.

The stratum lucidum, which is considered to be a subdivision of the stratum corneum by some histologists, is a thin layer containing highly refractile eosinophilic cells in which the process of keratinization is well advanced. The nucleus and many of the cytoplasmic organelles become disrupted and disappear as the cell becomes filled with the intracellular protein keratin. The stratum lucidum is evident only in thick skin.

The stratum corneum is the surface layer. Cells in this layer no longer possess a nucleus or other organelles. The plasma membrane is thickened and coated on its outer surface, at least in its deepest layers, by glycolipid; the interior of the cells is filled with keratin. The stratum corneum varies considerably in thickness, being greatest in thick skin and increasing in thickness when continually exposed to friction. It is chiefly the thickness of the stratum corneum that accounts for the difference in thickness between the epidermis of thick and thin skin.

Dermis

The junction between the dermis and epidermis presents an extremely uneven boundary when observed with the light microscope. Sections of skin cut perpendicular to the surface reveal numerous finger-like connective tissue protrusions called ***dermal papillae.*** These papillae project into the undersurface of the overlying epidermis (Figs. 14.1 and 14.2). They are complemented by what appear to be a series of similar epidermal projections or evaginations, called ***epidermal ridges*** or ***rete ridges,*** which project into the dermis. However, in sections cut in a plane parallel to the surface of the skin and through the dermal papillae, the epidermal ridges fail to exhibit profiles indicative of finger-like projections. Rather, the epider-

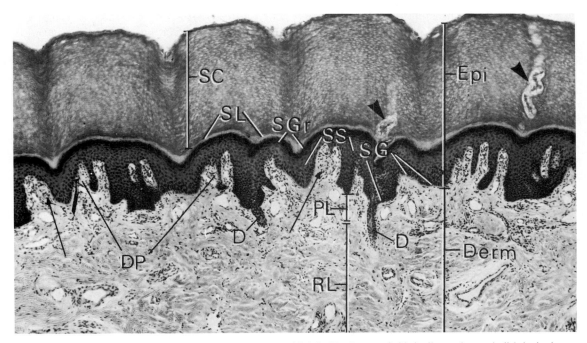

Figure 14.2. Light micrograph showing the layers of thick skin (human). Note the extremely thick stratum corneum (SC), and under this a thin pale layer, the stratum lucidum (SL). Other layers of the epidermis (Epi) are similar to those of thin skin, namely the stratum basale or germinativum (SG), the stratum spinosum (SS), and the stratum granulosum (SGr). In two locations marked by **arrowheads**, ducts of sweat glands can be seen as they spiral through the epidermis. Only a portion of each duct has been included in the plane of section. The dermis (Derm) contains papillae (DP) that are more pronounced than those of the thin skin. In several locations, **arrows** point to Meissner's corpuscles. These are sensory receptors and appear as oval bodies within the dermal papillae (DP). Again notice the greater cellularity of the papillary layer (PL) and the fact that collagen fibers of the reticular layer (RL) are thicker than those of the papillary layer. In two locations, portions of ducts (D) of sweat glands are seen where they enter the epidermis. At the sites where the ducts of the sweat gland enter the epidermis are epidermal down growths known as **interpapillary pegs**. × 65.

mal tissue, as seen in this plane, appears as a continuous sheet of epithelium, containing within it circular islands of connective tissue. These islands represent cross-sections of the true finger-like dermal papillae as they project into the epidermis. At sites where there is increased mechanical stress, the epidermal ridges, or rete ridges, are much deeper (the epithelium simply being thicker), and the connective tissue papillae are longer. Thus, the dermal papillae create a more extensive interface between dermis and epidermis.

In thick skin, dermal ridges are present in addition to the dermal papillae. The dermal ridges are true ridges. In effect, they are linear elevations of the connective tissue that protrude into the undersurface of the epidermis. The ridges tend to have a parallel arrangement with the dermal papillae occurring between them. These ridges form a distinctive pattern that is unique for each individual; on the surface of the skin, they are reflected as the familiar "fingerprint" and other linear patterns.

To strengthen the attachment of the epidermis to the underlying connective tissue, the basal cells of the epidermis exhibit several special features that are evident at the electron microscope level. First, the basal cell exhibits a pattern of irregular cytoplasmic protrusions. This increases the attachment surface between the cell and its subjacent basal lamina. Second, a series of attachment sites, namely, *hemidesmosomes,* are present along the basal plasma membrane of the basal cell. The hemidesmosome is structurally identical to the desmosome except that there is no adjacent cell with a complementary device; hence, the name *hemidesmosome.* The hemidesmosomes instead seem to attach to the basal lamina by means of very fine *anchoring filaments* that extend from the inner leaflet of the plasma membrane at the site of hemidesmosomes to the basal lamina, thus, further enhancing the attachment of the epidermal cells to the basal lamina. Beneath the basal lamina are numerous fibrils, referred to as *anchoring fibrils,* that are found concentrated mostly in the areas beneath the hemidesmosomes. They extend from the substance of the basal lamina into the dermis where, presumably, they enhance the attachment of the basal lamina to the connective tissue.

In examining the full thickness of the dermis at the light microscopic level, one can recognize a division into two structurally distinct layers, the **papillary layer** and the **reticular layer.** The papillary layer consists of loose connective tissue. It is located immediately under the epidermis and is separated from it by the basal lamina. The papillary layer is a relatively thin layer extending into (and, thus, also constituting) the dermal papillae and ridges. It contains blood vessels that serve, but do not enter, the epidermis. It also contains nerve processes, some of which terminate in the dermis and some of which penetrate the basal lamina to enter the epithelial compartment. The reticular layer is deep to the papillary layer and consists of dense connective tissue. It is considerably thicker

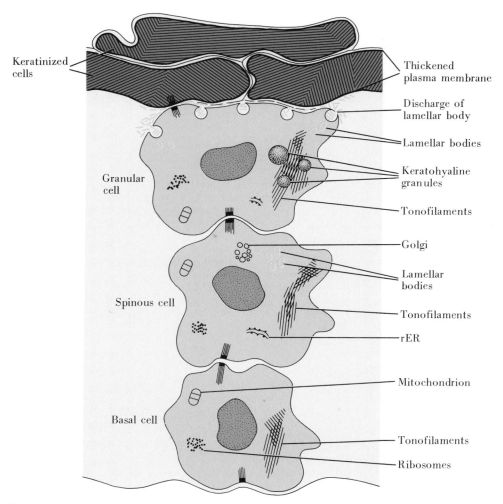

Figure 14.3. Schematic diagram of keratinocytes of epidermis. The keratinocytes in this figure reflect different stages of the life of the cell as it passes from the basal layer through the spinous and granular layers to the surface keratinized layer. The basal cell begins the synthesis of tonofilaments; these are grouped into bundles and seen with the light microscope as tonofibrils. The basal cell contains free ribosomes active in the synthesis of tonofilaments. The cell enters the spinous layer where the synthesis of tonofilaments continues. Also in the upper part of the spinous layer, the cells begin the production of keratohyaline granules and glycolipid containing lamellar bodies. Within the granular layer, lamellar bodies are discharged by the cell; the remainder of the cell cytoplasm contains numerous keratohyaline granules in close association with tonofilaments. The surface cells are keratinized; they contain a thickened plasma membrane and bundles of tonofilaments in a specialized matrix. (From Matoltsy AG, Parrakal PF: In Zelickson AS (ed): *Ultrastructure of Normal and Abnormal Skin.* Philadelphia, Lea & Febiger, 1967.)

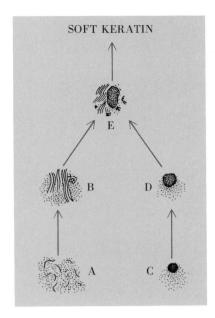

SOFT KERATIN

Figure 14.4. Outline of steps leading to the formation of soft keratin as seen with an electron microscope. Tonofilaments are produced by activity of ribosomes. **(A).** The tonofilaments then group as bundles **(B)**, which are visible with the light microscope as tonofibrils. Somewhat later, keratohyaline granules are also produced by ribosomes **(C)** and **(D)**; at this time the keratohyaline granules are surrounded by a rim of ribosomes. Finally, the tonofilaments (tonofibrils) react with the keratohyaline granules **(E)**, which provide a matrix for the fibrils. (From Reith EJ, Rhodin JG: *Fundamentals of Keratinization.* New York, McGraw-Hill, 1962.)

than the papillary layer and, as already mentioned, varies in thickness in different parts of the body. Histologically, the reticular layer can be identified as the layer of dermis that contains thicker collagen fibers and fewer cells than the loose connective tissue of the papillary layer.

Eccrine sweat glands, hair follicles, and associated sebaceous glands develop as downgrowths of the epidermis. The sweat glands and hair follicles extend from the epidermis through the dermis and, usually, into the underlying subcutaneous tissue. The secretory portion of the sweat gland and the deepest part of the hair follicle are usually located in the subcutaneous tissue. The sebaceous glands empty into the upper third of the hair follicle and are located in the dermis.

CELLS OF THE EPIDERMIS

There are four cell types in the epidermis: the *keratinocyte,* the *melanocyte,* the *Langerhans cell,* and the *Merkel cell.*

Keratinocytes

The keratinocytes are the most numerous cells in the epidermis. They are the cells that become keratinized (Fig. 14.3) and that synthesize the water barrier. In the stratum basale, the keratinocyte contains rough endoplasmic reticulum (rER), mitochondria, a small Golgi apparatus, numerous free ribosomes, and 10-nm intermediate filaments called *tonofilaments.* The cytoplasm displays basophilia when viewed with the light microscope due to the presence of numerous free ribosomes.

As the cells enter and move through the stratum spinosum, the synthesis of tonofilaments continues and the filaments become grouped into bundles sufficiently thick to be visualized with the light microscope. These bundles are called *tonofibrils.* The cytoplasm becomes eosinophilic due to the staining reaction of the tonofibrils that fill more and more of the ctyoplasm.

In the upper reaches of the stratum spinosum, the keratinocyte begins the synthesis of *keratohyaline granules* and *lamellar bodies.* The keratohyaline granules are synthesized by free ribosomes and, during their formation, small keratohyaline granules are surrounded by ribosomes (Fig. 14.4). As their synthesis continues, they fill much of the cell. Those cells that have accumulated large numbers of keratohyaline granules constitute the layer called the stratum granulosum. The keratohyaline granules contain a substance that combines with the tonofibrils converting them into keratin.[1] The actual keratinization process is relatively rapid; it occurs between the time the cell leaves the stratum granulosum and enters the stratum corneum. The transformation of the cell from the stratum granulosum into a keratinized cell also involves the breakdown of the nucleus and other organelles and the thickening of the plasma membrane. Finally, now in the stratum corneum, there is a timed desquamation of the surface keratinized cells. This process occurs in those cells of the stratum corneum that have accumulated acid phosphatase.

---

[1] The keratin of the surface epidermal cells is called *soft keratin* in contrast to the *hard keratin* of hair and nails.

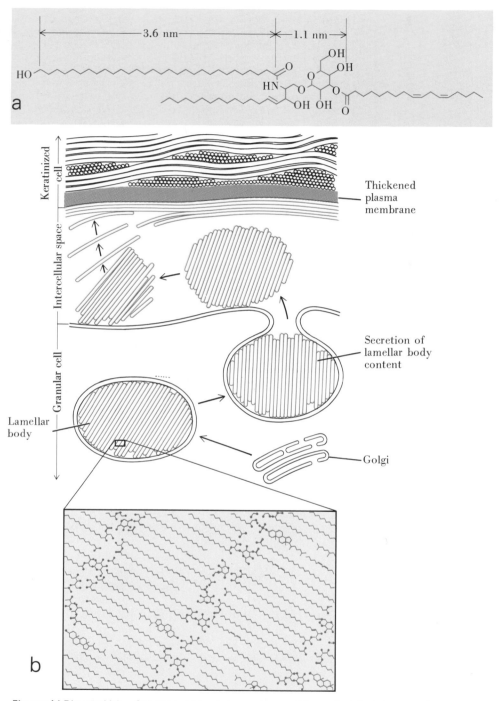

Figure 14.5(a and b). Scheme of acylglucosylceramide molecule **(a)** present in lamellar bodies. This molecule along with other lipid molecules make up the lamellae of the lamellar bodies **(b)**. The lamellar bodies, produced by an intracellular pathway involving the Golgi, are finally discharged by the cell, where they function in the intercellular space as a water barrier. The lamellar arrangement of lipid molecules is depicted in the intercellular space just below the thickened plasma membrane of the keratinized cell. Filaments of the keratinized cell are shown in both longitudinal and cross-section. (Based on Wertz P, Dowling D: *Science* 217:1262, 1983.)

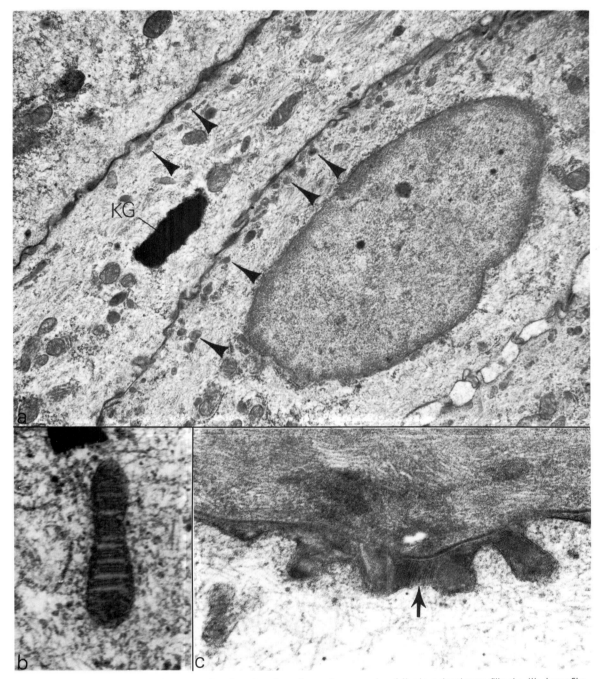

Figure 14.6(a). Electron micrographs showing keratinocytes, much of their cytoplasm filled with tonofilaments. One cell exhibits a keratohyaline granule (KG). Near the plasma membrane closest to the surface (upper left), two of the cells display lamellar bodies **(arrowheads). (b)** A lamellar body at higher magnification; **(c)** Part of a keratinized cell and the underlying keratinocyte. Between the cells is the lamellar material from the lamellar bodies that has been discharged into the intercellular space **(arrow).** (Courtesy of Dr. A. I. Farbman, 1984.)

This hydrolytic enzyme is thought to participate in the exfoliation of these keratinized cells.

At the same time that the keratinocytes produce keratin, they also produce a glycolipid that functions as a water barrier (Fig. 14.5). The glycolipid is packaged within the cell as membrane-bound *lamellar bodies* (or membrane-coating granules, MCG). The lamellar bodies are produced by an intracellular pathway involving the Golgi apparatus and then are discharged into the intercellular space by the cells of the stratum granulosum (Fig. 14.6). The glycolipid spreads to fill the intercellular space, forming a barrier to water. The significance of this water barrier can be illustrated by noting that a major life-threatening factor in severe burns is the loss of body fluid. The intercellular space of epidermal cells below the level of the water barrier contains extracellular fluid that is in equilibrium with the interstitial fluid on the connective tissue side of the basal lamina and this interstitial fluid of the connective tissue, in turn, is in equilibrium with the plasma of the blood. Thus, loss of fluid from the skin due to absence of the water barrier ultimately reflects itself as a generalized fluid loss from the body.

Melanocytes

The color of an individual's skin is due to a number of factors including the presence of oxy-hemoglobin in the dermal vascular bed, which imparts a red hue. The color of the skin is further modified by the presence of carotenes, an exogenous pigment taken up from foods and concentrated in tissues containing fat. Certain minerals taken into the body through absorption or by digestion can also lead to pigmentation of the skin (for example, tatoo marks are made of inorganic pigments that are driven into the skin with needles and are ingested by macrophages). Endogenous pigments such as the degradation products of hemoglobin: iron-containing hemosiderin and iron-free bilirubin can impart color to the skin. Hemosiderin is a golden brown pigment; bilirubin is yellowish brown. Bilirubin is normally removed from the bloodstream by the liver and voided by way of the bile. Exogenous pigments, such as bilirubin, may demonstrate abnormal accumulations if the liver or other involved organ fails to function normally imparting a yellow color to the skin.

Color is also due to pigment in the epidermis. The chief pigment is melanin, a product of the melanocyte. Melanocytes are rounded cells with long dendritic processes located primarily in the stratum basale (Fig. 14.7). Special staining procedures are needed for their display with the light microscope. However, with the transmission electron microscope, they can be identified readily because they contain developing and mature melanin

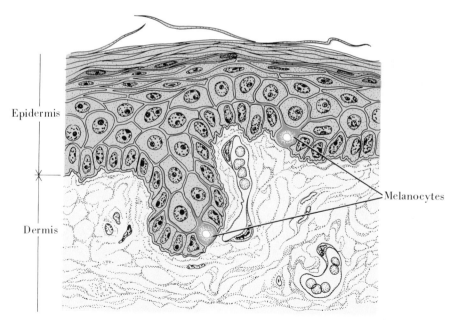

Figure 14.7. Diagram of thin skin showing two melanocytes in the stratum basale. The cells require special stains for their display. The melanocyte contains long dendritic processes that extend between other cells of the epidermis. (Based on Ham AH, Cormack DH: *Histology*, 8th ed. Philadelphia, JB Lippincott, 1979.)

granules (Fig. 14.8). The melanocytes do not establish desmosomal attachments with neighboring keratinocytes; and their numerous dendritic processes extend throughout the two lower layers of the epidermis.

The melanocytes produce melanin by a process that involves the transformation of tyrosine into 3,4-dihydroxyphenylalanine (DOPA) by the enzyme tyrosinase and the subsequent transformation of DOPA into melanin (melanosome melanization). The process of formation occurs in membrane-limited bodies called *melanosomes,* which are derived from the Golgi apparatus (Fig. 14.9). Mature melanosomes are transferred to keratinocytes by passing through the dendritic processes. This type of cell-to-cell transfer has been called *cytocrine secretion.* In Caucasians, the melanin is degraded by lysosomal activity of the keratinocytes. In Negroid skin, the melanosomes are more stable. Tanning of the skin after exposure to sunlight is due to the production of melanin.

In amphibians, melanin production is markedly influenced by melanocyte-stimulating hormone (MSH). Whereas the MSH has a well-defined role in lower forms, the action of this hormone in the human is not entirely understood. However, it should be noted that increased pigmentation of the skin in the human does occur in certain hormone

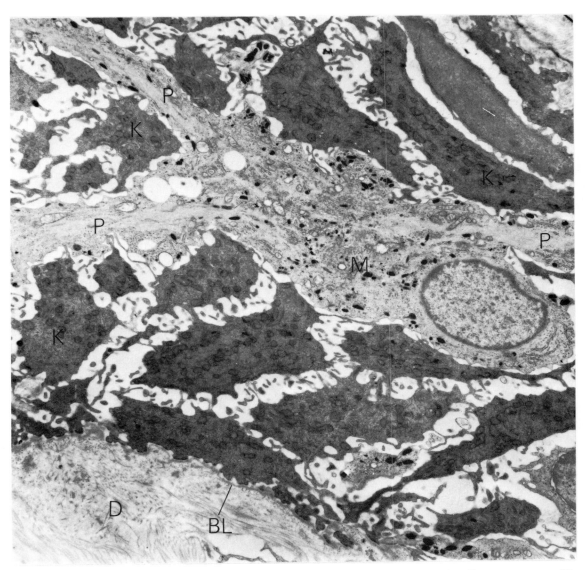

Figure 14.8. Electron micrograph of a melanocyte (M) showing melanin granules. Three processes (P) can be seen extending between the neighboring keratinocytes (K). The basal lamina (BL) marks the boundary between the epithelium and the dermis (D). × 5,800. (Courtesy of Dr. B. Munger, 1984.)

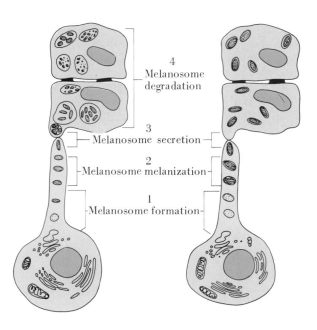

Figure 14.9. Formation of melanin pigment and secretion of pigment granules into keratinocytes. Melanocytes produce melanin within membrane-limited bodies called melanosomes **(1, 2)**. Secretion of melanosomes consists of their passage into neighboring keratinocytes **(3)**. In Negroid skin, the melanosomes remain discrete; in Caucasian skin, the melanosomes are degraded **(4)** through the intervention of lysosome-like organelles. (Based on Weiss L, Greep RO: *Histology,* 4th ed. New York, McGraw-Hill, 1977.)

imbalances, specifically Addison's disease. When tyrosinase activity is absent, melanin is not produced, causing a condition known as ***albinism.***

Langerhans Cell

The Langerhans cell, like the melanocyte, cannot be distinguished with certainty in routine hematoxylin and eosin (H&E)-stained paraffin sections. The nucleus stains heavily with hematoxylin and the cytoplasm is clear. With special techniques such as gold impregnation the Langerhans cell is seen to be located in the stratum spinousm and to possess dendrite processes, thereby resembling the stellate melanocyte. However, with the electron microscope, several distinctive features of the Langerhans cell are evident (Fig. 14.10). Its nucleus is characteristically indented in many places so that the nuclear profile is very uneven; it does not form desmosomes with neighboring keratinocytes; and it possesses characteristic granules that appear as rods, some of which may exhibit a bul-

bous expansion along their length. A striated band is present at the center of the rod.

The Langerhans cell was formerly thought to be related to the melanocyte, but it is now known that it plays an important role in the immune response as it is involved in the presentation of antigens to T-cells. As an antigen-presenting cell, the Langerhans cell is involved in the initiation of cutaneous contact hypersensitivity reactions (i.e., contact allergic dermatitis). The Langerhans cell most likely is derived from mesenchyme and has been added to the list of cells that constitutes the mononuclear phagocytic system.

Merkel Cell

The Merkel cell is a modified epidermal cell located in the stratum basale. It makes contact with neighboring epidermal cells by means of desmosomes. It contains numerous small, dense granules considered to be related to the catecholamine-containing granules of neural tissue (Fig. 14.11). The base of the Merkel cell is in contact with the expanded terminal disc of a nerve fiber, forming a special receptor that functions as a mechanoreceptor (Fig. 14.12).

NERVE SUPPLY TO THE SKIN (Fig. 14.12)

The skin contains numerous sensory receptors that are peripheral terminals of sensory neurons (see Fig. 14.12). The most numerous of these are *free nerve endings* in the epidermis; free nerve endings also occur in the dermis. The free nerve endings in the epidermis extend as far as the stratum granulosum; as was previously stated, they serve as nociceptors (pain receptors). Networks of free dermal nerve endings surround many hair follicles. The networks surrounding tactile hairs, such as cat's whiskers, are very extensive and serve as mechanoreceptors. Other nerve endings are enclosed in a capsule. These *encapsulated nerve endings* include Pacinian corpuscles, Meissner's corpuscles, and Ruffini endings. Merkel cells in the epidermis have already been described. In addition, the skin contains efferent nerve fibers that innervate the blood vessels, sweat glands, and smooth muscle associated with the sweat glands.

Pacinian Corpuscles

Pacinian corpuscles are large ovoid structures, measuring 1 mm or more in their long axis. They contain the termination of a myelinated nerve fiber. Once within the corpuscle, only the initial part of the nerve fiber retains its myelin cover; the ter-

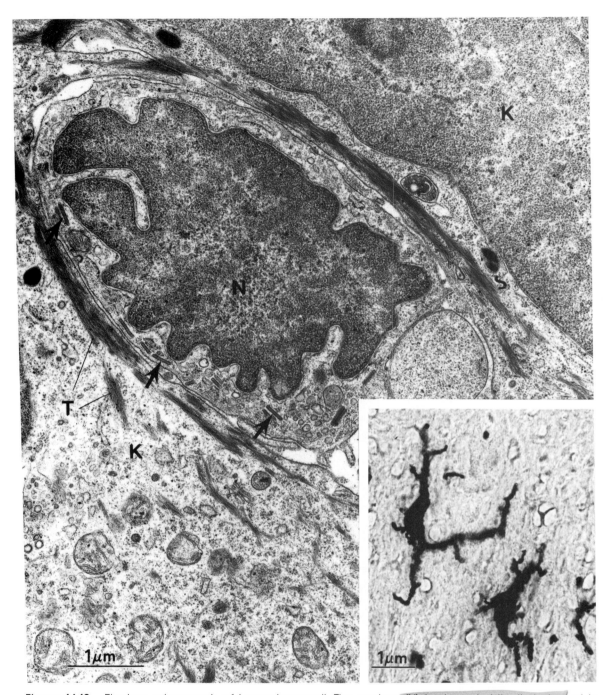

Figure 14.10. Electron micrograph of Langerhans cell. The nucleus (N) is characteristically indented in many places and the cytoplasm contains distinctive rod-shaped bodies **(arrows)**. Note the tonofilaments (T) in adjacent keratinocytes (K), but the absence of these filaments in the Langerhans cell. In the light micrograph **(inset)**, the dendritic nature of the Langerhans cell can be seen by application of a special stain. × 19,600; **inset,** × 1,200. (Courtesy of Dr. C. Squier, 1984.)

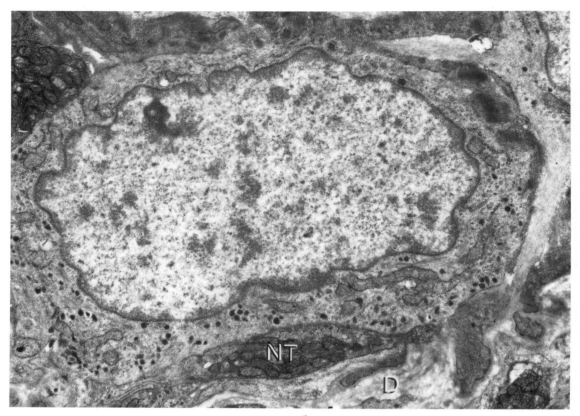

Figure 14.11. Electron micrograph of Merkel cell (MC). The cell has small granules in the cytoplasm, and it makes contact with a peripheral terminal (NT) of a neuron. The dermis (D) is in the lower part of the illustration. × 14,450. (Courtesy of Dr. B. Munger, 1984.)

minal part of the fiber is unmyelinated. The nerve fiber occupies an axial position within the corpuscle. It is surrounded by layers, or lamellae, of flat cells that are continuous with the endoneurium. Between the flattened cells are spaces considered to be filled with fluid. In sections, the Pacinian corpuscle bears some resemblance to the cut face of an onion. Pacinian corpuscles are pressoreceptors. They are found in the connective tissue of the skin, especially skin that has great sensitivity such as the fingertips, in the hypodermis, and, in general, in connective tissue throughout the body.

Meissner's Corpuscles

Meissner's corpuscles are found in the dermis of the skin, being especially numerous in the fingers and toes. They are generally cylindrical in shape, measuring about 150 μm in their long axis. They consist of supporting cells, which are thought to be modified Schwann cells, and the unmyelinated terminal or terminals of afferent nerve fibers. The supporting cell and the nerve fiber zigzag through the corpuscle. Meissner's corpuscles are tactile receptors. They are located immediately under the epidermis.

Ruffini Endings

Ruffini endings are rounded, somewhat fusiform structures, measuring up to 1 mm in length. They are found in skin and joints. A single, large-diameter myelinated fiber enters the capsule and there it branches into many unmyelinated twigs. These unmyelinated nerve fibers intertwine with collagen fibers also present within the nerve endings. Other spaces within the capsule are considered to be fluid-filled.

HAIR

Hairs are keratinized filaments that develop from an invagination of the epidermis called the *hair follicle.* They are present over almost the entire body, being absent from the sides and palmar surfaces of the hands, from the sides and plantar surfaces of the feet, from the lips, and from the region around the urogenital orifices. In some lo-

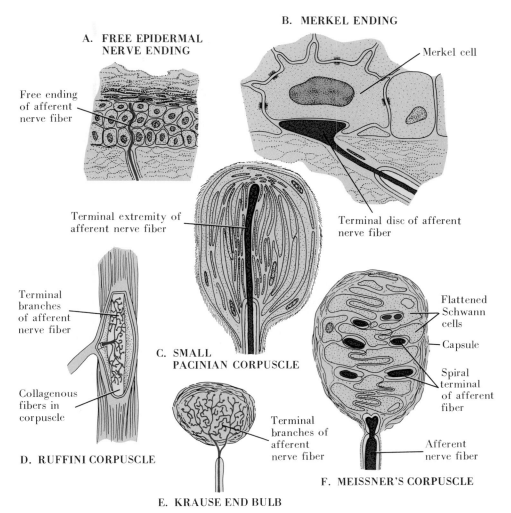

A. FREE EPIDERMAL NERVE ENDING

Free ending of afferent nerve fiber

B. MERKEL ENDING

Merkel cell

Terminal disc of afferent nerve fiber

Terminal extremity of afferent nerve fiber

C. SMALL PACINIAN CORPUSCLE

Terminal branches of afferent nerve fiber

Collagenous fibers in corpuscle

D. RUFFINI CORPUSCLE

E. KRAUSE END BULB

Terminal branches of afferent nerve fiber

Flattened Schwann cells

Capsule

Spiral terminal of afferent fiber

Afferent nerve fiber

F. MEISSNER'S CORPUSCLE

Figure 14.12. Diagram of the sensory receptors in the skin. **C, D, E,** and **F** are encapsulated endings, surrounded by a capsule of connective tissue. (Based on Ham AW, Cormack DH: *Histology,* 8th ed. Philadelphia, JB Lippincott, 1979.)

cations, hairs are influenced by sex hormones to a noticeable degree. For example, in the male, thick pigmented facial hairs begin to grow and develop at puberty into a mustache and beard; in both the male and female, pubic hairs and axillary hair begin to develop at puberty; and in the male, the hairline tends to regress with age, sometimes leading to baldness. Color of the hair is due to melanin pigments.

Hairs grow in cycles. A period of growth in which a new hair develops is followed by a period of rest in which the hair is lost. In young rodents, the hair cycles are synchronized so that waves of hairs in the growth phase move over the body surface followed by periods of rest. In humans, the growth occurs in a mosaic pattern, that is, it is not synchronized with the growth of neighboring hairs.

Structure of Hair Follicle

The hair follicle varies in histological appearance according to whether it is in the growing or resting stage. Because the growing follicle shows the full-blown structure, it will be described (Fig. 14.13). The outermost part of the hair follicle is a downgrowth of the epidermis called the ***external root sheath.*** At its deepest point, the hair follicle forms a bulb-like expansion and this is invaginated by connective tissue to form a connective tissue papilla. Whereas the external root sheath is several cells thick over most of the length of the follicle, it is only one cell thick over the bulb. Other cells forming the bulb, including those that surround the connective tissue papilla, are called the ***matrix.*** About two-thirds of the distance from the bulb to the neck of the follicle, cells from the external root

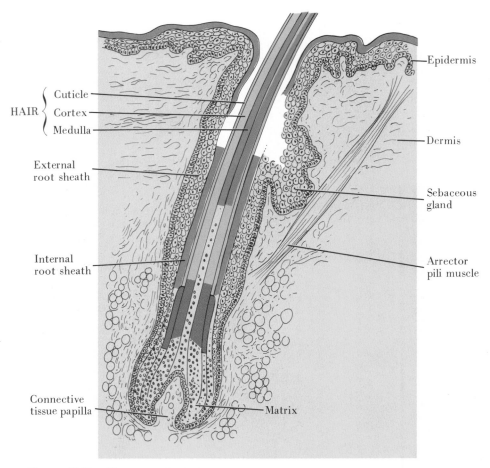

HAIR { Cuticle / Cortex / Medulla

External root sheath

Internal root sheath

Connective tissue papilla

Epidermis

Dermis

Sebaceous gland

Arrector pili muscle

Matrix

Figure 14.13. Diagram of a hair in a hair follicle, showing the distribution of soft (medium magenta) and hard (pale magenta) keratin and the keratogenous zone (dark magenta) in which the keratin of the hair is produced. (Based on Leblond, CP: *Ann NY Acad Sci* 53:464, 1951.)

sheath grow outward to form a *sebaceous gland.* Every hair follicle is joined to a sebaceous gland and the gland secretes its product into the space around the hair. From here, the secretion reaches the skin surface.

The matrix of the bulb consists of dividing cells that differentiate into keratin-producing cells of the hair and the *internal root sheath.* The internal root sheath is a multilayered cellular covering that surrounds the deep part of the hair. Both the hair and the internal root sheath have three layers. The hair consists of the medulla, cortex, and cuticle; the internal root sheath consists of the cuticle, Huxley's layer, and Henle's layer. Keratinization of the hair and internal root sheath occurs in a region called the *keratogenous zone* shortly after the cells have left the matrix. By the time the hair emerges from the follicle, it is entirely keratinized as hard

keratin. The internal root sheath, now consisting of soft keratin, does not emerge from the follicle with the hair, but is dissolved at about the level where the sebaceous glands pour their secretions into the follicle.

The hair follicle is surrounded by a connective tissue sheath and attached to the connective tissue sheath is a bundle of smooth muscle called the *arrector pili muscle.*

SEBACEOUS (OIL) GLANDS

The sebaceous glands develop as an outgrowth of the external root sheath of the hair follicle, usually several glands to one follicle. They secrete an oily substance called *sebum* that coats not only the hair, but also the surface of the skin. Sebum is produced as a holocrine secretion, that is, the entire cell becomes filled with the fatty product, the cell undergoes progressive disruption and then necrosis as the product fills the cell, and ultimately, both product and cell debris are discharged from the gland. New cells are produced by mitotic activity of cells at the periphery of the gland. These cells, at the periphery of the sebaceous gland, are the basal cells. They are adjacent to a basal lamina just as are the basal cells of the epidermis. These basal sebaceous cells contain smooth and rough endoplasmic reticulum, free ribosomes, glycogen, mitochondria, a Golgi, but few lipid droplets (Fig. 14.14). Desmosomes join them to neighboring cells. As the basal cells begin to produce the lipid product, the sER increases in amount and the increase is construed to reflect an active role of the sER in the production of lipid product. As the cells become filled with numerous lipid droplets separated by thin partitions of cytoplasm, they move away from the basal layer. Ulti-

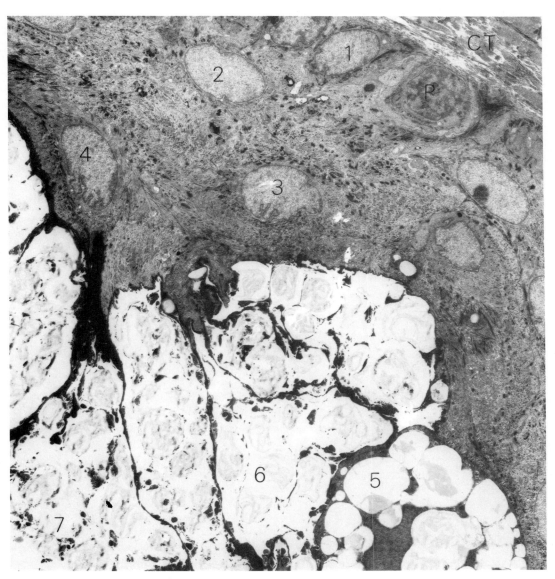

Figure 14.14. Electron micrograph of sebaceous gland. Gland cells **(1)** close to the connective tissue (CT) are small and undifferentiated. Among these cells are dividing cells—one of which (P) appears to be in early prophase. From this peripheral position the cells move toward the opening of the gland **(2, 3, 4)** and produce sebum. The oily produce is reflected in the cytoplasm first as small lipid droplets **(5)**, which gradually fuse **(6)** and constitute the product of the gland. The cells perish **(7)** during the secretion. (Courtesy of Dr. B. Munger, 1984.)

mately, as already indicated, the entire cell and its product are discharged into the upper portion of the hair follicle.

At the time of puberty, there is an increase in male sex hormone in both male and female. This is sometimes associated with production of sebaceous cells and sebum substantially greater than normal. The excessive accumulation of sebum in the glands gives rise to the condition called **acne.**

SUDORIFEROUS (SWEAT) GLANDS

Eccrine Sweat Glands

Sudoriferous (sweat) glands are of two types, designated as **eccrine** and **apocrine.** Eccrine sweat glands are distributed over the entire surface of the body except at a relatively few locations such as the lips and external genitalia. They are not associ-

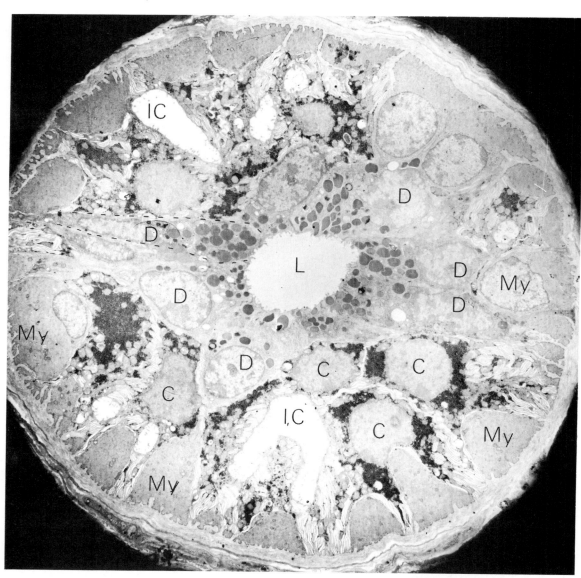

Figure 14.15(a). Electron micrograph of eccrine sweat gland showing myoepithelial cells (My) and two distinctive gland cell types, dark cells (D) and clear cells (C). The apical portion of the dark cell is broad; it faces the lumen (L) of the gland and contains numerous secretory granules. The boundary of one dark cell has been marked by **dashes.** The clear cell is more removed from the lumen of the gland. Its base rests on the myoepithelial cells or directly on the basal lamina. Most of the free surface of the clear cell faces an intercellular canaliculus (IC). Clear cells contain numerous mitochondria, extensive infoldings of the plasma membrane, and large numbers of glycogen granules. The glycogen appears as the dark material in the electron micrographs. (Courtesy of Dr. J. Terzakis.)

ated with hair follicles and, indeed, are especially numerous in thick skin devoid of hair.

The eccrine sweat gland is a simple coiled tubular gland. The secretory portion of the gland is located deep in the dermis or in the upper portion of the hypodermis. Three cell types are present in the glandular portion of the gland: *myoepithelial cells, clear cells,* and *dark cells.* Myoepithelial cells move secretions out of the gland by contraction.

They contain numerous contractile filaments that stain readily with eosin. The myoepithelial cells are directly adjacent to the basal lamina, and their location along with the eosinophilic staining of the cytoplasm, makes them readily identifiable in routine H&E-stained paraffin sections. The clear cells and dark cells are the secretory components of the gland. The dark cells are adjacent to the lumen and the clear cells are located between the dark

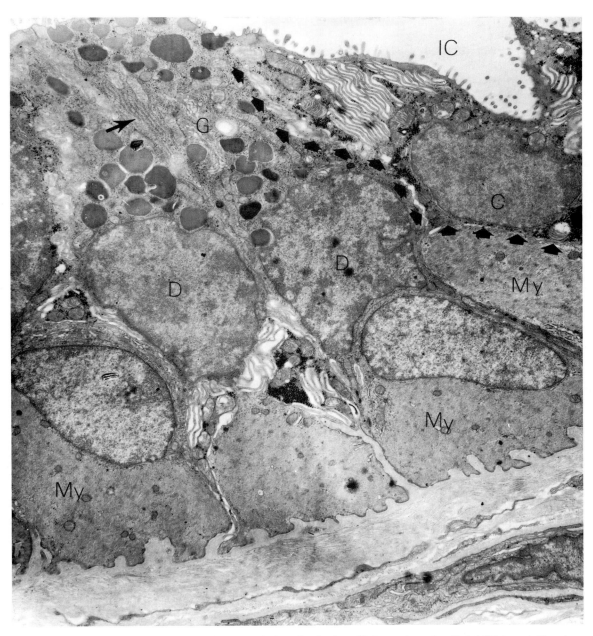

Figure 14.15 (b). At higher magnification the dark cells display rER **(arrow)** and a Golgi (G) in addition to the secretory granules. The clear cells show large amounts of folded membrane, mitochondria, and glycogen. The myoepithelial cells (My) contain large amounts of contractile filaments. The boundary of the clear cell in the upper right is marked by the short stubby **arrows.** (Courtesy of Dr. J. Terzakis.)

and the myoepithelial cells. With the electron microscope, the dark cells are seen to contain abundant rER and granules with a glycoprotein content; they are thought to secrete mucopolysaccharide (Fig. 14.15). The clear cells, on the other hand, show no secretory granules and only small amounts of rER. They do, however, contain numerous glycogen granules, mitochondria, and sER, and their surface is expanded by the presence of surface folds and microvilli. Between adjacent cells there are intercellular canaliculi that lead to the lumen of the gland. The features of the clear cells suggest that they are the cells that produce the watery secretion of sweat.

The duct of the sweat gland consists of stratified cuboidal epithelium. The duct begins as a coiled element in the same nest as the coiled secretory portion of the gland. It passes through the dermis as a gentle spiral and then continues to spiral through the epidermis. The cells of the duct are smaller and appear darker than cells of the secretory portion of the gland; the duct has a smaller diameter than the secretory portion. These features can be used to distinguish the duct from the secretory portion in a histological section.

The eccrine sweat glands produce a watery solution low in protein and containing varying amounts of sodium chloride, urea, uric acid, and ammonia. Thus, the eccrine sweat gland serves in part as an excretory organ. Many factors determine the composition of sweat. Sometimes an alteration in the composition of sweat indicates a diseased state. For example, elevated sodium levels can serve as a test for cystic fibrosis in field studies. In pronounced uremia, when the kidneys are unable to rid the body of urea, concentrations of urea increase in sweat and, after the water evaporates, crystals may be discernible on the skin, especially on the upper lip; these include urea crystals and are called urea frost.

The eccrine sweat glands play a major role in temperature regulation through the cooling that results from the evaporation of sweat.

Apocrine Sweat Glands

Apocrine sweat glands are widespread in many animal species, but have limited distribution in the human. They are found in the axilla, the areola and nipple of the mammary gland, the circumanal region, and in association with the external genitalia. They develop from the same downgrowth of epidermis that gives rise to the hair follicles above the opening of the sebaceous glands. Ceruminous glands of the ear canal and glands of Moll in the eyelid are also apocrine glands.

The apocrine glands are coiled tubular glands; they may be branched. The secretory portion of the gland is deep in the dermis or, more often, in the upper region of the hypodermis. It differs in several respects from the secretory portion of the eccrine gland. The most obvious difference, readily noted in H&E-stained paraffin sections, is the wide lumen (see Atlas section, Plate 61). It contains only one type of secretory cell; the cell may be cuboidal or low columnar, and its cytoplasm stains with eosin. Myoepithelial cells are also in the secretory portion of the gland, situated adjacent to the basal lamina. The duct portion of the gland resembles the duct of the eccrine gland. However, instead of emptying its contents on the surface of the skin, the duct opens into the hair follicle at the level above the duct of the sebaceous gland.

Apocrine glands produce a secretion that contains protein. The secretions of the glands vary with the anatomical location. In the axilla, the glands produce a proteinaceous milky fluid containing organic compounds, including steroid. In many mammals, similar glands produce pheromones, chemical signals used in marking territory, courtship, and maternal as well as social behavior. These glands are responsive to the sex hormones and they develop at puberty. In addition, the axillary apocrine glands of the female undergo cyclic changes that parallel the menstrual cycle.

Innervation of Sweat Glands

Both eccrine and apocrine sweat glands are innervated by the sympathetic portion of the autonomic nervous system. However, the eccrine sweat glands are stimulated by cholinergic transmitters (usually identified with the parasympathetic component of the autonomic system), whereas the apocrine glands are stimulated by adrenergic transmitters. The eccrine glands respond to heat and to nervous strain. In response to such acute stress, there is rapid expression of perspiration on the palms of the hands and forehead. The apocrine glands respond to emotional and sensory stimuli, but not to heat.

NAILS

The nails are keratinized plates, slightly curved, covering the dorsal surface of the terminal portions of the fingers and toes. The nail or, more properly, the **nail plate,** rests on the **nail bed.** The bed consists of epithelial cells that are continuous with the stratum basale and stratum spinosum of the epidermis (see Atlas section, Plate 63). The proximal part of the nail, referred to as the *root,* is buried in a fold of skin. The cells of the nail bed that are under the root of the nail constitute the *matrix.* The cells of the matrix divide, migrate toward the root of the nail, and, at the root, differentiate and produce the keratin of the nail. The constant addition of new cells and their production of keratin accounts for the growth of the nail. As it grows, it "slides" over the nail bed. The keratin of the nail is hard keratin, like that of the hair cortex.

As already noted, keratohyaline granules are not involved in the formation of hard keratin. Viewed from above, a crescent-shaped light area is seen near the root of the nail. This is the *lunula.* It is a reflection of the partially keratinized cells in this region of the nail. The edge of the skin fold covering the root of the nail is called the *eponychium,* or the *cuticle;* the epidermal thickening that joins to the free edge of the nail plate on its undersurface is the *hyponychium.*

PLATE 58. Skin I

The skin, or integument, consists of two main layers: the *epidermis,* comprised of stratified squamous epithelium that is keratinized, and a *dermis,* comprised of connective tissue. Under the dermis is a layer of loose connective tissue called the *hypodermis.* This is also generally referred to as the subcutaneous tissue and, by gross anatomists, as the superficial fascia. Typically, over most of the body, the hypodermis contains large amounts of adipose tissue, particularly in the adequately nourished individual.

The epidermis gives rise to nails, hairs, sebaceous glands, and sweat glands. Also, in the palms of the hands and the soles of the feet, the epidermis gives rise to an outer keratinized layer that is substantially thicker than over the other parts of the body. Accordingly, the skin over the palms of the hands and soles of the feet is referred to as *thick skin,* in contrast to the skin over other parts of the body, which is referred to as *thin skin.* It should be noted that in thick skin there are no hairs.

A sample of thick skin is shown in **Figure 1.** The epidermis **(Ep)** is at the top; the remainder of the field consists of the dermis, in which a large number of sweat glands **(Sw)** can be observed. Although the layers of the epidermis are examined more advantageously at higher magnification (e.g., **Fig. 3**), it is easy to see even at this relatively low magnification that about half of the thickness of the epidermis consists of a distinctive surface layer that stains lighter than the remainder of the epidermis. This is the keratinized layer. The dome-shaped surface contours represent a cross-section through the minute ridges on the surface of thick skin that produce the characteristic fingerprints. [The layers of the epidermis in thick skin are (1) the stratum basale; (2) the stratum spinosum; (3) the stratum granulosum; (4) the stratum lucidum; and, on the surface, (5) the stratum corneum, the keratinized layer.]

The dermis displays sweat glands **(Sw),** blood vessels **(BV),** and adipose tissue **(AT).** The ducts of the sweat glands **(D)** extend from the glands to the epidermis. One of the ducts is shown as it enters the epidermis at the bottom of an epithelial ridge. It will pass through the epidermis in a spiral course to open onto the skin surface.

KEY

AT, adipose tissue	**SGl,** sebaceous gland
BV, blood vessels	**SGr,** stratum granulosum
D, duct of sweat glands	**SS,** stratum spinosum
De, dermis	**Sw,** sweat gland
Ep, epidermis	**arrowhead,** inset,
HF, hair follicle	granules in cell of
P, pigment	stratum granulosum
SB, stratum basale	**arrows,** inset,
SC, stratum corneum	"intercellular bridges"

Fig. 1, × 45	**Fig. 3,** × 320; (inset, ×
Fig. 2, × 60	640); all human

A sample of thin skin is shown in **Figure 2.** In addition to sweat glands, thin skin contains hair follicles **(HF)** and their associated sebaceous glands **(SGl).** Each sebaceous gland opens into a hair follicle. Oftentimes, as in this tissue sample, the hair follicles and the glands, both sebaceous and sweat, extend beyond the dermis **(De)** and into the hypodermis. Note the blood vessels **(BV)** and adipose tissue **(AT)** in the hypodermis.

The layers of the epidermis are shown at higher magnification in **Figure 3.** The cell layer that occupies the basal location is the stratum basale **(SB).** It is one cell deep. Just above this is a layer, several cells in thickness, referred to as the stratum spinosum **(SS).** It consists of cells that have spinous processes on their surface. These processes meet with spinous processes of neighboring cells, and together, they appear as intercellular bridges **(arrows, inset).** The next layer is the stratum granulosum **(SGr),** whose cells contain keratohyalin granules **(arrowhead, inset).** On the surface is the stratum corneum **(SC).** This consists of keratinized cells—cells that no longer possess nuclei. The keratinized cells are flat and generally adherent to other cells above and below without evidence of cell boundaries. The pigment in the cell of the stratum basale is melanin; some of this pigment **(P)** is also present in connective tissue cells of the dermis.

PLATE 58

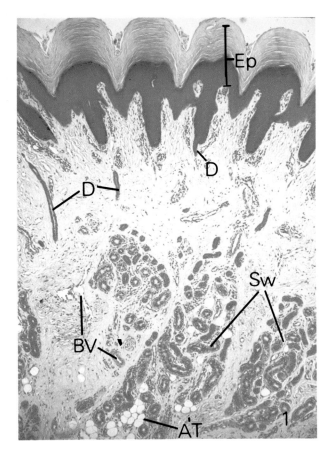

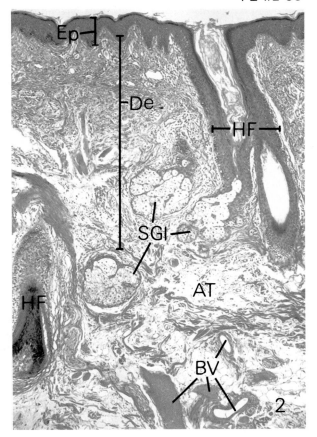

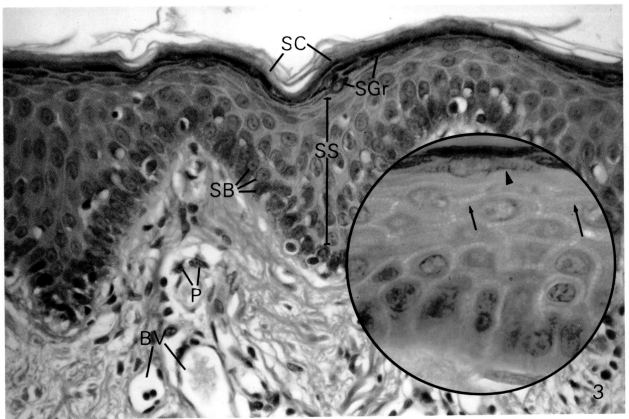

PLATE 59. Skin II

The epidermis contains four distinctive cell types: keratinocytes, melanocytes, Langerhans cells, and Merkel cells. Keratinocytes are the most numerous of these cells; they are generated in the stratum basale and move toward the surface. As they do so, they produce the intracellular protein keratin and the special extracellular lipid that serves as a water barrier in the upper reaches of the epidermis. Histologically, the keratinocytes are the cells that show spinous processes in the stratum spinosum. The other three cell types are not readily identified in H&E paraffin sections. However, the product of the melanocyte is evident in H&E sections and this is considered in the first two figures of this plate.

The skin contains pigment, called melanin, which protects the tissue against ultraviolet light. This pigment is chiefly in the epidermis; it is formed by melanocytes that then pass the pigment to the keratinocytes. The pigment is present in greater amounts in Negroid skin than in Caucasian skin, and this can be seen by comparing Caucasian skin (**Fig. 1**) and Negroid skin (**Fig. 2**). The epidermis and a small amount of the dermis are shown in each figure. Whereas the deep part of the Negroid skin contains considerable pigment, the amount of pigment in Caucasian skin is insufficient to be noticeable at this magnification. Cells for producing the pigment are present in both skin types and in approximately equal numbers. After prolonged exposure to sunlight, pigment would also be produced in sufficient amount to be seen in Caucasian skin.

In routine H&E-stained paraffin sections of Caucasian skin, such as the sample in **Figure 1**, the melanocytes are among the cells that appear as small, rounded, clear cells (**CC**) mixed with the other cells of the stratum basale. However, it needs to be emphasized that not all clear cells of the epidermis are melanocytes. For example, Langerhans cells may also appear as clear cells, but they are located more superficially in the stratum spinosum. Merkel cells may also appear as clear cells, thus making it difficult to identify these three cell types with certainty.

In Negroid skin (**Fig. 2**), most of the pigment is in the basal portion of the epidermis, but it is also present in cells progressing toward the surface and within the non-nucleated cells of the keratinized layer. The **arrows (Fig. 2)** indicate the melanin pigment in keratinocytes of the stratum spinosum and

in the stratum corneum. In Caucasian skin, the melanin is broken down before it leaves the upper part of the stratum spinosum. Thus, pigment is not seen in the upper layers of the epidermis.

Figure 3 is included in the plate because it shows certain features of the dermis, the connective tissue layer of the skin. It is divided into two layers, the papillary layer (**PL**) of loose connective tissue and the reticular layer (**RL**) of more dense connective tissue. The papillary layer is immediately under the epidermis; it includes the connective tissue papillae that project into the undersurface of the epidermis. The reticular layer is deep to the papillary layer. The boundary between these two layers is not demarcated by any specific structural feature except for the change in the histological composition of the two layers.

The specimen in **Figure 3** was stained with H&E and also with a procedure to display elastic fibers (**EF**). They are relatively thick and conspicuous in the reticular layer (see also inset), where they appear as the dark-blue profiles, some of which are elongate whereas others are short. In the papillary layer, the elastic fibers are thinner and relatively sparse (**arrows**). The **inset** shows the typical eosinophilic staining of the thick collagenous fibers in the reticular layer. Although the collagenous fibers at the lower magnification of Figure 3 are not as prominent, it is nevertheless possible to note that they are thicker in the reticular layer than in the papillary layer. Finally, realizing that many of the small dark-blue profiles in the reticular layer represent oblique and cross-sections through elastic fibers and not nuclei of cells, it should be evident that the papillary layer is more cellular than the reticular layer.

KEY

CC, clear cells
EF, elastic fibers
PL, papillary layer
RL, reticular layer

arrows (Fig. 2), pigment in different layers of epidermis
arrows (Fig. 3), delicate elastic fibers

Fig. 1, × 300
Fig. 2, × 300

Fig. 3, × 200; all human

PLATE 59

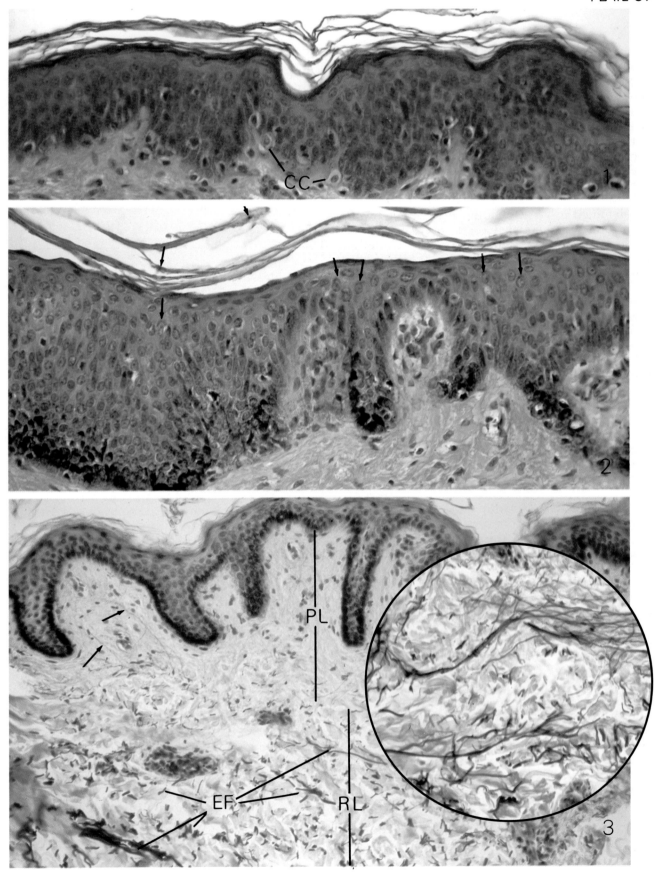

PLATE 60. Eccrine and Apocrine Sweat Glands

Sweat glands are of two types, designated as apocrine glands and eccrine glands. Apocrine glands have a limited distribution; in the human they are found in the axilla, anogenital region, and the mammary areola. Apocrine sweat glands are large, tubular structures that are sometimes branched. They empty into the upper portion of the hair follicle and they produce a product that becomes odoriferous after being secreted. The apocrine sweat is important in lower animals, serving as a sex stimulant and as a marker of territory. Apocrine glands develop at puberty under the influence of sex hormones. They also respond to nerve stimulation, but not to heat. In addition to the apocrine glands, which are obviously sweat glands, two additional types of glands, namely, the ceruminous glands of the external ear and the glands of Moll in the eyelids, are also classified as apocrine glands.

Eccrine sweat glands in the human are distributed over the entire body surface except for the lips, glans penis, inner surface of the prepuce, clitoris, and labia minora. The eccrine sweat glands are especially numerous in the thick skin of the hands and feet.

Figure 1 is a section of adult skin showing both apocrine and eccrine sweat glands. The apocrine sweat glands **(aSG)** are easily identified by virtue of the large lumen of their secretory portion. This histological feature is in striking contrast to the small lumen displayed by the secretory portion of the eccrine sweat gland **(SG).** Coincidentally, the apocrine sweat gland is close to a hair follicle **(HF).** As already mentioned, the apocrine gland opens into the upper portion of a hair follicle. The two small circular areas are examined in the larger circular **insets** to show the cell types of the apocrine gland at higher magnification. Note that the **small circular area** on the **left** includes a tangential section through one of the glandular units.

The secretory portion of the apocrine sweat gland consists of a single secretory cell type and myoepithelial cells. These can be seen in the **circular inset** on the **right.** The epithelial cells are either cuboidal or columnar, and, if columnar, they typically display granules **(G)** in their apical cytoplasm. The myoepithelial cells are in the basal portion of the epithelial cell layer. Nuclei of myoepithelial cells are elongate and, when cut in cross-section, they appear as rounded nuclear profiles in the base of the epithelial cell layer **(arrow, right circular inset).** On the other hand, when seen in different planes of section, the profiles of myoepithelial cell

nuclei may appear more elongate as they are in the **left circular inset (arrows).** This **inset** also shows the cytoplasmic portion of the myoepithelial cells **(arrowheads)** of an adjacent glandular unit.

Eccrine sweat glands are shown at higher magnification in **Figure 2.** Typically, a section includes profiles of both the secretory portion of the gland **(SG)** and profiles of the duct portion **(D).** The secretory portion of the gland consists of a double layer of cuboidal epithelial cells and peripherally, along the basal lamina, a conspicuous layer of myoepithelial cells. The duct portion of the gland has a narrower outside diameter than the secretory portion; however, the lumen of the duct portion is typically narrower than that of the gland. Occasionally, the duct may be distended **(asterisk).** The **oval inset** shows where a secretory unit **(SG)** continues into the ductal unit **(D).** The duct has been cut as it turns so that in the upper part of the inset the duct is seen essentially in cross-section, whereas in the middle part of the inset it has been cut in a more or less longitudinal plane. Moreover, where the duct has been cut longitudinally, the lumen is not in the plane of section. The duct consists of a double layer of small cuboidal cells and no myoepithelial cells. In addition, there is an acidophilic staining associated with the apical portion of the duct cells that are adjacent to the lumen. This is evident in the duct seen in the **oval inset** and it can be contrasted readily with the absence of such staining in the apical region of the secretory cells **(SG),** also seen in the **oval inset.**

PLATE 60

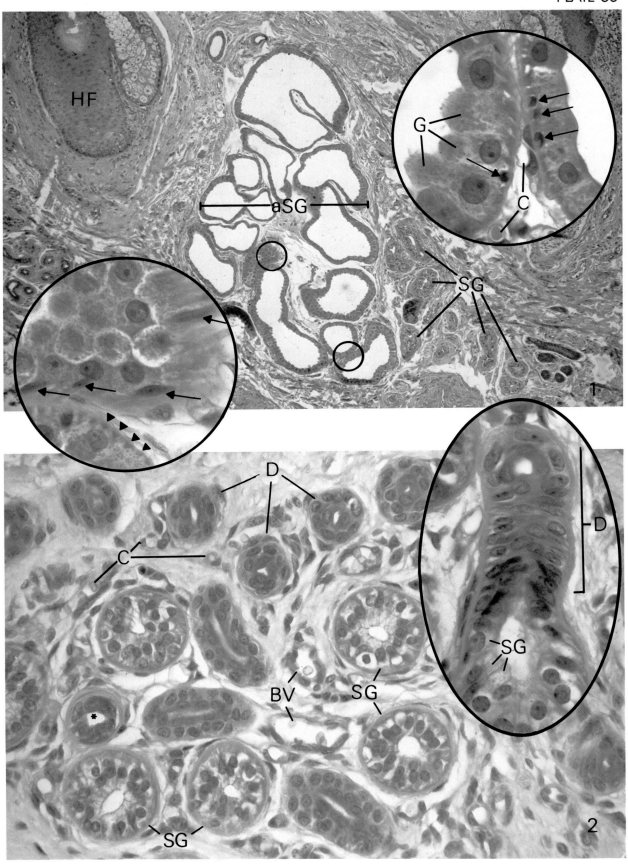

PLATE 61. Sweat and Sebaceous Glands

This section through a sweat gland **(Fig. 1)** shows five profiles of the ductal portion **(D)** and two profiles of the secretory portion **(SG).** The larger secretory segment is through a region either just below or above where a U turn was made; therefore, it shows two luminal profiles, one going up, the other down, or vice versa. The lumens of both the ductal and the secretory unit are marked by **asterisks.**

The glandular unit of the eccrine sweat gland contains two epithelial cell types and myoepithelial cells **(M). Arrowheads** show small cross-sections of myoepithelial cell cytoplasm; **arrows** show where more elongate profiles of myoepithelial cytoplasm are evident. The epithelial cells are of two types, designated as dark cells and clear cells. Unfortunately, the characteristic dark cytoplasmic staining of the dark cells is not evident unless special precautions are taken to preserve the secretory granules in their apical cytoplasm. Nevertheless, it should be noted that the dark cells are closer to the lumen, whereas the light cells are closer to the base of the epithelial layer, making contact with either the basal lamina or, more frequently, the myoepithelial cells. In addition, the clear cells are in contact with intercellular canaliculi. Several such intercellular canaliculi are shown in the secretory units **(small arrows). Figure 1** again shows that the duct consists of two layers of small cuboidal cells.

Sebaceous glands develop from the epithelial cells of the hair follicle and they discharge their secretion into the follicle and from here it reaches the skin surface. The sebaceous secretion is rich in lipid, and this is reflected in the cells of the sebaceous gland. A section of a sebaceous gland and the related hair follicle is shown in **Figure 2.** At this level, the hair follicle consists of the external root sheath **(RS)** surrounding the hair shaft. The seba-

KEY

BC, basal cells
CT, connective tissue
D, duct of eccrine sweat glands
eRS, junction between sebaceous gland and external root sheath
M, myoepithelial cell
RS, external root sheath of hair follicle
Seb, sebaceous gland
SG, secretory component of eccrine sweat gland

arrowheads, myoepithelial cell cytoplasm (X.S.)
arrows, myoepithelial cell cytoplasm (L.S.)
asterisk, lumens of glands
small arrows, intracellular canaliculi
numbers, Figure 3, see text

ceous gland **(Seb)** appears as a cluster of cells, most of which display a washed-out or finely reticulated cytoplasm. This is due to the fact that these cells contain numerous lipid droplets, and the lipid is lost by dissolution in fat solvents during the routine preparation of the H&E paraffin section. The opening of the sebaceous gland through the external root sheath **(eRS)** and into the hair follicle is shown in the lower right of **Figure 2.** The same sebaceous gland is depicted at higher magnification in **Figure 3,** and it is labeled with **numbers** to show a series of cells, each filled with increasingly greater amounts of lipid and each progressively closer to the opening of the gland into the hair follicle. The sebaceous secretion includes the entire cell and, therefore, cells need to be replaced constantly in the functional gland. Cells at the periphery of the gland are basal cells **(BC).** Dividing cells in the basal layer replace those that are lost with the secretion.

PLATE 61

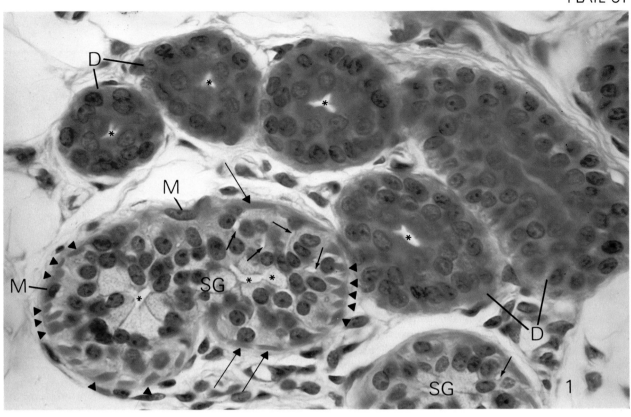

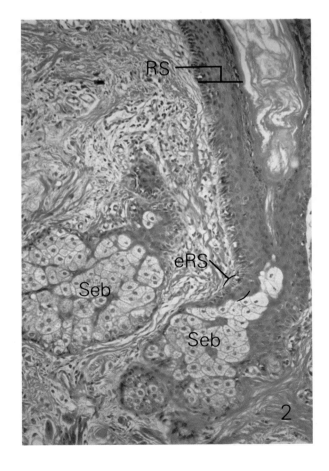

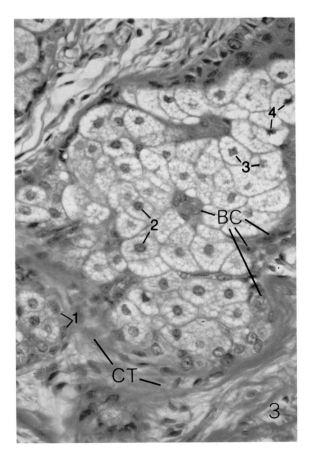

PLATE 62. Integument and Sensory Organs

The specimen shown in **Figure 1** is a section of thick skin showing the epidermis (**Ep**) and the dermis (**De**) and, under the skin, a portion of the hypodermis (**Hy**). Again to be noted is that the thickness of the epidermis is due largely to the thickness of the stratum corneum. Most of this layer is only lightly stained; at the surface, the staining is more intense. Also to be noted are the thick collagenous fibers in the reticular layer of the dermis and the greater cellularity of the papillary layer of the dermis. Finally, note the presence of some sweat glands in the upper part of the hypodermis. The duct (**D**) of one gland has been labeled.

The main feature of this specimen, as shown in **Figure 1,** is that it depicts those sensory receptors that can be recognized in a routine H&E-stained paraffin section. They are the Meissner's corpuscle (**MC**) and the Pacinian corpuscles (**PC**). Meissner's corpuscles are in the upper part of the dermis, immediately under the epidermis. These corpuscles are small and sometimes difficult to identify at low magnification; however, their location is characteristic. Knowing where they are located is a major step in finding the Meissner's corpuscles in a tissue section. Structures suspected of being Meissner's corpuscles should then be examined at higher magnification, and this will be done in **Figure 3.**

Pacinian corpuscles (**PC**) are shown in the upper part of the hypodermis. Again, this location is characteristic although they are often more deeply located. These corpuscles are large, slightly oval structures and even at low magnification, a layered, or lamellated, pattern can be discerned. At the higher magnification in **Figure 2,** the concentric layers, or lamellae of the Pacinian corpuscle (**PC**) can be seen to be due to flat cells. These are fibroblast-like cells and, while not evident within the tissue section, these cells are continuous with the endoneurium of the nerve fiber. The space

KEY

BV, blood vessels
D, ducts of sweat glands
De, dermis
Ep, epidermis
Hy, hypodermis

MC, Meissner's corpuscles
N, nerve bundles
PC, Pacinian corpuscles

asterisks, nerve fiber in center of Pacinian corpuscle

between the cellular lamellae is wide, and it contains mostly fluid. The neural portoin of the Pacinian corpuscle travels longitudinally through the center of the corpuscle. In this specimen, the corpuscles have been cross-sectioned; an **asterisk** has been placed in two of the corpuscles to mark the centrally located nerve fiber. **Figure 2** also shows the duct (**D**) of a sweat gland, some nearby blood vessels (**BV**), and two nerve bundles (**N**).

The two Meissner's corpuscles that were labeled in **Figure 1** are shown at higher magnification in **Figure 3.** To be noted is the direct proximity of the corpuscle to the undersurface of the epidermis. The section depicts the long axis of the corpuscles. A Meissner's corpuscle consists of an axon (sometimes two) taking a zigzag course from one pole of the corpuscle to the other. The nerve fiber terminates at the superficial pole of the corpuscle. Supporting cells are continuous with Schwann cells of the nerve and also take a zigzag route through the corpuscle. Consequently, as seen in **Figure 3,** the nerve fibers and supporting cells are oriented approximately at right angles to the long axis of the corpuscle. Meissner's corpuscles are particularly numerous near the tips of the fingers and toes.

PLATE 62

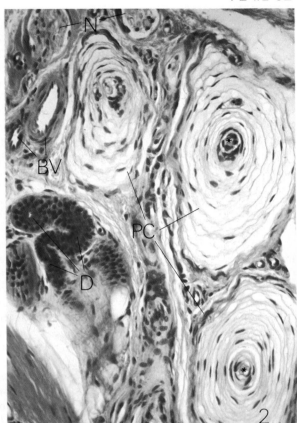

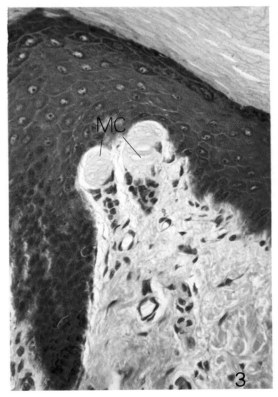

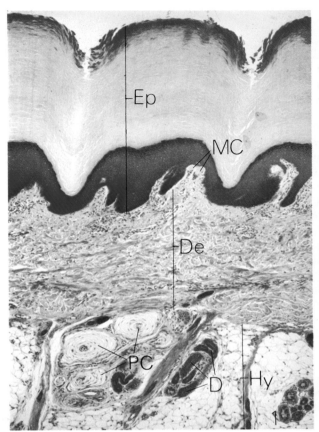

PLATE 63. Hair Follicle and Nail

The growing end of a hair follicle consists of an expanded bulb of epithelial cells that is invaginated by a papilla (**HP**) of connective tissue (**Fig. 1**). The epithelial cells surrounding the papilla at the very tip of the follicle are not yet specialized; they constitute the matrix, the region of the hair follicle where cell division occurs. As the cells leave the matrix, they form cell layers that will become the shaft of the hair and the inner and outer root sheaths of the hair follicle.

The cells that will develop into the shaft of the hair are seen just to the right of the expanded bulb. They constitute the cortex (**C**), medulla (**M**), and cuticle (**asterisks**) of the hair. The cells of the cortex become keratinized. This layer will come to constitute most of the hair shaft as a thick cylinder. The medulla forms the centrally located axis of the hair shaft; it does not always extend through the entire length of the hair and is absent from some hairs. The cuticle consists of overlapping cells which ultimately lose their nuclei and become filled with an amorphous material. The cuticle covers the hair shaft like a layer of overlapping shingles.

The root sheath (**RS**) has two parts: the outer root sheath, which is continuous with the epidermis of the skin, and the inner root sheath, which extends only as far as the level where sebaceous glands enter the hair follicle. The inner root sheath is further divided into three layers: Henle's layer, Huxley's layer, and the cuticle of the inner root sheath. These layers are seen in the growing hair follicle and are shown at higher magnification in the circular inset with the **numbers 1 to 4: 1**—cells of the outer root sheath; **2**—Henle's layer; **3**—Huxley's layer; **4**—cuticle of the inner root sheath. Number **5** points to the future cuticle of the hair.

Many of the cells of the growing hair follicle contain pigment that contribute to the color of the hair. Most of this pigment is inside the cell (**inset**); however, in very dark hair some pigment is also extracellular.

The connective tissue surrounding the hair follicle forms a distinct layer referred to as the sheath, or dermal sheath (**DS**), of the hair follicle.

A nail is a keratinized plate located on the dorsal aspect of the distal phalanges. A section

KEY

B, bone
C, cortex
D, dermis
DS, dermal sheath
EP, epiphyseal plate
Epon, eponychium
HP, dermal papilla of hair follicle
Hypon, hyponychium
asterisks, cuticle of hair
M, medulla
N, nail or nail plate
NM, nail matrix
NR, nail root
PC, Pacinian corpuscles
RS, root sheath
SL, stratum lucidum
numbers, 1—external root sheath; 2—Henle's layer; 3—Huxley's layer; 4—cuticle of inner root sheath; 5—future cuticle of the hair

Fig. 1, × 300   **Fig. 2,** × 12 (inset × 440); all human

through a nail plate is shown in **Figure 2.** The nail itself (**N**) is difficult to stain. Under the free edge of the nail is a boundary layer, the hyponychium (**Hypon**), which is continuous with the stratum corneum of the adjacent epidermis. The proximal end of the nail is overlapped by skin, and here there is a junctional region called the eponychium (**Epon**), which is also continuous with the stratum corneum of the adjacent epidermis. Under the nail is a layer of epithelium, the posterior portion of which is referred to as the nail matrix (**NM**). The cells of the nail matrix function in the growth of the nail. Together, the epithelium under the nail and the underlying dermis (**D**) constitute the nail bed. The posterior portion of the nail, covered by the fold of skin, is the root of the nail (**NR**).

The relationship of the nail to other structures in the fingertip is also shown in **Figure 2.** The bone (**B**) in the specimen represents a distal phalanx. Note that in this bone there is an epiphyseal growth plate (**EP**) at the proximal extremity of the bone, but not at the distal extremity. Numerous Pacinian corpuscles (**PC**) are present in the connective tissue of the palmar side of the finger. Also seen to advantage in this section is the stratum lucidum (**SL**) in the epidermis of the thick skin.

PLATE 63

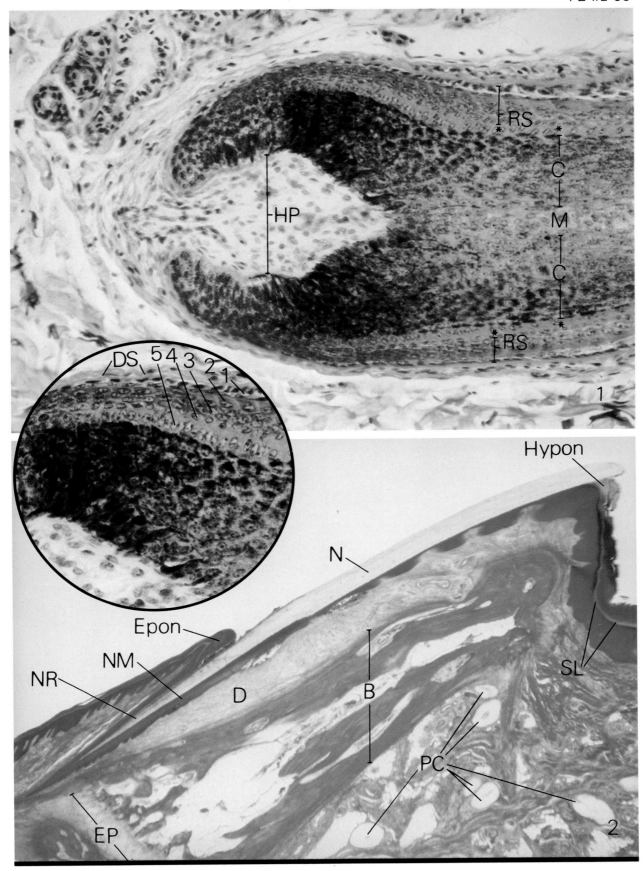

RS

C

M

C

RS

HP

DS 5 4 3 2 1

Epon

NM

NR

D

N

B

PC

Hypon

SL

EP

1

2

Digestive System I: Oral Cavity and Pharynx

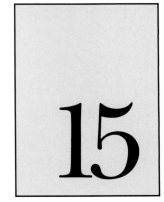

The digestive system consists of the alimentary canal and its associated glands, namely, the salivary glands, pancreas, liver, and gallbladder. In passing through the alimentary canal, food is broken down physically and chemically and ultimately solubilized so that the degraded products can be absorbed. Absorption occurs chiefly through the wall of the small intestine. Undigested food and other substances within the alimentary canal, such as mucus, bacteria, desquamated cells, and bile pigments, are excreted as the feces.

After preliminary maceration, moistening, and formation into a bolus by the action of the structures of the oral cavity and the salivary glands, the food passes rapidly through the pharynx and esophagus. (It should be noted that the rapid passage of food through the pharynx keeps it clear for the passage of air.) The food passes more slowly through the gastrointestinal tract and, during its transit through the stomach and small intestine, the major alterations associated with digestion, solubilization, and absorption occur.

The digestive system will be considered in three chapters that deal, respectively, with (I) the oral cavity and pharynx; (II) the esophagus and gastrointestinal tract; and (III) the liver, gallbladder, and pancreas.

ORAL CAVITY

The oral cavity is divided into a vestibule and an oral cavity proper. The **vestibule** is just internal to the lips and cheeks, extending as far as the teeth. The **oral cavity proper** is behind the teeth, having a roof comprised of the hard and soft palates, and a floor from which the tongue projects. Posteriorly, the oral cavity opens into the oropharynx; the boundary between the two is called the **fauces**. His-

tologically, the oral cavity can be divided into three general areas according to the functional demands of its mucous membrane: (1) the masticatory mucosa, (2) the general nonmasticatory, or lining, mucosa, and (3) the specialized mucosa.

Masticatory Mucosa

The masticatory mucosa is present on the gingiva and the hard palate (Fig. 15.1). It is firmly bound to the underlying bone and it does not stretch or does so only minimally. Masticatory mucosa consists of stratified squamous epithelium and a connective tissue layer, the lamina propria. This layer is comparable to the dermis of the skin in that there is a papillary layer of loose connective tissue and a reticular layer of more dense connective tissue.

The stratified squamous epithelium of the masticatory mucosa is generally keratinized (Fig. 15.2). In some places, particularly in the gingiva, the epithelium may be parakeratinized and sometimes also nonkeratinized. The **keratinized epithelium** consists of four layers: stratum basale, stratum spinosum, stratum granulosum, and a stratum corneum. These layers are similar to those of the epidermis of skin except that a stratum lucidum is not found in the oral mucosa. **Parakeratinized epithelium** is similar histologically to keratinized epithelium except that the cells in the stratum corneum retain their nuclei. Thus, in parakeratinized epithelium, the surface layer stains intensely with eosin and, in addition, the keratinized cells display flat, pyknotic nuclei. In nonkeratinized stratified squamous epithelium, the surface cells retain nuclei, but the cytoplasm of the surface cells does not stain intensely with eosin.

The junction between eipthelium and lamina propria is characterized by numerous deep papil-

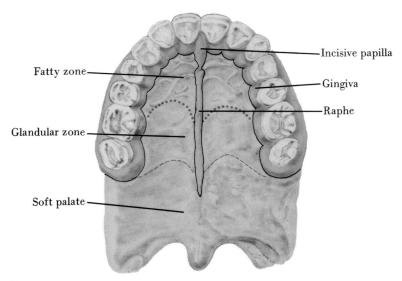

Figure 15.1. Roof of oral cavity proper. The hard palate, containing bone, is bisected into right and left halves by a raphe. Anteriorly, the hard palate contains fatty tissue in the submucosa; posteriorly, there are mucous glands within the submucosa. Neither the raphe nor the gingiva contains a submucosa; instead the mucosa is attached directly to bone. The soft palate has muscle instead of bone in its substance and glands continuous with those of the hard palate in the submucosa. (Based on Bhaskar SN (ed): *Orban's Oral Histology and Embryology,* 9th ed. St. Louis, CV Mosby, 1980, p. 284.)

lary projections of connective tissue into the undersurface of the epithelium; the connective tissue papillae account for the designation of this layer as papillary. The presence of papillae at the interface between the epithelium and lamina propria is thought to contribute to the relative immobility of the masticatory mucosa. At the ultrastructural level, the interface between epithelium and lamina propria is also irregular. In addition, the electron microscope shows special fibrils, called *anchoring fibrils,* which enhance the stability of the epithelial-connective tissue interface. The loose connective tissue of the papillae contains capillaries and nerve fibers. Some of the nerve fibers extend into the epithelium as naked intraepithelial sensory nerve endings. Some papillae also contain Meissner's corpuscles.

In certain places, as indicated in Figure 15.1, the hard palate contains a distinct submucosa; elsewhere, the mucosa is attached directly to bone. The areas of direct mucosal attachment to bone are along the perimeter of the hard palate where it meets the gingiva and along a midline band called the *raphe.* The submucosa in the anterior portions of the hard palate contains adipose tissue; the submucosa in the posterior portion of the hard palate contains glands. The glands in the submucosa of the hard palate are continuous with those of the

soft palate and, like them, they are mucous glands. The submucosa of the hard palate contains thick collagenous fibers that extend as bands from the mucosa to the bone (Fig. 15.3). These contribute to the relative immobility of the palatine mucosa. The gingiva, also part of the masticatory mucosa, is considered after the section on teeth.

Lining Mucosa

The lining mucosa is found on the lips, cheeks, alevolar mucosa, floor of the mouth, undersurface of the tongue, and soft palate. This mucosa covers the musculature of lips, cheeks, and tongue; bones (alveolar mucosa); and glands. It is relatively distensible and it adjusts to the movements of the underlying muscles.

The lining mucosa consists of stratified squamous epithelium and lamina propria. Generally, the epithelium is nonkeratinized, although in some places it may be parakeratinized. However, the epithelium of the vermilion border of the lip is keratinized. The nonkeratinized lining epithelium is thicker than keratinized epithelium (see Atlas section, Plate 71). It consists of three layers: stratum basale, stratum spinosum, and stratum superficiale, that is, the superficial or surface layer. The cells of the mucosal epithelium are similar to those

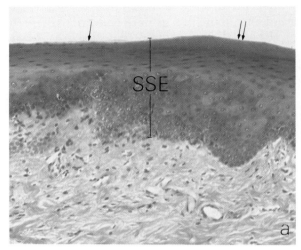

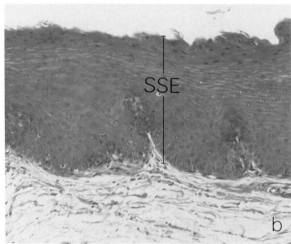

Figure 15.2. Light micrographs showing stratified squamous epithelium (SSE) and connective tissue of the mucosa of the hard palate (human). On the right side of **(a)**, the epithelium is keratinized and the flattened surface cells **(double arrows)** are devoid of nuclei. On the left side of the same figure, the flattened surface cells **(single arrow)** display the same staining characteristics as the keratinized cells, except that they retain their nuclei: they are parakeratinized. **(b)** Another area from the same specimen of the hard palate. The stratified squamous epithelium is nonkeratinized.

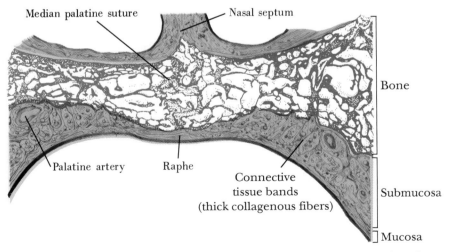

Figure 15.3. Frontal section through hard palate. Connective tissue bands traverse the submucosa and join the mucosa to the periosteum of the bone in the hard palate. Note the absence of a submucosa at the raphe. (Based on Bhaskar SN (ed): *Orban's Oral Histology and Embryology,* 9th ed. St. Louis, CV Mosby, 1980.)

of the epidermis of the skin, namely, keratinocytes, Langerhans cells, melanocytes, and Merkel cells.

The lamina propria contains connective tissue papillae that project into the undersurface of the epithelium. As in the masticatory mucosa, a basal lamina separates the epithelium from the connective tissue; nevertheless, some nerve fibers penetrate the basal lamina and enter the epithelium to function as naked nerve receptors. Meissner's corpuscles are also present in some papillae. The connective tissue papillae of the lining mucosa are not nearly as numerous nor as deep as those found in the masticatory mucosa. Indeed, the sharp contrast between the numerous deep papillae of the gingiva and the shallow and few papillae of the alveolar muscosa allows for a ready identification of the two different regions in a histological section (see Fig. 15.19).

A submucosa is present in most regions of the oral cavity that are covered by lining mucosa, an exception being the undersurface of the tongue. In the lips and cheeks, the submucosa contains bands of collagen and elastic fibers that bind the mucosa to the underlying muscle. It is felt that the elasticity of this submucosal connective tissue, as well as the elasticity of the lamina propria, prevents excessive folding of the mucosa, which could lead to injury while chewing if such folds were caught between the teeth. The submucosa contains the minor salivary glands of the lips, tongue, and cheeks. However, the buccal glands often extend into the substance of the buccinator muscle and sometimes they are found on the outer surface of the muscle. An unusual feature of buccal mucosa is the occasional presence of isolated sebaceous glands, without an associated hair. These sebaceous glands are found just lateral to the corner of the mouth and they are visible as small white areas, called *Fordyce spots.*

The submucosa of the entire oral cavity contains the larger blood vessels, lymphatic vessels, and nerves, all of which, in turn, supply the subepithelial neurovascular networks of the lamina propria.

TONGUE AND SPECIALIZED MUCOSA

The dorsal surface of the tongue is divided anatomically into two parts, an anterior two-thirds and a posterior one-third, by the *sulcus terminalis* (Fig. 15.4). This sulcus is in the form of a shallow V with its apex directed posteriorly. The apex coincides with the location of a depression or pit called the *foramen cecum.* This is a developmental remnant of the thyroglossal duct, and it marks the surface area from which, at an early developmental period, the epithelium grew downward to form the thyroid gland. Remnants of the duct may persist and form cysts or a small mass of lingual thyroid tissue.

The region of the tongue behind the sulcus terminalis is referred to as the *root,* or *base,* of the tongue. It contains numerous oval and rounded elevations that mark the presence of the lingual tonsils. These contain lymph nodules typically with germinal centers; and epithelial crypt may be associated with the tonsil. Lymphocytes invade much of the overlying stratified squamous epithelium so that the boundary between epithelium and connective tissue is obscured. Elsewhere, where lymph nodules are not present, the mucosa displays the general properties of lining mucosa. There is no distinct submucosa. The posterior lingual salivary glands extend into the muscle layer that constitutes the main mass of the tongue; they are mucous glands.

Lingual Papillae

Anterior to the sulcus terminalis, the tongue contains numerous papillae creating a specialized mucosa (Fig. 15.4). The three main types are *filiform,* *fungiform,* and *circumvallate papillae.* A fourth type located at the edges of the tongue are the *foliate papillae.* Although in adult humans they may be poorly defined in many cases, those that are well developed appear as a series of linear ridges separated by a series of grooves. A section cut at a right angle to these papillae appears as a series of folds in which taste buds are located in the facing walls of the neighboring papillae (See Atlas section, Plate 65, Fig. 1).

Of the three main types, the filiform papillae are the most numerous; they are also the smallest. They consist of a connective tissue core covered by stratified squamous keratinized epithelium. The filiform papilla tapers to a point that is aimed backward. In longitudinal sections through a filiform papilla, the convex dorsal surface typically has a shoulder of epithelium at its anterior base. These papillae are distributed over the entire dorsal surface of the anterior portion of the tongue and they contain no taste buds (See Atlas section, Plate 64, Fig. 1).

Fungiform papillae are mushroom-shaped projections on the dorsal tongue surface, singly interspersed among the filiform papillae. Normally they are just visible at the gross level, appearing as small red spots. (They appear white in Figure 15.4 because the specimen is from a cadaver and the blood that ordinarily shows through the thin epithelial surface of the papilla has drained from the

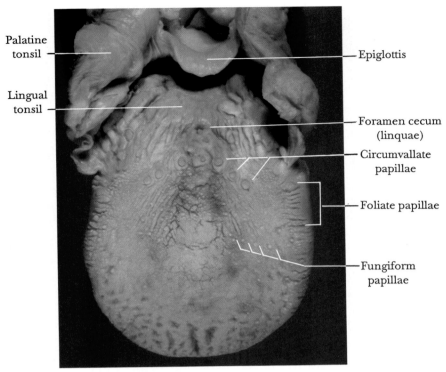

Palatine tonsil

Lingual tonsil

Epiglottis

Foramen cecum (linquae)

Circumvallate papillae

Foliate papillae

Fungiform papillae

Figure 15.4. Photograph of a human tongue. Circumvallate papallae are positioned as a V separating the anterior two-thirds of the tongue from the posterior third. Fungiform and filiform papillae are on the anterior portion of the dorsal tongue surface; the uneven contour of the posterior tongue surface is due to lingual tonsils. The palatine tonsil is at the junction between the oral cavity and the pharynx. (Speciman courtesy of Dr. G. Von Hagens.)

site.) Fungiform papillae contain a connective tissue core and a stratified squamous epithelial surface. Taste buds are present on their dorsal surface, but may be absent in a given section. There is a disease called *familial dysautonomia* and, interestingly, one of the physiological defects in this disease is the inability to taste. This is associated with the absence not only of taste buds, but also of fungiform papillae. The absence of fungiform papillae in the newborn, a relatively simple clinical determination, is an indicator of the disease.

There are approximately 7 to 9 circumvallate papillae arranged in the form of a "V" just anterior and roughly parallel to the sulcus terminalis. These papillae are large and round when viewed from above (Fig. 15.4). They are surrounded by a deep trench. The core of the circumvallate papilla consists of connective tissue and this is covered with stratified squamous epithelium. The epithelium that forms both walls of the trench contains numerous taste buds (see Atlas section, Plate 65, Fig. 2). Ducts of lingual glands open into the bottom of the trench surrounding the circumvallate

papilla. These are the *von Ebner's glands;* they are serous secreting glands.

The undersurface of the tongue has properties of the lining mucosa. However, as already noted, it contains no submucosa. It presents a smooth contour, without any notable surface specializations. The epithelium is thinner than that of the dorsal surface and usually nonkeratinized. However, it may exhibit a parakeratinized or, in some instances, a keratinized epithelium. The connective tissue of the mucosa is similar to that of the dorsal surface, but the papillae, although numerous, do not extend as deep into the epithelium.

Taste Buds

Taste buds are present on fungiform, circumvallate, and foliate papillae. They are also present in the mucous membrane of the pharynx, particularly on the epiglottis. In a histological section, the taste bud appears as a plump, oval, pale-staining body whose long axis extends through the full thickness of the epithelium (Fig. 15.5). The apex of

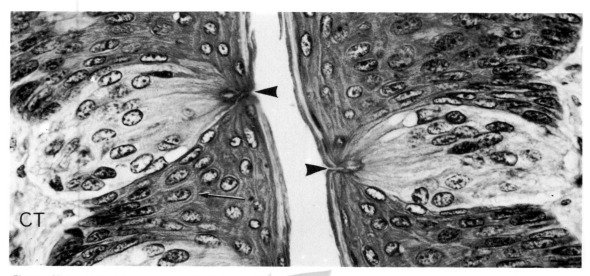

Figure 15.5. Light micrograph of taste buds. The taste buds appear as the light oval structures extending through the full thickness of the epithelium from the connective tissue (CT) to the surface. Here the taste bud opens at the surface by means of a small pore (**arrowheads**). Although three cell types are present in the taste bud, their specific identification in routine paraffin sections is not realistic. Note the intercellular "bridges" between the cells in the stratified squamous epithelium (**arrow**). × 640.

the taste bud just reaches the epithelial surface, having access to the oral cavity through a small opening in the epithelium called the *taste pore.*

Three types of cells are present in the taste bud (Fig. 15.6). Two of these are elongate and extend from the basal lamina to the taste pore; they are the *supporting* and the *sensory* or *neuroepithelial cells.* Near the taste pore the cells taper, and each cell sends microvilli through the taste pore. A third type of cell, the *basal cell,* is located at the periphery of the taste bud near the basal lamina. It is thought to give rise to the other two cells types, whose average life span has been calculated to be about 10 days.

At the taste pore, the microvilli are surrounded by an amorphous, dense substance. This is thought to be a secretory product of the supporting cells since similar material is seen in these cells. Nerve fibers penetrate the basal lamina of the taste bud and make contact with the neuroepithelial cells. These nerve fibers are contained in the facial (VII) nerve, glossopharyngeal (IX) nerve, and vagus (X) nerve. A more detailed description of the overall nerve supply of the tongue is given below.

Muscles of the Tongue

The substance of the tongue contains striated muscle. The muscles are both extrinsic (having one attachment outside of the tongue) and intrinsic (confined entirely to the tongue without external attachment). Generally the groups of muscle fibers are arranged in three planes, each at approximate right angles to the other two planes. This arrangement of muscle fibers is found only in the tongue and allows for easy histological identification of this tissue as lingual muscle. Variable amounts of adipose tissue are found between the muscle fiber groups.

Nerve Supply

The nerve supply to the tongue is complex, involving several cranial nerves. The musculature of the tongue is innervated by the hypoglossal (XII) nerve. Special sensation (taste) for the anterior two-thirds of the tongue is served by the facial (VII) nerve, and for the posterior one-third by the glossopharyngeal (IX) nerve. General sensation for the anterior two thirds is served by the trigeminal (V) nerve and for the posterior one-third by the glossopharyngeal (IX) nerve. In addition, the tongue has both a sympathetic and parasympathetic innervation for blood vessels and glands. Cell bodies of neurons (ganglion cells) are often seen within the tongue. These belong to postganglionic parasympathetic neurons, and they are destined for the minor salivary glands within the tongue. (Sympathetic postganglionic neurons have their cell body in the superior cervical ganglion.)

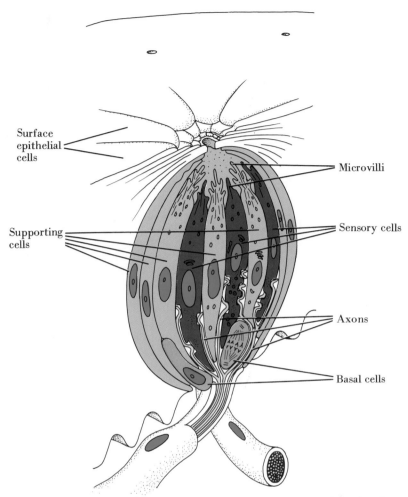

Figure 15.6. Taste bud showing supporting, sensory, and basal cells. One of the basal cells is in the process of dividing. Nerve fibers terminate about the sensory cells. (Based on Warwick, R, Williams PL: *Gray's Anatomy,* 35th British ed., 1973.)

TOOTH AND SUPPORTING STRUCTURES

In the human, there are 10 deciduous teeth in each jaw: a central incisor, lateral incisor, canine, and two molar teeth one each side. These are replaced over a period of years by 16 permanent teeth: a central incisor, lateral incisor, canine, two premolar teeth, and three molar teeth on each side. The premolar teeth and molar teeth have more than one root; the incisor and canine teeth have one root each. Types of teeth vary in number of roots and general shape, but all teeth contain the same tissues, and these can be illustrated by the consideration of a tooth with a single root (Fig. 15.7).

The central portion of the tooth consists of a *pulp cavity* that contains soft tissue called the *dental pulp.* The pulp cavity is surrounded by a relatively thick layer of mineralized tissue, the *dentin,* except where the pulp cavity opens to the exterior of the tooth via an *apical foramen* in its root. Blood vessels and nerves pass through the apical foramen in reaching or leaving the pulp cavity. The dentin is covered by two different mineralized tissues. The part of the tooth that projects into the oral cavity is covered by *enamel;* the part of the tooth imbedded in the jaw is covered by *cementum.* These parts of the tooth are called the *crown* and *root,* respectively. Both clinical and anatomical crowns are defined (see Fig. 15.7). The clinical crown is the part of the tooth that appears in the oral cavity; the anatomical crown is the part of the tooth that is covered by enamel.

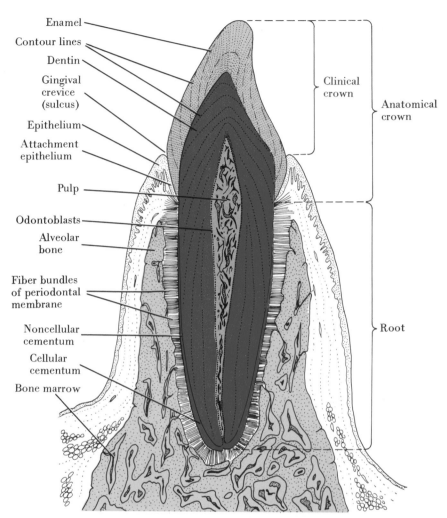

Enamel
Contour lines
Dentin
Gingival crevice (sulcus)
Epithelium
Attachment epithelium
Pulp
Odontoblasts
Alveolar bone
Fiber bundles of periodontal membrane
Noncellular cementum
Cellular cementum
Bone marrow

Clinical crown
Anatomical crown
Root

Figure 15.7. Schematic diagram of a tooth embedded in the jaw. The three mineralized components of the tooth are dentin, enamel, and cementum. The central soft core of the tooth is the pulp. The periodontal ligament (membrane) contains bundles of collagenous fibers that bind the tooth to the surrounding alveolar bone. The clinical crown of the tooth is the portion which projects into the oral cavity; the anatomical crown is the portion of the tooth covered by enamel. (Based on Ham AW, Cormack DH: *Histology,* 8th ed. Philadelphia, JB Lippincott, 1979.)

The tooth is fastened to the surrounding bone by collagenous fibers that are part of the *periodontal ligament* (membrane). The space in the bone that accommodates the tooth is called the *alveolus* and the bone to which the periodontal fibers (collagenous) are attached is called *alveolar bone.* The crown and root meet at the *neck,* or *cervix,* of the tooth, and here, epithelium of the oral mucosa contacts the tooth to form a dentogingival junction. The oral mucous membrane attaching to the tooth also attaches firmly to the crest of the alveolar bone and this firmly attached mucous membrane is called the *gingiva.*

Histological Features of the Tooth Tissues

Because certain parts of the tooth are highly mineralized, sections of teeth are prepared by methods similar to those used to prepare sections of bone, namely, by means of ground sections and by means of stained demineralized sections. The ground section is most often used to study an extracted, or exfoliated, tooth. As in the preparation of bone, the ground section displays mineralized tissue, but destroys soft tissue, while demineralization removes mineral and retains soft tissue. De-

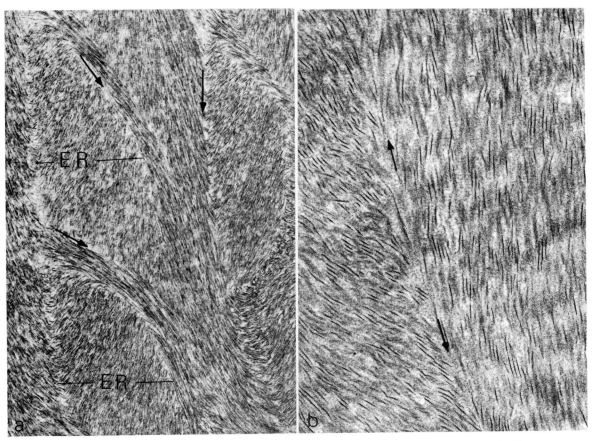

Figure 15.8. Electron micrograph of young enamel. **(a)** Enamel rods (ER) are cut obliquely. The **arrows** mark the boundaries between adjacent rods (× 14,700). **(b)** Parts of two adjacent rods are seen at higher magnification (× 60,000). **Arrows** mark the boundary between the two rods. The dark needle-like objects are young apatite crystals; the substance between the apatite is the organic matrix of the developing enamel. As the enamel matures, the apatite crystals grow and the bulk of the organic matrix is removed.

mineralized sections have the advantage that they can be used to view a section of a tooth in situ and, thus, to reveal the relationship of the tooth to the adjacent supporting structures. However, in routinely demineralized sections of a mature tooth, the enamel is dissolved and lost. Diagrams of a tooth showing features of both enamel and soft tissues are composite diagrams that combine the data derived from both ground and demineralizd sections.

Enamel

Enamel is a cell-free extracellular tissue. It is approximately 96 percent mineral in the mature tooth. Histologically, the enamel consists of *rods* (Fig. 15.8), or *prisms,* bound together by interprismatic substance. The rods extend through the thickness of the enamel from the dentinoenamel junction to the enamel surface (Fig. 15.9). Also seen in a longitudinal ground section are lines roughly at right angles to the direction of the enamel rods. These *contour lines of Retzius* reflect the incremental pattern of enamel formation (see Fig. 15.7).

Enamel is an extracellular product of enamel organ cells. Although the enamel of an erupted tooth is devoid of cells, it is not a static tissue. Erupted enamel is under the influence of the salivary glands through their production of saliva without which the enamel is subject to decay.

Enamel Formation (Amelogenesis). Enamel is produced by the *ameloblasts* with the close cooperation of other enamel organ cells (the overall aspects of enamel organ histology are considered in Atlas section, Plate 70). The major stages of amelogenesis are the period of matrix production, or the secretory stage, and the period of maturation. Several transitional and substages can also be identified.

In the formation of mineralized tissues of the tooth, dentin is produced first. Then, partially

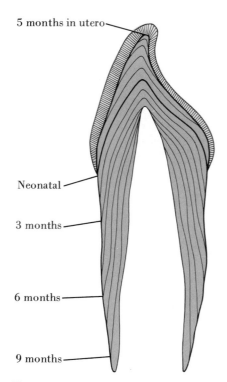

Figure 15.9. Schematic diagram of partially formed tooth. The enamel is depicted to show rods extending from the dentinoenamel junction to the surface of the tooth. Although the full thickness of the enamel is formed, the full thickness of the dentin has not yet been established. The contour lines within the dentin show the extent to which the dentin has developed at a particular time as labeled in the illustration. Note that the pulp cavity in the center of the tooth becomes smaller as the dentin develops. Contour lines showing increments of enamel development also exist but are not shown in this figure. They are depicted in Figure 15.7. (Based on Schour I, Massler M: *J Am Dent Assoc* vol. 23, 1936.)

mineralized enamel matrix (see Fig. 15.8) is deposited directly on the surface of the previously formed dentin. The cells producing this partially mineralized organic matrix are referred to as *secretory ameloblasts.* These cells produce an organic proteinaceous matrix by activity of the rough endoplasmic reticulum (rER), Golgi apparatus, and secretory granules. The secretory ameloblasts continue to produce enamel matrix until the full thickness of the future enamel is achieved. Maturation of the partially mineralized enamel matrix involves the removal of organic material as well as continued influx of calcium and phosphate into the maturing enamel. Cells involved in this second stage

of enamel formation are referred to as *maturation ameloblasts.* They function primarily as transport epithelium, moving substances into and out of the maturing enamel. Maturation ameloblasts are formed by a reorganization of secretory ameloblasts. Calcium enters the maturing enamel in cycles, and maturation ameloblasts undergo cyclical alterations in their morphology that correspond to the cyclical entry of calcium into the enamel.

Secretory ameloblasts are narrow, highly polarized, columnar cells (Fig. 15.10). They are di-

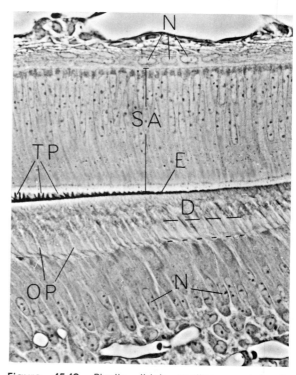

Figure 15.10. Plastic thick section, unstained, viewed with phase contrast optics showing enamel organ cells and odontoblasts as they begin to produce enamel (E) and dentin (D), respectively. Young enamel is deposited by secretory ameloblasts (SA) onto the previously formed dentin. The enamel appears dark in the illustration. On the left, the enamel surface displays a characteristic picket fence pattern due to the sharp contrast between the lightly stained Tomes' processes (TP) of the secretory ameloblasts and the darkly stained young enamel product that partly surrounds the cellular processes. The upper N marks nuclei of cells constituting the stratum intermedium layer. Other enamel organ cells are not labeled. The lower N marks nuclei of odontoblasts in the basal pole of the cell. The apical pole of the odontoblast cell body extends as far as the **broken line** composed of short segments. At this point, odontoblastic processes (OP) continue from the cell body through the predentin (unlabeled) and into the dentin. The **broken line** composed of long segments marks the boundary between predentin and dentin.

rectly adjacent to the developing enamel. At the apical pole of the cell is a process, **Tomes' process,** which is surrounded by the developing enamel. A cluster of mitochondria in the basal extremity of the cell accounts for the eosinophilic staining of this region in hematoxylin and eosin-stained (H&E) paraffin sections. Adjacent to the mitochondria is the nucleus; in the main column of cytoplasm are the rER, Golgi, secretory granules, and other cell elements. Junctional complexes are present at both apical and basal extremities. Contractile filaments are joined to these junctional complexes and these are believed to move the secretory ameloblast over the developing enamel. The rod produced by the ameloblast follows in the wake of the cell. Thus, in mature enamel, the direction of the enamel rod is a record of the path taken earlier by the secretory ameloblast.

At their basal poles, the secretory ameloblasts are adjacent to a layer of enamel organ cells called the **stratum intermedium.** The plasma membrane of these cells and that of the basal pole of the ameloblasts is positive for alkaline phosphatase, an enzyme presumably active in calcification. Stellate enamel organ cells are external to the stratum intermedium and separated from the adjacent blood vessels by basal laminae.

The main histological feature that marks the cycles of maturation ameloblasts is the presence of a striated, or ruffled, border (Fig. 15.11). Maturation ameloblasts with a striated border occupy about 70 percent of a specific cycle and those that are smooth-ended are about 30 percent of a specific cycle. Cells adjacent to the maturation ameloblasts are stellate; they are referred to as papillary cells (there is no stratum intermedium during enamel maturation). The main feature of maturation ameloblasts and the adjacent papillary cells is the presence of numerous mitochondria. This is indicative of cellular activity that requires large amounts of energy and is a reflection of the fact that the maturation ameloblasts (and the adjacent papillary cells) function as transport epithelium.

The matrix of developing enamel contains three major proteins: **amelogenins, enamelins,** and **tuft protein**; mature enamel contains enamelins and tuft protein. Accordingly, it is concluded that amelogenins are removed during enamel maturation. Tuft protein is located near the dentinoenamel junction. It is present in enamel tufts and accounts for the fact that the enamel tufts are hypomineralized, that is, they have a higher percentage of organic material than the remainder of the mature enamel. The maturation of the developing enamel results in the continued mineralization of enamel so that it becomes the hardest substance in the body.

Probably the most distinctive feature of enamel is the large size of its hydroxyapatite crystals. They are considerably larger than hydroxyapatite crystals of other mineralized tissues of the body. The components of biological hydroxyapa-

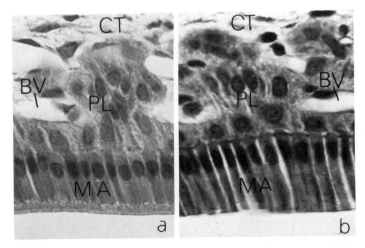

Figure 15.11. Light micrographs of maturation ameloblasts (MA): demineralized H&E, paraffin sections. The maturing enamel has been lost owing to action of the demineralizing solution, and the space below the ameloblasts previously occupied by the enamel appears empty. Maturation ameloblasts with a striated border are shown in **(a)**, and smooth-ended maturation ameloblasts are shown in **(b)**. At the basal pole of the maturation ameloblasts are the cells of the papillary layer (PL). A stratum intermedium is no longer present during the maturation process. BV, blood vessels; CT, connective tissue.

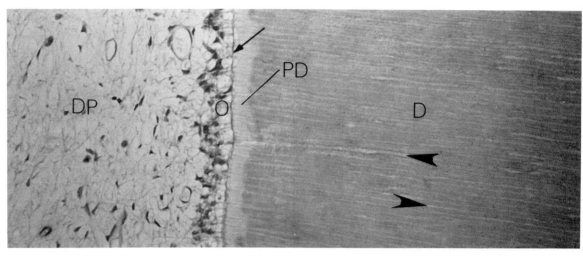

Figure 15.12. Light micrograph of human tooth, decalcified, stained with H&E. On the left is the dental pulp (DP), the soft tisue core of the tooth which resembles embryonic connective tissue, even in the adult tooth. Dentin (D) is on the right; two **arrowheads** indicate the dentinal tubules in dentin which contain the odontoblastic processes. The odontoblasts (O) are adjacent to the unmineralized dentin called the predentin (PD). At their apical extremities, the odontoblasts form junctional complexes which separate the predentin from the lateral intercellular space of the odontoblasts. This boundary, formed by the junctional complexes of the odontoblasts, appears as a membrane (**arrow**), due in large part to microfilaments within the odontoblasts which are attached to the junctional complexes. × 200.

tites are not stoichiometric with respect to the theoretical formula, $Ca_{10}(PO_4)_6(OH)_2$. For example, hydroxyapatite contains numerous trace elements, some of which are incorporated into the crystal at the time of tooth formation and others after the tooth has erupted. This is the case with the fluoride ion, which can be incorporated by topical application of fluoride solutions or in toothpaste. The fluoride increases the resistance of enamel to caries.

Dentin

The bulk of the tooth substance consists of dentin. It is immediately under the enamel in the crown and under the cementum in the root; it forms the thick, mineralized wall of the pulp cavity. Dentin is approximately 70 percent mineral hydroxyapatite) and 30 percent organic material. The bulk of the organic material, as much as 90 percent, consists of collagen; the remainder consists of other proteins, including phosphoproteins, and glycosaminoglycans. Because of the relatively high organic content of dentin, extremely useful knowledge of dentin structure can be obtained from both demineralized and ground sections.

The cells associated with dentin are called *odontoblasts.* These cells have cylindrical cell body and a long cytoplasmic extension, the *odontoblastic process.* The cell body is located at the surface of the dentin (actually, the predentin; see Fig. 15.10), and the odontoblastic process extends into the dentin. The space containing the odontoblastic

process is the *dentinal tubule.* These tubules containing the odontoblastic process extend through the full thickness of the dentin.

In demineralized paraffin sections of a tooth, the matrix of the dentin (Fig. 15.12) stains with eosin; the elongated dentinal tubules are roughly parallel to each other, and according to the plane of section, they appear elongate, oval, or circular. The cell body of the odontoblast contains a profusion of organelles found in collagen-producing cells, namely, a large amount of rER, a large Golgi apparatus, secretory granules, mitochondria, and related vesicles (Fig. 15.13). Less conspicuous are the microtubules and cytoplasmic filaments. The Golgi apparatus contains a collagen precursor which is filamentous in form. The orderly arrangement of granules (interpreted as containing calcium) on the filaments of certain Golgi vesicles accounts for their designation as *abacus bodies* (Fig. 15.14). The abacus bodies become more condensed as they mature into the secretory granules. The young odontoblastic process (Fig. 15.15) is broad where it joins the cell body and quickly tapers to a gradually narrowing cylinder. It contains chiefly microtubules, cytoplasmic filaments, secretory granules, and vesicles. Mitochondria are also sometimes seen in the process.

At the apical pole of the odontoblast cell body, a junctional complex joins neighboring odontoblasts, evidently creating a microcompartment that separates the predentin from the lateral intercellular space. The junctional complex does not create a

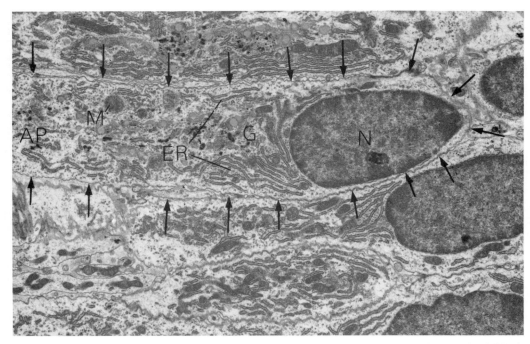

Figure 15.13. Electron micrograph of odontoblasts. The plasma membrane of one odontoblast has been marked with **arrows**. The cell contains a large amount of rough endoplasmic reticulum (ER) and a large Golgi (G). The odontoblastic process is not shown; it would extend from the apical pole (AP) of the cell. The black objects in the Golgi region are abacus bodies. The tissue has been treated with pyroantimonate, which forms a black precipitate with calcium. N, nucleus; M, mitochondria.

complete seal since it allows for the passage of small bundles of collagen fibers *(von Korff's fibers)* during the early formation of dentin, and it allows for the passage of nerve fibers.

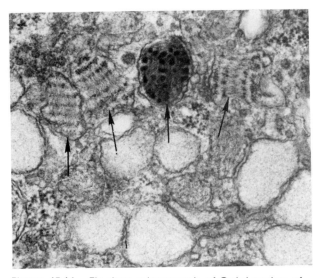

Figure 15.14. Electron micrograph of Golgi region of odontoblast showing numerous large vesicles. Abacus bodies **(arrows)** contain parallel arrays of filaments and these are studded with granules.

Dentinogenesis. Dentin is the first mineralized component of the tooth to be deposited. It is formed by odontoblasts, and during the formation of the very outermost dentin, referred to as mantle dentin, also by subodontoblastic cells which produce von Korff's fibers. The odontoblasts differentiate from cells at the periphery of the dental papilla. The progenitor cells have the appearance of typical mesenchymal cells, that is, they contain little cytoplasm. During their differentiation into odontoblasts, cytoplasmic volume and organelles characteristic of collagen-producing cells increase. The cells form a layer at the periphery of the dental papilla, and they secrete the organic matrix of dentin, called **predentin,** at their apical pole (the end of the cell away from the dental papilla). As the thickness of the predentin increases, the odontoblasts move or are displaced centrally (see Fig. 15.9). A wave of mineralization follows the receding odontoblasts, and this mineralized product is the dentin. As the cells move centrally, the odontoblastic process becomes increasingly long, its greatest length being surrounded by the mineralized dentin. In newly formed dentin, the wall of the dentinal tubule is simply the edge of the mineralized dentin. With time, the dentin immediately surrounding the dentinal tubule becomes more highly mineralized; this more mineralized sheath

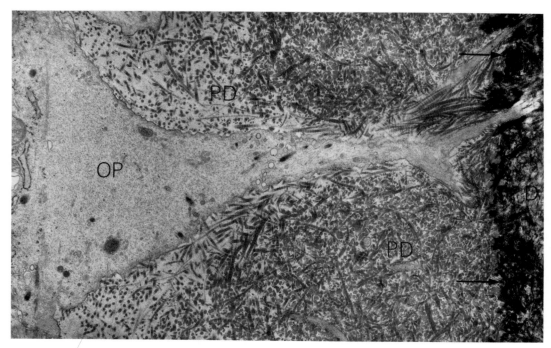

Figure 15.15. Electron micrograph of odontoblastic process (OP) of young odontoblast. The process extends through predentin (PD) and into dentin (D). Profiles in predentin are collagen fibrils, smaller near the cell body of the odontoblast and larger at the mineralization front **(arrows)**.

of dentin is referred to as the ***peritubular dentin.*** The remainder of the dentin is then referred to as the ***intertubular dentin.***

Ground and demineralized sections of dentin show incremental lines, called ***incremental lines of von Ebner,*** which reflect the cyclical patterns of cellular activity during dentin formation (see Fig. 15.9). Certain lines called ***lines of Owen*** are more pronounced. The line of Owen that forms at the time of birth is referred to as the ***neonatal line.*** These lines are much like the growth rings of a tree; they can be used in some cases to identify when certain unusual substances, such as lead, have been incorporated into the tooth. The investigation of these lines might prove to be useful in forensic medicine, especially with new developments in analytical scanning electron microscopy. From the point of view of developmental biology, von Ebner lines of dentin (and the lines of Retzius of enamel) serve to show where odontoblasts (and ameloblasts) were positioned at a particular time in the development of the tooth.

Dental Pulp

The dental pulp has a shape that approximates the shape of the tooth. It is contained within the pulp cavity, bounded by the mineralized dentin. The dental pulp decreases in size as dentin formation continues (see Fig. 15.9). In the adult tooth, the pulp cavity and the size of the dental pulp are their smallest, and extensions of the pulp into the cusps of the crown, called ***pulpal horns,*** are more pronounced. Pulpal horns have a high concentration of nerve fibers, and the dentin over the pulpal horns has a higher number of dentinal tubules which contain nerve fibers.

Histologically, the dental pulp consists of odontoblasts at its perimeter (these are also identified as the cells associated with dentin), fibroblasts, macrophages, mast cells, and migrating cells from the blood (see Fig. 15.12). In the uninflamed pulp, the fibroblasts are the most numerous of these cells. They are stellate in shape and contain little cytoplasm in the perinuclear region. The extracellular components of the dental pulp include collagen fibrils arranged in small bundles, but no elastic fibers, and large amounts of ground substance (proteoglycans, with many of the glycosaminoglycans containing sulfate groups).

The pulp cavity contains blood vessels and nerves that enter and leave the pulp as a bundle through the apical foramen. The neurovascular bundle travels to the crown of the tooth where neural and vascular networks form under the odontoblasts. Nerve fibers from the neural networks contact the cell body of some odontoblasts; others pass for a short distance into the dentinal tubules where they contact the odontoblastic process. Because the tooth is especially sensitive at the

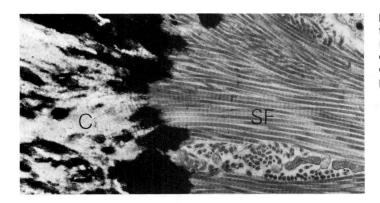

Figure 15.16. Electron micrograph of Sharpey fiber (SF) extending from periodontal ligament (right) into the cementum (C). The Sharpey fiber consists of collagenous fibrils. Those within the cementum are mineralized; those within the periodontal ligament are not mineralized.

dentinoenamel junction where nerve fibers have not been observed, models to explain sensation of the tooth invoke the intermediary of the odontoblast as a receptor and also the fluid in the dentinal tubule as a factor in tooth pain. Whereas the nerve fibers within the dentin clearly subserve pain and have their cell bodies in the trigeminal ganglion, other nerve fibers within the dental pulp belong to the autonomic nervous system. These are fibers with cell bodies in the superior cervical ganglion and they subserve vascular responses.

Capillary loops from the vascular networks enter the layer of odontoblasts. These capillaries are fenestrated and surrounded by a basal lamina. Lymphatic vessels have been described in the dental pulp, but their identification is difficult.

Cementum

The cementum is a mineralized tissue that covers the roots of teeth.[1] It begins at the cervix of the tooth where the enamel terminates. In most instances, the cementum overlaps the edge of the enamel for a short distance; less often the enamel and cementum do not actually meet, and a narrow region of dentin is exposed at the cementoenamel junction. At the other end of the tooth the cementum often extends on the dentinal surface into the apical canal for a variable but short distance. In several respects, cementum is a bone-like tissue. Its mineral content is about 45 to 50 percent, close to that of bone; its organic and water content is about 50 to 55 percent. As with bone, the main organic component is collagen; proteoglycans are also present in substantial amount. As with all the other mineralized tissues of the body, hydroxyapatite, containing trace elements, is the mineral form.

In some locations cementum contains *cementocytes* in lacunae; this cementum is called *cellular*

cementum. The cells contain numerous processes within canaliculi radiating from the lacunae. In contrast to bone, the canaliculi do not appear to interconnect throughout the cementum. In other regions, the cementum contains no cells; this is the *noncellular cementum.* The major difference between bone and cementum is that cementum is avascular, whereas bone is vascular. Another point to note is that under normal circumstances cementum is not resorbed during physiological movement, or drift, of a tooth. Thus, during tooth movement, the adjacent alveolar bone is resorbed, but the cementum is not. During shedding of deciduous teeth, however, the cementum is resorbed along with dentin by osteoclast-like cells.

The primary function of cementum is to provide for the attachment of collagen fibers of the periodontal ligament. Those collagen fibers that extend from the periodontal ligament into the cementum are called *Sharpey's fibers* (Fig. 15.16). The arrangement is similar to that of Sharpey's fibers in bone.

A relatively rare hereditary disease called *hypophosphatasia* involves premature loss of the anterior deciduous teeth. The exfoliated teeth are practically devoid of cementum.

Periodontal Ligament

The periodontal ligament is the fibrous connective tissue joining the tooth and its surrounding bone. The ligament is also called the *periodontal membrane,* but neither of these terms describes its structure and function adequately. The periodontal ligament provides for attachment, support, bone remodeling (during movement of a tooth), nutrition of adjacent structures, proprioception, and tooth eruption. The first two of these functions are the most apparent.

A histological section of the periodontal ligament shows it to contain areas of both dense and loose connective tissue. The dense connective tissue contains collagen fibers and fibroblasts that are

[1] Continuously growing teeth, such as the incisor teeth of rodents and the molar teeth of rabbits, have a layer of enamel over part of the unerupted portion of the tooth.

elongate and parallel to the long axis of the collagen fibers (Fig. 15.17). The fibroblasts move back and forth, leaving behind a trail of collagen fibers. Periodontal fibroblasts have also been shown to contain internalized collagen fibrils that are digested by the hydrolytic enzymes of the cytoplasmic lysosomes. These observations indicate that not only do the fibroblasts produce collagen fibrils, but they also resorb collagen fibrils, thereby adjusting continuously to the demands of tooth movement.

The areas of loose connective tissue contain blood vessels and nerve endings in addition to the cells and thin collagenous fibrils.

The periodontal ligament contains longitudinally disposed fibers, designated *oxytalan fibers.* They are attached to bone or cementum at one end and possibly to bone or cementum at the other end. Some are attached to blood vessels. Oxytalan fibers stain with special elastic stains; ultrastructurally, they resemble developing elastic fibers, their chief structural component being the microfibril characteristic of developing elastic fibers.

Near the cementum the periodontal ligament contains remnants of the epithelial root sheath. These remnants of epithelium are called the *epithelial rests of Malassez.*

Alveolar Process

The alveolar process contains sockets, or *alveoli,* for the roots of the teeth. A thin layer of compact bone, the *alveolar bone proper,* forms the wall of the alveoli (see Fig. 15.7); it is the bone to which the principal fibers of the periodontal ligament are attached. The remaining parts of the alveolar process are designated as *supporting bone.* They include the cortical plates of the alveolar process, each of which consists of compact bone and spongy bone. The cortical plate fuses with the crest of the alveolar bone proper on the lingual and labial faces of the alveolus.

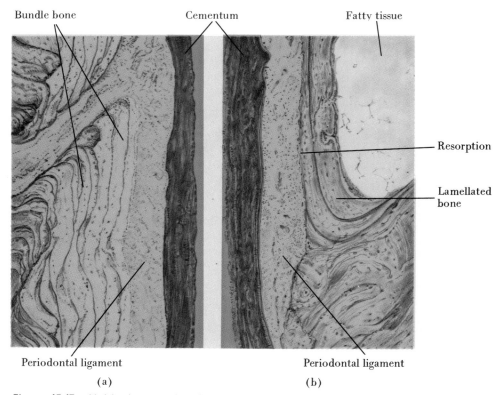

(a)   (b)

Figure 15.17. Light micrographs of periodontal ligament from two sides of a tooth that is moving to the right. Each figure shows cementum, periodontal ligament, and alveolar bone. The other parts of the tooth are not shown. The scalloped edge of the bone (right) is indicative of bone resorption; the layered pattern of bone (left) is indicative of bone formation. As the tooth moves to the right, bone in the path of the tooth is resorbed and, at the same time, bone is deposited in the wake of the tooth. The cells of the periodontal ligament function to provide constant and adjustable attachment of the tooth during this movement.

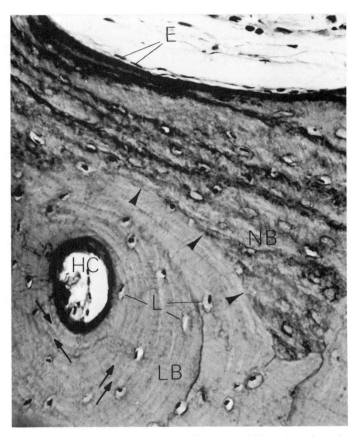

Figure 15.18. Light micrograph of lamellar (LB) and nonlamellar bone (NB); **arrowheads** mark the boundary between the two. The lamellar bone **(lower left)** shows concentric layering **(arrows)** of the matrix around a Haversian canal (HC). Lacunae (L) in the lamellar bone have a tendency to be oriented with their long axis parallel to the concentric lamellae. Dark objects in the lacunae are nuclei of osteocytes. The matrix of the nonlamellar bone does not display a similar layering: the osteocytes are more numerous than those in the lamellar bone and do not display any signs of preferential orientation. The marrow is in the upper part of the illustration and on the surface of the bone are flat lining bone cells that constitute the endosteum (E).

The alveolar bone proper is chiefly lamellar bone, but the surface of the bone also contains areas of nonlamellar **bundle bone** (Fig. 15.18), especially where new bone has been formed and where the collagen fibers of the periodontal ligament are attached. The surface of the alveolar bone proper typically shows regions of bone deposition and bone resorption. This is particularly noticeable where movement of a tooth is in progress. Bone in the path of the moving tooth shows numerous scalloped profiles indicative of resorption, whereas bone behind the moving tooth shows smooth layers of bone indicative of bone formation (see Fig. 15.17).

The loss of alveolar bone, especially at the alveolar crest, is regularly associated with periodontal disease. Also, a tooth that is not in functional occlusion with its opponent tends to lose its supporting bone.

Gingiva

The gingiva is the part of the oral mucous membrane commonly called the gums. It extends for a short distance from the teeth and is firmly attached to both the teeth and the underlying tissue. It is subject to considerable mechanical force during the biting and chewing of food, and its structure reflects features to resist such forces. The gingiva is lined by stratified squamous epithelium; this is usually parakeratinized, although it may also be keratinized or nonkeratinized.

An idealized diagram of the gingiva is shown in Figure 15.19. The junction between the epithelium and the underlying connective tissue is very irregular due to the numerous connective tissue papillae projecting into the undersurface of the epithelium. In contrast, the boundary between epithelium and connective tissue of the lining (non-masticatory) mucosa contains far fewer papillae and, thus, has a much smoother profile.

The part of the epithelium adherent to the tooth is called the **attachment,** or **junctional, epithe-**

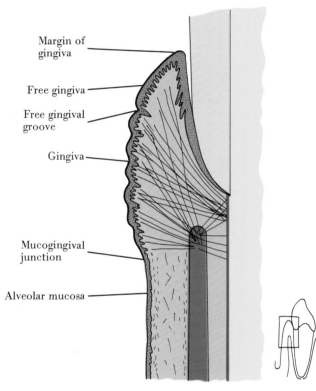

Figure 15.19. Schematic diagram of gingiva. The gingival epithelium is attached to the enamel of the tooth. Here the junction between epithelium and connective tissue is smooth. Elsewhere the gingival epithelium is deeply indented by connective tissue papillae and the junction between the two is irregular. The **black lines** represent collagen fibers from the cementum of the tooth and from the crest of the alveolar bone which extend toward the gingival epithelium. Note the shallow papillae in the lining mucosa (alveolar mucosa), which sharply contrast with those of the gingiva. The schematic diagram of gingiva corresponds to the **rectangular area** of the small diagram. (Based on Bhaskar SN (ed): *Orban's Oral Histology and Embryology,* 9th ed. St. Louis, CV Mosby, 1980, p. 290.)

lium. The epithelium also faces a shallow crevice of variable depth, the **gingival sulcus,** and this epithelium is called the **cervicular epithelium.** Then the epithelium makes a V turn and covers the gingiva as far as the lining mucosa. An imaginary line drawn horizontally from the bottom of the gingival sulcus to the surface of the gingiva marks the extent to the **free gingiva.**

In making contact with the tooth, the epithelial cells secrete a basal lamina-like material that serves as a glue on the tooth surface, and then the cells attach to the basal lamina material by hemidesmosomes. The basal lamina and hemidesmosomes together are referred to as the **epithelial attachment.** The attachment epithelium covers and is attached to the cementum in older individuals where passive tooth eruption and gingival recession cause the roots of the tooth to project into the oral cavity.

The term **periodontium** is applied to those tissues that are involved in attachment of the tooth to the jaw. These include the part of the gingiva facing the tooth, the cementum, the periodontal ligament, and the alveolar bone.

SALIVARY GLANDS

There are two groups of salivary glands; the **major salivary glands,** consisting of the parotid, submandibular, and sublingual glands, and the **minor salivary glands,** consisting of labial, buccal, molar (corresponding to buccal glands, but opposite the molar teeth), lingual, and palatine glands. The major salivary glands are large and have long ducts. Two of the major glands (parotid and submandibular) are located outside of the oral cavity, while the minor salivary glands are chiefly in the submucosa of different parts of the wall of the oral cavity.

The salivary glands all develop by the proliferation of a solid core of cells from the developing oral epithelium. The cord of cells grows into underlying mesenchyme, profuse branching occurs, and the terminal ends, or end pieces, of the cords form solid balls of cells (Fig. 15.20). Degeneration of the innermost cells of this branching network leads to the canalization of the cell cords, which become ducts, and of end-pieces, which become acini.

Most of the saliva is produced by the salivary glands. A smaller amount derives from the gingival sulcus, tonsillar crypts, and general transudation from the epithelial lining. One of the unique features of saliva is the large and variable volume produced. The volume (per weight of tissue) of saliva exceeds that of other digestive secretions by

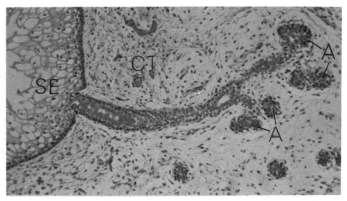

Figure 15.20. Light micrograph of developing salivary gland, H&E section. A cord of cells grows from the surface epithelium (SE) into the underlying connective tissue (CT); branching of the cord occurs; and the terminal ends of the branches develop into acini (A).

as much as 40 times. Perhaps this is related to the fact that saliva has many functions, only some of which are related to digestion.

Structural Features of Salivary Glands

Salivary glands consist of parenchymal and stromal components. The parenchyma is often likened to a bunch of grapes in which the branching stems represent ducts and the grapes represent the acini, the secretory portion of the gland. Despite the general structural similarity of salivary glands, there is considerable variation in the product of

different glands. This variation is reflected in the ultrastructural appearance of the secretory granules and in differences in histological and histochemical properties. It should be noted that the product of the salivary glands involves activity by all components of the gland, namely, acinar end pieces, ducts, and stromal cells.

The minimal physiological parenchymal unit of a salivary gland is referred to as a *salivon* (Fig. 15.21). It consists of an acinus and those duct segments that modify the acinar product. The acinus is composed of pyramidal secretory cells arranged about a central lumen and surrounded by myoepithelial cells. A basal lamina separates the

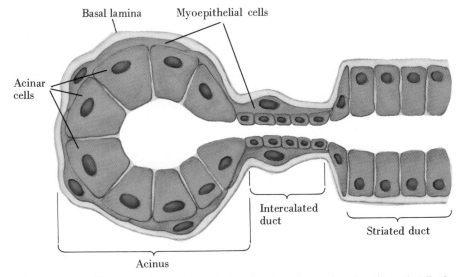

Figure 15.21. Diagram of a salivon, the basic physiological parenchymal unit of a salivary gland. This consists of the acinar cells, the surrounding myoepithelial cells, the intercalated duct, and the striated duct. (Based on Johnson LR (ed): *Gastrointestinal Physiology*, 2nd ed. St. Louis, CV Mosby, 1981, p. 47.)

secretory and myoepithelial cells from the adjacent connective tissue. The lumen of the acinus leads to a duct system that has three distinct segments: the **intercalated duct,** the **striated duct,** and the **excretory duct.** The cells of the intercalated duct are also surrounded by myoepithelial cells.

Acini are made up of either serous or mucous cells. In addition, some of the mucous acini have a cap of serous cells called **demilunes** because of their crescent appearance in certain plains of section. While serous acini are generally spherical, mucous end-pieces are sometimes more tubular. Nevertheless, the term acinus, which is from Latin meaning grape, is used to refer even to the more tubular mucous end-pieces. With respect to human salivary glands, the parotid gland consists only of serous acini (see Atlas section, Plate 67); the sublingual gland consists of mucous acini, many of which have serous demilunes (see Atlas section, Plate 68); and the submandibular gland contains a mix of both serous and mucous acini, the predominant type being serous (see Atlas section, Plate 66). The minor salivary glands are mucous, except for the glands in the tip of the tongue and the von Ebner's glands, which are serous. The latter empty into the trench of the circumvallate papillae.

Serous Cells. The serous cell contains, in addition to cytoplasmic components regularly found in cells, large amounts of rER, free ribosomes, a prominent Golgi, and numerous secretory granules (Fig. 15.22). The secretory granules are found in the apical cytoplasm and most of the other organelles in the basal or perinuclear location. The base of the serous cell may display infoldings of the plasma membrane and basilateral folds in the form of foot processes that interdigitate with similar processes of neighboring cells. Laterally, the neighboring cells are joined near their apical surface by junctional complexes (zonula occludens, zonula adherens, and possibly a macula adherens). A special feature of the salivary gland acinus is that the lumen may extend between neighboring cells as a narrow, serpentine canaliculus, extending almost to the basal lamina. The junctional complex is always located at the bottom of the canaliculus.

In H&E sections, the basal cytoplasm of the serous cell stains with hematoxylin due to the rER and the free ribosomes, whereas the apical region stains with eosin due in large part to the presence of secretory granules.

Mucous Cells. The mucous cell undergoes cycles of activity. During part of the cycle, mucus is synthesized and stored within the cell as mucinogen granules. The product is discharged, and then the cell begins to synthesize mucus again. After discharge of the mucinogen granules, the cell is difficult to distinguish from a serous cell. However, most of the mucous cells apparently contain large numbers of mucinogen granules in their apical cytoplasm. Because the mucinogen is lost in H&E-stained paraffin sections, the apical portion of the cell has an empty appearance. With the transmission electron microscope, the rER, mitochondria, and other components are seen chiefly in the basal portion of the cell; this part of the cell also contains the nucleus, which is typically flattened against the base of the cell (Fig. 15.23). The apical portion of the cell contains numerous mucinogen granules and a large Golgi apparatus, involved in the addition of large amounts of carbohydrate to a protein base. The mucous cells possess apical junctional complexes and intercellular canaliculi similar to those seen between serous cells. If serous demilunes are present, the canaliculi extend to serous cells of demilunes and serve as the delivery route for the secretions of these cells.

Myoepithelial Cells. Myoepithelial cells are contractile cells with numerous cell processes that embrace the basal aspect of the secretory cells of the acini. They are also present about the cells that make up the intercalated ducts. In both locations, the myoepithelial cells are instrumental in moving secretory products toward the excretory duct. Myoepithelial cells are sometimes difficult to identify in H&E sections. The nucleus of such a cell is often seen as a small, round profile near the basement membrane. The contractile filaments stain with eosin and are often recognized as a thin eosinophilic band in the region where the basement membrane is located. The cells are on the epithelial side of the basal lamina (Fig. 15.24).

Duct System. All salivary glands discharge their secretions into the oral cavity by means of excretory ducts. In addition, the major salivary glands contain striated and intercalated ducts.

Intercalated ducts are comprised of short cuboidal cells (see Atlas Section, Plate 66). In the simplest form, the cells contain no special ultrastructural features to suggest their function except for the presence of apical junctional complexes that separate the lumen of the duct from the lateral intercellular space. In some locations, the cuboidal cells contain mucinogen granules and the mucus becomes part of the secretion of the gland. Intercalated ducts are most prominent in those salivary glands, such as the parotid gland, in which the secretion is watery. In mucous-secreting glands, such as the sublingual gland, the intercalated ducts are extremely short and, thus, extremely difficult to identify.

Striated ducts are formed by columnar cells whose cytoplasm stains intensely with eosin and

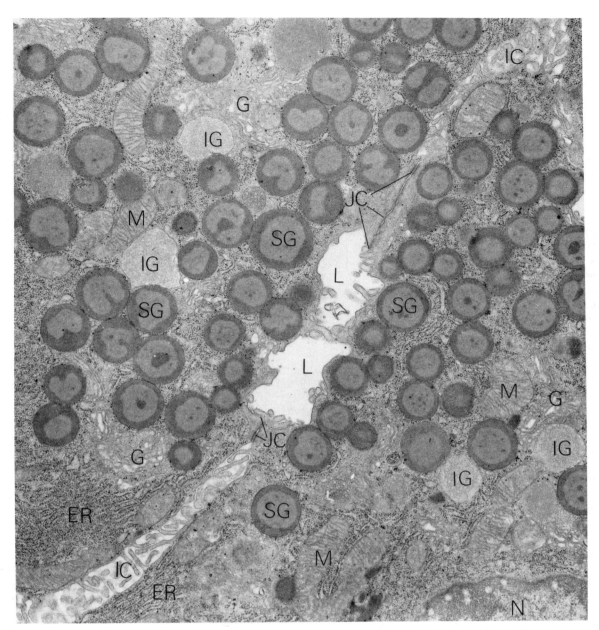

Figure 15.22. Electron micrograph showing the apical portion of parotid gland serous cells. The cells are polarized with their product, in the form of secretory granules (SG), near the lumen (L) of the acinus. The cells display rough endoplasmic reticulum (ER) and several Golgi profiles (G). Immature secretory granules (IG) are present close to the Golgi. At the apical pole of the cells are junctional complexes (JC). Branches from the lumen, called intercellular canaliculi (IC), showing numerous microvilli, extend between the cells. Their connection to the lumen is not seen in this micrograph. M. mitochondria; N, nucleus. × 15,000.

shows basal striations in routinely prepared H&E sections. The nucleus of the striated duct cell typically occupies a central (rather than basal) location within the cell (see Atlas section, Plate 67, Fig. 2). With the transmission electron microscope, the cell is shown to possess numerous, deep infoldings of the plasma membrane and elongate mitochondria adjacent to the infoldings. These structural fea-

tures, particularly the elongate mitochondria, account for the basal striations as seen with the light microscope. Laterally, the neighboring cells are joined by apical junctional complexes that effectively seal the lumen from the lateral intercellular space. Basally, the cell contains folds that interdigitate with basilateral folds of neighboring cells.

Excretory ducts are surrounded by larger

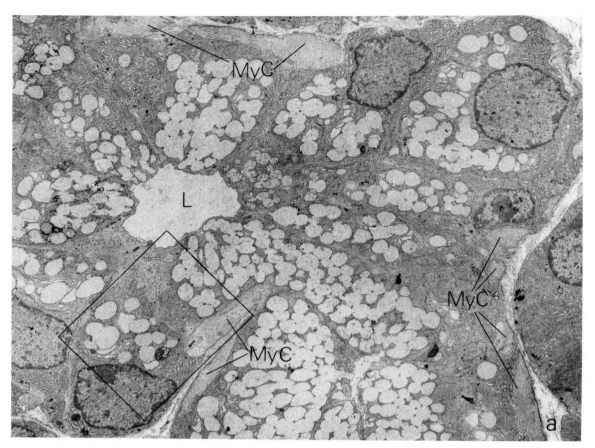

Figure 15.23(a). A lower-power electron micrograph of a mucous acinus. The mucous cells contain numerous micinogen granules. Many of the granules have coalesced to form larger irregular masses that will ultimately discharge into the lumen (L) of the acinus. Myoepithelial cell (MyC) processes are evident at the periphery of the acinus. A portion of one of the secretory cells and part of an underlying myoepithelial cell process **(rectangle)** is shown in Figure 15.23(b) at higher magnification. × 5,000.

amounts of connective tissue. The epithelium of small excretory ducts is pseudostratified columnar, and there may be some goblet cells among the columnar cells. The columnar cells stain with eosin, but somewhat less than those of the striated ducts. As the ducts increase in diameter, they become lined with stratified columnar epithelium, and as the ducts approach the oral epithelium, the largest ones may be lined with stratified squamous epithelium.

Connective Tissue. The connective tissue forms a stroma for the parenchymal part of the salivary gland. In the minor salivary glands, the connective tissue of the gland blends imperceptibly with the surrounding connective tissue. On the other hand, the major salivary glands are surrounded by a capsule of connective tissue of moderate density. Septa from the capsule divide the substance of the gland into lobules. These septa characteristically contain the large blood vessels and ducts. In both major and minor salivary

glands, the connective tissue that actually surrounds the acini and ducts is of the loose variety. This connective tissue contains a variety of cell types typically found in loose connective tissue, particularly lymphocytes and plasma cells (see Atlas section, Plate 67) that contribute antibodies to the saliva (namely, secretory IgA). The means by which the antibody gains access to the saliva is discussed below.

Blood Vessels and Nerves

Salivary glands are richly supplied with blood vessels. Those around striated ducts appear to be arranged parallel to the duct. Nerves of both the sympathetic and parasympathetic systems innervate the salivary glands; both systems stimulate the glands. Cell bodies of neurons in the vicinity of salivary glands belong to postganglionic parasympathetic neurons. The secretion due to parasympathetic stimulation is chiefly watery. Sympathetic stimulation yields a thicker saliva. Both systems

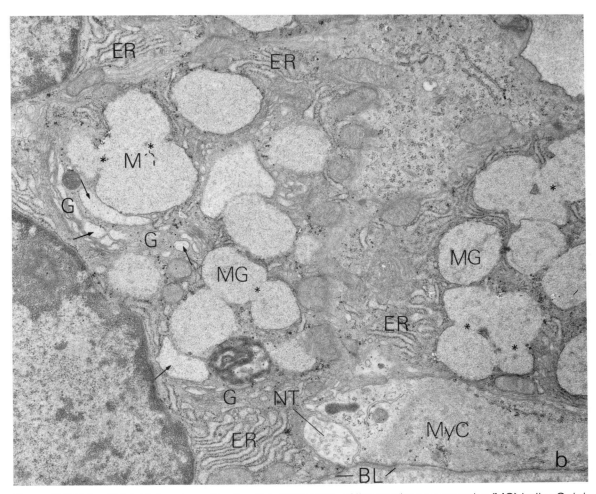

Figure 15.23(b). At this higher magnification the relationship of the mucinogen granules (MG) to the Golgi apparatus (G) and rough endoplasmic reticulum (ER) is evident. Note that some of the Golgi cisternae are somewhat enlarged **(arrows)** and contain a substance that resembles the mucinogen granules (MG). Also, note the nature of the coalescence of the mature mucinogen granules **(asterisks).** At the lower right a myoepithelial cell (MyC) process can be seen interposed between the surrounding basal lamina (BL) and the secretory epithelial cell. A nerve terminal (NT) lying in relation to the myoepithelial cell is also evident. × 15,000.

bring about vasodilation. However, sympathetic stimulation has a biphasic vascular effect causing first a vasoconstriction and then a vasodilation.

Saliva

Functions of Saliva. Saliva performs functions in several major areas: digestion, protection, and maintenance of the teeth. The digestive functions are accounted for by an enzyme, alpha amylase, which disrupts 1,4-glycosidic bonds of carbohydrates. Although relatively little digestion may occur in the oral cavity, the enzyme activity continues in the stomach and most of the dietary starch is digested to the disaccharide stage before reaching the duodenum. Saliva serves to lubricate the bolus and dissolve some of its constituents.

The protective functions include general protection of the oral cavity by buffering noxious stimuli. For example, the salivary gland secrete copiously just before one vomits, and the saliva neutralizes the regurgitated acid gastric juice. The saliva also contains antibacterial agents that reduce the activity of microbes in the oral cavity. Saliva also serves to clean the oral cavity.

Saliva plays several specific roles in maintaining the teeth. Calcium and phosphate of the saliva are instrumental in the posteruptive mineralization of newly erupted teeth and in the repair of white spot (precarious) lesions of the enamel. Proteins of the saliva cover the teeth with a protective coat called the **_acquired pellicle._** Antibodies and other antibacterial agents serve to retard bacterial

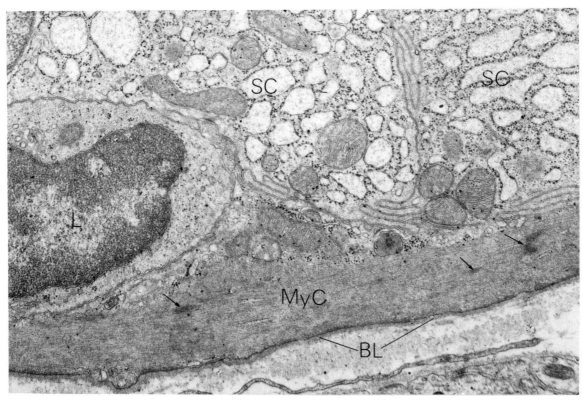

Figure 15.24. Electron micrograph showing the basal portion of two secretory cells (SC) from submandibal gland. A process of a myoepithelial cell (MyC) is also present. Again note the location of the myoepithelial cell on the epithelial side of the basal lamina (BL). The cytoplasm of the myoepithelial cell contains contractile filaments and densities **(arrows)** similar to those seen in smooth muscle cells. The cell on the left with the small nucleus is a lymphocyte (L). Having migrated through the basal lamina, it is thus also within the epithelial compartment. × 15,000.

action that otherwise would lead to tooth decay. Patients whose salivary glands are irradiated, as in the treatment of salivary gland tumors, fail to produce normal amounts of saliva so that these patients typically develop rampant caries.

Composition and Formation of Saliva. Saliva contains chiefly water, proteins (glycoproteins), and electrolytes (Table 15.1). It has a particularly high potassium content, but the potassium concentration decreases when the rate of salivary secretion is high. The loss of potassium may present a problem in noneating patients whose saliva drains externally, even temporarily, as in the case of a patient recovering from gross neck resection for the removal of a malignancy.

The initial secretion produced by the salivon contains sodium and potassium with osmolarity similar to that of plasma. As the saliva passes through the duct system, sodium is reabsorbed, so that the saliva become hypotonic. Striated ducts play a major role in the reabsorption of sodium, although some reabsorption also occurs in the larger extretory ducts. At the same time that so-

dium is being reabsorbed, potassium is secreted by duct cells into the saliva. The amount of potassium secreted does not match the amount of sodium reabsorbed and so the saliva remains hypotonic. As secretion rates increase, reabsorption of sodium appears to fall behind and the saliva becomes less hypotonic.

The synthesis of salivary immunoglobulin (IgA) is a two-step process. There is a significant difference between plasma IgA and salivary IgA. Plasma IgA exists chiefly as a monomer (sedimentation coefficient 7S) and to a lesser extent as a dimer (10S). The dimer consists of two 7S units joined by a J chain (Figure 15.25). Salivary IgA has a sedimentation coefficient of 11S and turns out to consist of a dimer in addition to a **secretory component.** Together, the dimer and the secretory component are referred to as **secretory IgA,** or **SIgA.** The synthesis of SIgA begins in plasma cells. These cells synthesize 7S IgA and the J chain and these then polymerize to form the dimer. These dimers are released by the plasma cells into the stroma of the salivary glands. The secretory com-

TABLE 15.1. Composition of Unstimulated Saliva

	MEAN (MG/ML)
Organic Constituents	
Protein	220.0
Amylase	38.0
Lysozyme	22.0
SIgA	19.0
IgC	1.4
IgM	0.2
Glucose	1.0*
Urea	20.0
Uric acid	1.5
Creatinine	0.1
Cholesterol	8.0
cAMP	7.0
Inorganic Constituents	
Sodium	15.0
Potassium	80.0
Thiocyanate	
Smokers	9.0
Nonsmokers	2.0
Calcium	5.8
Phosphate	16.8
Chloride	50.0
Fluoride	Traces (according to intake)

*Higher in patients with uncontrolled hyperglycemia.
Source: Modified from Jenkins GN: *The Physiology and Biochemistry of the Mouth,* 4th edition. Oxford, Blackwell Scientific Publications, 1978.

ponent is a glycoprotein synthesized by the glandular epithelium of the salivary glands. It is thought to move to the plasma membrane of the glandular epithelium and serve as a receptor that binds the dimeric IgA. The SIgA is then internalized (by pinocytotic vesicles) by the gland cells and secreted into the lumen as a secretory component of the saliva.

IgG and IgM are present in saliva only to a small degree. They are thought to gain entry into the saliva through the gingival sulcus.

PHARYNX

The pharynx serves both the respiratory and the digestive system as a passageway for air and food. The pharynx communicates anteriorly with the nasal and oral cavities and with the larynx and accordingly is divided into the nasopharynx, the oropharynx, and the laryngopharynx. Below the opening to the larynx, the pharynx is tubular; it continues into the esophagus inferiorly.

Parts of the pharynx are subject to abrasion by food that has not been extensively macerated; these parts are surfaced by nonkeratinized stratified squamous epithelium. Parts of the pharynx not subject to abrasion are lined by pseudostratified ciliated columnar epithelium that contains goblet cells. Under the lining epithelium, the lamina propria of the pharynx consists of connec-

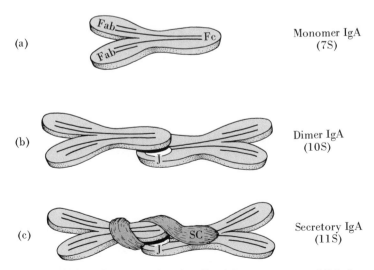

Figure 15.25. Diagram showing the **(a)** monomer and **(b)** dimer of IgA (products of plasma cells), with the J chain (J) joining the monomers. The secretory component (SC), a product of the epithelial cells, is added to the dimer to form **(c)** secretory IgA (SIgA). Fab and Fc indicate parts of basic antibody molecule. (Based on Shaw JH, et al.: *Textbook of Oral Biology.* Philadelphia, WB Saunders, 1978, p. 765.)

tive tissue that is best described as being fibroelastic because of the high content of elastic fibers. External to the fibroelastic connective tissue is the striated muscle of the pharyngeal constrictors and other pharyngeal muscles, and external to these is more connective tissue. The pharynx contains mucous glands near its junction with the esophagus. There is no distinct submucosa except in some of the areas where the pharynx forms lateral recesses.

The pharynx contains aggregates of lymph nodules that, because of their location, are designated as the *pharyngeal* and *palatine tonsils*. The palatine tonsils are at the fauces (the junction between the oral cavity and pharynx) and, thus, are also called the *fauceal tonsils*. Pharyngeal tonsils are within the roof of the pharynx. When these become enlarged, as they frequently do in childhood, they are called *adenoids*.

The auditory tube (eustachian tube) from the middle ear opens into the sides of the nasopharynx, not far from the molar teeth. Inflammation of the gingiva, which often occurs during tooth eruption, may cause pressure on the tube and an earache.

ATLAS PLATES

64–70

PLATE 64. Tongue I

The tongue is a muscular organ covered by mucous membrane. The mucous membrane consists of stratified squamous epithelium, keratinized in parts, resting on a loose connective tissue. The undersurface of the tongue is relatively uncomplicated. However, the mucosa of the dorsal surface is modified to form three types of papilla: filiform, fungiform, and circumvallate. These are located as follows: The circumvallate papillae form a V-shaped row that divides the tongue into a body and a root; the dorsal surface of the body, i.e., the portion anterior to the circumvallate papillae, contains filiform and fungiform papillae.

Figure 1 shows the dorsal surface of the tongue with the filiform papillae **(FilP).** They are the most numerous of the three types of papillae. Structurally they are bent conical projections of the epithelium, with the point of the projection directed posteriorly. These papillae do not possess taste buds and are comprised of stratified squamous keratinized epithelium.

The fungiform papillae are scattered about as isolated, slightly rounded, elevated structures situated among the filiform papillae. A fungiform papilla is shown in the **inset.** A large connective tissue core (primary connective tissue papilla) forms the center of the fungiform papilla, and smaller connective tissue papillae (secondary connective tissue papillae) project into the base of the surface epithelium **(arrowhead).** The connective tissue of the papillae is highly vascularized. Because of the deep penetration of connective tissue into the epithelium, combined with a very thin keratinized surface, the fungiform papillae appear as small red dots when the dorsal surface of the tongue is examined by gross inspection.

The undersurface of the tongue is shown in **Figure 2.** The smooth surface of the stratified squamous epithelium **(Ep)** contrasts with the irregular surface of the dorsum of the tongue. Moreover, the epithelial surface on the underside of the

KEY	

CT, connective tissue
Ep, epithelium
FilP, filiform papillae
M, muscle bundles
N, nerves
arrowhead, inset, Fig. 1,
  secondary connective
  tissue
	arrows, Fig. 1, isolated
	  connective tissue
	  papillae due to plane
	  of section

Figs. 1 and 2, monkey,
  × 65
  inset, × 130

tongue is usually not keratinized. The connective tissue **(CT)** is immediately deep to the epithelium, and deeper still is the striated muscle **(M).**

The numerous connective tissue papillae that project into the base of the epithelium, both ventral and dorsal surfaces, give the epithelial-connective tissue junction an irregular profile. Often these connective tissue papillae are cut obliquely and then appear as small islands of connective tissue within the epithelial layer **(arrows, Fig. 1).**

The connective tissue extends as far as the muscle without change in character and no submucosa is recognized. The muscle is striated **(M)** and is unique in its organization: the fibers travel in three planes. Therefore, most sections will show muscle fibers cut longitudinally, at right angles to each other, and in cross-section. Nerves **(N)** that innervate the muscle are also frequently observed in the connective tissue septa between the muscle bundles.

The surface of the tongue behind the vallate papillae (the root of the tongue) contains lingual tonsils (not shown). These are similar in structure and appearance to the palatine tonsils illustrated in the Atlas section, Plate 50.

PLATE 64

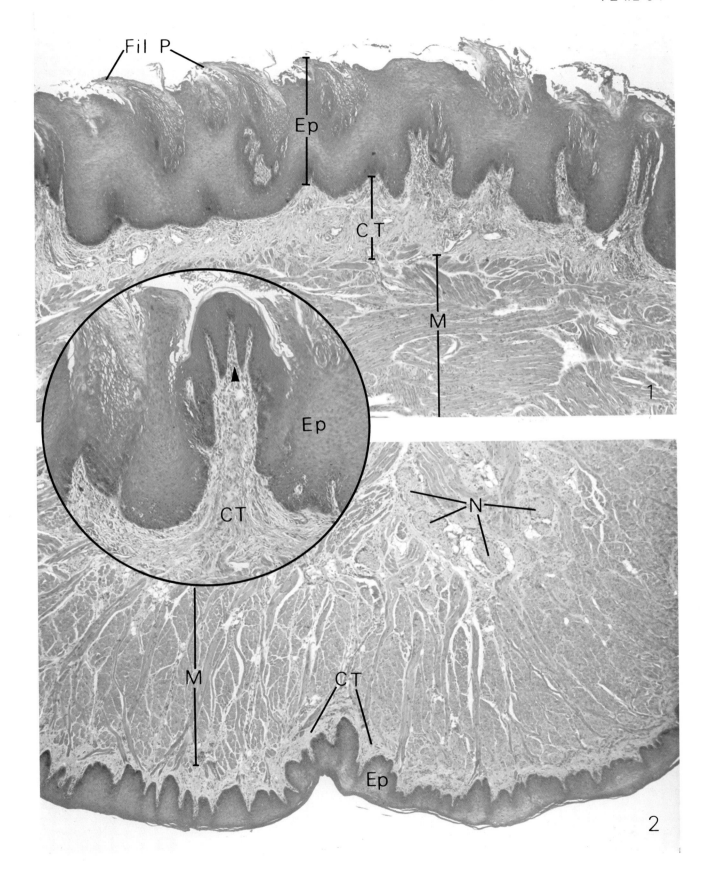

Fil P

Ep

CT

M

1

Ep

CT

N

M

CT

Ep

2

PLATE 65. Tongue II

The sides of the tongue contain a series of vertical ridges that bear taste buds. When these ridges are cut at right angles to their long axis, they appear as a row of papillae (**Fig. 1**). These ridges are called *foliate papillae.* Foliate papillae are not always conspicuous in the adult human tongue, but are quite evident in the infant tongue. They can immediately be distinguished from fungiform papillae in a section because they appear in rows whereas fungiform papillae appear alone. Moreover, numerous taste buds (**TB**) are present on adjacent walls of neighboring foliate papillae. In contrast, fungiform papillae have taste buds on the dorsal surface. The foliate papillae are covered by stratified squamous epithelium that is usually not, or is only slightly, keratinized. The part of the epithelium (**Ep**) that is on the free surface of the foliate papillae is thick and has a number of secondary connective tissue papillae (**arrowheads**) projecting into its undersurface.

The connective tissue within and under the foliate papillae contains serous type glands (**Gl**), called *von Ebner's glands,* which open via ducts (**D**) into the cleft between neighboring papillae. [In addition to von Ebner's glands, which are entirely of the serous type, the tongue contains mixed (serous and mucous) glands near the apex and mucous glands in the root (not illustrated).]

The dense patches (**arrows**) within the connective tissue consist of accumulations of round cells, namely lymphocytes, in the form of a diffuse lymphatic tissue. They are typically seen just below the clefts of the papillae.

Of the true papillae found on the dorsal surface of the tongue—filiform, fungiform, and circumvallate (vallate)—the circumvallate are the largest. About 7 to 11 of these form a "V" between the body and root of the tongue. *Circumvallate papillae* are covered by stratified squamous epithelium, which may be slightly keratinized. Each circumvallate papilla (**Fig. 2**) is surrounded by a trench or cleft. Numerous taste buds (**TB**) are on the lateral walls of the papillae; moreover, the tongue epithelium facing the papilla within the cleft may contain some taste buds. The dorsal surface of the papilla is rather smooth; however, nu-

merous secondary connective tissue papillae (**arrowheads**) project into the underside of the epithelium. The deep trench surrounding the circumvallate papillae and the presence of taste buds on the sides rather than on the surface are features that distinguish circumvallate from fungiform papillae.

The connective tissue near the circumvallate papillae contains many serous type glands (**Gl**), von Ebner's glands, which open via ducts (**D**) into the bottom of the trench.

The taste buds extend through the full thickness of the stratified squamous epithelium (**inset**) and open at the surface at a small pore (**arrowheads**). The cells of the taste bud are chiefly spindle-shaped and oriented at a right angle to the surface. The nuclei of the cells are elongated and mainly in the basal two-thirds of the bud. At least three cell types are present in the taste bud; one is a special receptor cell, the sensory or neuroepithelial cell. Nerve fibers enter the epithelium and terminate in close contact with the sensory cells of the taste bud, but they cannot be identified in routine H&E preparations. Other cell types in the taste bud include the supporting cells and the basal cells. The latter sometimes exhibit mitotic figures (**asterisk**), and give rise to the other cell types.

PLATE 65

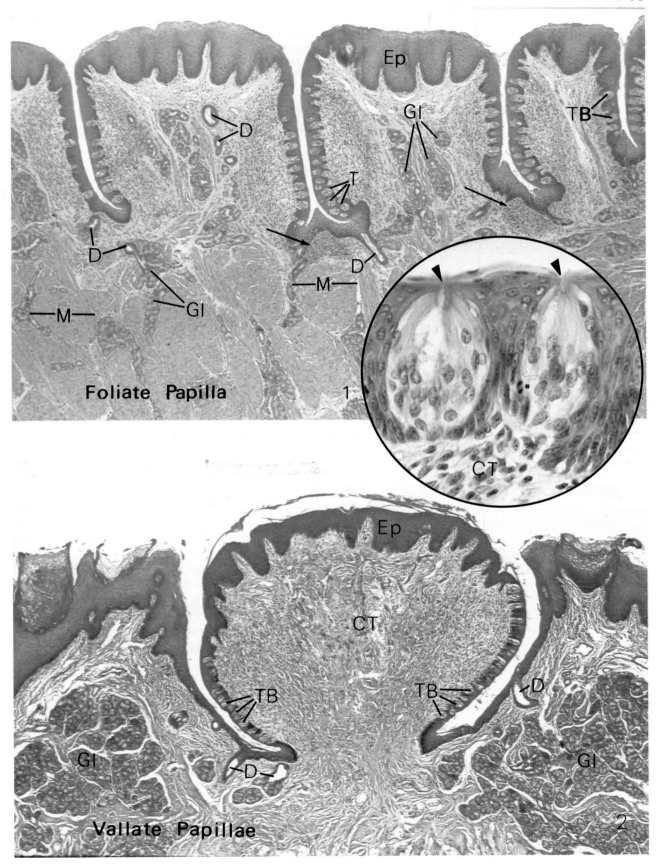

Foliate Papilla 1

Vallate Papillae 2

PLATE 66. Submandibular Gland

The salivary glands are compound (branched) tubuloacinar glands. The secretory unit is the acinus, which is made up of either serous cells (serous acini) or mucous cells (mucous acini). Generally, serous cells can readily be distinguished from mucous cells in H&E preparations by the deep staining of the cytoplasm in contrast to the empty or washed-out appearance of the mucous cell—a characteristic feature due to loss of the stored mucinogen granules within the cell during tissue preparation. A second distinguishing feature relates to nuclear shape. The nuclei of mucous cells are typically flattened against the base of the cell, whereas nuclei of serous cells are rounded.

The submandibular glands contain both serous and mucous acini (**Fig. 1**). In humans, the serous components predominate. The **rectangle** in the **upper right** of **Figure 1** reveals a cluster of mucous acini (**MA**). The mucous-secreting cells of the acini are readily discernible at this low magnification due to their light staining. The remainder of the field is comprised largely of serous acini (**SA**). A few adipose cells (**A**) and various ducts (**ED, StD,** and **ID**) are also evident in the field.

When examined at higher magnification, as in **Figure 2,** the individual mucous cells exhibit distinct cell boundaries. Their nuclei are flattened (except those that are tangentially sectioned). In contrast, the cytoplasm of the serous cells stains deeply and the nuclei appear ovoid or round.

Serous cells are also found forming a cap known as a serous demilune (**SD**) on the periphery of many of the mucous acini. The cells of the serous demilune secrete via channels between the mucous cells, thereby allowing the secretory product to reach the lumen of the acinus and mix with the mucous secretion. It should be realized that some acini that appear to be of the serous type, and particularly those that appear as small spherical profiles, may actually be a demilune of a mucous acinus that has been cut in a plane that excludes the mucous cells from the section.

Associated with the acinar epithelium are myoepithelial cells. They are located in relation to the basal aspect of the secretory cells and rest on the basal lamina. However, myoepithelial cells are difficult to identify in salivary gland H&E-stained preparations, and none can be identified with assurance here.

The nature of the duct system of the submandibular gland is shown to advantage in **Figure 1.** The initial ducts leading from the acinus, the intercalated ducts (**ID**), are very small. They possess a flattened to cuboidal epithelium and exhibit a distinct lumen. Intercalated ducts in the submandibular gland (and also the parotid gland) tend to be relatively long; thus, they are frequently encountered in a section. They merge (**arrows**) to form the larger striated ducts (**StD**). These ducts have an epithelium of low to tall columnar cells and at high magnification show basal striations (see Atlas section, Plate 67). **Figure 2** provides a comparison between an intercalated duct (**ID**) and a small striated duct (**StD**) from the **rectangle** in **Figure 1.** Outside of the lobule the striated duct becomes the excretory duct (**ED,** upper left, **Fig. 1**). It is characterized by a wider lumen and a taller columnar epithelium. As the excretory ducts increase in size, the epithelium becomes pseudostratified and finally stratified in the main excretory ducts.

KEY

A, adipose cell
ED, excretory duct
ID, intercalated duct
MA, mucous acini
SA, serous acini
SD, serous demilune
StD, striated duct
arrows, Fig. 1, intercalated ducts joining to form a striated duct

asterisk, lumen of mucous acinus
rectangle, Fig. 1, cluster of mucous acini

Fig. 1, human, × 160   **Fig. 2,** human, × 400

PLATE 66

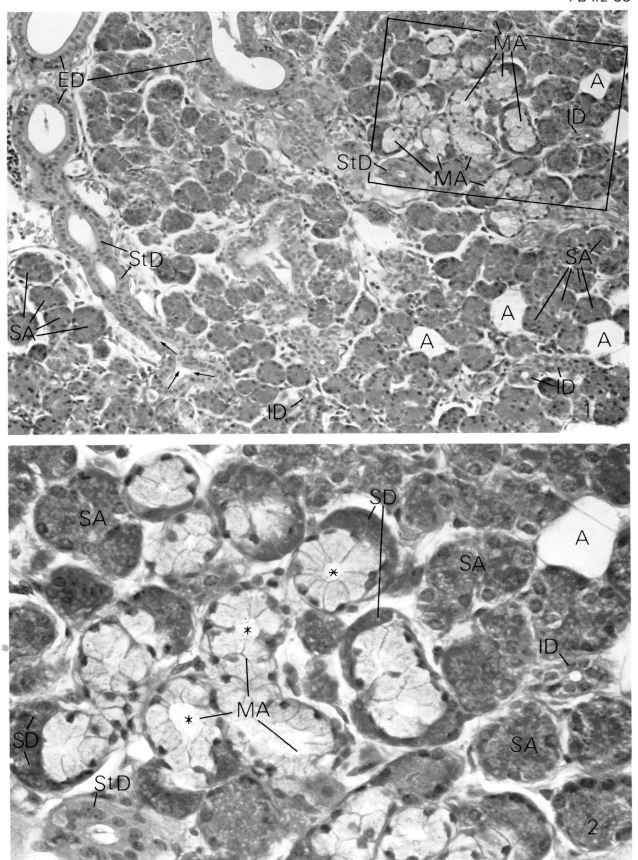

PLATE 67. Parotid Gland

The parotid gland in the human is comprised entirely of serous acini and their ducts (**Fig. 1**). However, numerous adipose cells (**AC**) are usually distributed throughout the gland. Both the serous acini and their duct system are comparable in structure and arrangement to these same components in the submandibular gland. Within the lobule, the striated ducts (**StD**) are readily observed. They exhibit a simple columnar epithelium. The intercalated ducts are smaller; at the low magnification of **Figure 1,** they are difficult to recognize. A few intercalated ducts (**ID**) are indicated. The lower portion of **Figure 1** reveals an excretory duct (**ED**) within a connective tissue septum (**CT**). The epithelium of this excretory duct exhibits two layers of nuclei and is either pseudostratified or possibly already a true stratified epithelium.

Figure 2 is from a glutaraldehyde, osmic-acid-fixed, plastic-embedded specimen stained with H&E. The serous cells are optimally preserved and reveal their secretory (zymogen) granules. They appear as the fine dot-like objects within the cytoplasm. The acinus in the upper right of the figure has been cut in cross-section and reveals the acinar lumen (**AL**). The **small rectangle** drawn in the acinus represents an area comparable to the electron micrograph shown as Figure 15.22. That the acini are not simple spheres but rather irregular elongate structures can be perceived from the large acinar profile to the left of the striated duct (**StD**). Also note that because of the small size of the aci-

KEY	
A, acinus	**ID,** intercalated duct
AC, adipose cell	**PC,** plasma cells
AL, acinar lumen	**S,** striations of duct cells
CT, connective tissue	**StD,** striated duct
ED, excretory duct	

| **Fig. 1,** (human), × 160 | **Fig. 2,** monkey, × 640 |

nar lumen and the variability in sectioning an acinus to reveal its lumen, it is seen infrequently.

A cross-sectional profile of an intercalated duct (**ID**) appears on the left of the micrograph: note its simple cuboidal epithelium. A single flattened nucleus is present at the top of the duct, and may represent a myoepithelial cell associated with the beginning of the duct system as well as the acini. The large duct occupying the center of the micrograph is a striated duct (**StD**). It is comprised of a columnar epithelium. The striations (**S**) that give the duct its name are readily evident. Also of significance is the presence of plasma cells (**PC**) within the connective tissue surrounding the duct. Again, it is these cells that play a role in the production of salivary immunoglobulins.

PLATE 67

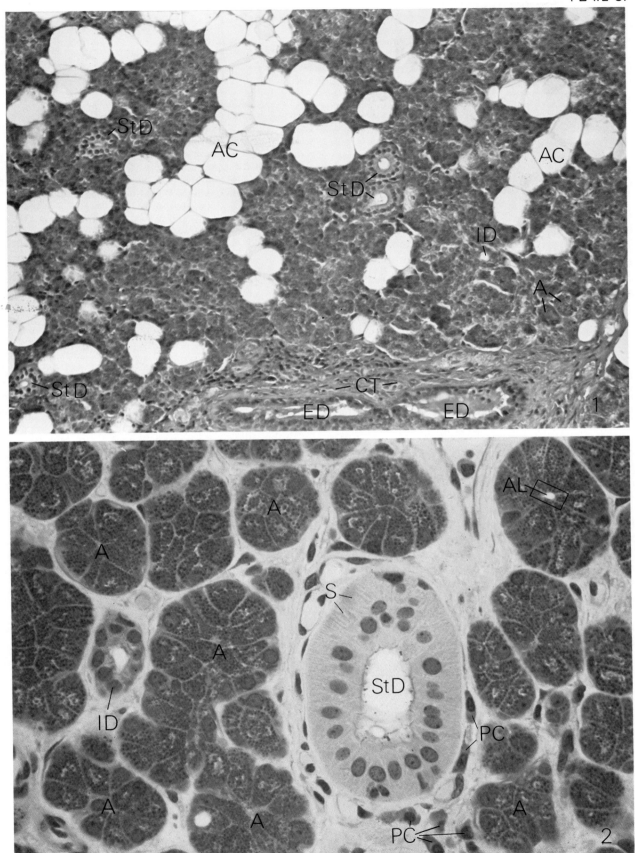

PLATE 68. Sublingual Gland

The sublingual gland resembles the submandibular gland in that it contains both serous and mucous elements. However, in the sublingual gland, the mucous acini predominate. **Figure 1** shows a sublingual gland at low power. The mucous acini (**MA**) are conspicuous due to their light staining. Critical examination of the mucous acini at this relatively low magnification reveals that they are not spherical structures, but rather elongate or tubular structures with branching outpockets. Thus, the acinus is rather large and much of it is usually not seen within the plane of a single section.

The serous component of the gland is comprised largely of demilunes, but occasional serous acini are present. (It should be realized, as already noted, that some of the serous demilunes may be sectioned in a plane that does not include the mucous component of the acinus, thus giving the appearance of a serous acinus.)

The ducts of the sublingual gland that are observed in a section with the greatest frequency are the intralobular ducts. They are the equivalent of the striated duct of the submandibular and parotid glands, but lack the extensive basal infolds and mitochondrial array that creates the striations. One of the intralobular ducts (**InD**) is evident in **Figure 1 (upper right)**. The area within the **rectangle** includes part of this duct and is shown at higher magnification in **Figure 2**. Note that, through a fortuitous plane of section, the lumen of a mucous acinus (**MA**) is seen joining an intercalated duct (**ID**). The juncture between the acinus and the beginning of the duct, the intercalated duct (**ID**), is marked by the **arrowhead.** The intercalated duct is comprised of a flattened or low columnar epithelium similar to that seen in the other salivary glands. However, the intercalated ducts of the sublingual gland are extremely short and, thus, are usually difficult to find. The intercalated duct seen in this micrograph joins with one or more other intercalated ducts to become the intralobular duct (**InD**), which is identified by its columnar epithe-

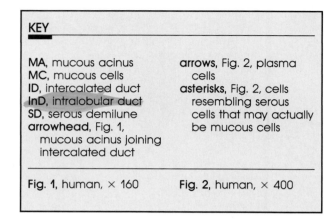

KEY

MA, mucous acinus
MC, mucous cells
ID, intercalated duct
InD, intralobular duct
SD, serous demilune
arrowhead, Fig. 1,
    mucous acinus joining
    intercalated duct

arrows, Fig. 2, plasma
    cells
asterisks, Fig. 2, cells
    resembling serous
    cells that may actually
    be mucous cells

Fig. 1, human, × 160   **Fig. 2,** human, × 400

lium and relatively large lumen. However, the point of transition from intercalated to interlobular duct is not recognizable in the micrograph because the duct wall has only been grazed and the shape of the cells cannot be determined.

Examination of the acini at the higher magnification of **Figure 2** also reveals the serous demilunes (**SD**). Note how they form a cap-like addition to the mucous end-pieces. The cytological appearance of the mucous (**MC**) and serous cells is essentially the same as that described for the submandibular gland. The area selected for this higher magnification also reveals isolated cell clusters (**asterisks**) that bear some resemblance to serous acini. It is likely, however, that these cells may actually be mucous cells that have either been cut in a plane parallel to their base and do not include the mucinogen-containing portions of the cell, or they are in a state of activity where, after depletion of their granules, the production of new mucinogen granules is not yet sufficient to give the characteristic "empty" mucous cell appearance.

An additional important feature of the connective tissue stroma is the presence of lymphocytes and plasma cells. Some of the plasma cells are indicated by the **arrows.** (The plasma cells are associated with the production of salivary IgA and are also present in the other salivary glands.)

PLATE 68

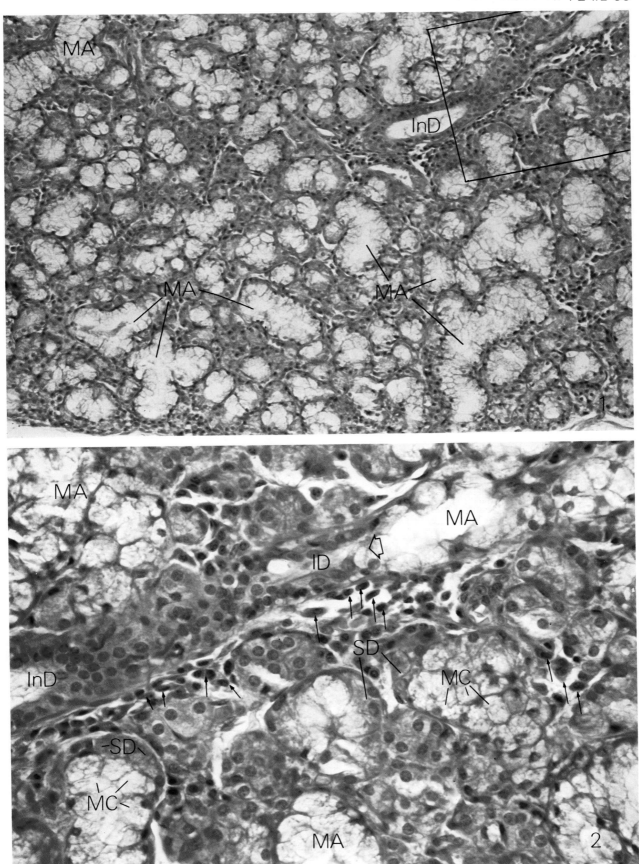

PLATE 69. Soft Palate

The soft palate is the posterior part of the roof of the mouth. Instead of bone, as in the hard palate, it contains striated muscle between the nasal and oral surfaces. During swallowing, the soft palate separates the nasopharynx from the oropharynx.

A section through the entire thickness of the soft palate is shown in **Figure 1.** From top to bottom, the following components can be recognized: (1) the epithelial **(Ep)** lining of the nasal surface (a small polyp **(P)** is connected by a stalk to the surface); (2) the lamina propria **(LP)** of nasal mucosa; (3) glands **(Gl)**; (4) striated muscle **(StM)**; (5) mucous glands **(MGl)**; (6) lamina propria **(LP)** of oral mucosa; and (7) epithelial **(EP)** lining of the oral surface.

The epithelium **(Ep)** lining the nasal surface consists of ciliated pseudostratified columnar cells **(Fig. 2).** Goblet cells **(GC)** are also present in this layer. The epithelium rests on a thick basement membrane **(BM).** The lamina propria **(LP)** is loose and cellular. It contains an aggregation of lymphocytes **(Lym)** and mixed seromucous glands. Some of the nuclei of the cells that make up these glands are oval in appearance **(arrows),** whereas others are flattened against the basal part of the cell. The glands may also invade the muscular layer (see **Fig. 1).**

The muscle of the soft palate is striated. Although striations are not evident at the magnification in **Figure 1,** it is possible on the basis of other characteristics (see Atlas section, Plate 72) to conclude that it is striated and not smooth. Connective tissue is between the muscle bundles.

The oral side of the soft palate contains numerous mucous glands. The nuclei of the mucous cells are pressed against the basal part of the cell **(arrowheads, Fig. 3),** thereby outlining the mucous alveoli. A duct **(D)** through which these glands empty their secretions onto the surface is seen in **Figure 3.**

The epithelium on the oral surface is stratified squamous. Numerous connective tissue papillae

KEY	
BM, basement membrane	**StM,** striated muscle
D, duct	**arrowheads,** flat nuclei of mucous cells
Ep, epithelium	**arrows,** Fig. 2, oval nuclei of serous cells
GC, goblet cells	
Gl, glands	**arrows,** Fig. 3, lymphocytes in epithelial layer
LP, lamina propria	
Lym, lymphocytes	**asterisks,** connective tissue papillae
MGl, mucous glands	
P, polyp	
Fig. 1, monkey, × 40	**Figs. 2 and 3,** monkey, × 160

(asterisks) project into the undersurface of the epithelium. The dark staining of the deepest part of the epithelium is due in part to the cytoplasmic staining of the basal cells. New cells that will migrate to the surface are produced in this layer. As the cells approach the surface, the nuclei become flattened and oriented in a plane parallel to the surface. The presence of nuclei in the surface cells indicates that the epithelium is not keratinized.

Stratified squamous epithelium is also present on the posterior edge and on part of the adjacent "nasal" surface of the soft palate. At some distance from the posterior edge, the stratified squamous epithelium is replaced by pseudostratified ciliated columnar epithelium. However, at the junction between the two, there is a narrow band of stratified columnar epithelium.

Stratified columnar epithelium does not have a wide distribution. It is present where stratified squamous epithelium meets columnar or pseudostratified columnar epithelium as, for example, in large ducts, in the larynx, at the junction of the naso- and oropharynx, and on the upper surface of the soft palate.

PLATE 69

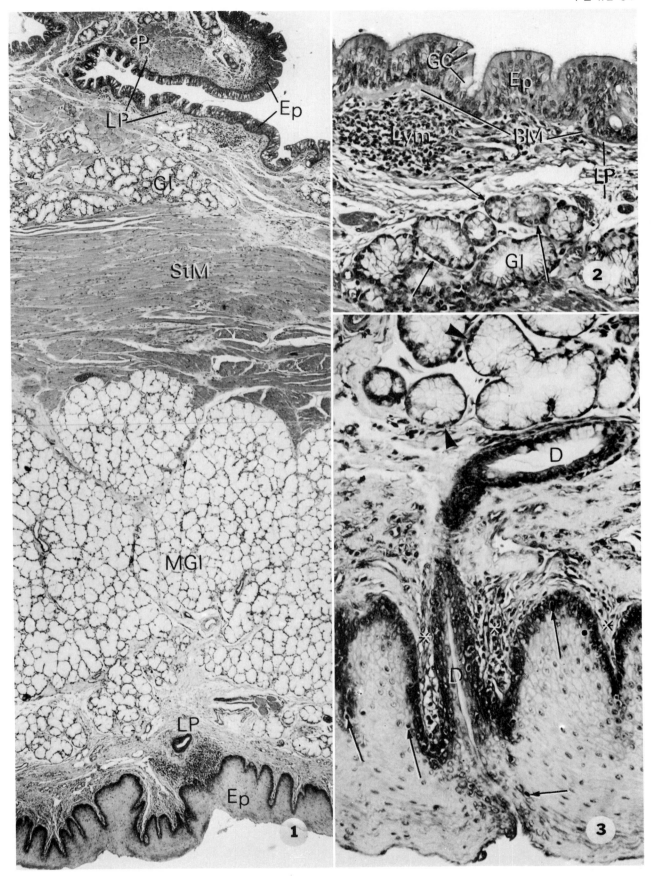

PLATE 70. Developing Tooth

During early fetal development, a plate of epithelium called the dental lamina grows into the underlying embryonic connective tissue (mesenchyme) from the oral epithelium. At regular intervals, where future teeth will be, the cells of the dental lamina proliferate and become the enamel organs.

The enamel organ (**EO**) appears as an expanded cell mass that has been invaginated by a connective tissue papilla, the dental papilla (**DP**) (**Fig. 1**). It is attached to the oral epithelium (**Ep**) by the dental lamina (**DL**). The junction between the enamel organ and the dental papilla assumes the shape of the future dentinoenamel junction before dentinogenesis or amelogenesis begins. The mesenchyme that surrounds the enamel organ and dental papilla forms a delicate fibrous sac called the dental sac (**DS**). This sac along with its contents is called the tooth germ (**TG**).

Figure 2 shows a tooth germ in which dentinogenesis and amelogenesis have just begun. The parts of the enamel organ are designated; the inner enamel epithelium (**A**) (these are called ameloblasts once they begin to form enamel), the stratum intermedium (**SI**), the stellate reticulum (**SR**), and the outer enamel epithelium (**OEE**). The dental papilla (**DP**) will become the future pulp cavity. At the periphery of the dental papilla are the columnar-shaped odontoblasts (**O**) that produce dentin (**D**). The enamel (**E**) is deposited by ameloblasts on the surface of the previously formed dentin.

Figure 3 shows a tooth, stained with toluidine blue, at a later stage of development. The enamel (**E**) is unstained; however, the ameloblasts (**A**), dentin (**D**), and odontoblasts (**O**) stain intensely. The most recently formed enamel and dentin are at the bottom of the figure. A serial section of this region, stained with H&E, is examined at higher magnification in **Figure 4**. The sequence of events that are shown in **Figure 4** (and in **Fig. 2**) are as follows: (1) cells of the enamel organ induce mesenchymal cells of the dental papilla to become odontoblasts; (2) the odontoblasts begin to pro-

---

KEY

A, ameloblasts
D, dentin
DL, dental lamina
DP, dental papilla
DS, dental sac
E, enamel
EO, enamel organ
Ep, oral epithelium

O, odontoblasts
OEE, outer enamel epithelium
Pd, predentin
SI, stratum intermedium
SR, stellate reticulum
TG, tooth germ

Fig. 1, pig, × 16
Fig. 2, dog, × 40
Fig. 3, rat, × 65
  inset, × 160

Fig. 4, rat, × 160
  inset, × 640

---

duce dentin; (3) when the ameloblasts are confronted with the dentin, they deposit enamel on the outer dentinal surface.

In the formation of dentin, an organic matrix containing collagenous fibers is produced by the odontoblasts. This calcifies to become dentin. The immediate product of the odontoblasts is called predentin (**Pd**). It stains less intensely than the dentin. The odontoblastic process (**inset, Fig. 4**) is contained in a dental tubule and both the process and its tubule extend through the entire thickness of the dentin.

In the early stages of amelogenesis, the ameloblasts secrete an organic matrix. Mineralization of this (as with the dentinal matrix) begins almost immediately. However, in teeth with a thin layer of enamel (e.g., rat), after the enamel reaches its full thickness it undergoes maturation. Organic material and water are removed and the enamel continues to mineralize to a greater extent than occurs anywhere else in the body. During maturation, the ameloblasts (**inset, Fig. 3**) acquire the characteristics of absorptive or transport cells. The maturation of enamel is a cyclical event marked by the cyclical entry of calcium into the maturing enamel.

PLATE 70

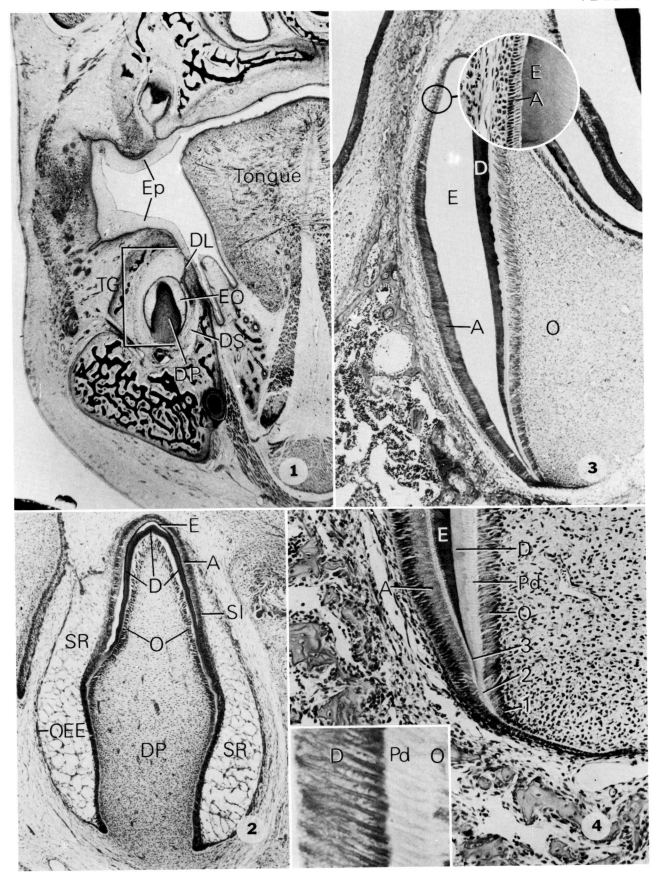

/

Digestive System II: Esophagus and Gastrointestinal Tract

From the esophagus to the rectum, the wall of the alimentary canal, or digestive tube, is comprised of four layers designated as the mucosa, the submucosa, the muscularies externa, and the serosa (Fig. 16.1). Where the digestive tube is directly adherent to the posterior abdominal wall or to other organs, there is an adventitia, or fibrosa, in place of a serosa. In other locations, the digestive tube is joined to the body wall by a mesentery or its derivatives. The mesentery serves as a route for blood vessels, lymphatic vessels, and nerves.

The *muscosa* is comprised of a lining epithelium, an underlying connective tissue designated as the lamina propria, and a muscularis mucosae. The epithelium differs throughout the alimentary canal, being especially adapted to the function and contents of the specific part of the tube. In all parts of the alimentary canal (more so in some than in others), the body is subject to the entry of foreign substances, both microbes and molecules, which are recognized as nonself and serve as antigens against which the body reacts. The numerous cells responding to these foreign substances are contained in the lamina propria, along with the usual resident connective tissue cells. They include lymphocytes, plasma cells, eosinophils, and other migrant cells from the blood. The lymphocytes and plasma cells are so numerous in the lamina propria of certain parts of the alimentary canal that this layer of the mucous membrane has been designated as diffuse lymphatic tissue by classical histologists. In addition, nodules of lymphatic tissue are found throughout the alimentary canal. The nodules may be confined to the mucosa, but more often, they extend into the submucosa. The diffuse lymphatic tissue and the lymphatic nodules are collectively referred to as the *gut-associated lymphatic tissue* (GALT). In the small intestine, aggregates of

nodules called Peyer's patches are usually located on the side of the tube opposite to the attachment of the mesentery. Aggregated nodules also occur in the appendix.

The *muscularis mucosae* consist of smooth muscle cells arranged as inner circular and outer longitudinal layers. These constitute the deepest part of the mucosa at the boundary between it and the submucosa.

The *submucosa* consists of moderately dense, irregular connective tissue. It contains the largest blood vessels of the alimentary canal. These send branches to the mucosa, to the muscularis externa, and to the serosa. The submucosa also contains lymphatic vessels and nerve plexuses. The nerve networks consist of sensory fibers and both parasympathetic and sympathetic fibers of the autonomic nervous system. Interspersed throughout the nerve networks are cell bodies (ganglion cells) of postganglionic parasympathetic neurons. The submucosal network of unmyelinated nerve fibers and ganglion cells constitute the *Meissner's plexus.*

The *muscularis externa* differs throughout the various parts of the alimentary canal and it will be considered as a special feature when each is described. Like the submucosa, it contains networks of nerve fibers and ganglion cells; these constitute the *myenteric plexus of Auerbach.*

The *serosa* is a serous membrane consisting of a single layer of simple squamous epithelial cells, the mesothelium, and a small amount of underlying connective tissue. The mesothelial cells contain microvilli on their free surface. The serosa is comparable to the viceral peritoneum of gross anatomy. It is continuous with the mesentery.

Histologically, the *mesentery* consists of a thin sheet of loose connective tissue, often with numerous fat cells. Through it, nerves, blood vessels, and

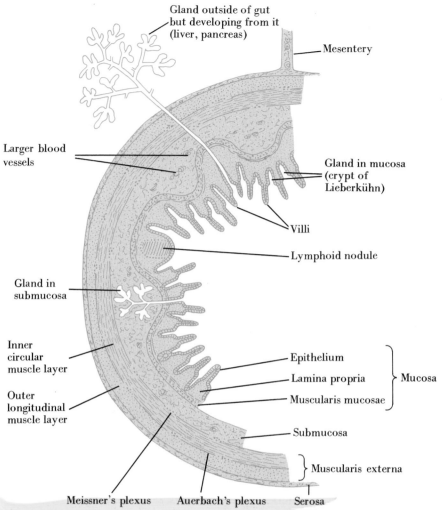

Figure 16.1. Diagram to show the four layers of the alimentary canal from the esophagus to the large intestine, namely, the mucosa, the submucosa, the muscularis externa, and the serosa (or adventitia). The specific example used shows the small intestine, and thus, the mucosa contains villi, which are not found in any other part of the alimentary canal. To be noted are: **(1)** glands in the mucosa, found throughout the tube except sparingly in the esophagus; **(2)** glands in the submucosa, found in the esophagus and duodenum of the small intestine; and **(3)** extramural glands, which empty only into the duodenum of the small intestine. Meissner's and Auerbach's plexuses are nerve plexuses. These along with blood vessels reach the digestive tube via the mesentery or similar sheets of peritoneum. However, where adventitia is present instead of a serosa, blood vessels and nerves reach the wall of the digestive tube from the adjacent connective tissue. (Based on Ham AW, Cormack DH: *Histology,* 8th ed. Philadelphia, JB Lippincott, 1979.)

lymphatic vessels course to and from the digestive tube. Each surface of the mesentery is covered by mesothelial cells. In some small laboratory animals, the mesentery is extremely thin and it can be viewed through a microscope by being spread on a slide (see Atlas section, Plate 10, Fig. 2; and Fig. 9.1.)

The digestive tube contains numerous intramural and several extramural glands that provide the tube with lubricating mucus, enzymes, water, and other substances. The intramural glands are within the mucosa and submucosa. They differ throughout the digestive tube and are described with the specific regions of the tube. The extramural glands are the pancreas, liver, and gallbladder. They empty their secretions into the first part of the small intestine, the duodenum.

ESOPHAGUS

The esophagus (Fig. 16.2) is a long muscular tube that continues from the pharynx and leads to the stomach. For most of its length it is in the thoracic cavity. The main function of the esophagus is to convey food and fluids from the pharynx to the stomach. This occurs during the act of swallowing.

Mucosa

The *mucosa* is lined by nonkeratinized, stratified squamous epithelium (in some animals, this epithelium is keratinized). The lamina propria is not unique, but the muscularis mucosae are thicker than in other parts of the digestive tube. The mucosa contains mucous glands in its uppermost re-

gion (these are sometimes missing) and in its lowermost region, near the stomach. The lowermost glands resemble those in the cardiac region of the stomach and are also called *cardiac glands.*

Submucosa

The *submucosa* contains mucous glands throughout its length; they are somewhat more numerous in the upper region of the esophagus. The submucosal glands are branched tubular glands, primarily producing mucus to lubricate the tube.

Muscularis Externa

The *muscularis externa,* in the upper third of the esophagus, consists of striated muscle and represents a continuation of the muscular layer of the pharynx. In the lower third, it is smooth muscle. The middle third contains both striated and

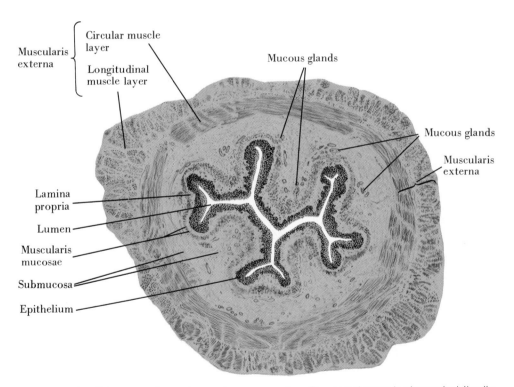

Figure 16.2. Diagram of esophagus in cross-section. The esophagus is characteristically collapsed, giving the lumen its branched appearance. The muscularis mucosa is relatively thick, thereby readily marking the extent of the mucosa. Mucosa glands are in the submucosa: their ducts, which empty into the lumen of the esophagus, have not been included in the plane of the section. Even at this relatively low magnification, it is possible to distinguish the circularly arranged muscle fibers from those which are longitudinally disposed (and therefore seen in cross-section). The adventitia is not included in the illustration; it is the connective tissue just external to the outer muscle layer. (After Sobotta, in Bloom W, Fawcett DW: *A Textbook of Histology,* 10th ed. Philadelphia, WB Saunders, 1975.)

smooth muscle, and can be regarded as a transition from one type to the other. The muscle is arranged in two layers, an inner circular and an outer longitudinal layer, an arrangement that is most evident in the lower part of the esophagus. The striated musculature at the beginning of the esophagus forms a sphincter, the *pharyngoesophageal sphincter.* This is actually the lowest part of the cricopharyngeus muscle. The lower esophageal sphincter is more of a physiological sphincter; no separate sphincter muscle can be identified at this site.

Adventitia

The *adventitia* of the esophagus consists of connective tissue that blends with the surrounding connective tissue in the neck and thorax. After entering the abdominal cavity, part of the esophagus is covered by a *serosa.*

Innervation of the Esophagus

Esophageal innervation is complex. The efferent supply to the muscle is by the vagus (X) nerve. The striated musculature in the upper part of the esophagus in innervated by somatic motor neurons of the vagus (from the nucleus ambiguus) without synaptic interruption. The smooth muscle of the lower part is innervated by visceral motor neurons of the vagus (from the dorsal motor nucleus) that synapse with postganglionic neurons whose cell bodies are in the wall of the esophagus.

STOMACH

The stomach is an expanded part of the digestive tube located directly under the diaphragm. It receives the bolus from the esophagus. Within the stomach, the food is mixed with digestive juices and churned into a thick mix called **chyme.** Digestion continues until ingredients are broken down enough to be passed into the intestine for further digestion and absorption. The stomach wall is impermeable to most materials, but alcohol and some water, salts, and drugs may be absorbed.

The gastric secretions include pepsin, intrinsic factor, mucus, electrolytes, and water. Among the electrolytes is hydrocholoric acid, which gives the gastric juice a low pH. In addition, the stomach produces a hormone, gastrin, and several other agents described below.

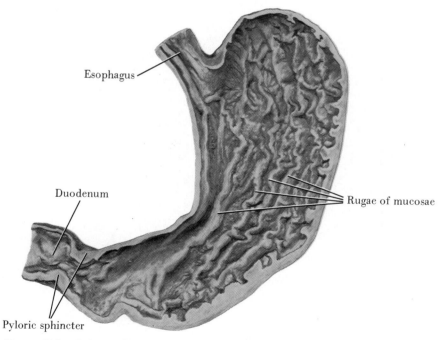

Esophagus

Duodenum

Rugae of mucosae

Pyloric sphincter

Figure 16.3.   Schematic drawing of the stomach. A small region of the stomach immediately adjacent to the entrance of the esophagus is the cardiac region; it contains the cardiac glands. A slightly larger region of the stomach leading toward the pyloric sphincter is the pyloric region, which contains the pyloric glands. The remainder of the stomach contains the fundic gastric glands; histologically this region of the stomach is designated the fundic region. (From Tortora G: 1983.)

The stomach is divided into three histologically distinct parts (Fig. 16.3): the *cardia (cardiac region),* near the esophageal orifice; the *pyloris (pyloric region),* leading to the pyloric sphincter (which guards the exit to the small intestine); and the *body* or *fundus (fundic region).* (Gross anatomists subdivide the body of the stomach into two regions. The fundic region is the one that extends above the level of a horizontal line drawn through the esophageal orifice; the body lies below this line). Throughout, the stomach has the same general structural plan, consisting of a mucosa, submucosa, muscularis externa, and a serosa.

Mucosa

The *mucosa* and the underlying submucosa of the empty stomach is thrown into a number of longitudinal folds, called *rugae.* A view of the inner surface also shows that smaller regions of the stomach mucosa are formed by shallow grooves that divide the stomach surface into irregular areas called *mamillated areas* (Fig. 16.4). The inner surface of the stomach contains numerous openings, the *gastric pits,* or foveolae which extend for a short distance into the mucosa. Glands within the stomach mucosa, the *gastric glands,* open into the bottom of the pits. The epithelium that lines the surface and the pits of the stomach is simple columnar. These columnar cells are designated *mucous surface cells.* Each cell possesses an apical cup of mucinogen granules, thereby converting the epithelium into a glandular sheet of cells (Fig. 16.5). The mucinogen granules are dissolved during the preparation of the tissue and, thus, the mucous cup appears empty and unstained in a routine hematoxylin and eosin (H&E) section. The nucleus and Golgi apparatus are below the mucous cup and, generally, the basal part of the cell contains only small amounts of rough endoplasmic reticulum (rER) that impart a light basophilia to the cytoplasm. The mucus produced by the mucous surface cells (and mucous cells of the glands) protects the stomach lining from damage due to acid and pepsin secreted by the gastric glands.

Gastric Glands

Gastric gland epithelium differs according to the type of gland in which it is contained. There are three types of gastric glands in the gastric mucosa: *cardiac glands* near the esophageal orifice; *pyloric glands* in the pyloric antrum; and *fundic,* or *gastric, glands* in the remainder of the mucosa.

Fundic Glands. Fundic glands (see Fig. 16.5) are the most numerous of the gastric glands. They

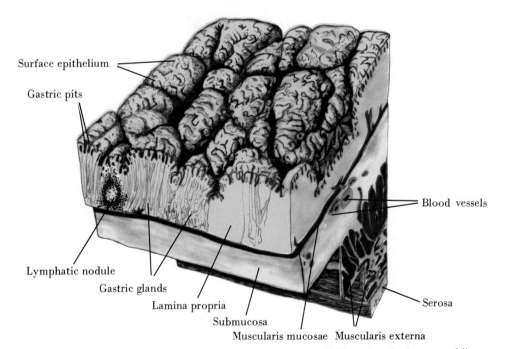

Figure 16.4. Three-dimensional diagram of stomach wall. The elevated areas of the mucosa are referred to as mamillated areas. Tubular depressions from the surface constitute the gastric pits; gastric glands open into the bottom of the pits. Note the lymphatic nodule in the mucosa. (Based on Braus H: *Anatomie der Menschen.* Berlin, Springer, 1924.)

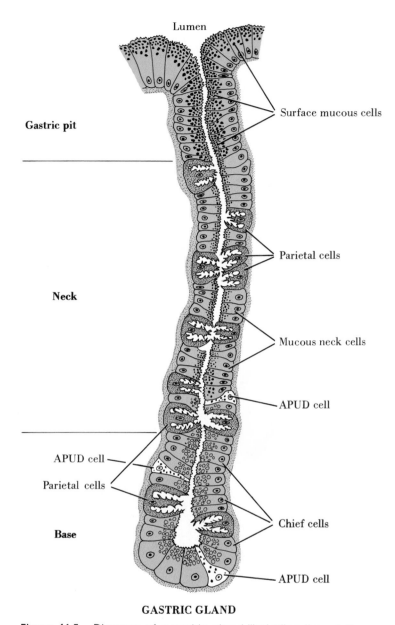

GASTRIC GLAND

Figure 16.5. Diagram of a gastric gland illustrating the relation-ship of the gland to the gastric pit. The neck region contains mucuous neck cells, parietal cells, and APUD cells. Undifferenti-ated cells (not illustrated) are located in the upper portion of the neck region. The base (or fundus) region contains parietal cells, chief cells and several different types of APUD cells. (Based on Ito S, Winchester RJ: Bat gastric mucosa. *J Cell Biol* 16:543, 1963.)

occur in the entire gastric mucosa except for the relatively small regions occupied by cardiac and pyloric glands. Three distinct cell types can be identified quite easily in H&E sections of fundic glands: mucous neck cells, parietal cells, and chief cells. In addition, the fundic glands contain undif-ferentiated cells and a variety of cells that belong to the group designated as amine percursor uptake decarboxylase (APUD) cells. (These cells are dis-cussed below under the heading of gastrointestinal hormones, APUD cells, and peptides.) The undif-ferentiated cells are located in the neck region of the gland; the APUD cells are scattered through-out.

Mucous neck cells are located just below the gastric pits, interspersed with parietal cells. They contain mucinogen granules in the apical cytoplasm. The mucinogen stains readily with special stains for mucosubstances and these stains show that the mucinogen differs from that of the mucous surface cells. However, in routine H&E sections, much of the mucinogen is lost. These cells possess a well-developed Golgi and scattered profiles of rER along with other organelles.

Parietal, or ***oxyntic,*** cells secrete hydrochloric acid and also, in the human, ***intrinsic factor.*** In sections the parietal cell is triangular, with its base adjacent to the basal lamina and its apex directed toward the lumen of the gland. The nucleus of the parietal cell is spherical and some cells are binucleate. The cytoplasm stains intensely and uniformly with eosin. This distinctive staining characteristic enables the parietal cell to be distinguished easily from other cells in the fundic glands. At the ultrastructural level, several unique features of cytological organization are evident (Fig. 16.6). These are the presence of intracellular secretory canaliculi that communicate with the lumen of the gland; numerous microvilli projecting from the surface of the canaliculi; a tubulovesicular system under the microvilli; and numerous mitochondria. In the resting cell, the tubulovesicular system predominates and microvilli are less numerous; upon stimulation and secretion of hydrochloric acid, the tubulovesicular system diminishes and microvilli become more numerous. Electron micrographs show connections between the two, leading to the conclusion that they are functionally interrelated in acid secretion. The large number of mitochondria indicates that the production of hydrochloric acid has a high energy requirement. Histamine, gastrin, and acetylcholine all stimulate acid secre-

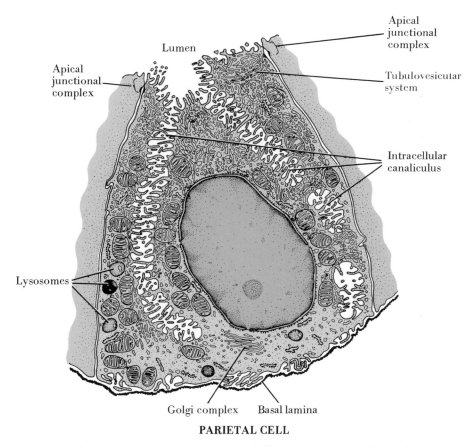

PARIETAL CELL

Figure 16.6. Diagram of a parietal cell. The cytoplasm of this cell stains intensely with eosin owing to the extensive amount of membrane comprising the tubulovesicular system (tubular endoplasmic reticulum) as well as mitochondria and the relatively small number of ribosomes. This cell produces the hydrochloric acid of gastric secretion. (Based on Lentz TL: *Cell Fine Structure.* Philadelphia, WB Saunders, 1971.)

tion and, presumably, there are receptors for these agents on the plasma membrane of the parietal cell.

In some species, chief cells secrete the intrinsic factor, but in the human this is a function of the parietal cells. The intrinsic factor is a glycoprotein ($\cong$55,000 D); it complexes with vitamin B_{12} in the stomach, a step necessary for subsequent absorption of the vitamin by the ileum. In achlorhydria, a condition characterized by the absence of parietal cells, intrinsic factor is not secreted, thereby leading to pernicious anemia. Because the liver has extensive reserve stores of vitamin B_{12}, the disease is often not recognized until long after the changes in the gastric mucosa takes place.

Chief cells are located in the deepest part of the fundic glands. They are typical protein-secreting cells (Fig. 16.7). The rER in their basal cytoplasm and secretory granules in their apical pole account for the basophilia and acidophilia, respectively. The basophilia in particular allows for easy identification of these cells in H&E sections. However, the acidophilia may be weak because the secretory granules are not always adequately pre-

served. Chief cells secrete *pepsin* in an inactive precursor form designated *pepsinogen.* Upon contact with the acid of the gastric juice, the pepsinogen is converted to pepsin, a proteolytic enzyme.

The gastric glands also contain APUD cells and undifferentiated cells. A number of APUD cell types have been described. All of them possess numerous small secretory granules that are discharged toward the connective tissue. The cells are located in the basal portion of the epithelial layer (Fig. 16.8), although some APUD cell types send a thin cytoplasmic extension to the lumen of the gland. In the preparation of routine H&E sections, the secretary granules are lost and, accordingly, the cells appear as small clear or relatively unstained areas of cytoplasm surrounding a basally located nucleus.

Cardiac Glands. Cardiac glands release their secretory product via short ducts into the gastric pits. The pits extend about a quarter of the distance to the muscularis mucosae. The glands are tubular and coiled (sometimes branched); they are made up mostly of mucus-secreting cells. Some un-

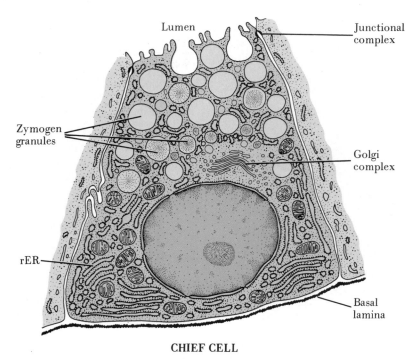

CHIEF CELL

Figure 16.7. Diagram of a chief cell. This cell produces the enzymes of the gastric secretion. The large amount of rER in the basal portion of the cell accounts for the intense basophilic staining seen in this region. Zymogen granules are not always adequately preserved and, thus, the staining in the apical region of the cell is somewhat variable. (Based on Lentz TL: *Cell Fine Structure.* Philadelphia, WB Saunders, 1971.)

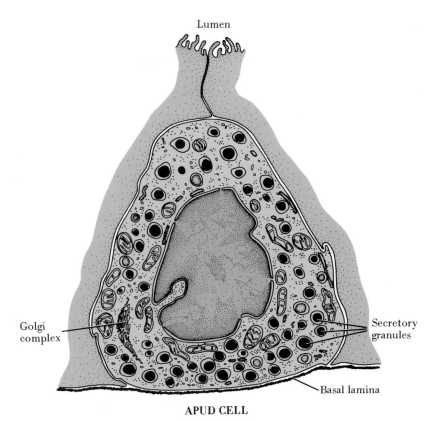

Lumen

Golgi
complex

Secretory
granules

Basal lamina

APUD CELL

Figure 16.8. Diagram of an APUD cell. This cell is diagrammed to show that it does not reach the epithelial surface. The secretory granules are regularly lost during the preparation of paraffin sections and, in the absence of other distinctive stainable organelles, the cell has more or less the appearance of a "clear cell"—that is, the nucleus appears to be surrounded by a small amount of clear cytoplasm in H&E-stained sections. (Based on Ito S, Winchester RJ: Bat gastric mucosa. *J Cell Biol* 16:574, 1963.)

differentiated cells are present in the neck or upper region of the gland. Scattered APUD cells are also present throughout the gland. Parietal cells are occasionally seen.

Pyloric Glands. Pyloric glands empty into gastric pits that are relatively long, extending through almost half the thickness of the pyloric mucosa. The glands are coiled, though not as extensively as those in the cardia of the stomach. Pyloric glands contain mucous cells, occasionally some parietal cells, APUD cells and undifferentiated cells. The latter are likewise restricted to the neck region. They produce mucus and gastrin.

The *lamina propria* of the stomach mucosa contains numerous cells of the immune system, migrant cells from the blood, and resident connective tissue cells. This tissue has the properties of diffuse lymphatic tissue due to the presence of numerous lymphocytes. The muscularis mucosae of the stomach consist of two thin layers of smooth muscle. However, the orientation of the layers is not always evident in histological sections.

Muscularis Externa

The *muscularis externa* of the stomach consists of three layers of smooth muscle: an outer longitudinal, a middle circular, and an inner oblique. The longitudinal layer is absent from much of the anterior and posterior stomach surfaces, and the circular layer is poorly developed in the paraesophageal region.

Submucosa and Serosa

The *submucosa* and *serosa* are typical of the description given previously for the alimentary canal in general.

FUNCTIONS OF GASTRIC MUSCULARIS EXTERNA

Three functions of the stomach depend upon its musculature:

1) to receive large volumes of ingested food and drink during a meal;

2) to mix the ingested food with gastric juices so that digestion can occur; and

3) to propel the gastric contents into the small intestines.

In considering gastric motility, the stomach is divided into an **orad portion** (the anatomical fundus and upper half of the body) and a **caudad portion** (the lower half of the body and the pyloric region). The orad region displays relatively little motility; it serves to receive the ingested food by a process termed **receptive relaxation.** This is under the control of neural (vagal) and humoral factors.

The caudad region displays peristaltic contractions that move in a caudad direction. The peristaltic wave moves more rapidly than the stomach contents and the overtaking peristaltic wave mixes and propels the gastric contents. The propulsion is in both an orad and caudad direction, but mostly in an orad direction. Because most of the gastric contents are propelled in an orad direction by the overtaking peristaltic wave, only a small amount of gastric contents enters the small intestines with each peristaltic wave.

When the stomach fails to empty properly, the subject complains of nausea, loss of appetite, and fullness. The most common cause of impaired emptying is an obstruction near the gastric outlet, as in gastric cancer and ulcer. Emptying of the stomach is regulated by the vagus, (X cranial) nerve. In some patients, surgical cutting of the vagus nerve may provide relief. In performing a surgical section of the vagus nerve, it also may be necessary to modify surgically the gastroduodenal junction in order to facilitate gastric emptying. Surgical sectioning of the vagus nerve is also used to decrease acid secretion in the treatment of patients with gastric ulcers. However, it is important to recognize that in the medical treatment of duodenal and gastric uclers, they are usually receptive to histamine H_2-receptor antagonists (such as cimetidine), which block receptors on parietal cells and inhibit acid secretion. However, stomal ulcers (in the jejunum) are often resistant to medical therapy. Vagotomy or more extensive gastrectomy is often necessary to decrease acid secretion of the stomach.

SMALL INTESTINE

The small intestine is a long tubular part of the alimentary canal. It is divided into three parts: duodenum, jejunum, and ileum. It receives chyme from the stomach and continues the solubilization and digestion of nutrients in preparation for their absorption. Most nutrients are absorbed by the small intestine.

The small intestine contains the four layers characteristic of the alimentary canal. However, the **mucosa** and **submucosa** are significantly modified at several levels of organization to increase the luminal surface area. Amplifications of the surface include plicae circulares (also known as the valves of Kirkring), villi, and striated border. The **plicae circulares** contain a core of submucosa (Fig. 16.9). The core projects as a narrow shelf from the main layer of the submucosa and is covered by the mucosa. Because of their generally circular arrangement, the plicae circulares are seen best in longitudinal section of the small intestine. However, they are sometimes seen also in cross- or slightly oblique sections because they may be oriented in a more longitudinal direction for short distances.

Villi are finger-like or leaf-like projections of the musosa (Fig. 16.10). They include an epithelial cover and an underlying lamina propria. Typically, each villus contains a centrally placed lymphatic capillary called a **lacteal.** The lacteal begins in the villus as a blind capillary and drains into larger lymphatic vessels in the submucosa. At times, such as after a meal when absorption is taking place, the lacteals are dilated and readily evident (Fig. 16.11). Otherwise, the lacteals are collapsed and are not evident in routine H&E sections.

Mucosa

The intestinal mucosa contains glands throughout its length. The **intestinal glands,** or **crypts of Lieberkühn,** are simple tubular glands that extend through the thickness of the mucous membrane and open into the intestinal lumen at the base of the villi (Fig. 16.10). The lining of the intestinal mucosa consists of simple columnar epithelium. Under the epithelium is the lamina propria. As in the stomach, the lamina propria contains numerous cells of the immune system (diffuse lym-

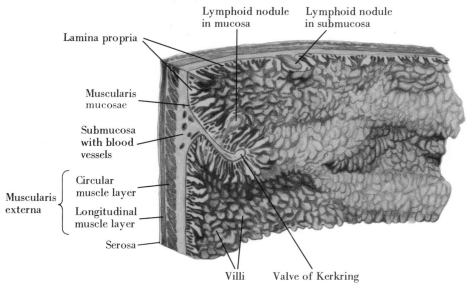

Figure 16.9. Diagram showing the wall of the small intestine in three dimensions. Note the valve of Kerkring (plica circulares), which has a core of submucosa covered by mucosa. The plicae are some of several structures that amplify the surface area of the small intestine. (Based on Braus H: *Anatomie der Menschen.* Berlin, Springer, 1924.)

phatic tissue) in addition to resident cells of the connective tissue. Throughout the small intestine, the mucosa contains isolated nodules of lymphatic tissue. In the more distal part, especially in the ileum and typically on the side of the small intestine opposite the mesenteric attachment, are the aggregations of nodules called **Peyer's patches** (see Atlas section, Plate 79).

The **muscularis mucosae** consist of two thin layers of smooth muscle cells, an inner circular and an outer longitudinal. Isolated smooth muscle cells extend from the muscularis mucosae through the lamina propria of the mucosa and into the villi.

Cells of the Intestinal Epithelium

Five cells types are present in the intestinal epithelium: enterocytes, goblet cells, APUD cells, Paneth cells, and undifferentiated cells. An additional specialized cell, the M cell, is located on the surface of the lymphatic nodules (see section on immune functions of alimentary canal). Moreover, lymphocytes are typically found within the epithelial layer.

The **enterocytes** are also referred to as **intestinal absorptive cells.** However, their function is not limited to absorption, and the more general term enterocyte appears to be more appropriate. They are tall columnar cells, with a basally positioned nucelus (Fig. 16.12). They contain numerous par-

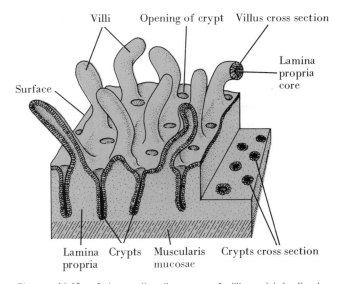

Figure 16.10. Schematic diagram of villi and intestinal crypts (glands). Note that the villi are projections into the lumen of the intestine. When cross-sectioned, they are seen to be surrounded by space of the lumen and possess a core of lamina propria. The crypts are depressions into the substance of the intestine. When cross-sectioned, they are seen to be surrounded by tissue comprising the lamina propria. (Based on Ham AW, Cormack DH: *Histology,* 8th ed. Philadelphia, JB Lippincott, 1979.)

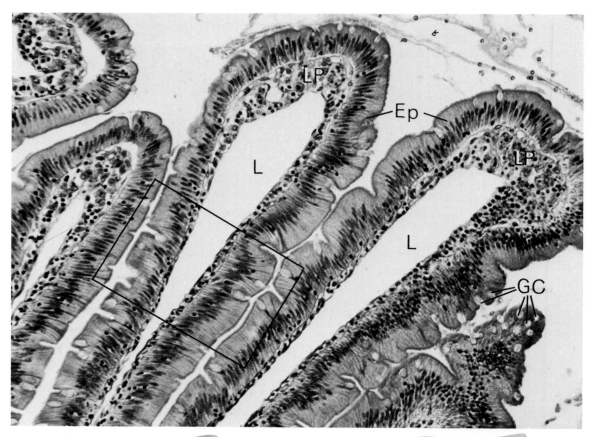

Figure 16.11. Light micrograph of villi. The surface of the villi consists of columnar epithelium (Ep). These are chiefly enterocytes with a striated border. Also evident in the epithelial layer are goblet cells (GC). Under the epithelium is a highly cellular connective tissue called the lamina propria (LP). The center of the villus contains a lymphatic capillary called the lacteal (L). When dilated, as they are in this specimen, they are easily identified. × 160.

allel microvilli at their apical surface, forming the **striated border** of light microscopy. A microvillus contains a core of microfilaments comprised of actin (Fig. 16.13). The actin microfilaments are anchored to the plasma membrane at the tip. The filaments extend into the terminal web, another network of microfilaments, immediately under the microvilli. The terminal web consists mostly of horizontally disposed microfilaments that insert into the zonula adherens of the apical junctional complex. Immunocytochemical studies show that the terminal web contains myosin in addition to actin. Below the terminal web, the apical cytoplasma contains a well-developed Golgi, numerous cisternae of rER, free ribosomes, mitochondria, and many vesicles and tubular profiles of the smooth endoplasmic reticulum (sER). The basal cytoplasm contains rER, free ribosomes, and mitochondria.

Enterocytes are organized so that they can function in the transport of fluid. They are joined at their apical poles by junctional complexes to neighboring enterocytes. These junctional complexes include occluding junctions that separate the lumen of the intestine from the lateral intercellular, or paracellular, space. The basal paracellular space is often dilated, particularly during fluid transport (see Atlas section, Plate 4). It is significant to note that the basilateral plasma membrane bordering the intercellular space contains ATPases associated with sodium from the cell into the space. The increased sodium concentration thus created within the intercellular space draws water osmotically from the cell and, in turn, from the lumen of the gut. When the intercellular space is minimal, the adjacent enterocytes show interdigitating folds of their plasma membranes.

Enterocytes are found chiefly on the villi and surface of the small intestine and, in lesser numbers, in the intestinal glands. Although their absorptive functions have been known for a long

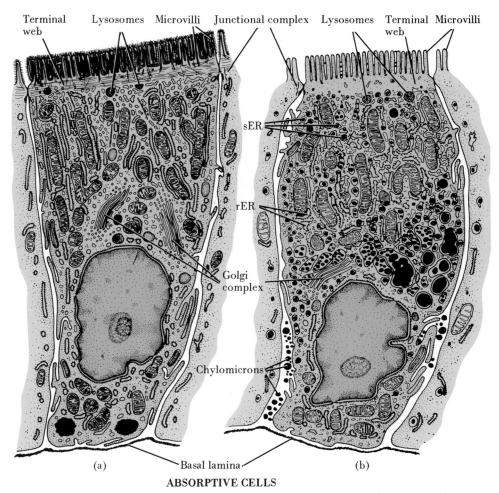

ABSORPTIVE CELLS

Figure 16.12. Diagram of an enterocyte **(a)** showing a striated border on its apical (luminal) surface and junctional complexes that seal the lumen of the intestine from the lateral intercellular space. The characteristic complement of organelles is depicted in the diagram. The cell in **(b)** shows the distribution of lipid during fat absorption as seen with the transmission electron microscope. Initially, lipid is seen in association with the microvilli of the striated border. The lipid is internalized and seen in vesicles of the sER in the apical portion of the cell. The membrane-bound lipid can be traced into the center of the cell, where some of the lipid-containing vesicles fuse, and then the lipid is discharged into the lateral intercellular space. The extracellular lipid, recognized as chylomicrons, passes beyond the basal lamina for further transport. (Based on Lentz TL: *Cell Fine Structure.* Philadelphia, WB Saunders, 1971.)

time, it is now known that they also synthesize digestive enzymes, some of which are located and function on the membrane of the striated border.

Goblet cells are interspersed among the other cells of the intestinal epithelium, being most numerous on the villi. As in other epithelia, the goblet cells produce mucus. Also, as in other epithelia, because water-soluble mucinogen is lost during preparation of a routine H&E section, the part of the cell that contained the mucinogen granules appears empty in the preparation. With the electron microscope, an extensive array of flattened Golgi saccules is seen to form a wide cup around the basal half of the mucinogen granules (Fig. 16.14). Basal to the wide cup portion of the goblet cell is a more narrow stem portion containing the nucleus, most of the rER, free ribosomes, and mitochondria.

Paneth cells are contained in the deepest part of the intestinal glands. They have ultrastructural features typical of cells that synthesize and secrete protein, namely, large amounts of well-organized

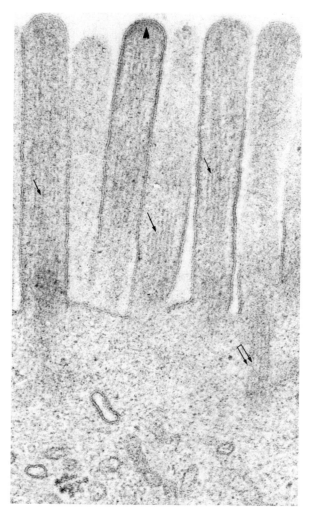

Figure 16.13. Electron micrograph of the microvilli that form the striated border of an enterocyte. The microvilli contain a core of longitudinally disposed microfilaments **(arrows).** The filaments, comprised of actin, are connected to the tip of the microvillus **(arrowhead)** and extend beyond the base of the microvillus **(double arrows)** into the terminal web region of the cell. × 85,000.

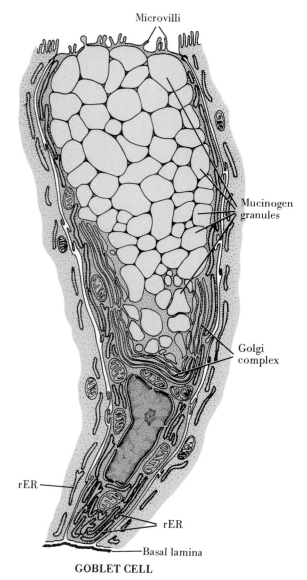

GOBLET CELL

Figure 16.14(a). Diagram of a goblet cell. The nucleus is in the basal pole of the cell. The major portion of the cell is filled with mucigen (mucinogen) granules forming the mucous cup that is evident with the light microscope. At the base and lower sides of the mucous cup are flattened saccules of the large Golgi apparatus. Other organelles are distributed throughout the remaining cytoplasm, especially in the perinuclear cytoplasm in the base of the cell. (Based on Neutra M, Leblond CP: *J Cell Biol* 1966.)

rER in the basal cytoplasm, and a well-developed Golgi and numerous large secretory granules in the apical cytoplasm. The apical granules stain intensely with eosin, thereby enabling these cells to be readily identified in H&E-stained sections (Fig. 16.15). Paneth cell granules contain lysozyme, an enzyme that digests the protective cell walls of certain groups of bacteria. The lysozyme granules are secreted in response to certain stimuli. Moreover, Paneth cells are able to phagocytose certain bacteria. The action of lysozyme and the special phago-

cytic activity of Paneth cells have led to the conclusion that they regulate the microbial flora of the intestines. Paneth cells are found in humans, monkeys, and some rodents, but not in rabbits, cats, and pigs.

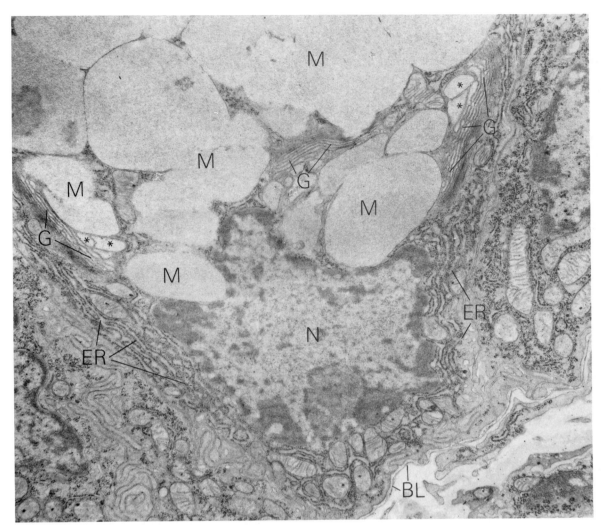

Figure 16.14(b). Electron micrograph of the basal portion of a goblet cell. The cell rests on the basal lamina (BL). The basal portion of the cell contains the nucleus (N), rough endoplasmic reticulum (ER), and mitochondria. Just apical to the nucleus are extensive Golgi profiles (G). As the mucous product accumulates in the Golgi cisternae, they become enlarged (asterisks). The large mucinogen granules (M) fill most of the apical portion of the cell and collectively constitute the "mucous cup" seen with the light microscope. × 15,000.

Submucosa

The *submucosa* of the small intestine consists of components described in the general description at the beginning of this chapter. In addition, the submucosa of the duodenum contains glands referred to as *Brunner's glands* (see Atlas section, Plate 77). These are mucus-secreting branched tubuloalveolar glands. The mucus secretion is discharged via ducts into the bottom of the intestinal glands. The cells of Brunner's glands possess features of zymogen-producing cells as well as mucus-producing cells. The cells exhibit numerous profiles of rER in the basal cytoplasm, a large supranuclear Golgi apparatus, and apical secretory granules that resemble, at least superficially, the zymogen granules of the pancreatic acinar cells. The secretion has been shown to be alkaline, viscous, and high in bicarbonate. These features suggest a protective role against the acid chyme that enters the duodenum from the stomach.

Muscularis Externa

The *muscularis externa* consists of an inner layer of circularly arranged smooth muscle cells and an outer layer of longitudinally disposed smooth muscle cells. The main components of Auerbach's plexus are located between these two muscle layers (Fig. 16.18). Two kinds of muscular contraction occur in the small intestine. Local contractions displace intestinal contents both proximally and distally are designated as *segmentation.* These contractions serve to circulate the chyme locally, mixing it with digestive juices and moving it

into contact with the mucosa for absorption. *Peristalsis,* the second type of contraction, moves the intestinal contents distally.

Serosa

The *serosa* corresponds to that given in the general description at the beginning of the chapter.

GASTROINTESTINAL HORMONES, APUD CELLS, AND PEPTIDES

The mucosa of the gastrointestinal tract produces four hormones (Table 16.1): secretin, gastrin, cholecystokinin (CKK), and gastric inhibitory peptide (GIP). In each case, the hormone is released into the bloodstream by the endocrine cells and, as it circulates throughout the body, it is bound by receptors on the plasma membrane of target cells. The endocrine cells of the gut are not grouped as clusters in any specific part of the gastrointestinal tract. Rather they are distributed singly throughout the gastrointestinal epithelium. Figure 16.16 shows the parts of the gastrointestinal tract from which the hormones are released into the blood.

The endocrine cells of the gastrointestinal tract and those of the pancreas are sometimes collectively grouped as the *GastroEnteroPancreatic (GEP) system.* In addition, the endocrine cells of the gastrointestinal tract are part of a larger group of cells designated as APUD *(Amine-Precursor Uptake Decarboxylase)cells* that produce not only gastrointestinal hormones but also paracrine substances. A paracrine substance differs from a hormone in that it diffuses locally to its target cell instead of being released into the bloodstream. A well-known substance that appears to act as a paracrine substance within the gastrointestinal tract and pancreas is *somatostatin.* This inhibits other gastrointestinal and pancreatic islet endocrine cells. APUD cells secrete a variety of regulator substances in other tissues and organs including respiratory epithelium, adrenal medulla, islets of Langerhans, thyroid gland (parafollicular cells), and pituitary gland.

In addition to the established gastrointestinal hormones there are several gastrointestinal peptides whose definite classification as a hormone or paracrine agent has not yet been established; these are designated as candidate, or putative, hormones. They and their actions are listed in Table 16.2.

Other local agents isolated from the gastrointestinal mucosa are neurotransmitters; these are released close to the target cell from a nerve ending. In addition to acetylcholine (not a peptide), peptides known to be in nerve fibers of the gastrointestinal tract are gastrin, VIP, and somatostatin. Thus, a particular peptide may be produced by

endocrine and paracrine cells and also be localized in nerve fibers.

At least 12 different cell types (APUD cells) have been identified with the electron microscope within the epithelium of the gastrointestinal tract as the sources of the hormones, paracrine substances, and candidate hormones. All the cells possess a broad base adjacent to the basal lamina. Some cells extend to the lumen where they display microvilli (for sampling the luminal contents ?), while others do not reach the lumen. All possess numerous small membrane-limited granules, mostly within the basal cytoplasm, and, where tested, these granules have been shown to contain an active peptide (Fig. 16.17). The granules discharge their product toward the basal lamina and subjacent connective tissue, and then the peptide diffuses locally to the target cell (paracrine) or into the bloodstream and through the blood vessels to the target cells (endocrine). The cells all display relatively little rER and small Golgi profiles.

Histologically, the cells appear as clear cells since there is not sufficient RNA to impart cytoplasmic basophilia (as in chief cells), there is not sufficient membrane to impart acidophilia (as in parietal cells), and the small granules are not adequately preserved in H&E paraffin sections. APUD cells are difficult to identify in routine H&E sections. In any attempt to do this, one should have a general idea about the frequency of these cells and, for gastric mucosa, this is shown in the Atlas section, Plate 75. Granules in some APUD cells can be displayed with silver staining procedures. These cells were originally designated as *argentaffin* or *argyophilic cells;* granules in other APUD cells can be displayed with bichromate solutions, and these were designated as *enterochromaffin cells.*

A clinical entity that has been identified as being the result of a tumor of a gastrointestinal endocrine cell is the *Zollinger-Ellison syndrome,* or *gastrinoma.* Excessive secretion by gastrin-producing cells of the pylorus (or by pancreatic islet cells) results in excessive secretion of hydrochloric acid by parietal cells. The excess acid cannot be adequately neutralized in the duodenum, thereby leading to duodenal ulcers with complications.

TABLE 16.1. Physiological Actions of Gastrointestinal Hormones*

| | HORMONES | | | |
ACTION	GASTRIN	CHOLECYSTOKININ (CCK)	SECRETIN	GASTRIC INHIBITORY PEPTIDE (GIP)
Acid secretion	S			I
Pancreatic bicarbonate ion secretion		S	S	
Pancreatic enzyme secretion		S	S	
Bile bicarbonate ion secretion		S	S	
Gallbladder contraction		S		
Gastric emptying		I		
Insulin release				S
Mucosal growth		S		
Pancreatic growth	S	S	S	

* S, stimulates; I, inhibits; blank spaces, not yet tested.
Source: Adapted from Johnson LR (ed): *Gastrointestinal Physiology,* 2nd edition. St. Louis, CV Mosby, 1981, p. 9.

TABLE 16.2. Candidate Hormones*

CANDIDATE HORMONE	ACTIONS
VIP (vasoactive intestinal peptide)	↓ Gastric secretion ↑ Insulin release ↑ Intestinal secretion ↑ Pancreatic bicarbonate ion secretion ↑ Glycogenolysis
Pancreatic polypeptide	↓ Pancreatic bicarbonate ion and enzyme secretion
Motilin	↑ Gastric motility ↑ Intestinal motility
Enteroglucagon	↑ Glycogenolysis

* ↑, stimulates; ↓, inhibits.
Source: Adapted from Johnson LR (ed): *Gastrointestinal Physiology,* 2nd edition. St. Louis, CV Mosby, 1981, p. 11.

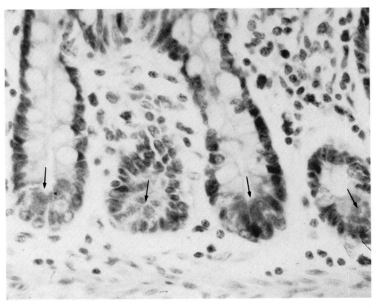

Figure 16.15. Light micrograph of intestinal glands showing Paneth cells. The specimen has been stained with H&E. Paneth cells are typically located in the bottom of the intestinal glands. The cytoplasm contains granules **(arrows)** that stain with eosin.

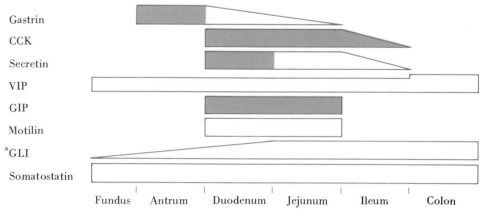

*Glucagon-like immunoactivity. Shaded portions — areas where physiological release occurs.

Figure 16.16.   Schema to show the distribution of gastrointestinal peptides. The solid green areas show where physiological release of gastrointestinal hormones occurs. CCK (cholecystokinin). VIP (vasoactive intestinal peptide), GIP (gastric inhibitory peptide), GLI (glucagon-like immunoactivity). (Modified from Johnson LR (ed): *Gastrointestinal Physiology*, 2nd ed. St. Louis, CV Mosby, 1981.)

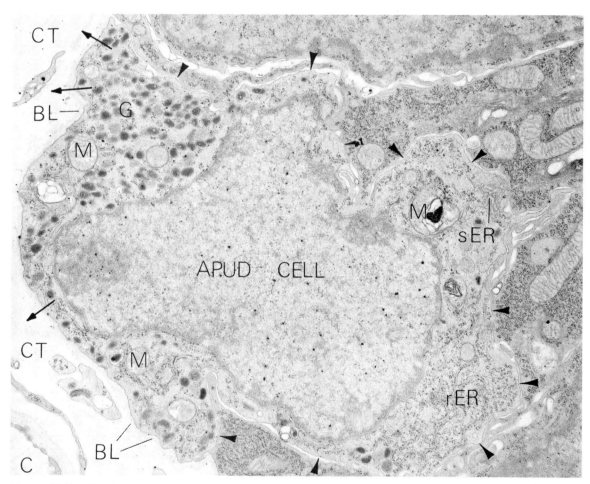

Figure 16.17.   Electron micrograph of an APUD cell of the colon. **Arrowheads** mark the boundary between the APUD cell and the adjacent epithelial cells. At its base the APUD cell is adjacent to the basal lamina (BL). This cell does not extend to the epithelial surface. Numerous secretory granules (G) in the base of the cell are secreted in the direction of the **arrows** across the basal lamina and into the connective tissue (CT). C, capillary; M, mitochondria; rER, rough endoplasmic reticulum; sER, smooth endoplasmic reticulum.

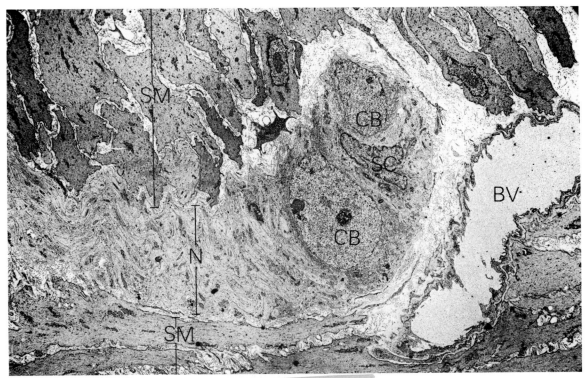

Figure 16.18. Electron micrograph of Auerbach's plexus in the small intestine. The plexus is located between the two smooth muscle (SM) layers of the muscularis externa. It consists of an extensive nerve network (N). Neuron cell bodies (CB) are also present as part of the network. A Schwann cell (SC) is also seen in proximity to the neuron cell bodies. BV, Blood vessel. × 3800.

DIGESTIVE AND ABSORPTIVE FUNCTIONS OF ENTEROCYTES

The plasma membrane of striated border microvilli plays a role in digestion as well as absorption. Digestive enzymes are anchored to the plasma membrane and their functional groups extend outward to become part of the glycocalyx. It should be noted that by this arrangement the end-products of digestion are close to the site for their absorption. Included among the enzymes are peptidases and disaccharidases. The plasma membrane of apical microvilli also contains the enzyme *enteropeptidase (enterokinase)*. This is particularly important in the duodenum where the enzyme converts trypsinogen into trypsin. Trypsin can then continue to convert additional trypsinogen into trypsin, and trypsin converts several other pancreatic zymogens into the active enzyme (Fig. 16.19). Thus, the enteropeptidase functions as the trigger that begins the cascade of reactions, which convert several zymogens to the active enzyme. A summary of digestion and absorption of the three major foods is outlined in the following paragraphs.

Triglycerides are digested into glycerol, monoglycerides, and long- and short-chain fatty acids. These are emulsified by bile salts and pass into the apical portion of the cell. Here the glycerol and long-chain fatty acids are resynthesized into triglycerides. The resynthesized triglycerides appear first in the apical vesicles of the sER (see Fig. 16.12), then in the Golgi (where they are converted into chylomicrons), and finally in vesicles that discharge the chylomicrons into the intercellular space. The chylomicrons are conveyed away from the intestines via lacteals. Short-chain fatty acids and glycerol take a different route. They leave the intestines via capillaries that lead to the portal veins and the liver.

The final digestion of carbohydrates is brought about by enzymes bound to the microvilli of the enterocytes (Fig. 16.20). Galactose, glucose, and fructose are conveyed to the liver by the vessels of the hepatic portal system. Some infants (also some adults) are unable to tolerate milk because of the absence of lactase. If given milk, they become bloated and suffer from diarrhea. The condition is alleviated if lactose (milk sugar) is eliminated from the diet.

The digestion and absorption of dietary protein are shown in Figure 16.21. The major end-products of protein digestion are amino acids and these are absorbed by the enterocytes. However, some peptides are absorbed and evidently broken down intracellularly. In one disorder of amino acid absorption (Hartnup's disease), free amino acids appear in the blood when the dipeptide is fed to patients, but not when the free amino acids are fed. This provides support for the conclusion that the absorption of dipeptides of certain amino acids is by a pathway different from that of the free amino acid.

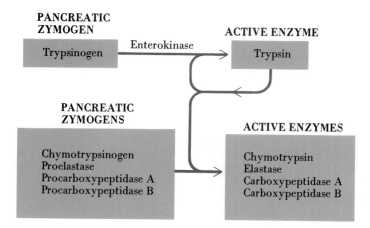

Figure 16.19. Schema to show the events in the activation of the proteolytic enzymes of the pancreas. The chain of events is triggered by enterokinase, which activates trypsinogen; in turn, trypsin activates other pancreatic zymogens, while at the same time it turns back to continue the activation of additional trypsinogen. (From Johnson LR (ed): *Gastrointestinal Physiology,* 2nd ed. St. Louis, CV Mosby, 1981.)

LARGE INTESTINE

The large intestine is comprised of the cecum, ascending colon, transverse colon, descending colon, sigmoid colon, rectum, and anal canal. The four layers characteristic of the alimentary canal are present throughout. However, neither plicae circulares nor villi are present.

Mucosa

The *mucosa* of the large intestine contains numerous straight tubular glands that extend through the full thickness of the mucosa. The glands consist of simple columnar epithelium, as does the intestinal surface from which they invaginate.

The major cell of the intestinal epithelium is the columnar absorptive cell. It has a thin striated border on its apical surface and ultrastructural features that generally resemble enterocytes of the small intestine. The columnar absorptive cell engages chiefly in water absorption, presumably by a mechanism similar to that described for the enterocyte. Although most nutrients are absorbed by

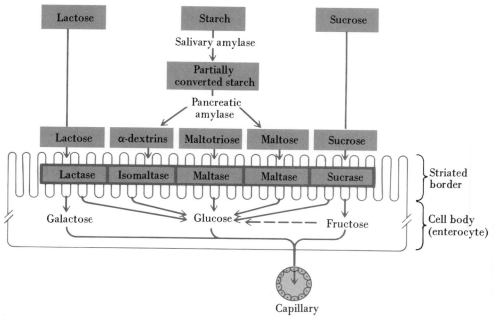

Figure 16.20. Schema to illustrate the digestion and absorption of carbohydrates by an enterocyte. Enzymes superimposed over the striated border are bound to the plasma membranes of the microvilli and act on their substrate in this location. The three absorbed monosaccharides are then passed through the enterocyte and into the underlying capillaries that lead to the portal vein, and via this vein to the liver. (From Johnson LR (ed): *Gastrointestinal Physiology,* 2nd ed. St. Louis, CV Mosby, 1981.)

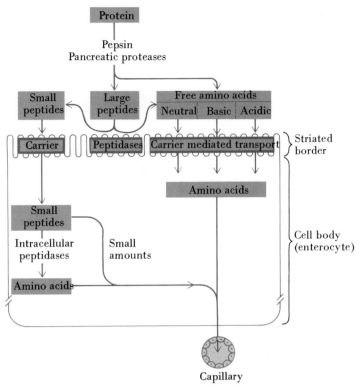

Figure 16.21. Schema to illustrate the digestion and absorption of protein by enterocyte. Free amino acids are absorbed into the cell; small peptides also enter the cell to be digested by intracellular peptidases; other peptidases are bound to the plasma membrane of the microvilli and act in this location as shown. (From Johnson LR (ed): *Gastrointestinal Physiology,* 2nd ed. St. Louis, CV Mosby, 1981.)

the small intestine, some absorption of nutrients also occurs in the large intestine, especially in the proximal part.

Goblet cells are more numerous in the large intestine than in the small intestine (Fig. 16.22). These produce mucus that lubricates the bowel, thereby allowing for easy passage of the increasingly more solid colonic contents. APUD and undifferentiated cells are present in the glands of the large intestine; Paneth cells are absent (except in the young). The lamina propria, muscularis mucosae, and submucosa are as in the small intestine. Isolated nodules of lymphatic tissue present in the mucosa usually extend into the submucosa.

Muscularis Externa

The *muscularis externa* differs from that of the small intestine in that, except for the rectum, the outer longitudinal layer of smooth muscle is arranged in three pronounced bands recognized at the gross level as the *teniae coli.* Between the teniae coli there is an extremely thin sheet of longitudinal smooth muscle. In the rectum, the outer longitudinal layer of smooth muscle is a uniformly thick layer, as in the small intestine.

The muscularis externa of the large intestine produces two major types of contraction: segmentation and peristalsis. The segmenting type of contraction is local and does not result in the propulsion of contents. The peristaltic contractions result in mass movements distally of colonic contents. The mass peristaltic movements do not occur frequently; in a healthy person, they occur only several times a day.

Submucosa and Serosa

The *submucosa* corresponds to the general description already given. Where the large intestine is directly in contact with other structures (as on much of its posterior surface), its outer layer is an adventitia; elsewhere, the outer layer is a typical serosa.

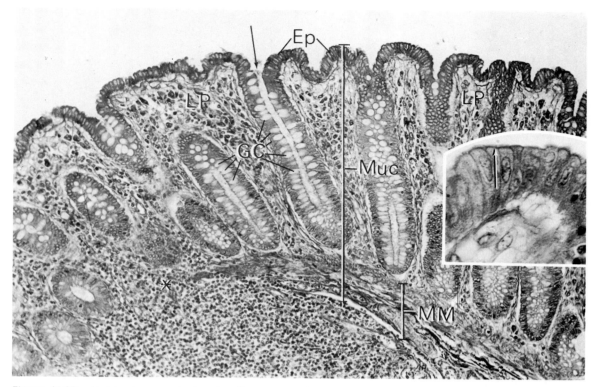

Figure 16.22. Light micrograph showing the mucosa (Muc) and part of the submucosa of the colon. The epithelium of the colonic surface is continuous with the straight, tubular intestinal glands **(arrow).** A highly cellular lamina propria (LP) is under the surface epithelium and around the glands. The **inset** shows the absorptive cells of the colonic surface. These cells possess a small striated border **(arrow).** Goblet cells (GC) are also present on the surface, but they are more numerous in the glands. In the vicinity of the **asterisk,** lymphocytes obscure the muscularis mucosa (MM).

Appendix

The appendix is a finger-like projection connected to the cecum of the large intestine. It has a relatively narrow lumen, often filled with debris, and a thick wall. The wall of the appendix resembles the wall of the large intestine except for some differences in the histological appearance (Fig. 16.23). These include a complete outer layer of longitudinal smooth muscle and the presence of a large number of lymph nodules positioned in both the mucosa and the submucosa. Because the lymph nodules disrupt the muscularis mucosae so frequently in extending into the submucosa, the muscularis mucosae typically appear as isolated lengths of smooth muscle.

Anal Canal

The anal canal is the terminal portion of the alimentary canal. It begins where the rectum suddenly narrows. The upper portion of the anal canal contains a number of vertical folds, called the **anal** (or **rectal**) **columns** (Fig. 16.24). These are pro-

nounced in the child, but not always well defined in the adult. The depressions between the anal columns are called **anal sinuses.** The sinuses may end rather abruptly at the lower end of the columns where the columns are joined by a small crescentic fold of mucosa termed the **anal valves.** The anal columns contain, in the submucosa, the terminal ramifications of the superior rectal artery and veins. Enlargements of the submucosal veins constitute internal hemorrhoids.

The mucosa in the upper portion of the anal canal is similar to that of the large intestine, containing straight, tubular, unbranched intestinal glands. Numerous goblet cells are found throughout the surface and glandular epithelium. In the region of the anal sinuses, **anal glands** extend into the submucosa and sometimes into the muscularis externa. These are branched, straight, tubular glands containing mucous cells. The duct of each gland consists of stratified columnar epithelium, and it opens into a small depression of the anal mucosa, called an **anal crypt.** The glands are important clinically because they may become in-

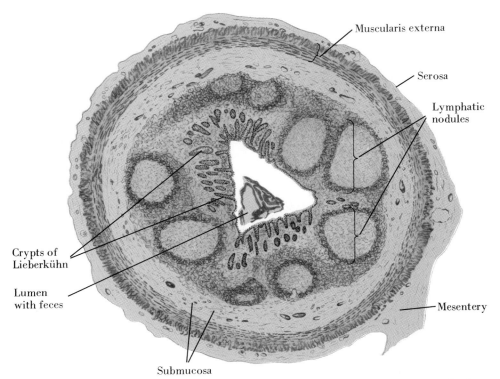

Muscularis externa

Serosa

Lymphatic nodules

Mesentery

Crypts of Lieberkühn

Lumen with feces

Submucosa

Figure 16.23. Diagram of a cross-section through the appendix. The appendix displays the same four layers as those of the large intestine except that the diameter of the appendix is much less. Typically, lymphatic nodules are seen around the entire appendix, often extending into the submucosa. (After Sobotta, in Bloom W, Fawcett DW: *A Textbook of Histology,* 10th ed. Philadelphia, WB Saunders, 1975.)

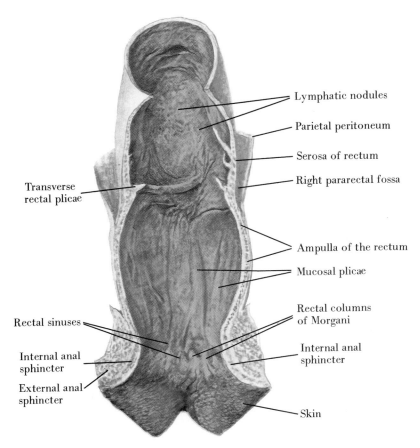

Lymphatic nodules

Parietal peritoneum

Serosa of rectum

Right pararectal fossa

Transverse rectal plicae

Ampulla of the rectum

Mucosal plicae

Rectal columns of Morgani

Rectal sinuses

Internal anal sphincter

Internal anal sphincter

External anal sphincter

Skin

Figure 16.24. Diagram of rectum and anorectal junction. The rectum is the terminal portion of the large intestine. The permanent plicae are transversely arranged. Characteristic mucosa of the large intestine extends as far as the rectal sinuses. Below the rectal sinuses, the epithelium is in transition to that of the skin, being first stratified columnar (or cuboidal) and then stratified squamous. (Based on Braus H: *Anatomie der Menschen.* Berlin, Springer, 1924.)

fected or form a cyst if a duct becomes occluded. The lower portion of the anal canal is surfaced by stratified squamous epithelium. Between the simple columnar epithelium of the upper portion and the stratified epithelium of the lower portion there is a variable amount of stratified columnar epithelium. The stratified squamous epithelium is continuous with that of the skin. In the skin of the circumanal region, there are large apocrine glands called *circumanal glands.*

The anal canal is surrounded by a complex group of sphincter muscles. The *internal sphincter* is formed by a thickening of the circular layer of the muscularis externa. There are several parts to the external sphincter; they are all striated muscle.

REPLACEMENT OF GASTROINTESTINAL EPITHELIUM

Cells of the gastrointestinal epithelium are regularly lost into the lumen of the digestive tube and replaced by the division of cells within the glands. In the stomach, undifferentiated cells are located in the neck of the glands, just below the crypts; these are the dividing cells. Some of the new daughter cells migrate upward into the gastric pits to become surface mucous cells. They have a life-span of 4 to 6 days. Other newly generated cells remain in the neck to become mucous neck cells and still others migrate down into the gland to become parietal, chief, and APUD cells. Cells in the glands live longer than those that migrate into the gastric pits.

In the small intestine, undifferentiated cells are located in the bottom half of the glands where they divide. Most give rise to enterocytes, some to goblet cells, and a few to APUD cells. As the enterocytes and goblet cells migrate upward, they become partially differentiated, but they continue to divide. The second round of divisions is augmentation divisions of committed cells; that is, cells committed to become enterocytes and goblet cells can still divide. Enterocytes and goblet cells survive for about 4 to 6 days. Other derivatives of cell division are the Paneth cells; they survive for a longer period, up to 4 weeks, and do not undergo augmentation divisions.

In the large intestine, undifferentiated cells are located in the lower half of the glands. They divide and give rise to columnar absorptive cells, goblet cells, and APUD cells. As in the small intestines, partially differentiated absorptive and goblet cells continue to divide (Fig. 16.25). Absorptive cells and goblet cells survive for 4 to 6 days; APUD cells survive longer.

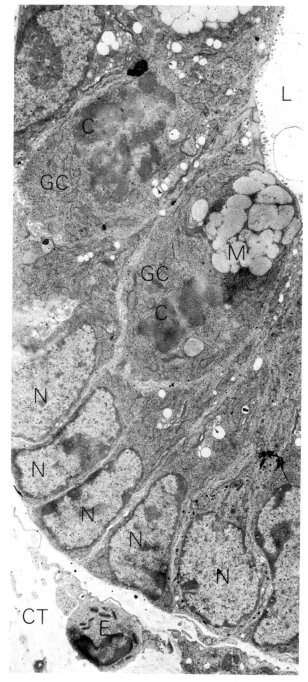

Figure 16.25. Electron micrograph of the intestinal mucosa. This electron micrograph demonstrates that certain cells of the intestine continue to divide even after they have begun to differentiate. Here, two goblet cells (GC) are shown in division. One of the goblet cells shows mucinogen granules (M) in its apical cytoplasm. The chromosomes (C) of the dividing cells are not surrounded by a nuclear membrane. Compare with the nuclei (N) of nondividing intestinal epithelium. The lumen of the gland (L) is on the right. CT, connective tissue; E, eosinophil. × 5000.

IMMUNE FUNCTIONS OF THE ALIMENTARY CANAL

Immunologists have learned that the gut-associated lymphatic tissue (GALT) is not only reactive, that is, it not only responds to antigenic stimuli, but that it functions in a monitoring capacity. This function has been partially clarified for the lymphatic nodules of the intestinal tract. The epithelium covering the nodules contains a special cell, the *M cell*, with distinctive surface microfolds or with thick microvilli. (These two surface configurations may reflect different functional variations of the apical cell surface.) The cells are readily identified with the scanning electron microscope because the thick microvilli and microfolds contrast sharply with the thinner microvilli that constitute the striated border of the adjacent enterocytes.

It has been shown with horseradish peroxidase (an enzyme used as an experimental marker in cell biology) that the M cells are able to pinocytose protein from the intestinal lumen, transport the pinocyteic vesicles through the cell, and discharge the protein by exocytosis into deep recesses of the adjacent extracellular space (Fig. 16.26). It is proposed that lymphocytes within the deeply recessed extracellular space sample the luminal protein, including antigen, and thus, have the opportunity to develop specific antibody against the antigen. The destination of these exposed lymphocytes has not yet been determined. Some apparently remain within the local lymphatic tissue, but others may be destined for other sites in the body such as salivary glands and mammary glands. It has already been noted that in the salivary gland, cells of the immune system (plasma cells) secrete IgA that are glandular epithelium then converts into secretory IgA (SIgA). Certain experimental observations suggest that antigen contact for the production of IgA by these plasma cells occurs in the lymphatic nodules of the intestines.

Radiation therapy and antimitotic drugs used in the treatment of cancer affect all dividing cells, not only dividing cancer cells, unless the cancer cells can be specifically targeted. Thus, although the gastrointestinal epithelial cells continue to slough off, during prolonged cancer therapy they are not replaced, and malabsorption and diarrhea result. When treatment is discontinued, the surface is repopulated with cells by division of stem cells that were quiescent during the therapy.

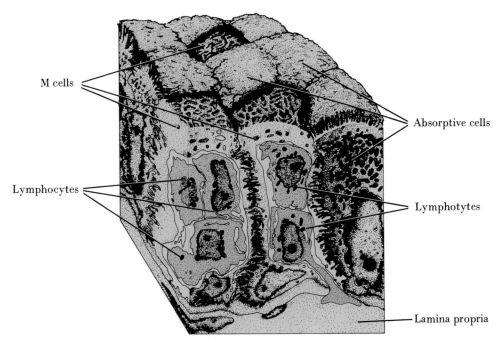

Figure 16.26. Diagram showing cells that cover a lymphatic nodule of the intestine. Some of these cells are typical of absorptive cells. Other cells display large blunt microvilli or blunt microridges (M cells). The M cells have deep recesses that contain lymphocytes. The M cells are considered to monitor intestinal contents and present antigen to the lymphocytes. (Based on Owen RC, Nemanic P (eds): *Scanning Electron Microscopy,* 1978.)

PLATE 71. Lip, A Mucocutaneous Junction

A sagittal section through the lip is shown in the low-power orientation photomicrograph on this page. It reveals the skin of the face, the red margin of the lip, and the transition to the oral mucosa of the mouth. The **numbered rectangles** indicate representative areas of each of these sites, which are shown at higher magnifications in **Figures 1, 3,** and **5,** respectively, on the adjacent plate. In examining the low-power orientation micrograph note the change in thickness of the epithelium from the exterior, facial portion of the lip (the vertical surface on the right) to the interior surface of the oral cavity (the surface beginning with the **rectangle numbered 5** and continuing down the left surface of the lip).

The epithelium **(Ep)** of the face **(Fig. 1)** is relatively thin and has the general features of thin skin found in other sites. Associated with it are hair follicles **(HF)** and sebaceous glands **(SGl).** The **circled area in Figure 1** is shown at higher magnification in **Figure 2.** The reddish brown material in the basal cells is the pigment melanin **(M),** and the dark blue near the surface is the stratum granulosum **(SG)** with its deep-blue-stained keratohyalin granules.

Figure 3 reveals the epithelium of the red margin of the lip to be much thicker than that of the face. The stratum granulosum is still present **(Fig. 4);** thus, the epithelium is keratinized. The principal feature that accounts for the coloration of the red margin in life is the deep penetration of the connective tissue papillae into the epithelium **(arrowheads, Fig. 3).** Note how thin the epithelium is where it overlies the papillae. The thinness of the epithelium at these sites in combination with the extensive vascularity of the underlying connective tissue, particularly the extensive venous vessels **(BV),** allows the color of the blood to show through the epithelium. The deep connective tissue papillae are more numerous than is suggested by the micrograph, where only two are apparent; the several other more shallow-appearing papillae have been cut in a plane that does not reveal their depth. The sensitivity of the red margin to stimuli such as light touch is due to the presence of an increased number of sensory receptors. In fact, each of the two deep papillae contains a Meissner's corpuscle, one of which **(MC),** is more clearly seen in **Figure 4.**

The transition from the keratinized red mar-

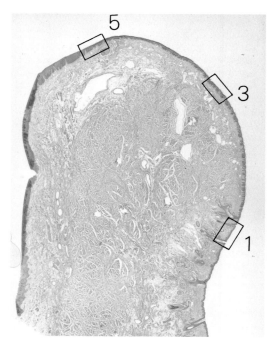

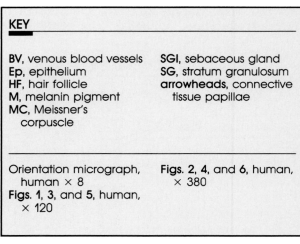

KEY

BV, venous blood vessels	**SGl,** sebaceous gland
Ep, epithelium	**SG,** stratum granulosum
HF, hair follicle	**arrowheads,** connective
M, melanin pigment	tissue papillae
MC, Meissner's	
corpuscle	

Orientation micrograph, human × 8	**Figs. 2, 4,** and **6,** human, × 380
Figs. 1, 3, and **5,** human, × 120	

gin to the fairly thick stratified squamous parakeratinized epithelium of the oral mucosa is evident in **Figure 5.** Note how the stratum granulosum suddenly ends. This is more evident at the higher magnification of **Figure 6.** Beyond the site where the stratum granulosum cells disappear, nuclei are seen in the superficial cells up to the surface **(arrows).** The epithelium is also much thicker at this point and remains so throughout the oral cavity.

PLATE 71

PLATE 72. Esophagus

The esophagus is a muscular tube that conveys food and other substances from the pharynx to the stomach. A cross-section of the wall of the esophagus is shown in **Figure 1.** The mucosa (**Muc**) consists of stratified squamous epithelium (**Ep**), a lamina propria (**LP**), and muscularis mucosae (**MM**). The boundary between the epithelium and lamina propria is distinct, though uneven owing to the presence of numerous deep connective tissue papillae. The basal layer of the epithelium stains intensely, appearing as a dark band that is relatively conspicuous at low magnification. This is due in part to the cytoplasmic basophilia of the basal cells. Also, the fact that the basal cells are small results in a high nuclear-cytoplasmic ratio that further intensifies the hematoxylin staining of this layer.

As in other stratified squamous epithelia, new cells are produced in the basal layer, from which they move to the surface. During this migration, the shape and orientation of the cells change. This change in cell shape and orientation is also reflected in the appearance of the nuclei. In the deeper layers, the nuclei are spherical; in the more superficial layers the nuclei are elongated and oriented parallel to the surface. The fact that nuclei can be seen throughout the epithelial layer, particularly the surface cells, indicates that the epithelium is not keratinized (**Fig. 2**). In some instances, the epithelium of the upper regions of the esophagus may be parakeratinized or more rarely keratinized.

As shown in **Figure 2,** the lamina propria (**LP**) is a very cellular, loose connective tissue containing many lymphocytes (**Lym**), small blood vessels, and lymphatic vessels (**LV**). The deepest part of the mucosa is the muscularis mucosae (**MM**). That location defines the boundary between mucosa and submucosa. The nuclei of the smooth muscle cells of the muscularis mucosae cells appear spherical because the cells have been cut in cross-section (**Fig. 2**).

The submucosa consists of irregular dense connective tissue that contains the larger blood vessels and nerves. No glands are seen in the submucosa of **Figure 1,** but they are regularly present throughout this layer and are likely to be included in the section of the wall. Whereas the boundary between the epithelium and lamina propria is striking, the boundary between the mucosa (**Muc**)

KEY	
Adv, adventitia	**Muc,** mucosa
Ep, stratified squamous epithelium	**SM,** smooth muscle
	StM, striated muscle
L, longitudinal layer of muscularis externa	**SubM,** submucosa
	arrows, Fig. 2, lymphocytes in epithelium
Lym, lymphocytes	
LP, lamina propria	
LV, lymphatic vessel	**asterisks, Fig. 1,** areas containing striated muscle in the muscularis externa
ME, muscularis externa	
MM, muscularis mucosae	
Fig. 1, monkey, × 60	**Fig. 2,** monkey, × 300 (inset. × 400)

and submucosa (**SubM**) is less well marked, though it is readily discernible.

The muscularis externa **ME**) as observed in **Figure 1** is comprised largely of smooth muscle, but it also contains areas of striated muscle. Although the striations are not evident at this low magnification, the more densely stained eosinophilic areas (**asterisks**) prove to be striated muscle when observed at higher power. Reference to the **inset,** which is from an area in **Figure 1** substantiates this identification. The **inset** shows circularly oriented striated and smooth muscle (**L**). The striated muscle stains more intensely with eosin, as seen in **Figure 1,** but of greater significance is the distribution and number of nuclei. In the midarea of the **inset,** numerous elongated and uniformly oriented nuclei are present; this is smooth muscle (**SM**). Above and below, few elongated nuclei are present; moreover, they are largely at the periphery of the bundles. This is striated muscle (**StM**); the cross-striations are just perceptible in some areas. The specimen shown here is from the middle of the esophagus, where both smooth and striated muscle are present. The distal third of the esophagus would contain only smooth muscle, whereas the proximal third would contain almost entirely striated muscle.

External to the muscularis externa is the adventitia (**Adv**) consisting of dense connective tissue.

PLATE 72

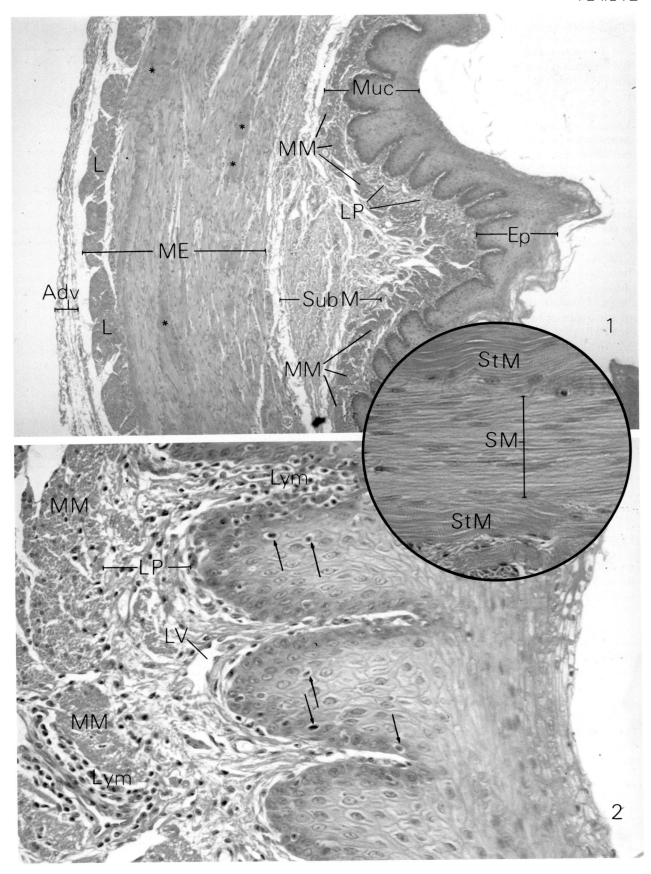

PLATE 73. Esophagus and Stomach, Cardiac Region

The junction between the esophagus and stomach is shown in **Figure 1**. The esophagus is on the right and the cardiac region of the stomach on the left. The **large rectangle** marks a representative area of the cardiac mucosa seen at higher magnification in **Figure 2**; the **smaller rectangle** shows part of the junction examined at higher magnification in **Figure 3**.

As noted in the previous plate, the esophagus is lined by stratified squamous epithelium **(Ep)** and it is indented on its undersurface by deep connective tissue papillae. When these are sectioned obliquely (as five of them have been), they appear as islands of connective tissue within the thick epithelium. Under the epithelium are the lamina propria and the muscularis mucosae **(MM)**. At the junction between the esophagus and the stomach **(Figs. 1 and 3)**, the stratified squamous epithelium of the esophagus ends abruptly and the simple columnar epithelium of the stomach surface begins.

The surface of the stomach contains numerous and relatively deep depressions called gastric pits **(P)**, or foveolae, which are formed by epithelium similar to and continuous with that of the surface. Glands **(Gl)** open into the bottom of the pits; they are cardiac glands. (The entire gastric mucosa contains glands. There are three types of gastric glands: cardiac glands, fundic glands, and pyloric glands. Cardiac glands are in the immediate vicinity of the opening of the esophagus; pyloric glands are in the funnel-shaped portion of the stomach that leads to the duodenum; fundic glands are throughout the remainder of the stomach.)

The cardiac glands and pits **(Fig. 1)** are surrounded by a very cellular lamina propria **(LP)**. At higher magnification **(Fig. 2)**, it can be seen that many of the cells of the lamina propria are lymphocytes and other cells of the immune system. Large numbers of lymphocytes **(L)** may be localized between the smooth muscle cells of the muscularis mucosae **(MM)** and, thus, the muscularis mucosae in these locations appear to be disrupted.

The columnar cells of the stomach surface and gastric pits produce mucus. Each surface and pit cell contains a mucous cup in its apical cytoplasm **(Fig. 3)**, thereby forming a glandular sheet of cells named mucous surface cells **(MSC)**. The content of the mucous cup is usually lost during the prepara-

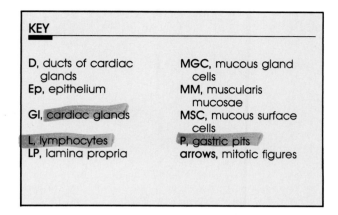

KEY

D, ducts of cardiac glands
Ep, epithelium
Gl, cardiac glands
L, lymphocytes
LP, lamina propria

MGC, mucous gland cells
MM, muscularis mucosae
MSC, mucous surface cells
P, gastric pits
arrows, mitotic figures

tion of the tissue and, thus, the apical cup portion of the cells appear empty in routine H&E paraffin sections such as the ones shown in this plate.

The epithelium of the cardiac glands also consists of mucous cells **(MGC)** **(Fig. 4)**. As seen in the photomicrograph, the nucleus of the gland cell is typically flattened, one side being adjacent to the base of the cell, the other side adjacent to the pale-staining cytoplasm. Again, mucus is lost during processing of the tissue and this accounts for the pale-staining appearance of the cytoplasm. While the cardiac glands are, for the most part, unbranched, some branching is occasionally seen **(Fig. 4)**. The glands empty their secretions via ducts **(D)** into the bottom of the gastric pits. The cells forming the ducts are columnar and the cytoplasm stains well with eosin. This makes it easy to distinguish the duct cells from mucous gland cells. Among the cells forming the duct portion of the gland are those that undergo mitotic division **(arrows, Figs. 2 and 4)** to replace both mucous surface and gland cells. Cardiac glands also contain APUD cells, but they are difficult to identify in routine H&E paraffin sections.

As mentioned previously, the cardiac glands are limited to a narrow region around the cardiac orifice. They are not sharply delineated from the fundic region of the stomach that contains parietal and chief cells. Thus, at the boundary, occasional parietal cells are seen in the cardiac glands.

In certain animals (e.g., ruminants and pigs), the anatomy and histology of the stomach are different. In these, at least one part of the stomach is lined with stratified squamous epithelium.

PLATE 73

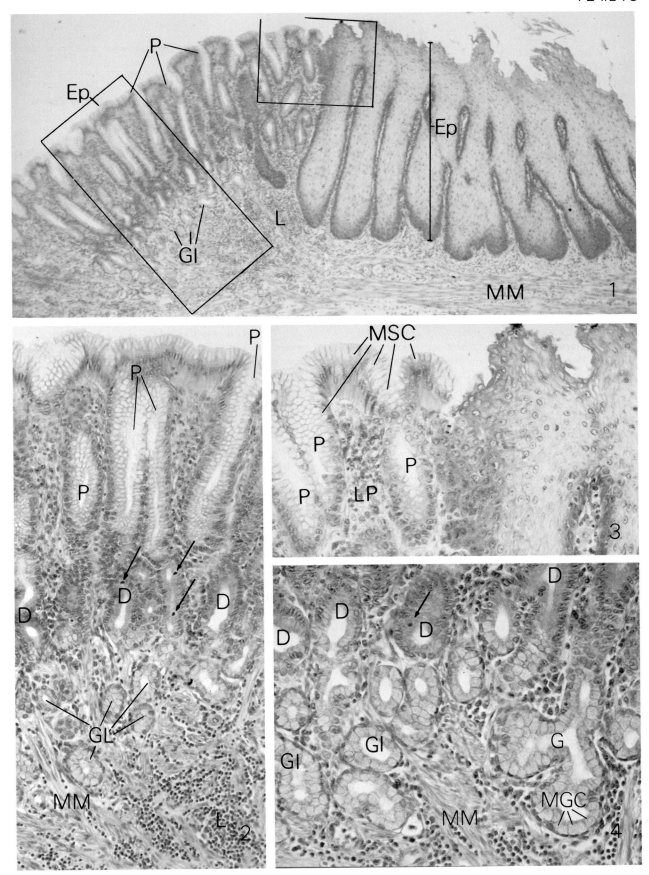

PLATE 74. Stomach I

The major extent of the stomach mucosa contains glands referred to as fundic glands and, from the vantage point of the histologist, the portion of the stomach with such glands in the mucosa is referred to as the fundic portion.

As with other parts of the gastrointestinal tract, the wall of the stomach (**Fig. 1**) consists of four layers: a mucosa (**Muc**), a submucosa (**SubM**), a muscularis externa (**ME**), and a serosa. The mucosa is the innermost layer and reveals three distinctive regions (**arrows**). The most superficial region contains the gastric pits; the middle region contains the necks of the glands, which tend to stain with eosin; and the deepest part of the mucosa stains most heavily with hematoxylin. The cells of these regions and their staining characteristics are considered in **Figure 1**, Atlas section, Plate 75. The cell types of the deep (hematoxylin staining) portion of the fundic mucosa are also considered in **Figure 3** of this plate.

The inner surface of the empty stomach is thrown into long folds referred to as rugae. One such cross-sectioned fold is shown in **Figure 1**. It consists not only of mucosa but also of submucosa (**asterisks**). The rugae are not permanent folds and they disappear when the stomach mucosa is stretched, as in the distended stomach. Also evident in **Figure 1** are the mamillated areas (**M**), which are slight elevations of the mucosa, much the same as cobblestones are elevated as they form the surface of a roadway. The mamillated areas consist only of mucosa without submucosa.

The submucosa and muscularis externa both stain predominantly with eosin—the muscularis a little darker. In addition, the smooth muscle of the muscularis externa gives an appearance of being homogeneous and uniformly solid. In contrast, the submucosa consisting of connective tissue may contain areas with adipocytes, and it contains numerous profiles of blood vessels (**BV**). The serosa is so thin that it is not evident as a discrete layer at this low magnification.

The junction between the cardiac and fundic regions of the stomach is shown in **Figures 2 and 3.** This junction can be identified histologically on the basis of the structure of the mucosa. The gastric pits (**P**), some of which are seen opening at the surface (**arrows, Fig. 2**), are similar in both regions, but the glands are different. The boundary between cardiac glands (**CG**) and fundic glands (**FG**) is marked by the **dashed line.**

KEY

BV, blood vessels

CG, cardiac glands
FG, fundic glands
L, lumen
LN, lymph nodule
M, mamillated areas
ME, muscularis externa

MM, muscularis
   mucosae
Muc, mucosa
P (Fig. 2), gastric pits
P (Fig. 3), parietal cells
SM, smooth muscle cells
SubM, submucosa

---

arrows (Fig. 1), three
   differently stained
   regions of fundic
   mucosa
arrows (Fig. 2), opening
   of gastric pits

asterisks, submucosa in
   ruga
dashed line, boundary
   between cardiac and
   fundic glands

The full thickness of the gastric mucosa is shown in **Figure 2,** as indicated by the presence of the muscularis mucosae (**MM**) deep to the fundic glands (**FG**). However, the muscularis mucosae under the cardiac glands are obscured by a large infiltration of lymphocytes forming a lymph nodule (**LN**).

Figure 3 provides a comparison between the cardiac and fundic glands at higher magnification. Consider first the cardiac glands (**CG**). These consist of mucous gland cells. They are comprised of simple columnar epithelium; the nucleus is in the most basal part of the cell and is somewhat flattened. The cytoplasm appears as a faint network of lightly stained material. The lumens (**L**) of the cardiac glands are relatively wide. Now consider the fundic glands (**FG**) to the left of the **dashed line.** The lumens of the fundic glands are small and only in certain fortuitously sectioned glands is a lumen readily seen. As a consequence, most of the glands appear to be cords of cells. Because this is a deep region of the fundic mucosa, most of the cells are chief cells. The basal portion of the chief cell contains the nucleus and extensive ergastoplasm—thus, its basophilia. The apical cytoplasm, occupied by secretory granules that were lost during the preparation of the tissue, stains poorly. Interspersed among the chief cells are parietal cells (**P**). These cells typically have a round nucleus that is surrounded by eosinophilic cytoplasm. Among the cells of the lamina propria are those with elongate nuclei. They belong to smooth muscle cells (**SM**).

PLATE 74

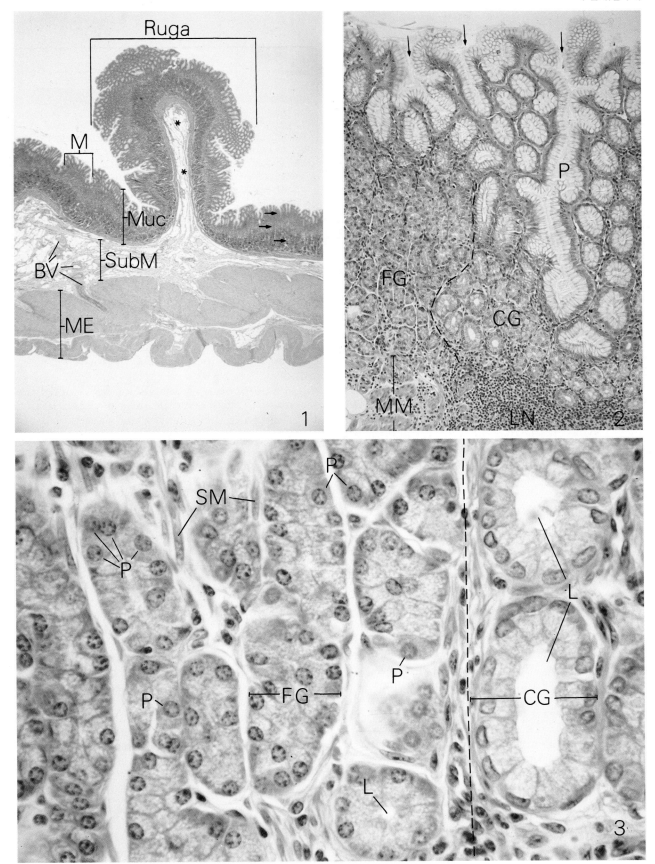

PLATE 75. Stomach II

Figure 1 shows an area of the fundic mucosa that includes the bottom of the gastric pits and the neck and deeper part of the fundic glands. It includes the areas marked by the **arrows** in **Figure 1** of the preceding plate. The mucous surface cells **(MSC)** of the gastric pits are readily identified because the mucous cup in the apical pole of each cell has an empty, washed-out appearance. Just below the gastric pits are the necks **(N)** of the fundic glands in which one can identify mucous neck cells **(MNC)** and parietal cells **(PC)**. The mucous neck cells produce a mucous secretion that is different from that produced by the mucous surface cells. As seen in **Figure 1,** the mucous neck cells display a cytoplasm that is lightly stained; there are no cytoplasmic areas that stain intensely nor is there a characteristic local absence of staining as in the mucous cup of the mucous surface cells.

Parietal cells are distinctive primarily because of the pronounced eosinophilic staining of their cytoplasm. Their nucleus is round, like that of the chief cell. Furthermore, the parietal cells tend to be located closer to the basal lamina of the epithelium than to the lumen of the gland because of its pear-like shape.

Figure 1, also reveals the signifiant characteristics of chief cells **(CC)**—namely, the round nucleus in a basal location; the ergastoplasm, deeply stained with hematoxylin (particularly evident in some of the chief cells where the nucleus has not been included in the plane of the section); and the apical, slightly eosinophilic cytoplasm (formerly occupied by the secretory granules).

APUD cells constitute the class of cells that can be displayed with special histochemical or silver-staining methods, but they are not readily evident in H&E sections. The distribution of cells demonstrable with special silver-staining procedures is shown in **Figure 3 (arrows).** Because of the staining procedure, these cells are properly designated as argentaffin cells. The mucous surface cells **(MSC)** in the section mark the bottom of the gastric pits and establish the fact that the necks of the fundic glands are represented in the section. The argentaffin (APUD) cells appear black in this specimen. The relatively low magnification permits the viewer to assess the frequency of distribution of these cells. At higher magnification **(Fig. 4),** it can be seen that the argentaffin cells **(arrows)** are al-

KEY

A, adipocytes	arrows, argentaffin cells
BV, blood vessels	MNC, mucous neck cells
CC, chief cells	MP, Meissner's plexus
GC, ganglion cells	MSC, mucous surface
ME, muscularis externa	cells
MM, muscularis	N, neck of fundic glands
mucosae	PC, parietal cells
arrowheads, nuclei of	SubM, submucosa
satellite cells	

Figs. 1 and 2, monkey, × 320	Fig. 3, × 160 Fig. 4, × 640

most totally blackened by the silver staining, although a faint nucleus can be seen in some cells. The silver stains the secretory product lost during the preparation of routine sections and, accordingly, in H&E-stained paraffin sections, the argentaffin cell appears as a clear cell. The special silver staining in **Figures 3 and 4** shows that many of the argentaffin cells tend to be near the basal lamina and away from the lumen of the gland.

Figure 2 shows the bottom of the stomach mucosa, the submucosa **(SubM),** and part of the muscularis externa **(ME).** The muscularis mucosae **(MM)** are the deepest part of the mucosa. The muscularis mucosae **(MM)** consist of smooth muscle cells arranged in at least two layers. As seen in the photomicrograph, the smooth muscle cells immediately adjacent to the submucosa have been sectioned longitudinally and display elongate nuclear profiles. Just above this layer, the smooth muscle cells have been cut in cross-section and they display rounded nuclear profiles.

The submucosa consists of connective tissue of moderate density. Also present in the submucosa are adipocytes **(A),** blood vessels **(BV),** and a group of ganglion cells **(GC).** These cells belong to Meissner's plexus **(MP).** The **circular inset** shows some of the ganglion cells **(GC)** at higher magnification. These "cells" are actually large cell bodies of parasympathetic neurons. Each cell body is surrounded by satellite cells intimately apposed to the neuron cell body. The **arrowheads** point to the nuclei of the satellite cells.

Amine Precursor Uptake Decarboxylase

PLATE 75

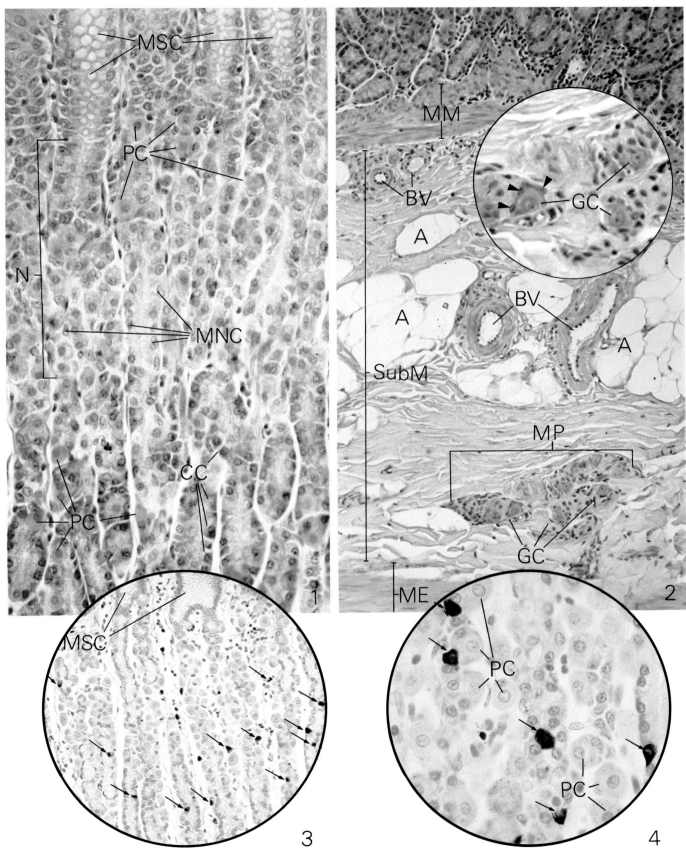

PLATE 76. Gastrodudodenal Junction

The junction between the stomach and the duodenum is shown in **Figure 1.** Most of the mucosa shown in the micrograph belongs to the stomach; it is the pyloric mucosa **(PMuc).** (The pyloric sphincter **(PS)** appears as a thickened region of the smooth muscle below the pyloric mucosa.) On the far right is the duodenal mucosa, the first part of the intestinal mucosa **(IMuc).** The area marked by the **rectangle** is shown at higher magnification in **Figure 2.** It provides a comparison of the two mucosal regions and also shows the submucosal glands and Brunner's glands.

The gastric and intestinal mucosa exhibit different histological characteristics. There are also distinctive features in the submucosa of the duodenum and in the muscularis externa of the stomach. These are evident in the low-magnification panoramic view afforded in **Figure 1** and they will be considered first.

The submucosa of the duodenum contains Brunner's glands. These are below the muscularis mucosae and, therefore, this structure serves as a useful landmark in identifying the glands. In the stomach **(Fig. 1),** the muscularis mucosae are readily identified as narrow bands of muscular tissue **(MM).** It can be followed toward the right into the duodenum, but then it is interrupted in the region between the two **asterisks.** Examination of this region at higher magnification **(Fig. 2)** reveals that in addition to intestinal glands **(IGl)** within the mucosa, there are also glands within the duodenal submucosa. These are Brunner's glands **(BGl).** Some of the glandular elements **(arrows)** can be seen to pass from the submucosa to the mucosa, thereby interrupting the muscularis mucosae **(MM).** The Brunner's glands empty their secretions into the duodenal lumen by means of ducts **(D).** In contrast, the pyloric glands **(PGl)** are relatively straight for most of their length **(Fig. 2),** but are coiled in the deepest part of the mucosa and are sometimes branched. They are restricted to the mucosa and empty into deep gastric pits. The boundary between the pits and glands is, however, hard to ascertain in H&E sections.

Figure 1 also shows the thickened region of the gastric muscularis externa where the stomach ends. This is the pyloric sphincter **(PS).** Its thickness, due mostly to the amplification of circular layer of smooth muscle of the muscularis externa, can be appreciated by comparison with the muscularis externa in the duodenum **(ME).**

With respect to the mucosal aspects of gastroduodenal histology, it has already been mentioned that the glands of the stomach empty into gastric

pits. These are depressions and, accordingly, when the pits are sectioned in a plane that is oblique or at right angles to the long axis of the pit, as in **Figure 2,** the pits can be recognized as being depressions because they are surrounded by lamina propria. In contrast, the inner surface of the small intestine has villi **(V).** These are projections into the lumen of slightly varying height. When the villus is cross- or obliquely sectioned, it is surrounded by space of the lumen, as is one of the villi shown in **Figure 2.** In addition, the villi have lamina propria **(LP)** in their core.

The **rectangular area** in **Figure 2** is considered at higher magnification in **Figure 3.** It shows how the epithelium of the stomach differs from that of the intestine. In both cases, the epithelium is simple columnar and the underlying lamina propria **(LP)** is highly cellular due to the presence of large numbers of lymphocytes. The boundary between gastric and duodenal epithelium is marked by the **arrow.** On the stomach side of the **arrow,** the epithelium consists of mucous surface cells **(MSC).** The surface cells contain an apical cup of mucus material that typically appears empty in an H&E-stained paraffin section. In contrast, the absorptive cells **(AC)** of the intestine do not possess mucus in their cytoplasm. Whereas goblet cells are found in the intestinal epithelium and are scattered among the absorptive cells, they do not form a complete mucous sheet. The intestinal absorptive cells also possess a striated border, which is shown in Atlas section, Plate 78.

PLATE 76

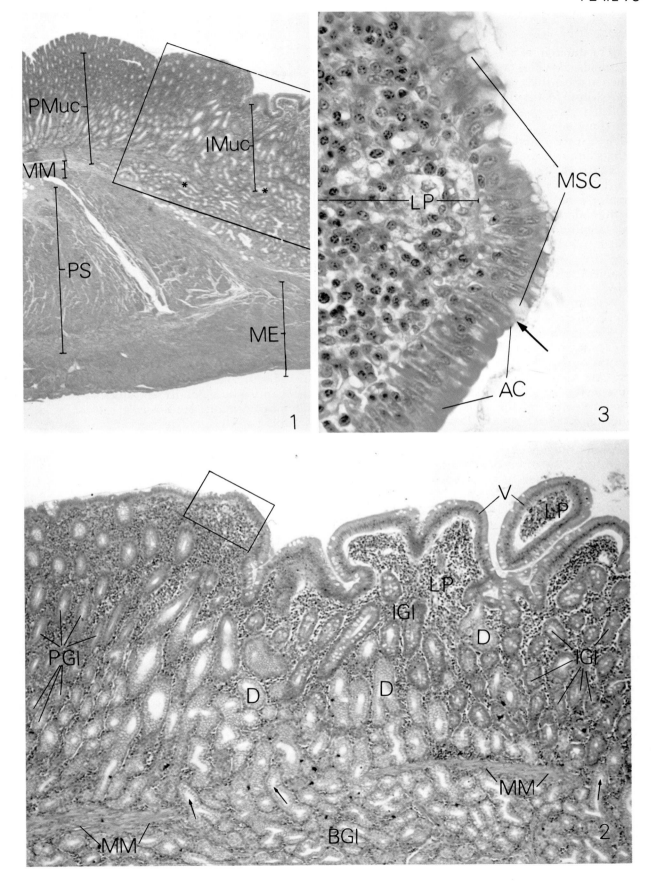

PLATE 77. Duodenum

The duodenum is the first and shortest part of the small intestine, measuring about 10 to 12 inches in man. It is adherent to the posterior abdominal wall in the human and is, therefore, immobile. It receives secretions (and other contents) from the stomach, pancreas, liver, and gallbladder, and, as already noted, it contains Brunner's glands in the submucosa.

Figure 1 shows a segment of the duodenal wall. The layers of the wall are, in order from the lumen: the mucosa (**Muc**), the submucosa (**SubM**), the muscularis externa (**ME**), and the serosa (**S**). Both longitudinal (**L**) and circular (**C**) layers of the muscularis externa can be distinguished. Although plicae circulares are found in the wall of the small intestine, including the duodenum, none is included in this photomicrograph.

A distinctive feature of the intestinal mucosa is the presence of finger-like and leaf-like projections into the intestinal lumen, called villi. Most of the villi (**V**) shown in **Figure 1** display profiles that correspond to their description as finger-like. However, one villus displays the form of a leaf-like villus (**asterisk**). The **dashed line** marks the boundary between the villi and the intestinal glands (also called crypts of Lieberkühn). The latter extend as far as the muscularis mucosae (**MM**).

Under the mucosa is the submucosa. It reveals the Brunner's glands (**BGl**). These are branched tubular or branched tubuloalveolar glands, whose secretory components, shown at higher magnification in **Figure 2,** consist of columnar epithelium. A duct (**D**) through which the glands open into the lumen of the duodenum is shown in **Figures 1 and 2,** where it is marked by an **arrow.**

The histological features of the duodenal mucosa are shown at higher magnification in **Figure 2.** Two kinds of cells can be recognized in the epithelial layer that forms the surface of the villus: enterocytes (absorptive) and goblet cells (**GC**). Most of the cells are absorptive cells. They have a striated border that will be seen at higher magnification in the following plate; their elongate nuclei are located in the basal half of the cell. Goblet cells are readily identified by the presence of the apical mucous cup, which appears empty. Most of the

---

KEY

BGl, Brunner's glands	**MM,** muscularis
C, circular (inner) layer	mucosae
of muscularis externa	**Muc,** mucosa
D, duct of Brunner's	**S,** serosa
gland	**SubM,** submucosa
GC, goblet cells	**V,** villi
IGl, intestinal glands	**arrow,** duct of Brunner's
(crypts)	gland
L, longitudinal (outer)	**asterisk,** leaf-like villus
layer of muscularis	**dashed line, Fig. 1,**
externa	boundary between
LP, lamina propria	base of villi and
ME, muscularis externa	intestinal glands

Fig. 1, monkey, × 120   **Fig. 2,** × 240

---

dark round nuclei also seen in the epithelial layer covering the villi belong to lymphocytes.

The lamina propria (**LP**) makes up the core of the villus. It contains large numbers of round cells whose individual identity cannot be ascertained at this magnification. However, it should be noted that these are mostly lymphocytes (and other cells of the immune system), which accounts for the designation of the lamina propria as diffuse lymphoid tissue. The lamina propria surrounding the intestinal glands (**IGl**) similarly consists largely of lymphocytes and related cells. The lamina propria also contains components of loose connective tissue and isolated smooth muscle cells.

The intestinal glands (**IGl**) are relatively straight and they tend to be dilated at their base. The base of the intestinal crypts contains Paneth cells. These cells possess eosinophilic granules in their apical cytoplasm. The granules contain lysozyme, a bacteriolytic enzyme thought to play a role in regulating intestinal microbial flora. The main cell type in the intestinal crypt is a relatively undifferentiated columnar cell. These cells are shorter than the enterocytes of the villus surface; they undergo mitosis and serve as the source of new cells for the intestinal epithelium. Also present in the intestinal crypts are goblet cells and APUD cells.

PLATE 77

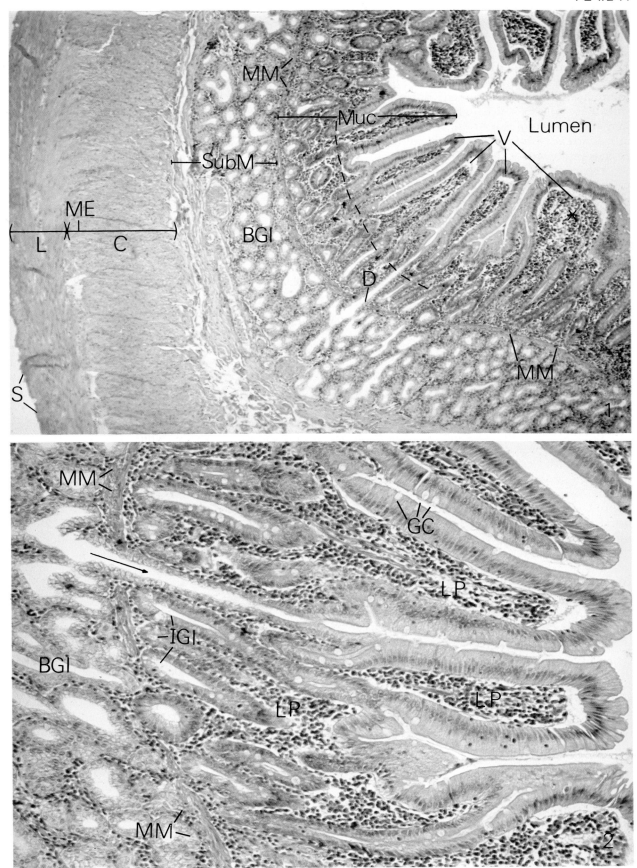

PLATE 78. Jejunum

Figure 1 is a longitudinal section of the jejunum showing the permanent circular folds of the small intestine, the plicae circulares (**PC**). These folds, or ridges, are arranged for the most part with their long axis at roughly right angles to the longitudinal axis of the intestine, therefore, the plicae shown here are cut in cross-section. The plicae circulares consist of mucosa (**Muc**) as well as submucosa (**SubM**). The broad band of tissue external to the submucosa is the muscularis externa (**ME**) and it is not included in the plicae. (The serosa cannot be distinguished at this magnification.)

Most of the villi (**V**) in this specimen have been cut longitudinally, thereby revealing their full length and also the fact that some are slightly shorter than others. The latter is considered to be due to the contraction of smooth muscle cells in the villi. Also seen in **Figure 1** are the lacteals (**L**), which in most of the villi are dilated. Lacteals are lymphatic capillaries that begin in the villi and play a role in the transport of certain dietary lipids from the small intestine.

Part of the plica marked by the bracket in **Figure 1** is shown at higher magnification in **Figure 2.** Note the muscularis mucosae (**MM**), the intestinal glands (**Gl**), and the villi (**V**). The boundary between the glands and villi is marked by the **dashed line.** Some of the glands are cut longitudinally, some are cut in cross-section, and most of the villi have been cut longitudinally. In conceptualizing the mucosal structure of the small intestine, it is important to recognize that the glands are epithelial depressions that project into the wall of the intestine, whereas the villa are projections that extend into the lumen. The glands are surrounded by cells of the lamina propria; the villi are surrounded by space of the intestinal lumen. The lamina propria with its lacteal occupies a central position in the villus; the lumen occupies the central position of the gland. Also note that the lumen of the gland tends to be dilated at its base.

Figure 3 shows the epithelium from portions of two adjacent villi at higher magnification. The epithelium consists chiefly of enterocytes. These are columnar absorptive cells, and typically exhibit a striated border (**SB**) at their apical surface. The dark band at the base of the striated border is due to the terminal web of the cell. The nuclei of the enterocytes have essentially the same shape, orien-

---

KEY

EC, endothelial cell	**dashed line,** boundary
GC, goblet cell	between villi and
Gl, intestinal gland	intestinal glands
(crypts)	**ME,** muscularis externa
L, lacteal	**MM,** muscularis
LP, lamina propria	mucosae
Ly, lymphocytes	**Muc,** mucosa
M, smooth muscle cell	**PC,** plica circulares
arrows, basal processes	**SB,** striated border
of enterocytes	**SubM,** submucosa
asterisks, basilateral	**V,** villi
intercellular spaces	

Fig. 1, monkey, × 22	**Fig. 3,** × 500
Fig. 2, × 60	

---

tation, and staining characteristics and, even if the cytoplasmic boundaries were not evident, the nuclei would be an indication of the columnar shape and orientation of the cells. The enterocytes rest on a basal lamina not evident in H&E-stained paraffin sections. The eosinophilic band (**arrow**) at the base of the cell layer, where one would expect a basement membrane, actually consists of flat lateral cytoplasmic processes from the enterocytes (see Atlas section, Plate 4). These processes partially delineate the basilateral intercellular spaces (**asterisks**) that are dilated, as can be seen here, during active fluid transport.

The epithelial cells with an expanded apical cytoplasm in the form of a cup are goblet cells (**GC**). In this specimen, the nucleus of almost every goblet cell is just at the base of the cup and a thin cytoplasmic strand (not always evident) extends to the basement membrane. The scattered round nuclei within the epithelium belong to lymphocytes (**Ly**).

The lamina propria (**LP**) and the lacteal (**L**) are located beneath the intestinal epithelium. The cells forming the lacteal are simple squamous epithelium (endothelium). Two nuclei of these cells (**EC**) appear to be exposed to the lumen of the lacteal; another elongate nucleus (**M**) slightly removed from the lumen belongs to a smooth muscle cell.

PLATE 78

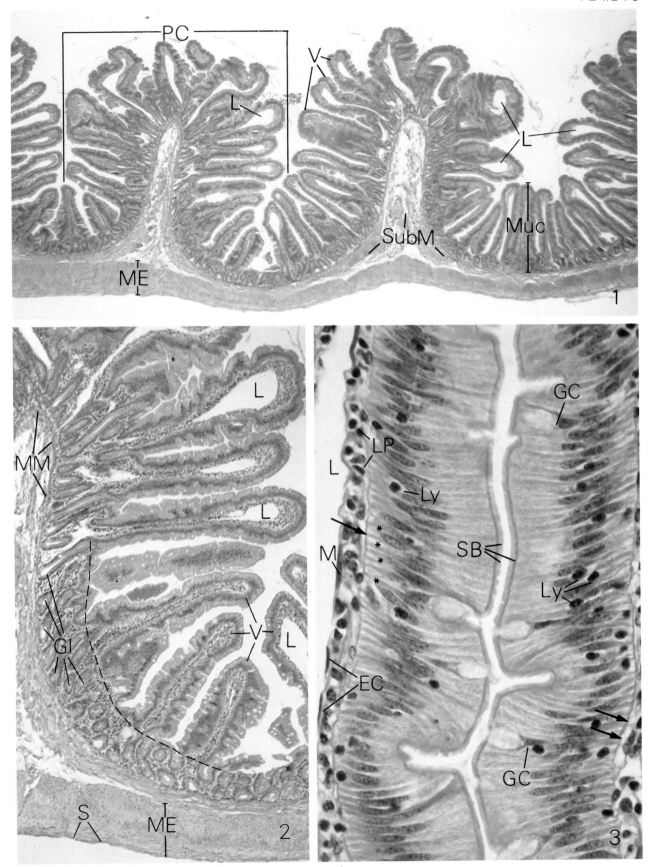

PLATE 79. Ileum

The ileum exhibits essentially the same histological features as those seen in the jejunum. The differences are chiefly in the degree to which certain features are present. For example, the villi occur frequently in the form of leaf-like structures, and lymphatic nodes forming Peyer's patches are present in greater frequency. For purposes of orientation, the submucosa (**SM**) and muscularis externa (**ME**) have been marked in the cross-section through the ileum shown in **Figure 1.** Just internal to the submucosa is the mucosa; external to the muscularis externa is the serosa. The mucosa reveals several longitudinally sectioned villi (**V**) that have been labeled and other unlabeled villi that can be identified easily on the basis of their appearance as islands of tissue completely surrounded by the space of the lumen. They are, of course, not islands because this appearance is due to the plane of section that slices completely through some of the villi obliquely or in cross-section, thereby isolating them from their base. Below the villi are the intestinal glands, many of which are obliquely or cross-sectioned and can be readily identified, as was done in the preceding plates, because they are totally surrounded by lamina propria.

There are about 8 to 10 projections of tissue into the intestinal lumen that are substantially larger than the villi. These are the plicae circulares. As already noted, plicae generally have circular orientation, but they may travel in a longitudinal direction for short distances and they may branch. In addition, even if all the plicae are arranged in a circular manner, if the section is somewhat oblique, the plicae will be cut at an angle, as appears to be the case with several plicae in **Figure 1.**

Sometimes, even in a cross-section through the intestine, a plica displays a cross sectional profile such as that shown in **Figure 2.** Note again that the submucosa (**SM**) constitutes the core of the plica. Although many of the villi in **Figure 2** present profiles (**V**) that would be expected if the villus were a finger-like projection, others clearly do not. In particular, one villus (marked with three **asterisks**) shows the broad profile of a longitudinally sectioned leaf-like villus. If this same villus were cut at a right angle to the plane shown here, it would appear much the same as the finger-like villus.

One of the distinctive features of the small intestine is the presence of single and aggregated lymph nodules in the intestinal wall. Isolated nodules of lymphatic tissue are common in the proxi-

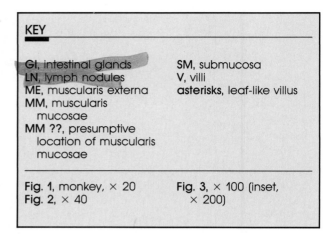

mal end of the intestinal canal. However, as one proceeds distally through the intestines, the lymph nodules occur in increasingly larger numbers. In the ileum, large aggregates of lymph nodules are regularly seen; they are referred to as Peyer's patches. Several lymph nodules (**LN**) forming a Peyer's patch are shown in **Figure 1.** The nodules are partly within the mucosa of the ileum and extend into the submucosa. Although not evident in the figure, the nodules are characteristically located opposite to where the mesentery connects to the intestinal tube.

Part of a lymph nodule and the overlying epithelium are shown at higher magnification in **Figure 3.** The lymphocytes and related cells are so numerous that they virtually obscure the muscularis mucosae. However, their location can be estimated as being near the presumptive label (**MM ??**) inasmuch as the muscularis mucosae are ordinarily adjacent to the base of the intestinal glands (**GI**). Moreover, upon examination of this area at higher magnification (**inset**), groups of smooth muscle cells (**MM**) can be seen separated by numerous lymphocytes close to the intestinal glands (**GI**). Clearly, the lymphocytes of the nodule are on both sides of the muscularis mucosae and, thus, within both the mucosa and the submucosa.

In places (**Fig. 3**), the lymph nodule is surfaced by the intestinal epithelium. Whereas the nature of the epithelium cannot be appreciated fully with the light microscope, electron micrographs (both scanning and transmission) have shown that among the epithelial cells are special cells, designated M cells, which sample the intestinal content (for antigen) and present this antigen to the lymphocytes in the epithelial layer.

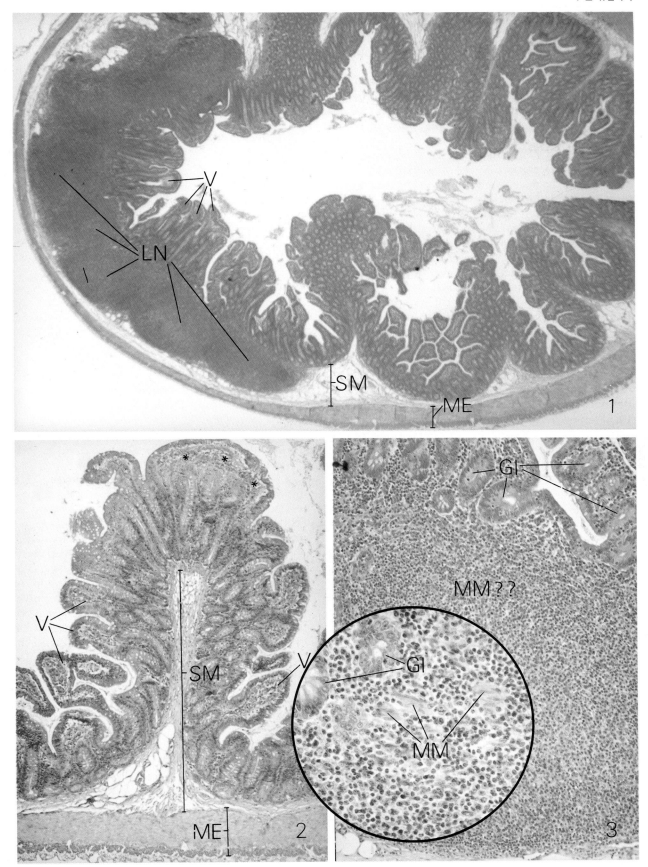

PLATE 79

PLATE 80. Colon

A cross-section through the large intestine is shown at low magnification in **Figure 1.** It shows the four layers that make up the wall of the colon: the mucosa (**Muc**), the submucosa (**SubM**), the muscularis externa (**ME**), and the serosa (**S**). Although these layers are the same as those in the small intestine, several differences should be noted. The large intestine has no villi, nor does it have plicae circulares. On the other hand, the muscularis externa is arranged in a distinctive manner and this is evident in the photomicrograph. The longitudinal layer [**ME(l)**] is substantially thinner than the circular layer [**ME(c)**] except in three locations where the longitudinal layer of smooth muscle is present as a thick band. One of these thick bands, called a tenia coli (**TC**), is shown in **Figure 1.** Because the colon is cross-sectioned, the teniae coli are also cross-sectioned. The three teniae coli extend along the length of the large intestine as far as, but not including, the rectum.

The mucosa, shown at higher magnification in **Figure 2,** contains straight, unbranched, tubular glands (crypts of Lieberkühn) that extend to the muscularis mucosae (**MM**). The **arrows** identify the openings of some of the glands at the intestinal surface. Generally speaking, the lumen of the glands is narrow except in the deepest part of the gland, where it is often slightly dilated (**asterisks, Fig. 3**). Between the glands (**Gl**) is a lamina propria (**LP**), which contains considerable numbers of lymphocytes and other cells of the immune system. Two **rectangles** mark areas of the mucosa that are examined at higher magnification in **Figures 3 and 4.**

The cells that line the surface of the colon and the glands are principally absorptive cells (**AC**) and goblet cells (**GC**). The absorptive cells have a thin striated border that is readily evident in **Figure 4** where the **arrows** show the opening of the glands. Interspersed among the absorptive cells are the globlet cells (**GC**). As the absorptive cells are followed into the glands, they become fewer in number while the goblet cells increase in number. Other cells in the gland are APUD cells, not easily identified in routine H&E-stained paraffin sections, and, in the deep part of the gland, are the undifferentiated cells that divide and, thus, serve

as the source of new cells. The undifferentiated cells are readily identified if they are undergoing division by virtue of the mitotic figures (**M**) that they display (**Fig. 3**).

Paneth cells are not usually seen in the crypts of the colon, although they are described as sometimes being present.

Figure 3 reveals the muscularis mucosae (**MM**) and the cells in the lamina propria (**LP**), many of which can be recognized as lymphocytes and others as plasma cells. The smooth muscle cells of the muscularis mucosae are arranged in two layers. Note that the smooth muscle cells marked by the **arrowheads** show rounded nuclei; however, other smooth muscle cells appear as more or less rounded eosinophilic areas. These smooth muscle cells have been cut in cross-section. Just above these cross-sectioned smooth muscle cells are others that have been cut longitudinally, and they display elongate nuclei and elongate strands of eosinophilic cytoplasm.

The submucosa consists of a rather dense irregular connective tissue (**Figs. 1 and 2**). It contains the larger blood vessels (**BV, Fig. 1**) and areas of adipose tissue (**A, Fig. 2**).

KEY	
A, adipose tissue	Muc, mucosa
AC, absorptive cells	S, serosa
BV, blood vessels	SubM, submucosa
GC, goblet cells	TC, tenia coli
Gl, intestinal glands	arrowheads, smooth
LP, lamina propria	muscle cells showing
M, mitotic figures	rounded nuclei
ME, muscularis externa	arrows, opening of
ME(c), circular layer of	intestinal glands
muscularis externa	asterisks, lumen of
ME(l), longitudinal layer	intestinal glands
of muscularis externa	
MM, muscularis	
mucosae	
Fig. 1, monkey, × 30	**Fig. 3,** × 525
Fig. 2, × 140	**Fig. 4,** × 525

PLATE 80

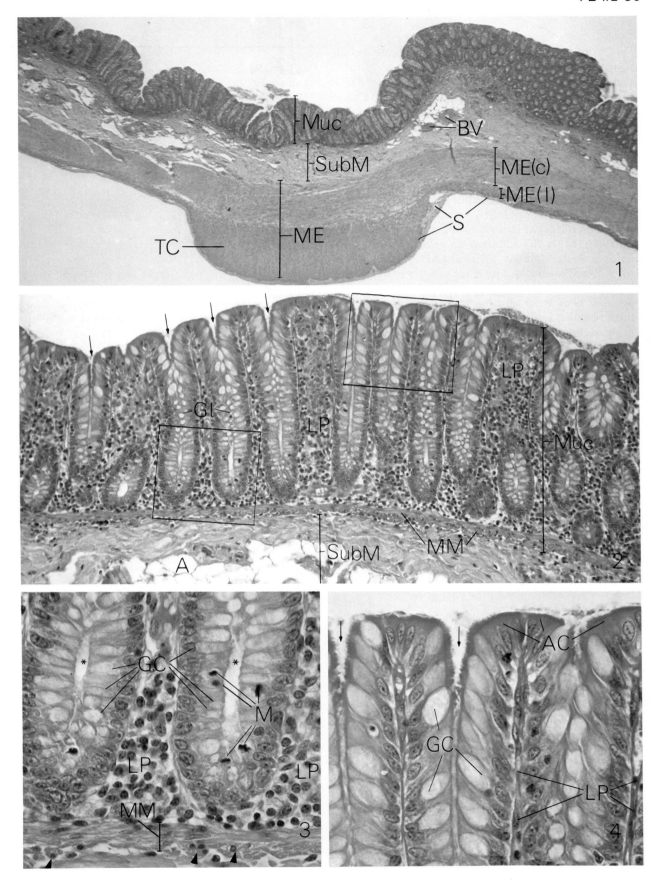

PLATE 81. Appendix

The appendix is a thin, finger-like process that is suspended from the cecum, the blind pouch from which the large intestine begins. The wall of the appendix is structured much like the small intestine, particularly the ileum, with its numerous lymphatic nodules. However, villi are not present, nor are there plicae circularis.

The wall of the appendix is illustrated in **Figure 1.** The lumen **(L),** mucosa **(Muc),** submucosa **(Subm),** muscularis externa **(ME),** and serosa **(S)** are shown. Like the mucosa of the large intestine, the mucosa of the appendix contains straight tubular glands **(Gl)** that extend as far as the muscularis mucosae **(MM, Fig. 2)** and are surrounded by a highly cellular lamina propria **(LP).** Most of the cells of the lamina propria are lymphocytes; however, other cells characteristic of lymphoid tissue are also present. Lymphocytes **(Lym)** may be so numerous in the mucosa and submucosa that they obscure the muscularis mucosae as done in other parts of the intestinal tract. The glands (crypts of Lieberkühn) contain large numbers of goblet cells and may contain occasional Paneth cells. APUD cells are slightly more numerous in each gland, on a relative basis, than they are in the small intestine. Absorptive cells are usually not present.

The submucosa **(Subm)** consists of a rather irregular connective tissue. The lymphatic nodules

occur chiefly in the submucosa and typically extend into the mucosa. As in the ileum, the nodules may obscure the submucosa. Some adipose tissue **(AT)** and two aggregations of lymphocytes **(Lym)** are shown in **Figure 1.** Although the dense connective tissue nature of the submucosa is readily evident in **Figure 1,** in other specimens the amount of lymphatic tissue may be sufficiently great to obscure the fibrous material as well.

The muscularis externa **(ME)** is comprised of an inner circular layer and an outer longitudinal layer of smooth muscle. External to the muscularis externa is the serosa **(S).**

KEY	
AT, adipose tissue	ME, muscularis externa
GI, glands	MM, muscularis
L, lumen	mucosae
LP, lamina propria	Muc, mucosa
Lym, lymphocytes	S, serosa
	Subm, submucosa
Fig. 1, human, × 40	Fig. 2, human, × 160

PLATE 81

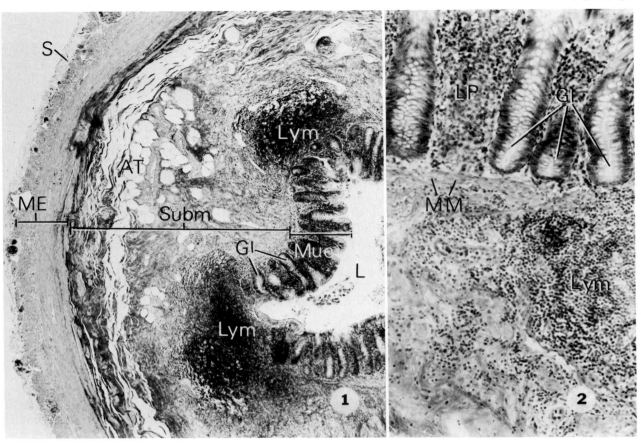

PLATE 82. Anorectal Junction

At the anorectal junction, there is a transition from the simple columnar epithelium of the intestinal mucosa to the keratinized stratified squamous epithelium of the skin. Between these two distinctly different epithelia there is a narrow region where the epithelium is first stratified columnar (or cuboidal) and then stratified squamous. In addition, the circularly arranged smooth muscle of the intestinal canal becomes thickened and serves as an internal anal sphincter.

A view of the anorectal junction is shown at low magnification in **Figure 1.** The mucosa characteristic of the large intestine is seen on the **upper left** of the micrograph. This region is the upper part of the anal canal and the intestinal glands are the same as those present in the colon. The muscularis mucosae (**MM**) are readily identified as the narrow band of tissue under the glands. Both the intestinal glands as well as the muscularis mucosae terminate within the **rectangular area** on the left of the field, and here, at the **diamond,** there is the first major change in the epithelium. This area will be considered at higher magnification in **Figure 2.** The **rectangular area** shown on the right includes the stratified squamous epithelium of the skin, and it will be examined at higher magnification in **Figure 3.**

Between the two **diamonds** in the **rectangular areas** shown in **Figure 1** is epithelium of the lower part of the anal canal. Under this epithelium, there is a lymph nodule (**LN**) that has a well-formed germinal center. As with other mucous membranes, isolated lymph nodules should not be construed to have fixed locations. Rather, they may or may not be present according to local demands.

Also, at this low magnification, note the internal anal sphincter muscle (**IAS**) that, as mentioned above, is the thickened, most distal portion of the circular layer of smooth muscle of the muscularis externa. Under the skin on the right is the external anal sphincter muscle (**EAS**). It is comprised of striated muscle fibers, which are seen in cross-section.

The junction between the simple columnar (**SC**) and the stratified (**St**) epithelium is marked with the **diamond** in **Figure 2.** The simple colum-

nar epithelium of the upper part of the anal canal contains numerous goblet cells and, as in the mucosa of the colon, this epithelium is continuous with the epithelium of the intestinal glands (**IG**). These glands continue to about the same point as the muscularis mucosae (**MM**). Characteristically, the lamina propria contains large numbers of lymphocytes. There is a particularly large number in the region marked **Lym.** For a further consideration of the stratified epithelium, an area marked by the **circle** is depicted at higher magnification in the **inset.** This shows that, in this specimen, the stratified epithelium is first cuboidal (**StC**) and then columnar (**StCol**).

The final change in epithelial type that occurs at the anorectal junction is shown in **Figure 3.** On the right is the stratified squamous epithelium of skin [**StS(k)**]. The keratinized nature of the surface is readily apparent. On the other hand, the stratified squamous epithelium (**StS**) below the level of the **diamond** is not keratinized, and nucleated cells can be seen all the way to the surface. Again, numerous lymphocytes (**Lym**) are in the underlying connective tissue and many have migrated into the epithelium in the nonkeratinized area.

PLATE 82

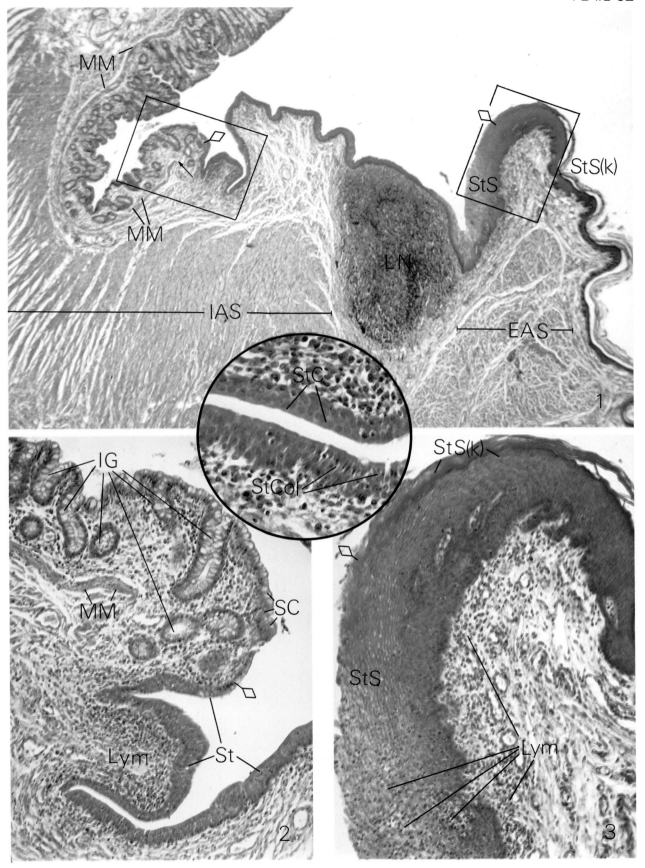

Digestive System III: Liver, Gallbladder, and Pancreas

17

LIVER

The liver is the largest mass of glandular tissue in the body. It is located in the upper right quadrant of the abdominal cavity and is unique among organs because, in addition to a supply of arterial blood from the hepatic arteries, it also receives a major supply of blood from veins of the digestive tube, pancreas, and spleen via the hepatic portal vein. Thus, the liver stands directly in the pathway of blood vessels that convey substances absorbed from the digestive tube. Whereas this position gives the liver the first chance to metabolize these substances, it also makes it the first organ to be exposed to toxic compounds that have been ingested. The liver has the ability to degrade toxic compounds, but it can be overwhelmed by these compounds and damaged. Within the liver, blood from branches of the hepatic artery and portal vein enters specialized capillaries called *sinusoids;* these vessels provide for the exchange of substances between the blood and liver parenchyma. The sinusoids lead to a venous network through which blood leaves the liver. The largest of these veins, the hepatic veins, empty into the inferior vena cava.

Both exocrine and endocrine functions are attributed to the liver by many authors. Although this is true, it should not be overlooked that the liver is also an organ engaging in metabolic conversions. The liver is classified as exocrine because one of its products (bile) is secreted through a system of ducts into the duodenum, and it is endocrine because most of its products are secreted directly into the bloodstream.

Some major functions of the liver parenchymal cell, the hepatocyte, are listed in Table 17.1. This table gives an overview of hepatocyte functions. It does not include specific enzymatic cataly-

sis of specific metabolic steps; functions of organelles that serve the cell, such as mitochondria in energy production and lysosomes in meeting needs of the hepatocyte; or functions whose significance in terms of body need is not yet clear.

The liver is divided into four lobes. These are evident on the surface and are important in gross anatomy, but they are not conspicuous in sections and, thus, are less important to the histology student. The site where the portal vein, hepatic artery, bile duct, nerves, and lymphatic vessels enter (or leave) the liver is called the *porta hepatis.* The portal vein, hepatic artery, and bile duct course together as a triad, called a *portal triad,* through the stromal ramifications of the liver.

The liver contains (1) the hepatocytes; (2) a stroma of connective tissue; (3) blood vessels, nerves, lymphatics, and ducts within the stroma; (4) sinusoids between plates of hepatocytes; (5) a surrounding capsule of fibrous connective tissue; and (6) a serous cover (visceral peritoneum) on the capsule where the liver is not directly adherent to the abdominal wall or organs.

Liver Lobule

The classical, structural, and functional unit of the liver is the liver lobule. It is shaped somewhat like a polyhedral prism and measures about 0.7×2.0 mm (Fig. 17.1). A cross-section of a lobule has the shape of a polygon, usually a hexagon; the portal triads are typically found at the angles of the polygon. The central structure of the lobule, traversing its long axis, is the *central vein.* Plates of hepatocytes radiate from the central vein to the perimeter of the lobule. The plates are one cell thick and are separated by the hepatic sinusoids, which are also radially arranged about the central vein. In the pig, the boundaries of the

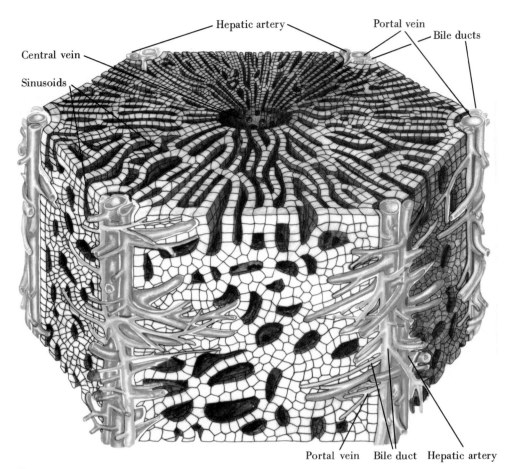

Figure 17.1. Liver lobule schematically diagrammed as a six-sided polyhedral prism with portal triads (hepatic artery, portal vein, and bile duct) at each of the corners. The vessels of the portal triads send distributing branches along the sides of the lobule and these branches open into the sinusoids. The long axis of the lobule is traversed by the central vein and this vessel receives blood from the sinusoids. Interconnecting sheets of hepatocytes are disposed in a radial pattern from the central vein to the perimeter of the lobule. (Based on Weiss L: *Histology*, 5th ed. New York, Elsevier, 1983.)

lobules are demarcated by connective tissue that is part of the hepatic stroma (Fig. 17.2). In the human and most other mammals there is no connective tissue boundary between lobules, and the plates of one lobule appear to be continuous with those of a neighboring lobule (see Atlas section, Plate 83, Fig. 1). The boundaries of the lobule can be approximated by finding a cross-sectioned central vein with radially disposed sinusoids and plates of hepatocytes, noting the position of the portal triads with respect to the central vein, and then joining the portal triads with imaginary lines to indicate the approximate boundaries of the lobule. The angular space that contains the portal triad and the surrounding connective tissue is called the *portal canal.* This canal is bordered by the outermost hepatocytes of the lobule. At the edges of the portal canal, between the connective tissue stroma

and the hepatocytes, is a small space called the *space of Mall.* This is thought to be a site where lymph originates in the liver.

Blood Vessels

The blood vessels that occupy the portal canals are called *interlobular vessels.* Only the interlobular vessels forming the smallest portal triads send blood into the sinusoids. The larger interlobular vessels branch into distributing vessels that are located at the periphery of the lobule and these send inlet vessels to the sinusoids (see Fig. 17.1). In the sinusoids, the blood flows centripetally toward the central vein. The central vein courses through the central axis of the liver lobule, becoming larger as it progresses through the lobule and empties into a *sublobular vein.* Several sublobular veins

TABLE 17.1. Major Functions of Hepatocytes

FUNCTION	MAIN ORGANELLE
Protein synthesis and secretion (albumin, prothrombin, fibrinogen)	rER, Golgi
Bile formation and secretion (recycling of many bile constituents to and from intestine)	sER
Metabolism of lipid-soluble drugs (including detoxification) and steroids (including cholesterol synthesis)	sER
Lipoprotein synthesis and secretion	rER, sER, Golgi
Carbohydrate metabolism	sER, cytosol (also rER in the newborn?)
Urea formation from ammonium ion (urea cycle)	Mitochondria, cytosol?

converge to form larger **hepatic veins** that empty into the inferior vena cava.

The **portal vein** and its branches within the liver have a structure typical of veins in general. The lumen is much larger than that of the artery associated with it. The **hepatic artery** has a structure typical of other arteries, that is, a thick muscular wall. In addition to providing arterial blood directly to the sinusoids, it provides arterial blood to the connective tissue in the larger portal canals. Capillaries in these larger portal canals return to the interlobular veins and, thus, the interlobular vein receives a supply of arterial blood before the vein empties into the sinusoid.

The **central vein** is a thin-walled vessel receiving blood from the hepatic sinusoids. The endothelial lining of the central vein is surrounded by small amounts of spirally arranged connective tissue fibers. Thus, the so-called central vein is actually the terminal venule of the system of hepatic veins. The sublobular vein, the vessel that receives blood from central veins, has a distinct layer of connective tissue fibers, both collagenous and elas-

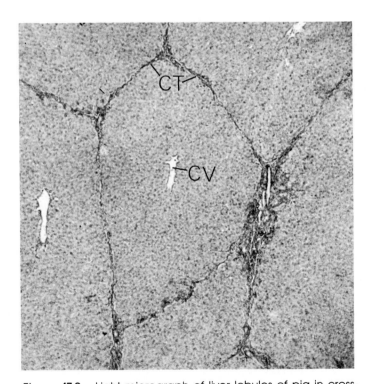

Figure 17.2. Light micrograph of liver lobules of pig in cross-section, showing the central vein (CV) and connective tissue (CT) surrounding the lobules. Some interlobular blood vessels can be seen in the connective tissue. At this relatively low magnification, the substance of the lobule appears as a uniform array of hepatocytes because their arrangement as sheets separated by sinusoids is difficult to discern.

tic, just external to the endothelium. The sublobular veins as well as the hepatic veins into which they drain travel alone. Being solitary vessels, they can be distinguished readily in a histological section from the portal veins that are members of a triad. There are no valves in hepatic veins.

The *sinusoid* is an irregularly dilated vessel whose caliber is larger than the diameter of regular capillaries. Sinusoids are lined by two kinds of cells: squamous cells similar to regular endothelium and Kupffer cells (Fig. 17.3). The endothelial cells have relatively few organelles. Still, pinocytotic vesicles are present, thereby suggesting pinocytotic activity as in other endothelial cells. Gaps are regularly observed between neighboring endothelial cells and the endothelial cells contain large fenestrae that lack a diaphragm. Also, the basal lamina surrounding the sinusoids is incomplete. (In some animals, such as sheep, goats, and calves, the endothelium of the sinusoids is continuous, there is a distinct basal lamina about the sinusoid, and fenestrae of the endothelial cells possess a diaphragm as in other endothelia.)

Kupffer cells are phagocytic; they are members of the mononuclear phagocytic system and are derived from monocytes. They contain a large amount of cytoplasm with organelles typical of those found in phagocytic cells. Often the cytoplasm contains fragments of red blood cells and iron in the form of ferritin, indicative of the cells' role in red blood cell breakdown. Kupffer cells are not joined to neighboring endothelial cells by junctional complexes and, in some micrographs, they can be seen to overlie the luminal surface of neighboring endothelial cells, as well as to span the lumen and even appear to occlude it partially.

Space of Disse

The *space of Disse* (perisinusoidal space) is interposed between the endothelium of the liver sinusoids and the hepatocytes (Fig. 17.4). As already mentioned, in most mammals the wall of the sinusoid is not complete; at best, there is an incomplete basal lamina and there is no ground substance external to the sinusoid. Thus, the soluble components of blood, but not cells, have ready access to the perisinusoidal space. Usually, two faces of each hepatocyte are in direct contact with the space of Disse. The numerous microvilli of the cell project into this space. The space of Disse serves as a route whereby the hepatocyte removes substances that derive from the blood and discharges certain products, which gain ready entry to the blood.

The space of Disse contains a small number of

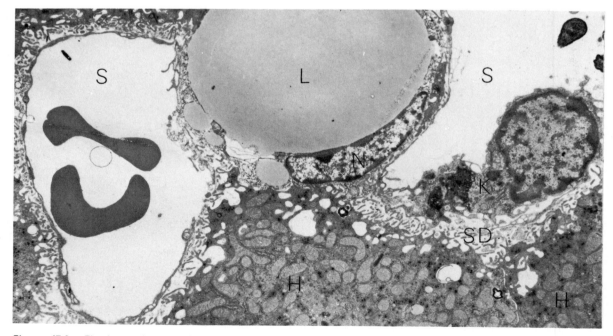

Figure 17.3. Electron micrograph showing two sinusoids (S), one of which displays a Kupffer cell (K). The other sinusoid is lined by thin cytoplasmic sheets that belong to endothelial cells. Surrounding each sinusoid is the space of Disse (SD), which contains numerous microvilli from the hepatocytes (H). Also seen in the space of Disse is a cell with a large lipid droplet. This is a lipocyte (L). Its nucleus (N) is shaped to conform to the curve of the lipid droplet. × 6600.

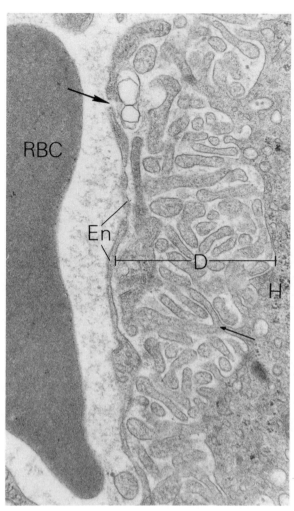

Figure 17.4. Electron micrograph showing space of Disse (D) between hepatocyte (H) and sinusoid. A gap **(large arrow)** separates the endothelial cells (En) that line the sinusoid. Such gaps allow for easy passage of small substances between the sinusoid and space of Disse. Numerous microvilli extend from the hepatocytes into the space of Disse. These are long and may branch **(small arrow)**. A red blood cell (RBC) is within the sinusoid. × 18,000. (Based on Bloom W, Fawcett DW: *A Textbook of Histology*, 10th ed. Philadelphia, WB Saunders, 1975.)

delicate collagen fibers that are displayed with classical silver staining procedures and, thus, have traditionally been designated as **reticular fibers.** These constitute the only stroma of the parenchymal portion of the liver lobule. This reticular stroma is continuous with the connective tissue in the portal space, or with the connective tissue that surrounds the lobule in the pig. The perisinusoidal reticular stroma is also continuous with the small amount of connective tissue surrounding the cen-

tral vein (terminal venule) in the center of the lobule. The space of Disse contains, at most, only a few fibroblasts (although some reports indicate that they are not present) and a cell capable of storing fat, the **lipocyte** (see Fig. 17.3). The relationship between the fibroblasts and lipocytes is not clear; it also has been suggested that they are different functional forms of the same cell.

In the fetal liver, the space between blood vessels and hepatocytes contains islands of blood-forming cells. In the adult in cases of chronic anemia, blood-forming cells may appear again.

Hepatocytes

The **hepatocyte** is the cell that makes up the cell plates of the lobule. Hepatocytes constitute about 80 percent of the cell population in the liver. The liver has a great number of functions, most of which are performed by hepatocytes. Thus, the cell has great functional diversity and this is regularly revealed in the cytological features of the cell.

The hepatocyte has a spherical nucleus, usually centrally placed. Many liver cell nuclei (over 50 percent) are polyploid, that is, they contain double (or more) the normal amount of DNA, and there is a correlation between nuclear size and the polyploid condition. In addition, many hepatocytes are binucleate; in these, the nuclei are the same size. Nuclei of hepatocytes contain one or more nucleoli and scattered clumps of chromatin (karyosomes) as well as a rim of perinuclear chromatin. The cytoplasm of the hepatocyte varies in appearance depending on several factors. In the well-fed individual, there are areas of ergastoplasm that display basophilia due to RNA. Also, there are irregular and round spaces in the cytoplasm, created by the loss of glycogen and lipid, respectively, during the preparation of the section. In contrast, in the fasted individual, where glycogen and lipid stores are depleted, there is reduction of ergastoplasm, and the cytoplasm stains rather uniformly with eosin. Generally, there are few lipid droplets in hepatocytes; however, they increase greatly after the ingestion of certain toxic substances.

The liver cell is polyhedral in shape; for convenience it will be described as having six surfaces, although there may be more. A schematic section of a cuboidal hepatocyte is shown in Figure 17.5. Two of its surfaces face the space of Disse. Two surfaces (and two surfaces parallel to the plane of the paper, one above and one below) show the plasma membrane facing its neighbor, and also facing a bile canaliculus. The bile canaliculus is a small canal formed by grooves in the two apposing cells. It contains microvilli from the hepatocyte. It

LUMEN OF SINUSOID

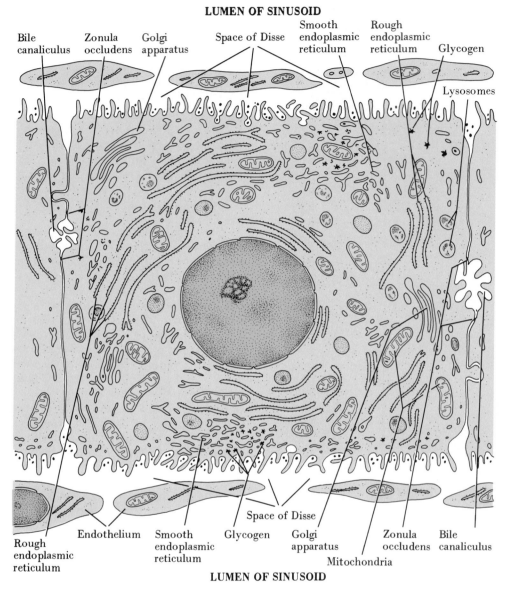

Figure 17.5. Schematic diagram of a hepatocyte showing representative cytoplasmic constituents. Two sides of the cell are shown facing sinusoids; two sides of the cell are shown facing bile canaliculi. Assuming that the cell is cuboidal in shape, the two additional sides of the cell, not shown, would also be facing bile canaliculi.

is sealed by zonulae occludentes, which prevent its contents from escaping into the adjacent intercellular space. The bile canaliculi form a ring about the hepatocyte (Fig. 17.6). They constitute a network which drains into small bile ducts, the *canals of Hering* (Fig. 17.7), and these, in turn, drain into the bile ducts of the portal canals. Thus, liver cells are organized for easy exchange of substances with the blood and for the discharge of bile through a system of canaliculi and ducts into the duodenum.

Electron micrographs of many hepatocytes show numerous organelles as depicted in Figure 17.8. Mitochondria are found throughout the cytoplasm. Profiles of rough endoplasmic reticulum (rER) and free ribosomes are present, and these correspond to the areas of basophilic staining observed with the light microscope. These basophilic areas are sites of protein synthesis. There are also areas of smooth endoplasmic reticulum (sER), and in places these are continuous with the rER. Glycogen is regularly found in liver cells, often in association with the sER. Typically, several Golgi

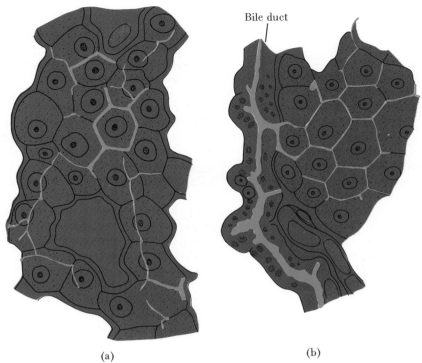

Bile duct

(a)   (b)

Figure 17.6. **(a)** Network of bile canaliculi demonstrated by intravenous injection of indigo carmine. Some bile canaliculi are clearly seen to form a band (green) about the hepatocyte. Thinner threads of dye show bile canaliculi just out of the main focal plane. (Special preparation fixed in potassium chloride formol; frozen section mounted in glycerine). **(b)** Bile canaliculi draining into duct. (Same type of preparation as in **a**.) (Based on Elias H: *Am J Anat* 85:379, 1949.)

areas are evident in a section and usually they are located in the vicinity of the bile canaliculi. Small, dense-appearing globules, 30 to 50 nm in diameter, are seen in dilated portions of the sER, in the dilated ends of some of the Golgi cisternae, and on occasion also in the dilated ends of cisternae of the rER. These are lipoprotein precursors that are synthesized by the hepatocyte and released into the blood. They play a role in the transport of lipids in the bloodstream. Also present in the cytoplasm, close to the bile canaliculi, are lysosomes. These are involved in organelle degradation and turnover within the hepatocyte; they are also increased in a number of pathological conditions, for example, in

Lipoproteins are multicomponent complexes of proteins and lipids that are involved in the transport of cholesterol and triglycerides. Cholesterol and triglycerides do not circulate free in the plasma because lipids on their own would be unable to remain in suspension. The association of the protein with the lipid-containing core makes the complex sufficiently hydrophilic to be suspended in the plasma.

Five classes of lipoproteins have been defined by their characteristic density, molecular weight, size, and chemical composition. These are, from largest and least dense to smallest and most dense: chylomicrons; very low density lipoproteins (VLDL); intermediate density lipoproteins (IDL); low density lipoproteins (LDL); and high density lipoproteins (HDL). (High levels of LDL are directly correlated with increased risk of developing cardiovascular disease; high levels of HDL or low levels of LDL have been associated with decreased risk). The lipoproteins serve a variety of functions in the cellular membranes and the transport and metabolism of lipids. Precursors of the lipoproteins are produced in hepatocytes. The lipid component is produced in the sER; the protein component in the rER. The lipoprotein complexes pass to the Golgi complex where secretory vesicles containing electron-dense lipoprotein particles bud off and then are released into the plasma at the cell surface bordering the space of Disse.

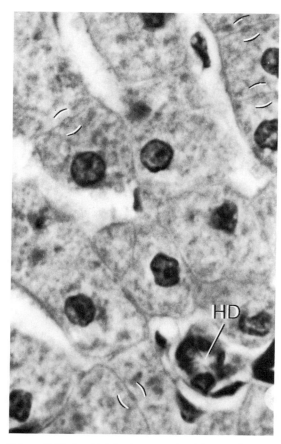

Figure 17.7(a). Light micrograph of liver cells and a small bile duct (HD). This duct is still surrounded by hepatocytes and is called a canal of Hering. The **brackets** mark cross-sectioned bile canaliculi. × 1240.

viral hepatitis and anoxia. Microbodies (peroxisomes) are present in liver cells; their functions are not yet understood. They have been implicated in disposing of hydrogen peroxide, gluconeogenesis, and metabolism of purines, alcohol, and lipids.

Nerves

The liver receives nerves from both sympathetic and parasympathetic parts of the autonomic nervous system. The nerves enter the liver at the porta hepatis and ramify through the liver in the portal canals along with the members of the portal triad. Sympathetic fibers are believed to innervate blood vessels; parasympathetic fibers are considered to innervate the large ducts (those that contain smooth muscle in their walls) and possibly blood vessels. Cell bodies of parasympathetic neurons are often seen near the porta hepatis.

Lymphatic Vessels

The liver produces a major part of the thoracic duct lymph. It differs in composition from lymph derived from the intestines in its high content of plasma proteins. Lymphatic vessels begin in the smallest portal canals. They are not found in the lobule itself. However, it is thought that lymph is formed from the fluid in the space of Disse and in the space of Mall. The lymphatic vessels of the portal canals communicate with lymphatic vessels of the capsule and, ultimately, large lymphatic vessels leave the liver through the porta hepatis. Some lymphatic vessels leave the liver with the hepatic veins. A third exit route for lymphatic vessels of the liver is through the bare area where the liver is in direct contact with the undersurface of the diaphragm.

Other Interpretations of Liver Structure

The description of the classic liver lobule, as given above, is most useful in understanding the structural organization of the liver and emphasizes the endocrine aspect of liver function. However, Rappaport and others have proposed a concept of organization based on the *liver acinus* as the functional unit of the liver (Fig. 17.9). The distributing vessels that lie at the border of two adjacent classic liver lobules constitute the morphological center of the liver acinus. These vessels actually supply the hepatocytes in each of the two adjacent classic lobules. The concept of the liver acinus is particularly useful in interpreting the gradient of metabolic activity that can be detected in zones of hepatocytes of adjacent classic lobules as shown in Figure 17.6. It is also useful in analyzing the progression of liver cirrhosis.

An older interpretation of liver organization, designated as the *portal lobule* (Fig. 17.10) has the bile duct as its morphological center and it emphasizes the exocrine function of the liver.

Liver Regeneration

Dividing cells are not usually seen in the normal liver. Nevertheless, the liver has impressive regenerative capabilities. In laboratory animals such as the rat, after surgical removal of two-thirds of the liver mass, the remaining cells can replace the original mass of liver tissue. In doing so, the normal lobulation is not restored. The liver can also regenerate new liver parenchyma after destruction due to toxic substances.

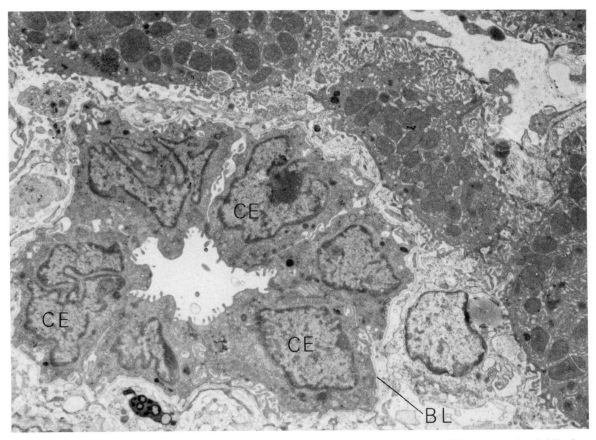

Figure 17.7(b). A terminal portion of a bile duct designated as a canal of Hering. The duct collects bile from the canaliculi between adjacent hepatocytes. The duct is close to the hepatocytes, but the actual connection between bile canaliculi and the canal of Hering is not shown. The duct is comprised of cuboidal epithelium (CE). BL, basal lamina. × 6000.

Bile Ducts

Bile is secreted by hepatocytes into the bile canaliculi. The canaliculi empty into small ducts at the outer portion of the liver lobule called the *ductules,* or *canals of Hering.* In turn, the canals of Hering drain into the intrahepatic bile ducts within the portal canals. The canal of Hering consists of cuboidal epithelium surrounded by reticular fibers (see Fig. 17.7a,b). The intrahepatic bile ducts are lined by cuboidal or low columnar epithelium. Increasing amounts of fibroelastic connective tissue surround the epithelium as the ducts become larger near the porta. Smooth muscle cells are present in the wall of the largest ducts.

The extrahepatic bile ducts are the *hepatic duct, cystic duct,* and *common bile duct* (Fig. 17.11). The hepatic duct conveys bile from the liver. It is joined by the cystic duct of the gallbladder and together these two form a common bile duct that leads to the duodenum. The common bile duct is joined by the pancreatic duct just before opening into the duodenum. The short common entry of these ducts is the *ampulla (ampulla of Vater).* Valves in the ampulla and the common bile duct *(the sphincter of Oddi)* control the flow of bile into the intestine.

GALLBLADDER

The gallbladder is a pear-shaped organ (see Fig. 17.11) that stores and concentrates bile. It is attached to the posterior-inferior surface of the liver. The gallbladder is a blind pouch that leads via a neck to the cystic duct. Through this duct it receives dilute bile from the hepatic duct and discharges concentrated bile into the common bile duct.

The wall of the gallbladder consists of a mu-

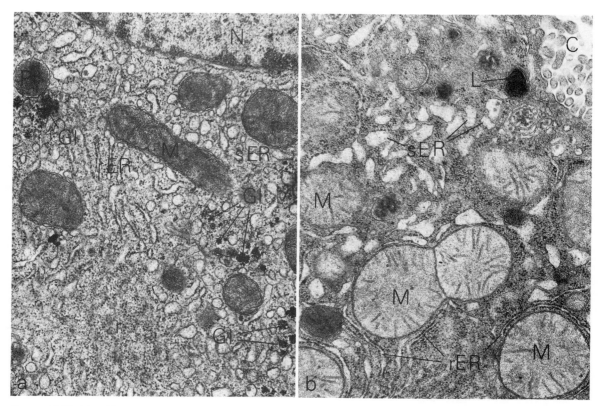

Figure 17.8(a,b). Electron micrographs showing **(a)** typical cytoplasmic constituents near the nucleus (N) of a hepatocyte. These include a peroxisome (P), mitochondria (M), glycogen (Gl), smooth endoplasmic reticulum (sER), and rough endoplasmic reticulum (rER). In one region, the membranes of the rER have been cut in a tangential plane showing the ribosomes (r) as they are positioned on the cytoplasmic face of the membrane. **(b)** A region of cytoplasm near the canaliculus (C). It includes a lysosome (L), mitochondria (M), and endoplasmic reticulum, both sER and rER. Note the numerous microvilli in the canaliculus. × 18,000.

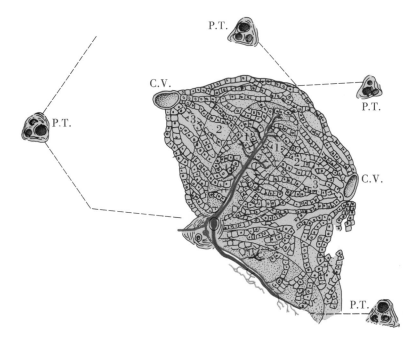

Figure 17.9. The liver acinus is another interpretation of liver organization. It consists of adjacent sectors of neighboring hexagonal fields partially separated by distributing blood vessels. The zones marked **1**, **2**, and **3** are supplied with blood that is most oxygenated and richest in nutrients in zone **1** and least so in zone **3**. The central veins (C.V.) in this interpretation are at the edges of the acinus instead of in the center as in the classical lobule. The vessels of the portal space, namely the portal triad (P.T.), are at some corners of the hexagon that outlines the cross-sectioned profile of the classical lobule. (Based on Rappaport AM, et al: *Anat Rec* 119: 11, 1954.)

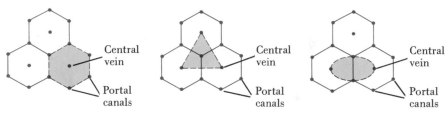

Figure 17.10. Comparison of different interpretations of liver structure. The classic lobule **(left)** has a central vein centrally positioned and portal canals at the edges of the cross-sectioned lobule. The portal lobule **(center)** has a portal canal in a central position and central veins at the edges of the cross-sectioned lobule. The liver acinus **(right)** has distributing vessels in the center and central veins at each pole of the cross-sectioned structure. (Based on Weiss L, Greep RO: *Histology,* 4th ed. New York, McGraw-Hill, 1977.)

cous membrane, a muscular layer, an adventitia, and a serous membrane (visceral peritoneum) except where it is attached to the liver. The mucosa consists of simple columnar epithelium and a lamina propria of loose connective tissue (Fig. 17.12). The muscularis consists of layers of smooth muscle with collagenous and elastic fibers between the

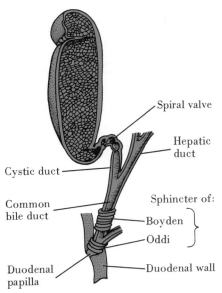

Figure 17.11. Schematic diagram of gallbladder and its ducts. The gallbladder is a blind pouch joined to a single cystic duct. Thickenings in this duct are called the spiral valve. The cystic duct joins with the hepatic duct and together they form a common bile duct that leads to the duodenum. At the entry to the duodenum, the common bile duct is joined by the pancreatic duct and together they enter the duodenum at the duodenal papilla. Sphincters guard the common bile duct (Boyden) and the common opening of this and the pancreatic duct (Oddi). (Based on Grant JCB: A *Method of Anatomy,* 4th ed. Baltimore, The Williams & Wilkins Co., 1948.)

layers. The adventitia is comprised of collagen and elastic fibers. The adventitial connective tissue also contains a rich lymphatic network. Nerves of the gallbladder are autonomic; cell bodies of parasympathetic neurons are found in the wall of the cystic duct.

The columnar epithelial cells have many small microvilli on their apical surface (Fig. 17.13). They contain numerous mitochondria throughout the cytoplasm; a Golgi apparatus is apical to the nucleus; rER is dispersed throughout the cell; and membrane-bound granules and pinocytotic vesicles are present in the apical cytoplasm. The mitochondria contribute to a light eosinophilic staining of the cytoplasm.

An apical junctional complex joins adjacent cells and separates the lumen of the gallbladder from the lateral intercellular (paracellular) space. The extent of the paracellular space varies according to the functional state of the mucosa, being greatly enlarged during the transport of water. In experimental studies in which the epithelial cells are induced to transport water, sodium is first actively transported into the paracellular space. This results in an increase in the osmotic pressure of fluid in the paracellular microcompartment; water is then drawn osmotically from the cell into the paracellular microcompartment causing it to become greatly enlarged. From here the water moves into the subjacent blood vessels. The increase in volume of the paracellular space during fluid transport is sufficient to be detected with the light microscope.

The mucosa of the gallbladder is thrown into numerous folds when the organ is empty, but only a few are present in the distended organ. Diverticulae of the mucosa, called ***Rokitansky-Aschoff sinuses,*** dip into the wall of the gallbladder. Sometimes these diverticulae extend into and through the muscular layer (see Atlas section, Plate 86, Fig. 4). They are lined by the same type of epithelium

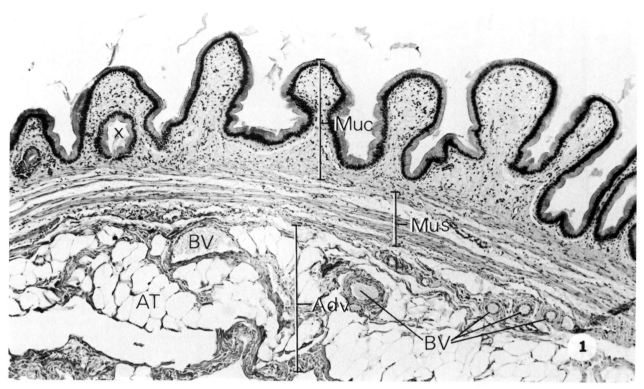

Figure 17.12. Light micrograph of gallbladder. The mucosa (Muc) consists of a lining of columnar epithelial cells and a lamina propria of loose connective tissue. Under this is a muscular layer (Mus) and external to the muscle is an adventitia with numerous adipocytes (AT) and blood vessels (BV). The portion of the bladder not attached to the liver will show a serosa instead of an adventitia. × 75.

as that which lines the inner surface of the organ. Near the neck of the gallbladder there are branched tubuloalveolar mucous glands. In (hematoxylin and eosin) (H&E)-stained sections, these can be distinguished readily from the epithelial outpouchings by the character of the epithelium. The mucous cells have an empty-appearing apical cytoplasm and flattened basal nuclei, whereas the absorptive cells in the outpouchings have an eosinophilic-staining cytoplasm and ovoid or tall nuclei.

In some individuals there are ducts, the **ducts of Luschka,** located in the connective tissue between the liver and the gallbladder near the neck. These connect with the cystic duct, not with the lumen of the gallbladder. They are histologically similar to the intrahepatic bile ducts and may be remnants of aberrant embryonic bile ducts.

The gallbladder responds to fat in the diet. The dietary fat causes the release of cholecystokinin from the small intestine. This hormone causes contractions of the muscular layer of the gallbladder and the resulting discharge of bile into the duodenum.

PANCREAS

The pancreas is an elongate gland that can be divided into a head, body, and tail. The **head** is an expanded portion that lies in the C-shaped curve of the duodenum (Fig. 17.14). It is joined to the duodenum by connective tissue. The centrally located **body** and tapering **tail** extend across the midline of the body toward the hilum of the spleen. The **pancreatic duct (duct of Wirsung)** extends through the length of the gland and empties into the duodenum via the **ampulla of Vater** (through which the common bile duct from the liver and gallbladder also enters the duodenum). In some individuals there is also an accessory pancreatic duct.

The pancreas is a mixed exocrine and endocrine gland. The exocrine units, or **acini,** are tubuloacinar glands, organized in principle much the same as salivary glands. As with salivary glands, their organization can be likened to a bunch of grapes, with the secretory acini comparable to the grapes and the system of ducts comparable to the stems.

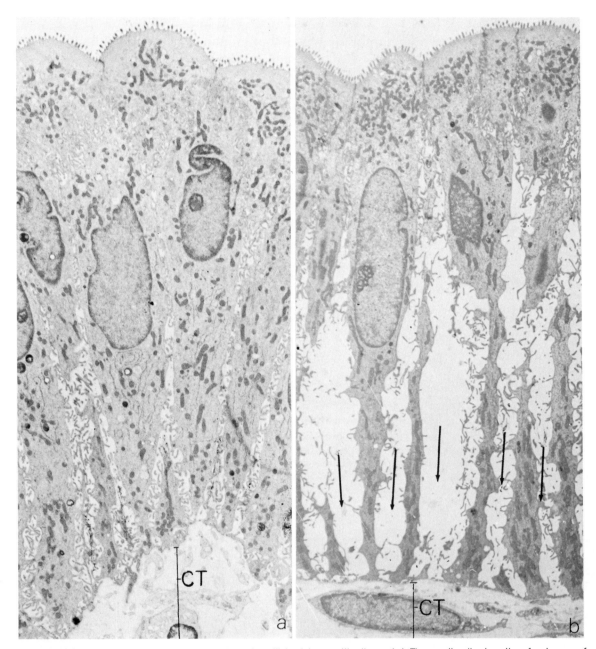

Figure 17.13(a,b). Electron micrographs of gallbladder epithelium. **(a)** The cells display the features of absorptive cells with microvilli on their apical surface. An apical junctional complex separates the lumen of the gallbladder from the lateral intercellular space. **(b)** During fluid transport, fluid enters the cell from the lumen of the gallbladder; the fluid is then pumped into the lateral intercellular space, and during active fluid transport this space becomes greatly distended **(arrows).** Fluid moves from the enlarged intercellular space across the basal lamina into the underlying connective tissue (CT) and then into blood vessels. The increase in lateral intercellular space during active fluid transport is sufficient to be evident with the light microscope. (Based on Kay G: 1966.)

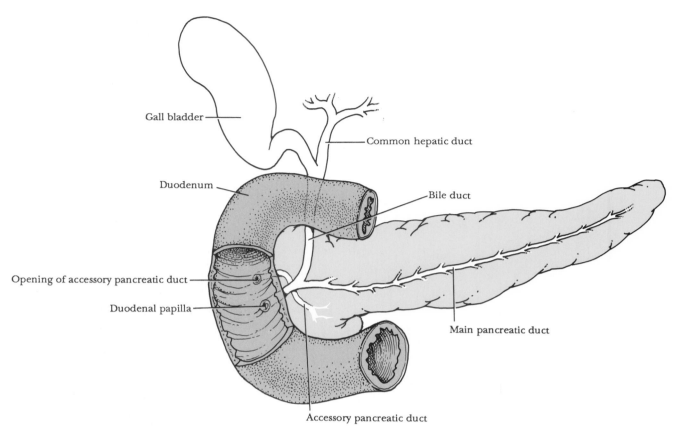

Figure 17.14. Diagram of pancreas, duodenum, and ducts. The main pancreatic duct traverses the length of the pancreas and enters the duodenum in company with the common bile duct. An accessory pancreatic duct is sometimes also present as shown. The site of duct entry is typically marked by a papilla. (Based on Grant JCB: *A Method of Anatomy*, 4th ed. Baltimore, The Williams & Wilkins Co., 1948.)

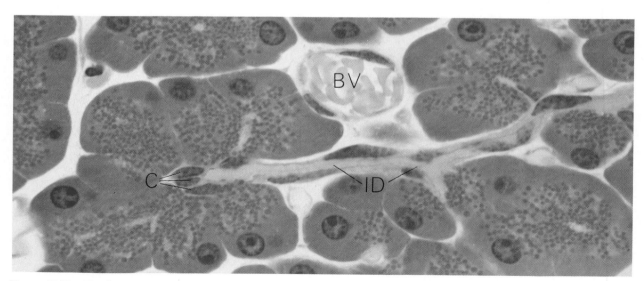

Figure 17.15. Plastic section (light micrograph) of a pancreatic acinus and the intercalated duct (ID) leading from it. The duct can be seen beginning within the acinus. The cells forming the duct within the acinus are known as centroacinar cells (C). BV, blood vessel.

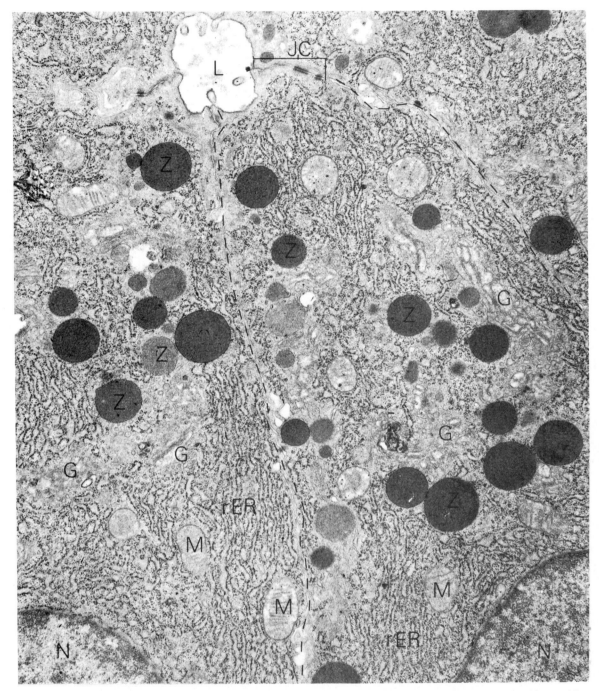

Figure 17.16. Electron micrograph of the apical cytoplasm of several pancreatic acinar cells. (One of the cells is outlined by the **broken line**.) Nuclei (N) of adjoining cells are evident at the bottom left and right of the micrograph. The apical cytoplasm contains rER, some mitochondria (M), the zymogen secretory granules (Z), and profiles of Golgi apparatus (G). At the apex of the cells a lumen is present into which the zymogen granules are discharged. A junctional complex (JC) is also evident near the lumen. × 20,000.

A thin layer of loose connective tissue surrounds the gland. From this outer layer of connective tissue, septa extend into the gland, dividing it into ill-defined lobules. Within the lobules, a stroma of loose connective tissue surrounds the parenchymal units. Between the lobules larger amounts of connective tissue surround the larger ducts, blood vessels, and nerve fibers. Moreover, in the connective tissue surrounding the pancreatic duct, there are small mucous glands that empty into the duct.

The endocrine units are called the *islets of Langerhans.* They are highly vascularized and, as with all endocrine glands, their product is conveyed to its target via the bloodstream. The islets vary in size from not much larger than several acini to those that are macroscopically visible. The islets are most prevalent in the tail of the pancreas.

Pancreatic Acini

The pancreatic acinus is a rounded structure comprised of generally pyramidal epithelial cells. These acinar cells produce the digestive enzymes of the pancreas. Pancreatic acini are unique among glandular acini in that the intercalated duct begins within the acinus (Fig. 17.15). The duct cells within the acinus are referred to as *centroacinar cells.* The base of the acinar cell contains the nucleus and a large region of ergastoplasm and, thus, the basal cytoplasm stains well with hematoxylin or basic dyes. The apical portion stains with eosin due to the presence of numerous zymogen granules. The centroacinar cells stain very lightly with eosin.

Ultrastructurally, the acinar cells display the features of a polarized synthetic-secretory cell (Fig. 17.16). The base of the cell contains many parallel cisternae of the rER with free ribosomes between the cisternae. These structures account for the basophilic staining of this region in H&E-stained paraffin sections. Mitochondria are generally small, located mostly between the cisternae of rER, but also elsewhere within the cell. The apical portion of the cell contains the Golgi and zymogen granules. The zymogen granules are most numerous in the resting gland. Microvilli extend from the apical surface of neighboring cells into the acinar lumen. The apical poles of the neighboring cells are joined by junctional complexes. The zonulae occludentes of these junctions separate the lumen of the acinus from the lateral intercellular space.

The centroacinar cell has a centrally placed nucleus and attenuated cytoplasm forming a squamous cell (Fig. 17.15). These cells are continuous with the short intercalated duct that lies outside the acinus. Squamous epithelium lines the intercalated ducts. These ducts lead into intralobular ducts that are lined with cuboidal or low

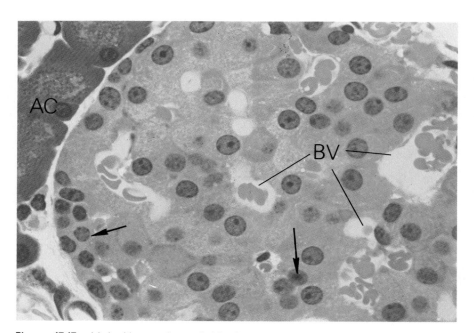

Figure 17.17. Islet of Langerhans, light micrograph. Identification of specific cell types without special stains is difficult. At best, one can identify small cells **(arrows)** at the periphery of the cell mass, that is, in proximity to the adjacent connective tissue, which are probably A cells. BV, blood vessels.

TABLE 17.2. Major Cell Types in Pancreatic Islets

CELL TYPE	PERCENTAGE	CYTOPLASMIC STAINING WITH MALLORY-AZAN	PRODUCT	GRANULES (TEM)
A	15–20	Red	Glucagon	About 250 nm; dense, eccentric core surrounded by light substance
B	60–70	Brownish orange	Insulin	About 300 nm; many with dense, crystalline (angular) core surrounded by light substance
D	5–10	Blue	Somatostatin	About 325 nm; homogeneous matrix

columnar epithelium. Larger ducts in the interlobular connective tissue are lined by columnar epithelium. These larger ducts also contain goblet cells and APUD cells.

The pancreas secretes about 1 liter of fluid per day. The acinar cells secrete a small volume of fluid rich in proteins; these are digestive enzymes. The cells of the small ducts produce a large volume of fluid rich in sodium and bicarbonate; the bicarbonate serves to neutralize acid in the duodenum.

The pancreatic secretion is regulated by hor-

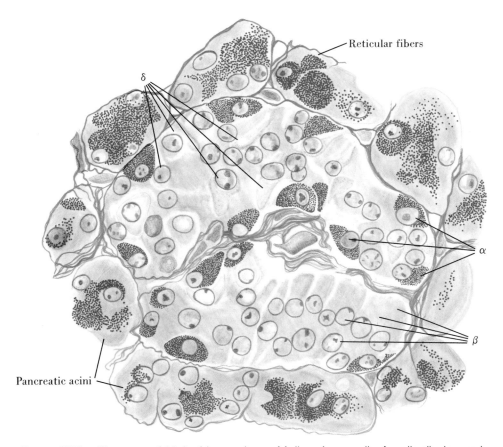

Figure 17.18. Diagram of islet of Langerhans, Mallory-Azan cells. A cells display red cytoplasmic staining; B cells (comprising most of the islet cells) display pale gray-green staining; and D cells show a blue cytoplasm.

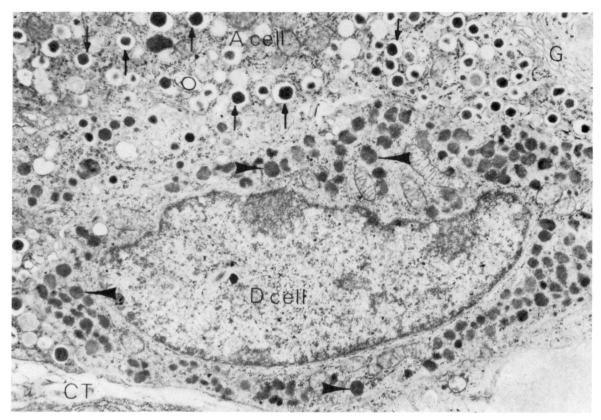

Figure 17.19. Pancreatic islet cells, electron micrograph. The cell in the upper part of the illustration is an A cell. It contains characteristic granules **(arrows)** showing a dense spherical core-surrounded by clear area and then a membrane. The A cell also displays a characteristically well-developed Golgi **(G)**. The cell in the bottom of the illustration is a D cell. It contains numerous membrane-bound granules of moderately low density **(arrowheads)**. CT, connective tissue. ×·15,000.

mones (see Tables 16.1 and 16.2) and autonomic innervation. Sympathetic nerve fibers are involved in regulation of pancreatic blood vessels. Parasympathetic fibers stimulate activity of acinar as well as centroacinar cells. Cell bodies of neurons occasionally seen in the pancreas belong to parasympathetic postganglionic neurons.

Islets of Langerhans

In H&E-stained section, the islets of Langerhans appear as clusters of pale-staining cells surrounded by more intensely staining pancreatic acini. It is not practical to try to identify the several cell types found in the islets in H&E sections (Fig. 17.17) However, after Zenker-formol fixation and staining by the Mallory Azan method, it is possible to identify three cell types designated A, B, and D cells (Table 17.2 and Fig. 17.18). The appearance of the granules allows the electron microscopist to distinguish major cell types. With the transmission

electron microscopy (Fig. 17.19), the islet cells have the general features of APUD cells.

In addition to the A, B, and D cells, which are colored in a distinctive manner with the Mallory Azan method, a small, unstained *clear cell* is also recognized. The clear cell may represent a number of cells or it may be a single cell with a diverse number of products. The clear cell (or cells) accounts for less than 5 percent of the islet cell population.

The islet cells produce two hormones, insulin and glucagon. Both have a direct effect on the level of glucose in the blood with insulin reducing the level and glucagon elevating it. The A cell also secretes several other products. Somatostatin, produced by the D cell, appears to function locally as a paracrine agent, inhibiting the production of hormones by A and B cells. In addition to insulin, glucagon, and somatostatin, islet cells produce many other products similar to those produced by APUD cells elsewhere.

ATLAS PLATES

83–87

PLATE 83. Liver I

The liver consists of large numbers of functional units called lobules. These are roughly cylindrical in shape with a venous channel, the central vein that courses through its long axis. Irregular interconnecting sheets, or plate-like arrangements of hepatic cells, radiate outward from the central vein and constitute the parenchyma of the lobule. Sinusoids separate the sheets of hepatic cells and empty into the central veins. In the human, the lobules are poorly delineated from their neighbors and it is often difficult to determine where one lobule ends and the next begins.

In the low-power view of the liver section shown in **Figure 1,** large numbers of hepatic cells appear to be uniformly disposed throughout the specimen. The hepatic cells are arranged in plates one cell thick, but when sectioned, they appear as interconnecting cords one or more cells thick according to the plane of section. The sinusoids appear as the light areas between the cords of cells, as in **Figure 2 (asterisks).**

Also present in **Figure 1** is a portal canal. It is a connective tissue septum carries the branches of the hepatic artery **(HA)** and portal vein **(pv),** bile ducts **(BD),** and lymphatic vessels and nerves. The artery and vein along with the bile duct are collectively referred to as a portal triad.

The hepatic artery and the portal vein are easy to identify because they are found in relation to one another within the surrounding connective tissue of the portal canal. The vein is typically thin-walled, and the accompanying artery is smaller in size and has a thicker wall. The bile ducts are comprised of a simple cuboidal or columnar epithelium, depending upon the size of the duct. They have the same general appearance as the ducts of most exocrine glands. Multiple profiles of the blood vessels and bile ducts may be evident in the canal due either to branching or to their passage out of the plane of section and then back in again.

The vessel through which blood leaves the liver is the hepatic vein. It is readily identified on the basis that it travels alone **(inset)** and that it is surrounded by an appreciable amount of connective tissue **(CT).** If more than one profile of a vein is present within this connective tissue, but no arteries or bile ducts are present, the second vessel

---

KEY

BD, bile duct
CT, connective tissue
CV, central vein
HA, hepatic artery

HV, hepatic vein
L, lymphatic nodule
PV, portal vein

---

asterisks, Fig. 2,
  blood sinusoids
dotted line,
  approximates the
  limits of a lobule

Fig. 1, human, × 85
  (inset, × 65)
Fig. 2, human,
  × 160.

---

will also be a hepatic vein. Such is the case in the **inset** where a profile of a small hepatic vein is seen just above the larger hepatic vein **(HV).**

The central veins **(CV** in **Figs. 1 and 2)** are the most distal radicals of the hepatic vein, and, like the hepatic vein, they also travel alone. Their distinguishing features are the sinusoids that penetrate the wall of the vein and the paucity of surrounding connective tissue. These characteristics are shown to advantage in the next plate.

At this point, it is well to re-examine **Figure 1** to define the boundaries of a liver lobule. A lobule is best identified when it is cut in cross-section. The central vein then appears as a circular profile and the hepatic cells appear as cords radiating from the central vein. A lobule fitting this general description is outlined by the **dotted lines** in **Figure 1.** The limits of the lobule are defined, in part, by the portal canal. In other directions the plates of the lobule do not appear to have a limit, that is, they have evidently joined and become contiguous with plates of adjacent lobules. However, one can estimate the dimensions of the lobule by approximating a circle with the central vein as its center and incorporating those plates that exhibit a radial arrangement up to the point that the radius of the circle will allow. In this case, the radial limit is set by the location of the portal canal. Similarly, the portion of the lobule in **Figure 2** shows a boundary by the presence of some very small bile ducts **(BD).** The location of these ducts serves as an indicator of the radius of the lobule as measured from the central vein.

PLATE 83

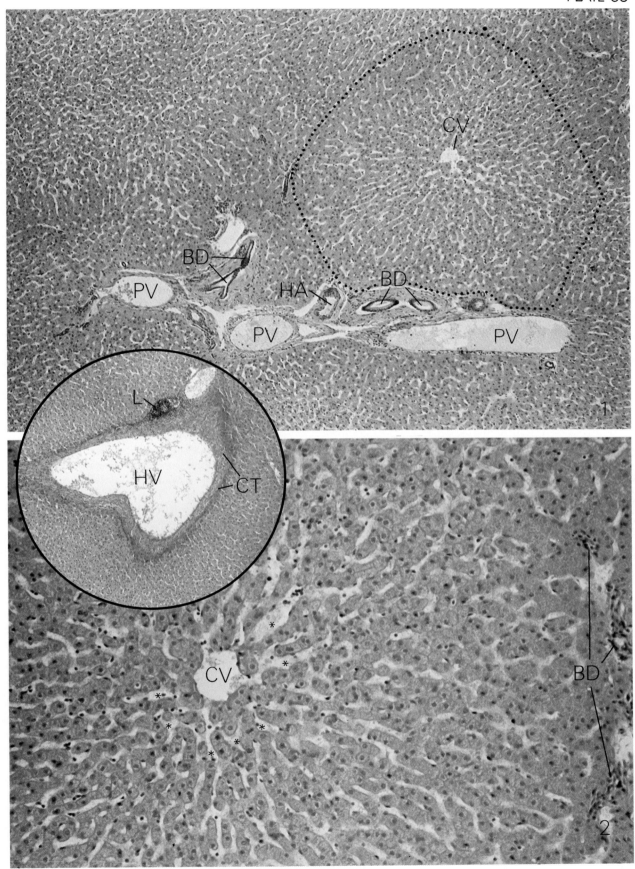

PLATE 84. Liver II

The central vein and surrounding hepatocytes from **Figure 2** of the preceding plate (plate 83) are shown at higher magnification here in **Figure 1.** The cytoplasm of the hepatocytes in this specimen exhibits a foamy appearance. This is due to extraction of glycogen and, to a lesser extent, lipid during preparation of the tissue. The boundaries between individual hepatocytes are discernable in some locations but not between those cells where the knife has cut across the boundary in an oblique plane. When cell boundaries are observed at higher magnification, frequently a very small circular or oval profile is observed midway along the boundary (see **inset**). Thesw profiles represent the bile canaliculi (**BC**).

The cells that line the sinusoids (**S**) show little, if any, cytoplasmic detail in H&E preparations. Kupffer cells (**KC**) are generally recognized by the shape of their nuclei; they appear ovoid and usually project into the lumen. The endothelial cell, in contrast, has a smaller, attenuated or elongated nucleus. Some nuclei of this description are evident in the micrograph. However, because occasional fibroblast nuclei are present in the space of Disse, it may not be possible to distinguish between the two cell types with any degree of assurance.

The termination of two of the sinusoids and their union with the central vein (**CV**) is indicated by the **curved arrows.** Note that the wall of the vein is strengthened by connective tissue, mostly collagen, which appears as the homogeneous eosin-stained material (**asterisks**). Fibroblasts (**F**) within this connective tissue (**F**) can be identified and distinguished from the endothelial cell (**En**) lining of the vein.

Figure 2 shows a plastic-embedded (glutaraldehyde-osmium fixed) liver specimen. In contrast to the H&E-stained preparation, this specimen demonstrates to advantage the cytological detail of the parenchymal cells and the sinusoids. The hepatocytes are deeply colored with toluidine blue, the dye employed to stain the specimen. Note that the cytoplasm exhibits irregular magenta masses (**arrows**). This is glycogen that has been retained by the fixation procedure and metachromatically stained by the toluidine blue. (Retention of the glycogen is due to the glutaraldehyde, the initial fixative employed in preserving the specimen.) Also evident are lipid droplets (**L**) of varying size

that have also been preserved and stained black by the osmium used as the secondary fixative. The quantity of lipid and glycogen are variable and, under normal conditions, reflect dietary intake. Careful examination of the hepatocyte cytoplasm also reveals small, punctate, dark-blue bodies contrasted against the lighter-blue background of the cell. These are the mitochondria. Another feature of this specimen is the clear representation of the bile canaliculi (**BC**) between the liver cells. They appear as empty circular profiles when cross-sectioned and as elongate channels (**lower right of figure**) when longitudinally sectioned.

Examination of the sinusoidal lining cells reveals two distinct cell types. The more prominent of the two is the Kupffer cell (**KC**). These cells exhibit a large nucleus and a substantial amount of cytoplasm. They tend to protrude into the lumen and sometimes give the appearance of occluding the vascular channel. Though a Kupffer cell may appear to span the lumen, it actually does not block the channel. The surface of the Kupffer cell exhibits a very irregular or jagged contour due to the numerous processes that provide the cell with an extensive surface area. The endothelial cell (**En**) has a smaller nucleus, attenuated cytoplasm, and a smooth surface contour. In this specimen the perisinusoidal space, the space of Disse, is just perceptible in some areas as a thin light band between the dark-stained hepatocytes and the ligher-stained cytoplasm of the endothelial and Kupffer cells. The nature of the space of Disse is more clearly revealed in the electron micrograph that follows.

PLATE 84

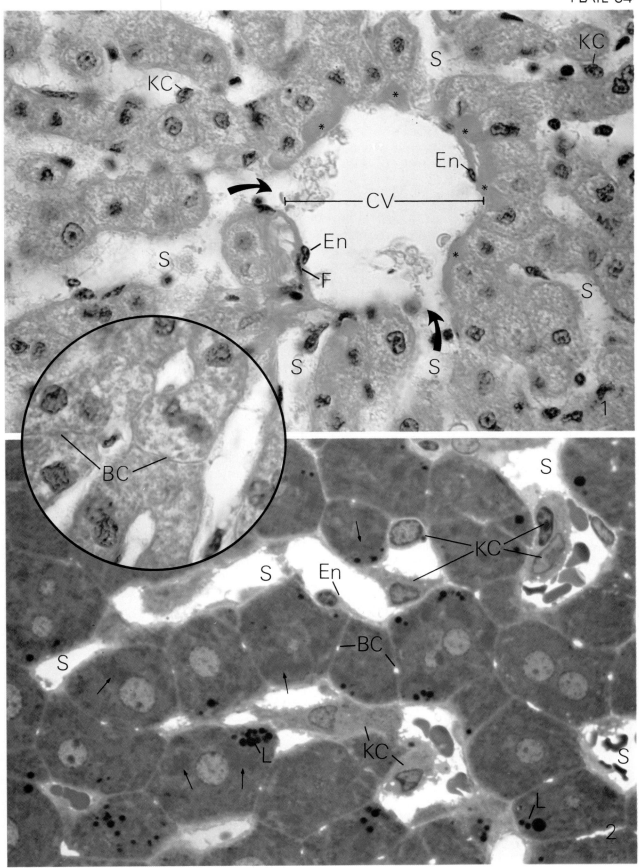

PLATE 85. Liver III, Electron Microscopy

A more detailed analysis of liver structural organization is provided by the accompanying electron micrograph, and it should also be compared with the plastic section, **Figure 2,** in the preceding plate (Atlas section, Plate 84). Shown in the electron micrograph are portions of two liver cords, which join one another in the upper left of the micrograph. A sinusoid **(S)** is seen between the two cords, but it turns out of the plane of section where the cords join. The nucleus of one of the hepatocytes is included in the section. This nucleus **(center)** displays the same characteristic, sparse heterochromatin distribution, as is seen in the hepatocyte nuclei included in the plastic section.

The cytoplasm displays numerous patches of glycogen particle aggregates **(G).** They correspond to the pink (metachromatic) stained areas in the toluidine blue specimen in Atlas section, Plate 84. Also, relatively conspicuous are the numerous ovoid mitochondria and profiles of rough endoplasmic reticulum **(ER).**

A few lipid droplets are also present. They appear as the relatively small spherical bodies **(L).** The amount of lipid in a given normal liver parenchymal cell may be quite variable. This is due, in part, to the plane of section through the cell (note the variation in the plastic section), as well as the location of the cells with respect to blood supply and dietetic conditions in general. The latter points also apply to the degree of glycogen storage in the parenchymal cells.

At this low magnification, the space of Disse **(D)** can be recognized as a narrow space containing small cytoplasmic processes or microvilli. The space of Disse is separated from the lumen of the sinusoid **(S)** by a thin endothelium, which, at higher magnifications, shows gaps of various sizes;

KEY

BC, bile canaliculus
D, space of Disse
ER, rough endoplasmic
reticulum

G, Golgi apparatus
KC, Kupffer cell
L, lipid droplet
S, sinusoid

Fig., mouse, 5100;
inset, 6000.

---

that is, one can detect open pathways between the space of Disse and the sinus lumen. The Kupffer cells **(KC)** can be seen forming a portion of the sinusoid wall. They seemingly substitute in places for the endothelial cells, but the bulk of the cell lies within the sinusoid lumen. The **inset** provides a better perspective of the Kupffer cell with its nucleus included in the plane of section. Note the presence of the secondary lysosomes. They appear as irregular, electron dense bodies within the cytoplasm of the Kupffer cell. Also note the numerous microvilli emanating from the liver parenchymal cell and projecting into the space of Disse.

The last feature of note in this micrograph is the two bile canaliculi **(BC),** which are seen on the left side of the micrograph. The boundaries between adjoining cells can just be made out at this low magnification and the site of the canaliculus is seen where the two adjoining membranes part to form this small canal.

PLATE 85

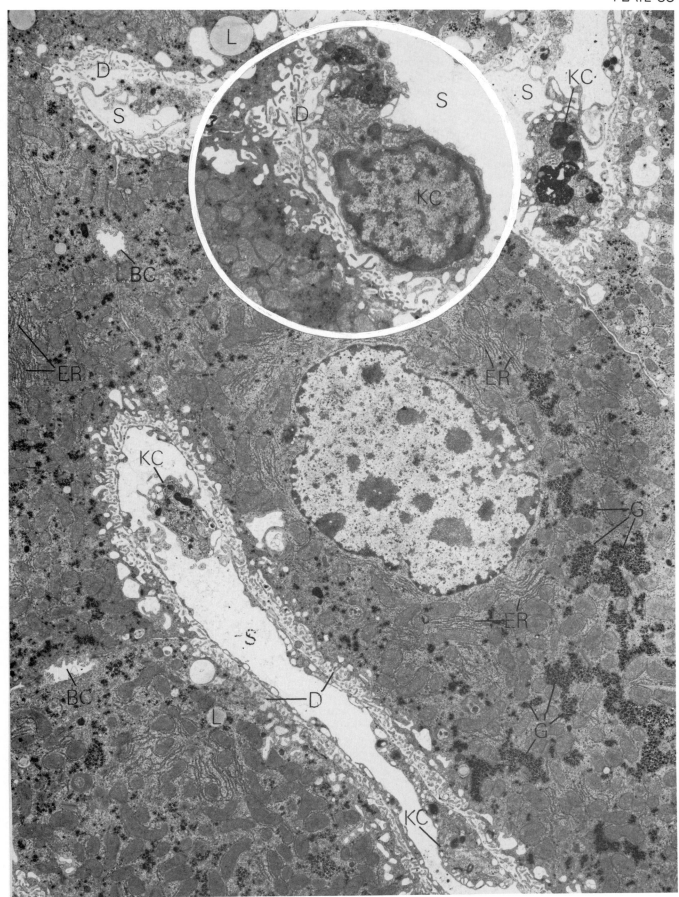

PLATE 86. Gallbladder

The gallbladder is a hollow, pear-shaped organ that concentrates and stores the bile. The full thickness of its wall is shown in **Figure 1.** It is comprised of a mucosa (**Muc**), muscularis (**Mus**), and an adventitia (**Adv**), or on its free surface (not shown), a serosa. The mucosa (**Fig. 2**) consists of a simple columnar epithelium (**Ep**) resting on a lamina propria of loose, irregular connective tissue (**CT**). The muscularis consists of interlacing bundles of smooth muscle (**SM**). The adventitia (**Fig. 1**) consists of irregular, dense connective tissue through which the larger blood vessels (**BV**) travel and more peripherally varying amounts of adipose tissue (**AT**).

The mucosa is thrown into numerous folds that are particularly pronounced when the muscularis is highly contracted. This is the usual histological appearance of the gallbladder unless, of course, steps are taken to fix and preserve it in a distended state. Occasionally, the section cuts through a recess in a fold and the recess may then resemble a gland (**arrows**). The mucosa, however, does not possess glands except in the neck region where some mucous glands are present (see below).

The epithelial lining (**Fig. 2, Ep**) of the gallbladder consists of absorptive cells. They have certain characteristics that may assist one in identifying the gallbladder and distinguishing it from other organs such as the intestines. Only one cell type is present in the epithelial layer (**Fig. 2 and 3**). These are tall columnar cells; the nuclei are in the basal portion of the cell. The cells possess a delicate apical striated border. However, this is not always evident in routine H&E-stained sections. The cytoplasm stains rather uniformly with eosin. This is related to its absorptive function and is in contrast to the staining of cells that are engaged in the production of protein. Lastly, with respect to its absorptive function, the epithelial cells frequently exhibit intercellular spaces at their basal aspect (**Fig. 3, arrows**). This is a feature associated with the transport of fluid across the epithelium and, as previously noted, it is also commonly seen in intestinal absorptive cells.

The lamina propria underlying the epithelium is usually relatively cellular. In this specimen, in addition to the presence of lymphocytes (**L**), a relatively common finding, there are also a large

number of plasma cells (**PC**) present within the lamina propria (**Fig. 3**). (The high concentration of plasma cells suggests a chronic inflammation.) Another feature of note is the presence of several glands and gland-like profiles (**GI**) other than those seen in the mucosa and already noted. These are readily apparent in **Figure 1.** Two of these structures, marked by **asterisks** in **Figure 1,** are shown at higher magnification in **Figure 4.** The smaller of the two structures is comprised of mucous cells (**MC**) and represents a section through a mucous gland. This specimen was taken from a site near the neck of the gallbladder where mucous glands are present. Note the characteristic flattened nuclei at the base of the cell and the light-staining or foamy appearance of the cytoplasm, features characteristic of mucous-secreting cells. In contrast, the epithelium of the large gland-like profile that is only partially included in the micrograph has rounded or ovoid nuclei. This epithelial-lined structure is not a true gland but represents an outpouching or evagination of the mucous membrane, which extends into and often through the thickness of the muscularis. These outpouchings are known as Rokitansky-Aschoff sinuses. Their role or significance, if any, is unknown. (Some authorities contend that they result from disease, but they are also found in small numbers in gallbladders that appear normal in all other respects).

KEY

Adv, adventitia
AT, adipose tissue
BV, blood vessel
CT, connective tissue, lamina propria
Ep, epithelium
GI, gland or gland-like structure
L, lymphocytes

Muc, mucosa
Mus, muscularis
MC, mucous cells
PC, plasma cells
SM, smooth muscle
arrows, Fig. 1, recess in luminal surface
arrows, Fig. 3, intercellular spaces

Fig. 1, × 45
Fig. 2, human, × 325
Fig. 3, human, × 550
Fig. 4, human, × 550

PLATE 86

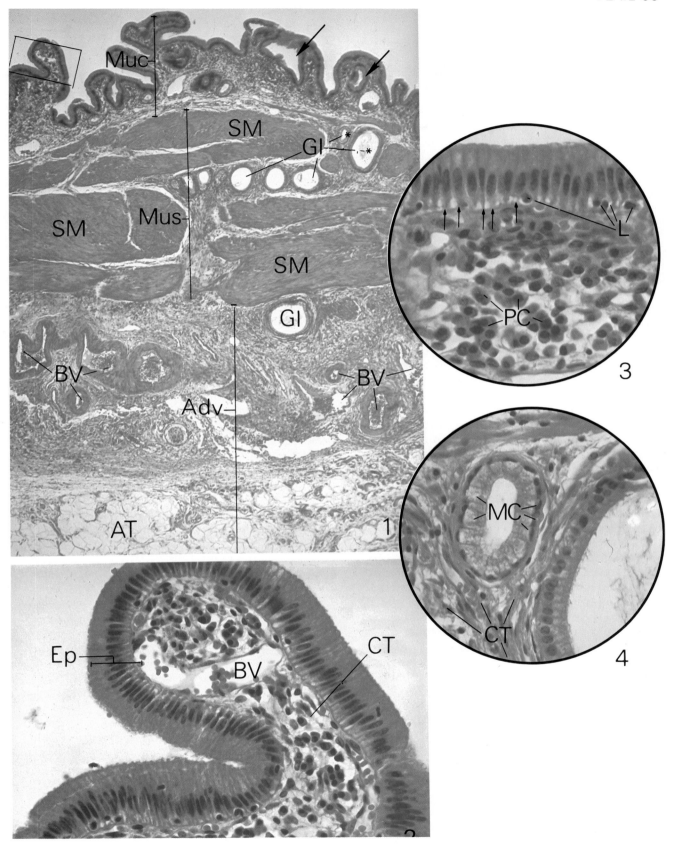

PLATE 87. Pancreas

The pancreas is an elongated gland with a head nestled in the C-shaped bend of the duodenum, a body, and a tail extending across the back of the abdomen. It is a mixed gland containing both an exocrine component and an endocrine component. The exocrine component is a compound tubuloacinar gland with a branching network of ducts that convey the exocrine secretions to the duodenum of the small intestines. The endocrine component is comprised of the islets of Langerhans; these discharge their secretions (hormones) into the local blood vessels, which, in turn, convey the hormones to the respective target tissue. Some secretions, referred to as paracrine secretions or parahormones, are also produced by the islets. Paracrine secretions act locally by diffusing to their target cells.

The pancreas is surrounded by a delicate capsule of moderately dense connective tissue. Septa from the capsule divide the pancreas into lobules, one of which is shown in **Figure 1,** bounded by connective tissue (**CT**). Larger blood vessels (**BV**) travel within the connective tissue septa; nerves also travel in the septa, but they are infrequently seen. Within the lobule are the numerous acini that comprise the exocrine component, larger intralobular ducts (**InD**), smaller intercalated ducts (not readily evident at the low magnification of **Fig. 1,** but considered at higher magnification in **Fig. 2**), and islets of Langerhans (**IL**). Also within the lobule are the small blood vessels and the connective tissue serving as a stroma for the parenchymal elements of the gland.

Figure 1 shows an islet of Langerhans (**IL**) among the far more numerous acini. (Islets are most numerous in the tail of the pancreas and fewest in the head). Cells within the islets are arranged as irregular cords. In routine H&E-stained paraffin sections, it is not possible to identify the various cell types within the islets. However, it should be noted that B cells are the most numerous; these produce insulin. The next most numerous are A cells; these produce glucagon. Examination of the **inset** shows numerous capillary vessels (**arrows**). The labels **A** and **B** are not intended to identify specific cells but rather to show those parts of the islets where A and B cells are found in greatest number.

Acini of the pancreas consist of serous type cells. In sections (**Fig. 2**), the acini present circular and irregular profiles. The lumen of the acini is small and only in fortuitous sections through an

acinous is the lumen included (**asterisks).** The nucleus is characteristically in the base of the cell and adjacent to the nucleus there is a region of intense basophilia. This is the ergastoplasm (**Er**) and it reflects the presence of rER that is active in the synthesis of pancreatic enzymes. Some acini reveal a centrally positioned cell with cytoplasm that shows no special staining characteristics in H&E-stained paraffin sections. These are centroacinar cells (**CC**). They are the beginning of the intercalated ducts.

Figure 2 is particularly well-suited for the consideration of intercalated ducts. This done best by noting first the cross-sectioned intralobular duct (**InD**). The latter consists of cuboidal epithelium. (There are no striated ducts in the pancreas). Leading to the intralobular duct is an intercalated duct (**ID**), which is seen in cross-section at the furthest distance from the intralobular duct and then, in longitudinal section, in the center of the illustration as it travels toward the intralobular duct. The lumen is readily evident where the intercalated duct is cross-sectioned but not readily evident where it is seen in longitudinal section. This is because the plane of section cuts chiefly through the cells rather than the lumen. As a consequence, **Figure 2** provides a good view of the nuclei of the duct cells. They are elongate with their long axis oriented in the direction of the duct. In addition, they display a staining pattern similar to that of centroacinar cells but different from that of nuclei of the parenchymal cells.

Once the cells of the intercalated duct have been confidently identified in one part of the section, their staining characteristics and location can be used to identify the intercalated ducts in other parts of the lobule, several of which are marked (**ID**).

498

PLATE 87

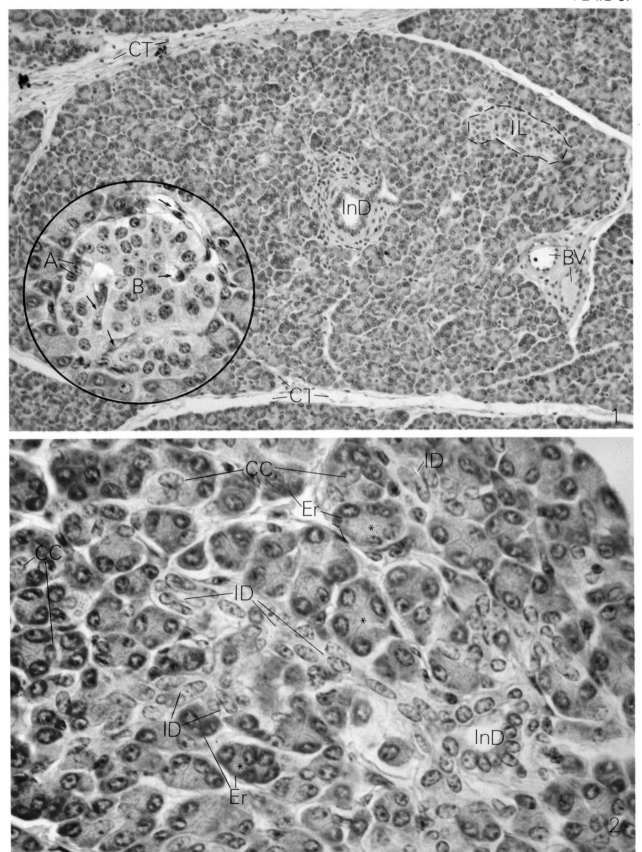

Respiratory System

18

The respiratory system consists of the lungs and a series of air passages leading to and from the lungs. As the air passages continue within the lung, they branch into increasingly smaller tubes until the very smallest air spaces, called *alveoli,* are reached (Fig. 18.1). The branching structure is commonly referred to as the bronchial tree.

The passages of the respiratory tract are divided into the *conducting portion* and the *respiratory portion.* The conducting portion consists of the nasal cavities (and during forced breathing also the oral cavity), the pharynx, the larynx, the trachea, the bronchi, and the bronchioles. While passing through the conducting portion of the respiratory tract, the air is conditioned: it is warmed, moistened, and freed of particulate matter. Mucus plays a major role in this conditioning. Not only does it moisten and warm the air, but it also traps particles that were not trapped by hairs in the nasal cavities. The mucus also prevents the dehydration of the underlying tissues. Mucus covers almost the entire luminal surface of the conducting passages and is constantly produced by goblet cells and other mucus-secreting glands in the walls of the passages. The secretions of the mucous glands are augmented by secretions of serous glands. The mucus is moved toward the pharynx by means of coordinated sweeping movements of cilia and is then swallowed or expectorated.

The respiratory portion is that portion of the tract in which gas exchange occurs between air and the blood. The respiratory portion consists of the respiratory bronchioles, the alveolar ducts, the alveolar sacs, and the alveoli.

Blood vessels enter the lungs with the bronchi and branch into successively smaller vessels and, ultimately, the smallest blood vessels come into intimate contact with the alveoli. This relationship between pulmonary capillaries and alveolar air spaces is the structural basis for the main function of the respiratory system—gas exchange in the lungs. The relationship is strikingly illustrated in the histological appearance of a lung section.

Parts of the respiratory system also serve other functions. For example, the olfactory mucosa serves as a receptor for smell and the larynx serves in phonation. Both of these activities take advantage of the air movement that is a consequence of respiration.

NASAL CAVITIES

The two nasal cavities are separated by a septum. Each cavity is divided into three parts: a vestibule, an olfactory segment, and a respiratory segment (Fig. 18.2). Air spaces within some of the bones that form the walls of the nasal cavity communicate with the respiratory segment. These air spaces are called *the paranasal sinuses.*

Vestibule

The *vestibule* is the short chamber just internal to the external nasal orifice. It is continuous with the skin of the face and is lined by stratified squamous epithelium. Numerous hairs within the vestibule filter our large particulate material before the air passes into the rest of the cavity. The wall of the vestibule contains cartilage.

Olfactory Mucosa

The roof of the nasal cavity and, to a variable extent, the contiguous medial and lateral walls form the *olfactory segment* of the nasal cavity and is lined by *olfactory mucosa.* In humans, only a small

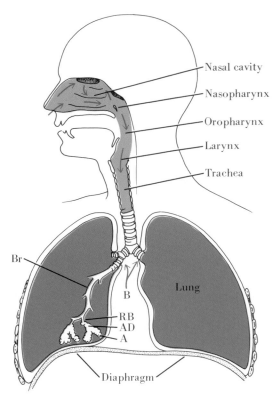

Figure 18.1. Respiratory passages. The nasal cavities, nasopharynx, oropharynx, larynx, trachea, bronchi (B), and bronchioles (Br) are the conducting portion of the respiratory passages. Gas exchange occurs between the blood and air spaces of the respiratory bronchioles (RB), alveolar ducts (AD), and terminal alveoli (A). (After Grant JCB: *A Method of Anatomy,* 4th ed. Baltimore, Williams & Wilkins, 1948.)

portion of the lateral and medial walls are comprised of olfactory mucosa, but in certain animals large parts of the walls are olfactory in addition to the roof. The olfactory epithelium is modified to serve as the receptor for smell. It contains three main cell types (Fig. 18.3): (1) olfactory cells (bipolar primary olfactory neurons); (2) sustentacular cells; and (3) basal cells

Olfactory cells possess on their apical surface long cilia that lie parallel to the surface of the epithelium in the fluid secretion of the mucous membrane. The cilia are thought to be nonmotile. The base of the bipolar neuron gives rise to a long nonmyelinated axonal process that leaves the epithelial layer, enters the underlying connective tissue, and joins axons of other bipolar neurons to form the olfactory nerves.

Sustentacular cells are columnar supporting cells. They contain numerous microvilli on their free surface and they are active metabolically.

Their support to the olfactory cells is thought to be not only physical but also metabolic. The sustentacular cell is the most numerous of the cell types in the olfactory epithelium. The nuclei of the sustentacular cells are more apically positioned than nuclei of receptor and basal cells.

Basal cells are more or less rounded cells located close to the basal lamina. They partly sheathe the first portion of the axon of the olfactory cell that extends from the epithelium to the underlying connective tissue (see Fig. 18.3).

Olfactory epithelium also contains a cell present in much smaller numbers called the *brush cell.* Brush cells, characterized by the presence of large, blunt apical microvilli, form synaptic contact with nerve fibers in the epithelium. In the case of the olfactory epithelium, these nerve fibers belong to the trigeminal (V) nerve that serves general sensation rather than olfaction. The implication is that brush cells are involved with general sensation of the olfactory mucosa.

The connective tissue under the olfactory epithelium contains *glands of Bowman.* These are branched tubuloalveolar glands that empty their secretions via ducts onto the olfactory surface. The connective tissue also contains numerous unmyelinated olfactory nerves, some myelinated nerves, blood vessels, and numerous lymphatic vessels (Fig. 18.4). The character of the connective tissue remains essentially the same from beneath the epithelium to the supporting bone.

Respiratory Mucosa

The *respiratory segment* (see Fig. 18.2) of the nasal cavity is below the olfactory segment and is lined with *respiratory mucosa.* The medial, or septal, wall is smooth, but the lateral wall is uneven due to the presence of shelf-like projections called *turbinates,* or *conchae.* The projections increase the surface area of the respiratory mucosa and contribute to its efficiency in modifying the inspired air. The epithelium covering the respiratory portion is pseudostratified columnar and it is ciliated. The main cell types are *ciliated cells, goblet cells,* and *basal cells* (see Fig. 18.6). *Brush cells* similar to those in the olfactory mucosa are also present, but in smaller number. In laboratory animals, the epithelium varies considerably. (For example, in different parts of the respiratory mucosa of the mouse the following kinds of epithelium occur: simple cuboidal, stratified cuboidal with and without cilia, ciliated columnar, and ciliated pseudostratified columnar with goblet cells.) In the human, there are sometimes changes from ciliated pseudostratified columnar epithelium to

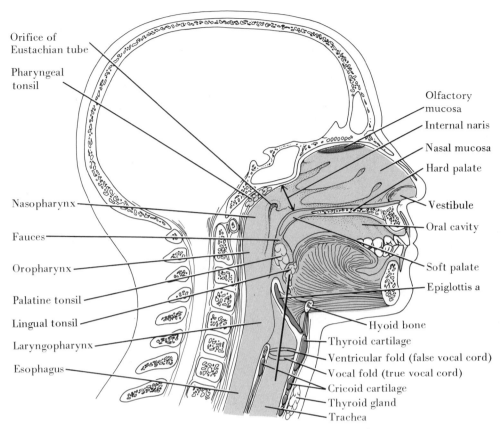

Orifice of
Eustachian tube

Pharyngeal
tonsil

Olfactory
mucosa

Internal naris

Nasal mucosa

Hard palate

Nasopharynx

Vestibule

Oral cavity

Fauces

Oropharynx

Soft palate

Palatine tonsil

Epiglottis a

Lingual tonsil

Hyoid bone

Laryngopharynx

Thyroid cartilage

Ventricular fold (false vocal cord)

Vocal fold (true vocal cord)

Esophagus

Cricoid cartilage

Thyroid gland

Trachea

Figure 18.2. Diagram of sagittal section of head showing the relationship of the pharynx to the respiratory and digestive systems. The pharynx, its three parts labeled, is located posteriorly. It serves both systems. The unlabeled vertical line drawn through the larynx corresponds to the cutting plane of the histological section shown in Figure 18.5. Note that the upper part of the section includes that part of the tongue which contains the lingual tonsils. The plane also obviously transects the epiglottis and laryngeal folds; lateral to the laryngeal folds is the thyroid cartilage (open in back), and below the folds is the ring-like cricoid cartilage (G. Tortora, 1983.)

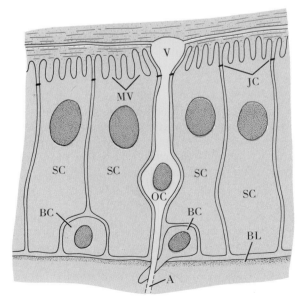

Figure 18.3. Major cell types of the olfactory mucosa. These are sustentacular cells (SC), olfactory cells (OC), and basal cells (BC). The olfactory cell is the receptor cell; it has an expansion, the olfactory vesicle (V), from which long nonmotile cilia extend, and it sends an axon (A) into the connective tissue that joins with axons of other olfactory cells to form the olfactory nerves. The basal cell (BC) extends beyond the basal lamina (BL) to enclose the first part of the olfactory axon. JC, junctional complex; MV, microvilli.

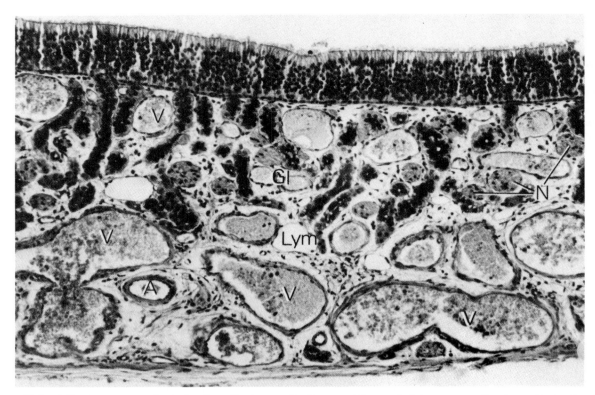

Figure 18.4. Olfactory mucosa includes the olfactory epithelium and the underlying connective tissue that extends as far as the bone (not shown). The illustration shows numerous blood vessels (artery, A, and veins, V), lymphatic vessels (Lym), nerves (N), and Bowman's glands (Gl). × 160.

other types, such as stratified squamous, especially on the rounded, more exposed portions of the turbinates. These alterations of the epithelium are referred to as *metaplasia,* that is, the abnormal transformation of one type of fully differentiated adult cell into a different type of adult cell. These cellular changes are considered to be controlled and adaptive.

The connective tissue of the respiratory mucous membrane is richly vascularized with venous networks capable of becoming greatly engorged with blood to facilitate heat exchange (the warming of inspired air when it is very cold). The connective tissue also contains branching tubuloalveolar glands with mucous and serous cells. These secrete onto the surface of the respiratory mucosa. The mucous membrane rests directly on the bone tissue that forms the walls of the nasal cavities. Attempts to separate the mucous membrane typically result in the separation of all the soft tissue as far as the bone. Accordingly, the soft tissue is sometimes referred to as a *mucoperiostium* to indicate that part of this mucous membrane also functions as the periostium of the underlying bones.

The *paranasal sinuses* are large air spaces within the frontal bone, ethmoid bone, sphenoid bone, and maxilla. They open into the nasal cavity. The epithelial lining of the sinuses is similar to that of the respiratory mucosa, namely, ciliated pseudostratified columnar epithelium with goblet cells. The underlying connective tissue contains glands similar to those of the respiratory mucosa. Coordinated ciliary activity moves the secretions of the sinuses to the nasal cavities.

PHARYNX

The pharynx, connecting the nasal cavities to the larynx, serves as a passageway for air and food and provides a resonating chamber for speech. The structure of the pharnyx is described in Chapter 15 on the digestive system.

LARYNX

The larynx is a box-like structure between the pharynx and the trachea (Fig. 18.2). It serves as a conduit for air going into and out of the lungs and it also serves as the organ of phonation. It has a cartilaginous framework consisting of nine pieces of hyaline cartilage, the largest of which is the *thyroid cartilage.* This is an unpaired cartilage easily felt in the upper part of the neck and it moves conspicuously during swallowing. Two other large unpaired cartilages are the *epiglottis* and the *cricoid cartilage.* The epiglottis is a leaf-like cartilage serving as a flap that prevents food from entering the larynx during swallowing. The epiglottis contains elastic cartilage allowing it to bend easily and it is covered by stratified squamous epithelium. The cricoid cartilage is a ring-like cartilage perched above the C-shaped cartilages of the trachea. Two other cartilages, the paired pyramidal *arytenoid cartilages,* are essential to the functioning of the larynx.

The fundamental feature of the larynx is the presence of *vocal folds.* The vocal folds are oriented in an anteroposterior direction and define the lateral boundaries of the opening (glottis) of the larynx. They are attached to the thyroid cartilage anteriorly and to the arytenoid cartilages posteriorly. The arytenoid cartilages form joints with the cricoid cartilage on which they can pivot according to the pull of muscles. The muscles that are attached both at their origin and insertion to the cartilages of the larynx are responsible for generating tension in the vocal folds and for opening and closing the glottis; these are the *intrinsic laryngeal muscles.* Other muscles connect the larynx to surrounding structures and they move the larynx during deglutition (the act of swallowing); these are the *extrinsic muscles.* When air passes through the glottis, the vocal folds are made to vibrate by the passing air. The vibrations are altered by altering the tension placed on the vocal folds and by altering the degree of glottal opening. The alteration of the vibrations produces sounds of different pitch.

A frontal section through the larynx shows the vocal folds in cross-section (Fig. 18.5). Above each vocal fold is an elongate recess called the *ventricle* and above this is another fold of mucous membrane, the *ventricular fold.*

The surface of the vocal folds (and most of the epiglottis) consists of stratified squamous epithelium (see Atlas section, Plate 89). The connective tissue oriented in an anteroposterior direction under the stratified squamous epithelium of the vocal fold is the *thyroarytenoid ligament.* It contains some elastic fibers. The muscle adjacent to this ligament and oriented in the same way is the *vocalis muscle.* Elsewhere, the laryngeal surface consists of ciliated pseudostratified columnar epithelium, containing chiefly ciliated cells, basal cells, and goblet cells in varying numbers, scattered through different parts of the epithelium. The

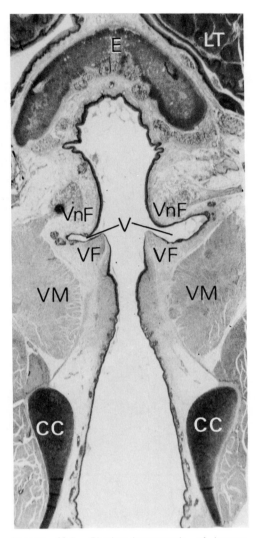

Figure 18.5. Photomicrograph of larynx sectioned in a plane marked by the line in Figure 18.2. The roof of the larynx contains the epiglottis (E). Above this is a small space of the oral cavity and then, above this, part of the tongue. The posterior portion of the tongue contains lingual tonsils (LT). The objects of main interest within the larynx are the vocal fold (VF), seen in cross-section, above which are the ventricles (V) and, above these, the ventricular folds (VnF). The vocalis muscle (VM) is under the vocal folds. The cricoid cartilage is marked (CC).

connective tissue of the larynx contains mixed mucoserous glands secreting onto the surface via ducts.

TRACHEA AND BRONCHI

The trachea extends from the larynx to about the middle of the thorax where it divides into two bronchi, the ***primary bronchi.*** C-shaped rings of hyaline cartilage stacked one upon the other form the framework of the trachea and keep it open. Fibroelastic tissue and smooth muscle, called the ***trachealis muscle,*** bridge the gap between the free ends of the C at the posterior of the trachea. The bronchi have essentially the same structure except that upon entering the lungs, the C-shaped rings are replaced by plates of hyaline cartilage. The bronchi divide into smaller branches, but retain the same histological features.

Structure

The trachea and bronchi consist of four layers: a mucous membrane (ciliated pseudostratified

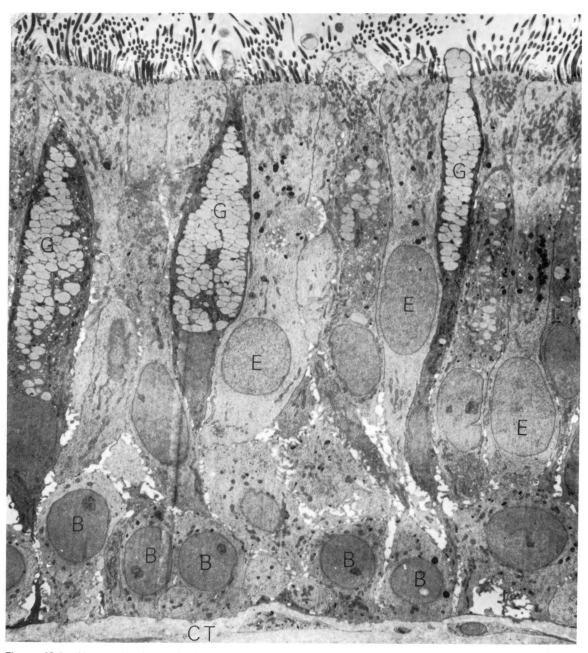

Figure 18.6. Human trachea, electron micrograph. The three main cell types of this respiratory epithelium are ciliated epithelial cells (E) extending to the surface, where they possess cilia; goblet cells (G), with mucinogen granules; and basal cells (B), which are confined to the basal portion of the epithelial layer near the connective tissue (CT). × 1800. (Courtesy of J. Rhodin, 1974.)

columnar epithelium and a lamina propria), a submucosa, a cartilaginous smooth muscle layer, and an adventitia.

Ciliated, Goblet, and Basal Cells. The tracheobronchial epithelium contains three common cell types and two less common types. The three common cell types are those regularly associated with ciliated pseudostratified columnar epithelium, namely, *ciliated cells, goblet cells,* and *basal cells* (Figs. 18.6 and 18.7). The ciliated cells are distributed throughout the conducting passages of the respiratory tract and extend into the respiratory bronchioles beyond the extent of the goblet cells. By the coordinated sweeping motion of the cilia, the ciliated cells move the mucus coat from the furthest reaches of the air passages toward the pharynx. In effect, these cells provide a "ciliary escalator" that serves as an important protective mechanism for removing small inhaled particles from the lungs. Goblet cells are interspersed among the ciliated cells. They produce a mucous secretion, which is added to that of the submucosal glands of the conducting passages. Basal cells are confined to the vicinity of the basal lamina; they do not reach the surface of the epithelial layer. They are the source of new cells as replacement of other cell types is needed.

Brush and Dense Core Granule Cells. The two less common cell types are the *brush cell* and the *dense core granule cell* (also called the *small granule cell* or the *argyrophilic cell;* Fig. 18.8 (a,b). Brush cells contain large, blunt microvilli. These cells have been found in close association with nerve fibers, and, as in the olfactory mucosa, they are thought to be related to a sensory function. The function of the small granule cells is not well understood. They also have been found in groups in association with nerve fibers. They form *neuro-*

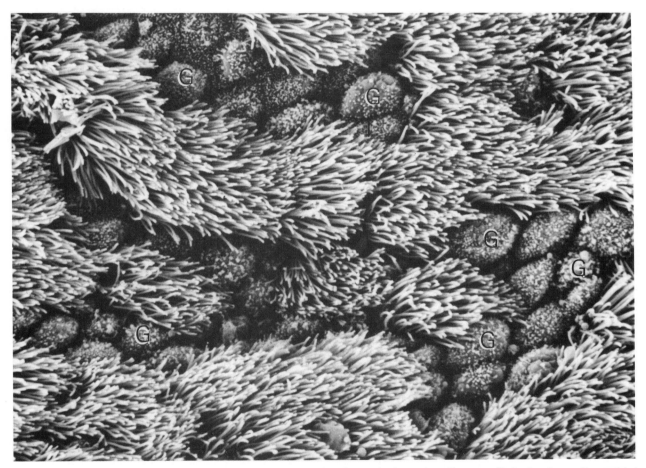

Figure 18.7. Scanning electron micrograph of the luminal surface of a bronchus. The nonciliated cells are the goblet cells (G). Their surface is characterized by small blunt microvilli that give a stippled appearance to the cell at this low magnification. The cilia of the many ciliated cells occupy the remainder of the micrograph. Note how they are all synchronously arrayed, i.e., uniformly leaning in the same direction, appearing just as they were when fixed at a specific moment during their wave-like movement.

Figure 18.8(a). A brush cell between pulmonary type I and II cells in a lung alveolus. Large blunt microvilli (MV) are distinctive features of the brush cell. The cytoplasm typically shows a Golgi (G), lysosomes (L), filaments (F), mitochondria (M), and glycogen (Gl). JC, junctional complex; BL, basal lamina; N, nucleus.

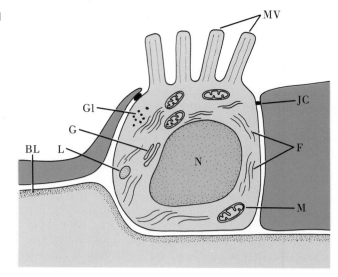

Figure 18.8(b). A dense core granule cell between two Clara cells, as in a terminal or respiratory bronchiole. The cell contains small granules (Gr), most of which are basal to the nucleus (N). In addition to the granules, the most conspicuous organelles of the cell are filaments (F), rough-surfaced endoplasmic reticulum (rER), a Golgi (G), and mitochondria (M). A nerve terminal (NT) is adjacent to the cell. JC, junctional complex; BL, basal lamina.

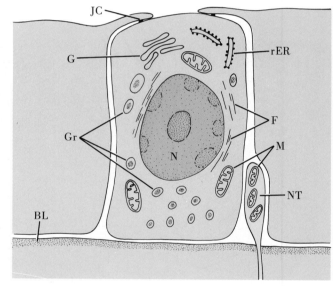

epithelial bodies that are thought to function in the reflexes regulating the airway or vascular caliber. The small granule cells are especially numerous in the lungs of the human fetus and newborn, suggesting that they might release vasoactive substances associated with the vascular adjustments needed for the onset of breathing at the time of birth.

In addition to the cell types referred to previously, intermediate cell types are also present in the respiratory epithelium of the trachea and bronchi; these are considered to be developing ciliary cells or goblet cells that have discharged their mucus.

Connective Tissue. The lamina propria of the trachea and bronchi is loose connective tissue, rich in elastic fibers. Hematoxylin and eosin-stained (H&E) paraffin sections do not reveal any definitive boundary between the lamina propria and the submucosa, but the boundary is marked by an elastic layer that is revealed with special elastic stains. The submucosa contains mixed seromucous glands that open by means of short ducts to the epithelial surface. In the posterior portion of the trachea, the glands are sometimes located external to the muscle layer.

BRONCHIOLES

As the bronchi branch into smaller tubes, the walls gradually lose some of their components. Generally speaking, when cartilage and submucosal glands are no longer present in the walls, the conducting passages are called bronchioles. In these, the epithelium is similar to the tracheobronchial epithelium, namely, ciliated pseudostratified columnar, with the three main cell types and the two less common cell types. In addition to the mucous membrane, smooth muscle is now the major component of the wall.

Terminal Bronchioles

Just before reaching the respiratory portion of the tract, the bronchioles are called ***terminal bronchioles.*** The most numerous cell type (Fig. 18.9) of terminal bronchioles are the ciliated cells and ***Clara cell.*** Also present in much smaller numbers are small granule cells and brush cells, the functions of which are considered to be the same as similar cells in the tracheobronchial epithelium. The Clara cells (Fig. 18.10) are nonciliated; the apex of these cells is dome-shaped and it is the site for the discharge of granular contents that are surface-active agents. Clara cells display the ultrastructural features of secretory cells: they possess basal rough endoplasmic reticulum (rER), a laterally or apically placed Golgi apparatus, apical granules that stain for protein, and numerous smooth endoplasmic reticulum (sER) profiles in the apical cytoplasm. The secretion of Clara cells is surface active, but it is different from that of alveolar type II cells (see below). Goblet cells are not present in terminal bronchioles of the healthy lung. However, they are found in smokers, a metaplasia, presumably as a response to smoke irritants.

Respiratory Bronchioles

The respiratory bronchiole is the first part of the respiratory tract in which gas exchange occurs. The walls of respiratory bronchioles consist of

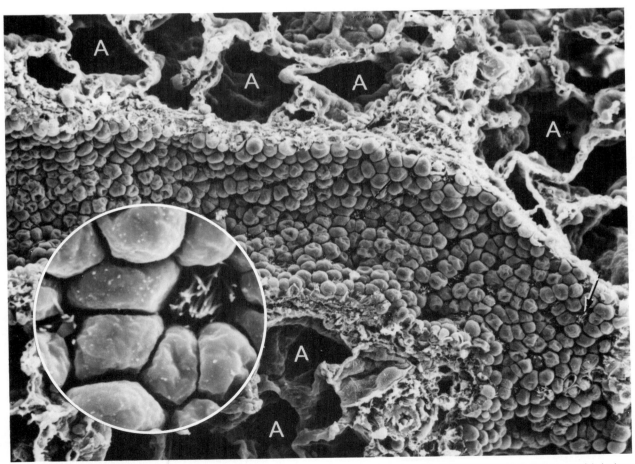

Figure 18.9. Scanning electron micrograph of a terminal bronchiole and surrounding alveoli (A). The bronchiole has been broken open in a longitudinal plane and shows the apical surface of the lining Clara cells. In various areas, isolated, ciliated cells are present; the cilia **(arrows)** are barely perceptible at this magnification. The **inset** shows some of the Clara cells at a higher magnification with the cilia of a ciliated cell clearly visible. Note the relatively few cilia present on these small cells.

Figure 18.10. A Clara cell between bronchiolar epithelial cells. The nucleus (N) is in a basal location;
rough-surfaced endoplasmic reticulum (rER), a Golgi
(G), and mitochondria (M) are chiefly in the basal
and paranuclear location; smooth-surfaced endoplasmic reticulum (sER) and secretory granules (SG)
are chiefly in the apical cytoplasm. One of the secretory granules is shown discharging its contents onto
the surface of the cell. JC, junctional complex; BL,
basal lamina.

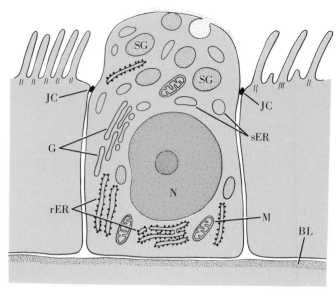

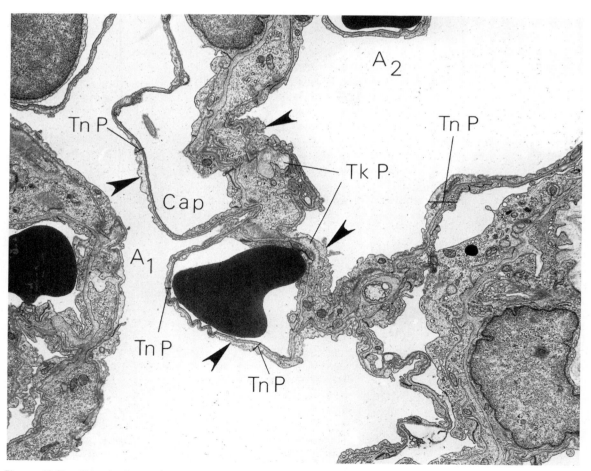

Figure 18.11. This electron micrograph shows two alveolar spaces A₁ and A₂ and the intervening septal wall
(marked by the **facing arrowheads**). The septal wall contains capillaries (Cap), some of which reveal red
blood cells. The septal wall displays thin portions (ThP) and thick portions (TkP). These can be seen in the
higher magnification shown in Figure 18.14.

cuboidal or columnar epithelium interrupted by alveoli. Because of the alveoli, part of the wall is able to engage in gas exchange. The initial segments between the alveoli consist of ciliated cells and Clara cells. Further along the respiratory bronchiole the ciliated cells are no longer present and the Clara cells are the chief epithelial cell type. Occasional small granule cells and brush cells are also present. A small amount of connective tissue and smooth muscle lie under the cuboidal epithelium. This layer contains interlacing bundles of smooth muscle and elastic fibers.

ALVEOLAR DUCTS, ALVEOLAR SACS, AND ALVEOLI

Alveoli are the small air sacs with thin walls that allow for the ready diffusion of gases between the air space and the blood. Alveoli are small polyhedral chambers open on one side to the common air space of the lung. Some alveoli that are arranged along a common linear air tract form a passageway referred to as an ***alveolar duct,*** much the same as cubicles along a corridor might be completely open on one side to the corridor (see Atlas section, Plate 91, Fig. 3). Near the termination of the alveolar duct, clusters of alveoli share a common opening to the alveolar duct. Such a cluster of alveoli is referred to as an ***alveolar sac.*** (Sometimes a small alveolar sac is found along the length of the alveolar duct.)

Alveolar Wall

The aeveolar wall is a partition or septum between two alveoli (Figure 18.11). On each air surface, the alveolar septum is covered by three kinds of epithelial cells: the alveolar (pneumonocyte) type I cell; the alveolar (pneumonocyte)

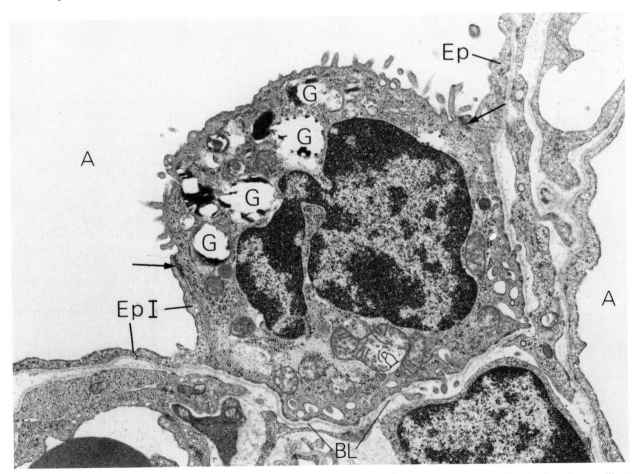

Figure 18.12. Electron micrograph of a type II alveolar cell. The cell has a dome-shaped apical surface with a number of short microvilli present at its periphery and a relatively smooth-contoured apical center. The lateral cell margins are overlain to a variable degree by the type I alveolar cells (EpI) and are joined to the type II cell by occluding junctions **(arrows).** Both cell types reset on the basal lamina (BL). The granules (G) in this specimen are largely dissolved but their lamellar character is shown to advantage in Figure 18.13.

type II cell; and the brush cell. The *alveolar type I cell* covers about 95 percent of the alveolar surface. This is the squamous pulmonary epithelial cell; it is also called the *small alveolar cell.* Its cytoplasm is so thin that it cannot be resolved from the components of the septal wall with the light microscope.

The *alveolar type II cell* is also called by several other names including the *great alveolar cell* and the *septal cell.* It is a cuboidal cell, located chiefly at septal junctions where its cytoplasm can be seen to bulge into the air space (Fig. 18.12). Alveolar type II cells are about as numerous as type I cells, but they cover only about 2 to 5 percent of the alveolar surface because of their cuboidal rather than squamous shape. The alveolar type II cell exhibits an usual type of secretory granule in its apical cytoplasm. With the electron microscope the granules appear as lamellar bodies (Fig. 18.13). The lamellae are stacked with a very regular periodicity, a characteristic of phospholipids. Moreover, freeze fracture studies show that the lamellae are

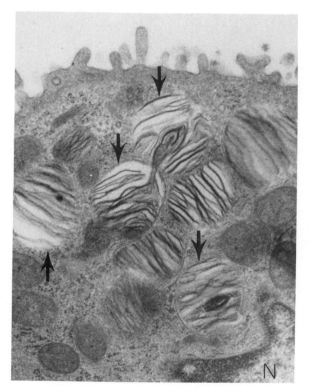

Figure 18.13. A higher power electron micrograph showing the secretory granules and their typical lamellar pattern. The granules are comprised of the precursors of pulmonary surfactant. (Courtesy of A. Mercuria, 1984.)

devoid of membrane-associated particles. The lamellar bodies are discharged by exocytosis from the alveolar type II cells. The liberated secretory product, composed chiefly of phospholipids, is known as *pulmonary surfactant.* This substance spreads as a monomolecular layer or film over the luminal surface of the alveolar cells. The surfactant coating reduces the attractive forces between the water molecules at the surface of the film; thereby decreasing the surface tension. This activity of the surfactant makes it easier for the adjacent alveolar walls to spread apart and prevents the collapse of the alveoli (atelectasis). In order for the newborn to take its first breath of air, it is essential that an adequate surfactant content is present in the alveoli to overcome the surface tension holding the alveolar walls together. Type II cells have also been shown to be active in the repair of alveolar epithelium after experimentally induced injury in laboratory animals.

Brush cells are found only infrequently in alveolar epithelium. Their ultrastructure and function are presumed to be similar to those of brush cells found in the other passages of the respiratory system. Brush cells are not readily identified with the light microscope.

All cells forming the alveolar epithelium are joined by zonula occludens that enable the cells to form a barrier between the air space and the other components of the septal wall. It should be noted that surfactant is secreted by septal cells onto the air side of the alveolar epithelium.

While the alveolar septum is extremely thin, it nevertheless also contains a rich capillary network and connective tissue elements, namely, a framework of collagenous and elastic fibers and fibroblasts and macrophages. With the light microscope, these cells are generally difficult to distinguish from the alveolar epithelium, the problem being greatest in trying to distinguish between squamous pulmonary cells (alveolar type I) and cells of the capillary endothelium.

The alveolar macrophage is also called the *alveolar phagocyte* and the *dust cell.* It is somewhat unusual macrophage because it is found not only in the connective tissue of the alveolar septum, the usual site for a macrophage, but also on the alveolar surface where it scavenges the surface. Some macrophages, when filled with phagocytosed material, pass up the bronchial tree to the pharynx and then are disposed of by being swallowed. However, other macrophages remain within the connective tissue filled with phagocytosed material. Alveolar macrophages also phagocytose red blood cells that have gained access to the alveolar air sacs in heart failure. These macrophages come to be filled with yellow, iron-containing pigment, called **hemosiderin,** from the breakdown of hemoglobin. They are referred to by pathologists as "heart failure cells."

Alveolar-Capillary Complex

The alveolar epithelium and the capillary endothelium both rest on a basal lamina. It is possible to divide the alveolar-capillary complex into two portions a thin portion and a thick portion (Fig. 18.14). In the **thin portion,** the basal lamina of the alveolar epithelium and the capillary endothelium fuse. Thus, the barrier between alveolar air space and blood consists of surfactant, alveolar type I cell, fused basal lamina, and capillary endothelium. Diffusion of gases occurs mainly through the thin portion of the alveolar-capillary complex.

In the **thick portion,** each epithelium retains its own basal lamina, and, in addition, the connective tissue septum contains some fibers and cells. This thick portion is now thought to be the major site for passage of fluid into the alveolar air spaces. Although the relatively low blood pressure and the balance between hydrostatic pressure and osmotic pressure in the pulmonary capillaries favors the retention of fluid in the capillary (rather than its exit at the arterial end of the capillary and its return at the venous end as in the systemic circulation), fluid does regularly enter the air spaces. It becomes a conspicuous clinical problem in pulmonary edema. It is now felt that before fluid enters the air space, it accumulates in the interstitial spaces of the thick portion. Some of the fluid in the interstitium of the thick portion is removed by means of lymphatic vessels not in the alveolar septum, but in the adjacent terminal bronchioles where the lymphatics begin.

The separation of the alveolar wall into two portions, one specialized for gas exchange and the other able to accommodate increased amounts of tissue fluid, is regarded by lung biologists to be a beneficial arrangement inasmuch as unfortunate accumulations of pulmonary fluid in the alveolar walls need not interfere with gas exchange. The patient can still breathe without undue distress despite the presence of some pulmonary congestion.

Alveolar Pores (of Kohn)

Light microscopy suggests that the wall between adjacent alveoli are complete septa. However, it has long been claimed that pores exist in the alveolar walls that provide for communication between adjacent alveoli. The existence of these openings, the **pores of Kohn,** has now been confirmed with the scanning electron microscope. These openings have significance in certain pathological conditions where obstructive lung disease blocks the normal pathway of air to the alveoli. In effect, in the presence of obstructive lung disease, gas exchange is not proportionately diminished because collateral routes (for example, pores of Kohn) continue to supply the alveoli that have been cut off from their delivery of air by usual routes.

BLOOD SUPPLY

The major arterial supply to the lungs is by branches of the **pulmonary arteries.** The pressure in the pulmonary arteries is substantially less than in the systemic arteries. The branches of the pulmonary artery travel with the respiratory passages and deliver blood to the pulmonary capillaries in the alveolar walls. The oxygenated blood is collected by the pulmonary capillaries and leaves the lungs ultimately via the **pulmonary veins.** They are more removed from the respiratory passages.

A second set of arteries, the **supernumerary arteries,** also exist. The supernumerary arteries leave the pulmonary arteries and travel to the alveoli in the outer reaches of the lung tissue. They do not accompany the respiratory passages. These arteries are of considerable importance in that they serve as an ancillary route through which blood can be conveyed to pulmonary capillaries. Intravascular coagulation probably occurs even in otherwise healthy individuals and emboli formed by loosened clots can plug up pulmonary arteries as they branch and become smaller. The presence of an alternate set of arteries to the pulmonary capillaries minimizes the physiological insult that would result if only one set of arteries delivered blood to the pulmonary capillaries.

Each lung also receives one or two **bronchial arteries** from the aorta. These convey blood to the larger masses of connective tissues of the lung. They extend as far as the terminal bronchioles. Branches of the bronchial arteries then continue and open into the pulmonary capillaries. Thus, the bronchial (systemic) and pulmonary circulations anastomose roughly at the junction of the conducting and respiratory passages. This anastomosis has physiological significance in the fetus and in lung disease. In chronic inflammation and in neoplasms, there is a significant increase in the number and size of the bronchial arteries.

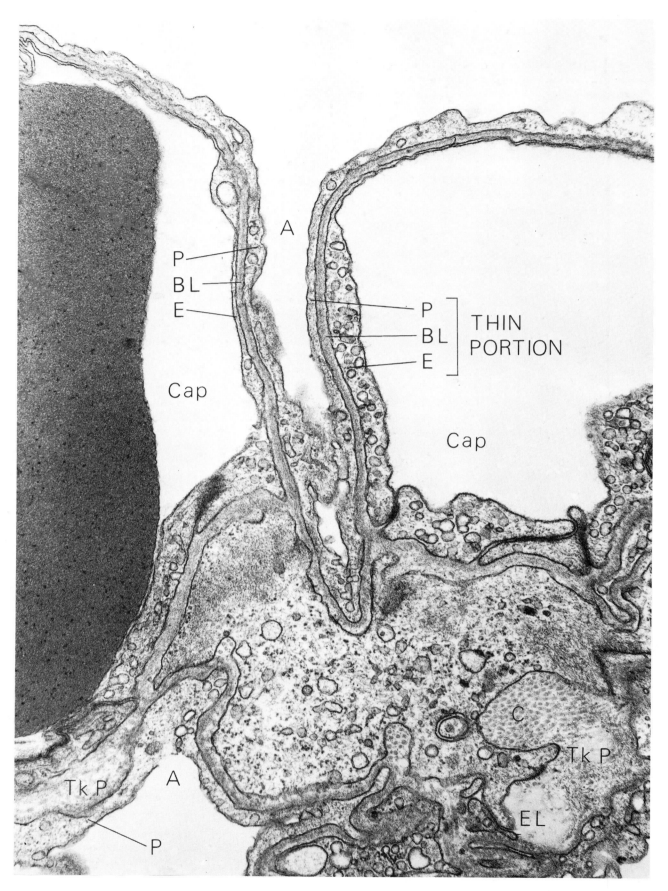

514

Bronchial veins drain only the connective tissue in the hilar region of the lungs. Most of the blood entering the lungs via the bronchial arteries leaves via the pulmonary veins.

LYMPHATIC VESSELS

Two sets of lymphatic vessels drain the lung. One set drains the substance of the lung following the route of the air passages to the hilus. Lymph nodes are present along the pathways of the larger lymphatic vessels. A second set of lymphatic vessels drains the surface of the lungs. Valves in the lymphatic vessels are unicuspid.

NERVES

The lungs are innervated by both sympathetic and parasympathetic systems. Receptors of various sorts serving the stretch reflex as well as those that monitor the quality of the air exist in the lung. However, they are not evident with the light microscope.

PLEURA

The surface of the lung is covered by a serous membrane that is referred to as visceral pleura. This consists of connective tissue and a surface of mesothelium.

Figure 18.14. Part of septal wall (electron micrograph) showing the alveolar capillary complex. The thin portion consists of a pneumonocyte I cell (P), capillary endothelium (E), and the fused basal lamina (BL) shared by both cells. In the thick portion (TkP), the pneumonocyte type I cell rests on a basal lamina, and under this is connective tissue in which collagen fibrils (C) and elastic fibers (EL) are readily evident. A, alveolar air space; Cap, capillary. × 33,000.

PLATE 88. Olfactory Mucosa

The olfactory mucosa is located in the roof and adjacent upper walls of the nasal cavity. It consists of a pseudostratified columnar epithelium that rests on a supporting connective tissue **(Fig. 1)**.

The olfactory epithelium contains three major cell types: receptor cells, sustentacular cells, and basal cells.[1] The surface is modified by the presence of cilia and other specializations. It is not possible to identify the various cell types on the basis of cytologic characteristics in H&E preparations. However, on the basis of location of the nuclei, some estimate is possible. A "cytoplasmic zone" without nuclei immediately under the surface **(Fig. 2)** can be distinguished from a "nuclear zone." The nuclei of sustentacular cells **(Sus)** are located in the most superficial part of the nuclear zone, immediately adjacent to the cytoplasmic zone. The nuclei of the basal cells **(Bas)** are located in the deepest part of the nuclear zone, immediately adjacent to the connective tissue. The broadest part of the nuclear zone contains the nuclei of the receptor cells **(Rec)**.

A receptor cell is a bipolar type of neuron that retains a surface location. It contains a distal process that extends from the perikaryon to the surface and, at the surface, it possesses a bulbous expansion, called the olfactory vesicle. This structure contains numerous cilia. The olfactory vesicle is not always evident in H&E preparations and is not clear in **Figure 2.** The proximal part of the receptor cell extends toward the basal region of the olfactory layer. Here it continues as a slender axon that along with the axons of other receptor cells, forms nonmyelinated nerve bundles **(N)** that proceed through the connective tissue, through the cribriform plate, and into the cranial cavity. The axons of the receptor cells are extremely slender and appear as dots in cross-section

---

[1] The brush cell is also present in the olfactory epithelium, but it is not recognizable in routine H&E preparations.

through the nerve. Nuclei of supporting cells are also evident within the nerve bundles.

The basal cells have only a small amount of cytoplasm that is confined to the vicinity of the nucleus and does not reach the surface. The sustentacular cells extend through the entire thickness of the epithelium. These cells do not contain cilia.

The connective tissue of the olfactory mucosa contains not only numerous bundles of the olfactory nerves, but also special glands called Bowman's glands **(Gl)**. These glands contain a pigment that stains intensely with hematoxylin. Ducts from the glands carry secretions to the mucosal surface. A number of these are seen just as they are about to penetrate the epithelium. Numerous blood vessels are present in the connective tissue.

The empty vessels with a flat epithelial lining are lymphatic vessels **(Lym)**. They can be distinguished from arteries **(A)** and veins **(V)** because their walls are extremely thin and also because they contain no blood cells. Although the absence of blood cells does not justify an identification of lymphatic vessels, the absence of cells in extremely thin-walled vessels is diagnostic, especially if all of the other vessels contain blood cells.

KEY

A, artery
Bas, basal cell nuclei
Gl, Bowman's glands
Lym, lymphatic vessel
N, nerve bundle

Rec, receptor cell nuclei
Sus, sustentacular cell nuclei
V, vein

| **Fig. 1,** cat, × 160 | **Fig. 2,** cat, × 640. |

PLATE 88

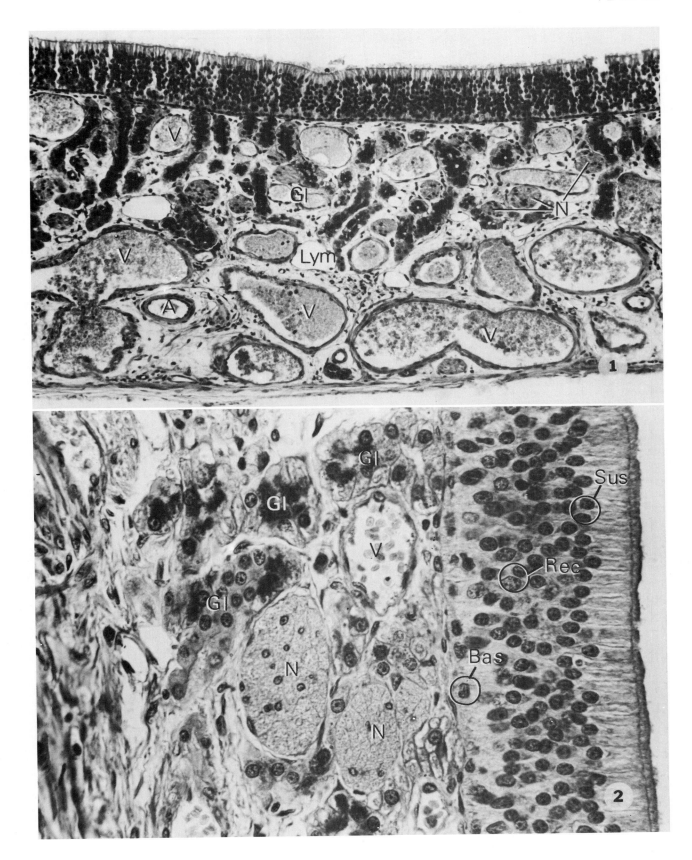

PLATE 89. Larynx

The larynx is the part of the respiratory passage that functions in the production of sound. It consists of a cartilaginous framework, to which muscles are attached, and a mucosal surface that varies in character in different regions. The muscles move certain cartilages with respect to others; in doing so, they bring about a greater or lesser opening of the glottis and a greater or lesser tension on the vocal folds. In this way, vibrations of different wavelengths are generated by the passing air, and sound is produced.

The vocal folds are ridge-like structures that are oriented in an anterposterior (ventraldorsal) direction. In frontal sections, the vocal folds **(VF)** are cross-sectioned, giving the appearance seen in **Figure 1.** The two vocal folds and the space between them constitute the glottis. Just above each vocal fold there is an elongated recess called the ventricle **(V)**, and above the ventricle there is another ridge called the ventricular fold **(VnF)** or sometimes the false vocal fold. Below and lateral to the vocal folds are the vocalis muscles **(VM).** Within the vocal fold there is a considerable amount of elastic material. However, it is usually not evident in routine H&E preparations. This elastic material is part of the vocal ligament. It lies in an anterposterior direction within the substance of the vocal fold and plays an important role in phonation.

The surfaces of a vocal fold and the facing ventricular fold within the **rectangle marked 2** are turned 90° clockwise and shown at higher magnification in **Figure 2.** Medially, both are lined by stratified squamous epithelium **(SSE).** Here, the contact between surfaces is considerable. Laterally, the surfaces consist of stratified columnar epithelium **(SCE).** The contact between these surfaces is less wearing. Small glands **(Gl)** are in the lamina propria of the laryngeal mucosa.

The **rectangle marked 3** is shown at higher magnification in **Figure 3.** It shows the junction between the stratified squamous epithelium **(SSE)** with its flat surface cells and the stratified colum-

nar epithelium **(SCE)** with its columnar surface cells. The lamina propria consists of loose connective tissue in which glands **(Gl)** are present.

Just below the portion of the larynx depicted in **Figure 1,** the epithelium changes again **(Fig. 4),** giving way, below, to a ciliated pseudostratified columnar epithelium **(PSE).** Note the cylinders of cytoplasm that clearly indicate the columnar nature of the surface cells. In the upper part of the figure the epithelium is stratified columnar; in the lower part of the figure it is pseudostratified columnar. This distinction is difficult to make from the examination of a single sample such as that shown in **Figure 4,** and other information is needed to make the assessment. The additional information in the illustration is the presence of cilia on the pseudostratified columnar epithelium; this epithelium is typically ciliated. Although not evident in the photomicrographs, it should be noted that stratified columnar epithelium has a very limited distribution, usually occuring between stratified squamous epithelium and some other epithelial types (e.g., pseudostratified columnar here or simple columnar at the anorectal junction.

The lamina propria in **Figure 4** is a loose cellular connective tissue, and it also shows some glands **(Gl).**

PLATE 89

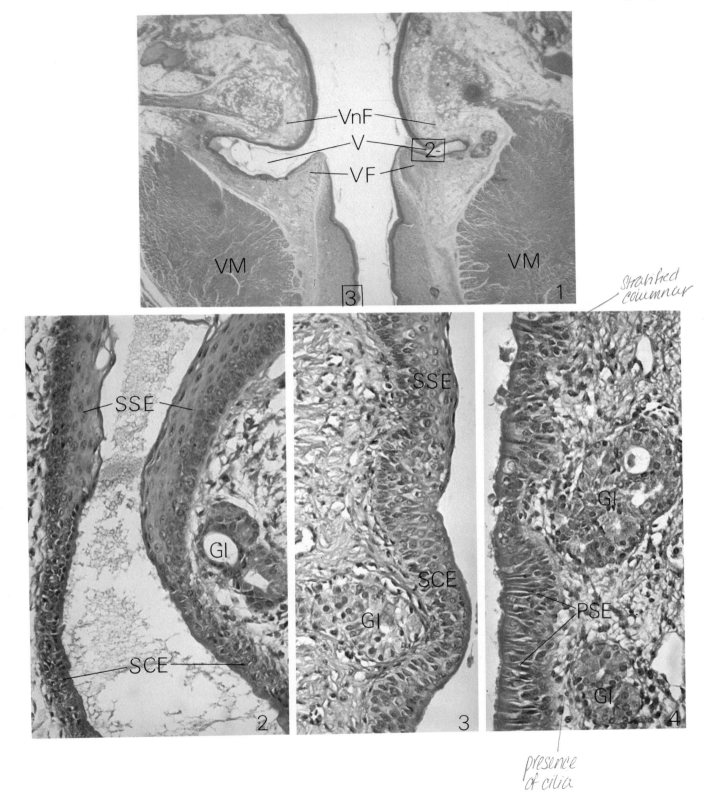

PLATE 90. Trachea and Bronchus

The trachea extends from the larynx to about the middle of the thorax, where it divides into two bronchi. Its primary function is to serve as a conduit for air. The lumen of the trachea is held open by a series of C-shaped hyaline cartilages that form the structural framework of the wall. Posteriorly, cartilage is lacking whereas smooth muscle and fibroelastic tissue are present.

The wall of the trachea consists of the following layers (see **Fig. 1**): from the inside (luminal surface) there is a mucosa **(Muc)**, a submucosa **(Submue)**, a cartilaginous layer **(Cart)**, and an adventitia **(Adv)**.

The **rectangle** in **Figure 1** outlines the area shown in **Figure 2** at higher magnification. The mucosa consists of ciliated pseudostratified columnar epithelium **(Ep)** resting on a highly elastic lamina propria **(LP)**. A division between the mucosa and submucosa is not evident in H&E sections, but the boundary **(double-headed arrow)** is marked by the presence of an elastic layer that is revealed with special elastic tissue stains. Seromucous glands **(Gl)** and their ducts **(Duct)** are present in the submucosa **(Fig. 2)**. Glands are also present in the posterior part of the trachea where there is no cartilage; here they often extend through the muscle layer into the adventitia.

Three major cell types are present in the tracheal epithelium: basal cells, ciliated columnar cells, and goblet cells **(Fig. 3)**. [Brush cells and dense core granule cells are also present, but they are not apparent in typical H&E preparations. The dense core granule cells (argyrophilic cells) are demonstrable with special silver stains]. The basal cells, located at the base of the epithelial layer, can be recognized by their spherical, densely staining nuclei **(N Bas)**, which are close to the basement membrane. These cells contain little cytoplasm.

The ciliated columnar cells extend from the basement membrane to the surface. The nuclei of these cells **(N Col)** are generally oval and tend to be located in the midregion of the cell. Moreover, they are somewhat larger and paler staining than the basal cell nuclei. At their free surface they contain numerous cilia that, together, give the surface a brush-like appearance. At the base of the cilia one sees a dense line. This is due to the linear aggregation of structures referred to as basal bodies located at the proximal end of each cilium.

Interspersed between the ciliated cells are mucus-secreting goblet cells **(GC)**. They appear empty because the mucus is lost during tissue preparation. Characteristically, the flattened nuclei are at the base of the mucous cup **(arrows)**.

Although basement membranes are not ordinarily seen in H&E preparations, a structure identified as such is regularly seen under the epithelium in the human trachea. Conspicuous because of its thickness, it is comprised of closely packed collagen fibrils that appear as a conspicuous layer beneath the epithelium and, thus, it is not a true basement membrane structure.

The trachea divides into two bronchi, one of which goes into each lung. The bronchi branch several times, decrease somewhat in diameter, and undergo certain structural changes **(Fig. 4)**. The large C-shaped cartilages are now replaced by smaller plates **(Cart)** that completely surround the bronchus. The connective tissue of the bronchus contains a large number of elastic fibers. However, the discrete elastic layer is replaced by smooth muscle **(SM)**, which now appears at the boundary between the mucosa and submucosa. The mucosa remains essentially the same, except for the presence of smooth muscle. The description of ciliated pseudostratified columnar epithelium given above also applies to the epithelium of the bronchi.

PLATE 90

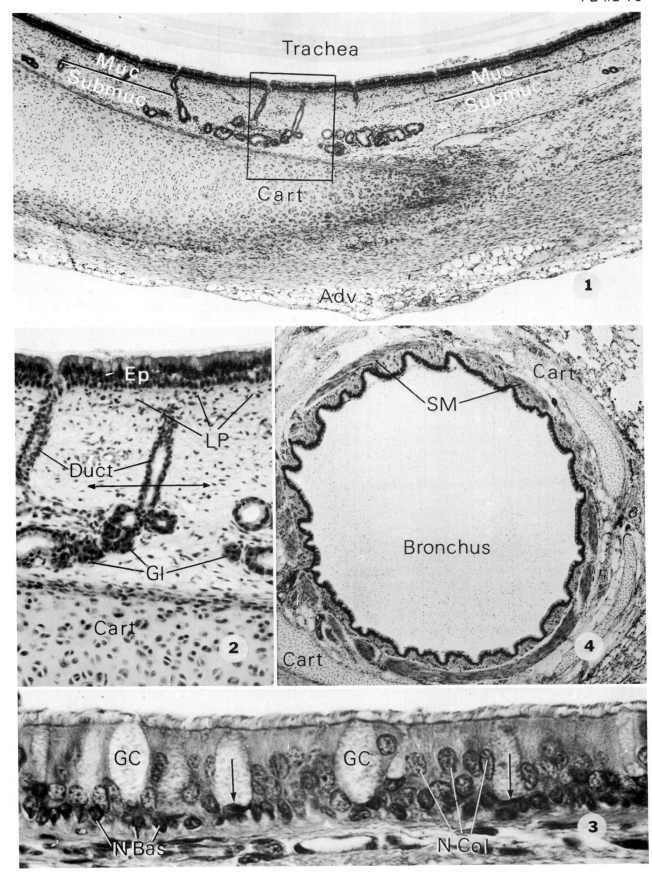

Trachea

Muc
Submuc

Muc
Submuc

Cart

Adv

1

Ep

LP

Duct

Gl

Cart

2

SM

Cart

Bronchus

Cart

4

GC

GC

N Bas

N Col

3

PLATE 91. Bronchiole and End Respiratory Passages

A bronchus enters each lung and then, within the lung, divides into smaller bronchi. As the bronchi become smaller, components of the wall are lost or changed in amount. Ultimately, the respiratory passage has distinctly different features from those of the bronchus and it is termed a bronchiole. Chief among the changes that lead to the formation of a bronchiole is the reduction and finally disappearance of cartilage. Among the other changes that occur are: the disappearance of submucousal glands; reduction in the number and finally disappearance of goblet cells; a change in pseudostratified columnar epithelium to ciliated columnar epithelium with some columnar cells that are nonciliated; and smooth muscle's occupation of a larger proportion of the bronchiolar wall.

A typical bronchiole is shown in **Figure 1.** Not uncharacteristically, blood vessels (**BV**) are adjacent to the bronchiole. The main features of the bronchiolar wall that are evident in the figure are bundles of smooth muscle (**SM**) and the lining epithelium (shown at higher magnification in Atlas section, Plate 92). Higher magnification would reveal the epithelium to be ciliated. The connective tissue is minimal and, at this low magnification, not conspicuous. Nevertheless, it is present and separates the muscle into bundles (that is, the muscle layer is not a single continuous layer). The connective tissue contains collagenous and some elastic fibers. Glands are not present in the wall of the bronchiole. Surrounding the bronchiole, comprising most of the lung substance, are the air spaces, or alveoli, of the lung.

In **Figure 2,** a short length of a bronchiole (**B**) is shown longitudinally sectioned as it branches into two respiratory bronchioles (**RB**). The last portion of a bronchiole, which leads into respiratory bronchioles, is called a terminal bronchiole. It is not engaged in exchange of air with the blood; the respiratory bronchiole does engage in air ex-

change. The place where the terminal bronchiole ends is marked by **arrows.** Not uncommonly, as shown in **Figure 2,** cartilage (**C**) is found in the bronchiolar wall where branching occurs. Blood vessels and a nodule of lymphocytes (**L**) are adjacent to the bronchiole.

The respiratory bronchiole has a wall that is comprised of two components: (1) one consists of recesses that have a wall similar to that of the alveoli and, thus, is capable of gas exchange; (2) the other has a wall formed by small cuboidal cells that appear to rest on a small bundle of eosinophilic material. This is smooth muscle surrounded by a thin investment of connective tissue. Both of these components are shown at higher magnification in the Atlas section, Plate 92.

The most distal component of the respiratory passage (**Fig. 3**) is the alveolus. Groups of alveoli clustered together and sharing a common opening are referred to as an alveolar sac (**AS**). Alveoli that form a tube are referred to as alveolar ducts (**AD**).

The outer surface of lung tissue is the serosa (**S**); it consists of a lining of mesothelial cells resting on a small amount of connective tissue. This is the layer that gross anatomists refer to as the visceral pleura.

522

PLATE 91

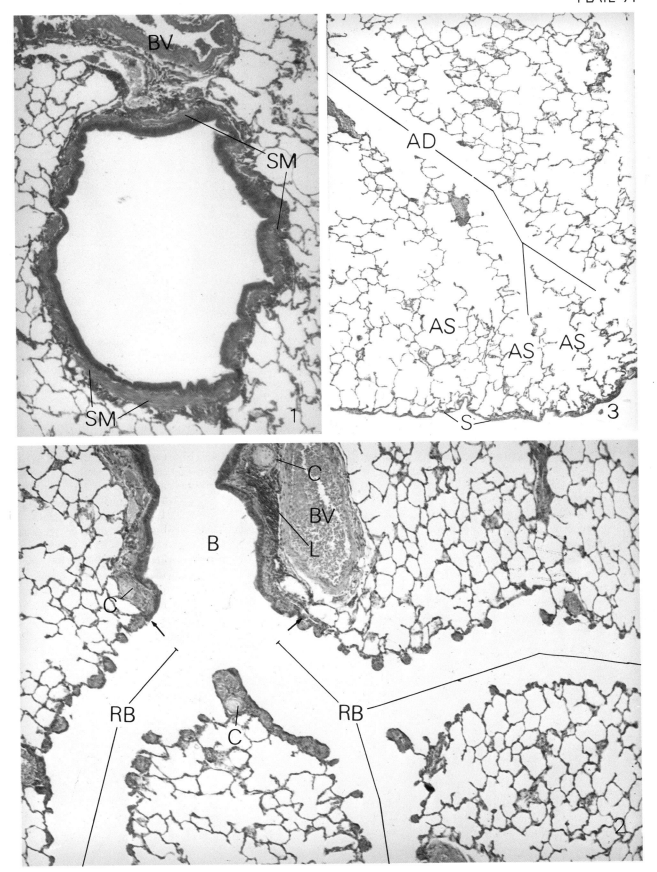

The histological features of the terminal bronchiolar wall are shown in **Figure 1.** The ciliated epithelium extends from the top of the figure to the **diamond.** This epithelium is ciliated pseudostratified columnar. Some basal cells are still present—therefore, the designation as pseudostratified columnar. Elsewhere, the epithelium might be ciliated simple columnar, and just before it becomes a respiratory brionchiole, the epithelium may include cuboidal or low columnar nonciliated cells. These nonciliated cells are Clara cells **(CC, Fig. 1,** beyond the **diamond).** Clara cells produce a surface-active agent that is instrumental in expansion of the lungs. The smooth muscle **(SM)** in the bronchiolar wall is organized in bundles; other cells under the epithelium and around the smooth muscle belong to the connective tissue.

The wall of a respiratory bronchiole is shown in **Figures 2** and **3.** The alveoli **(A)** are terminal air spaces; they are on the left in each of the two figures. The lumen of the respiratory bronchiole is on the right. Characteristically, the wall of the respiratory bronchiole consists of alternating thick and thin regions. The thick regions are similar to the wall of the bronchiole, except that cuboidal Clara cells instead of columnar epithelium form the surface. Thus, as seen in **Figure 2,** Clara cells **(CC)** are the surface lining cells of the thick regions, and smooth muscle bundles **(SM)** are under the Clara cells with a small amount of intervening connective tissue. The thin regions have a wall similar to the alveolar wall, and this will be considered below. The respiratory bronchiole shown in **Figure 3** is slightly more distal than the area seen in **Figure 2.** Structurally, it shows essentially the same features as those seen in **Figure 2** except that there are fewer Clara cells and the smooth muscle is somewhat thinner.

The alveolar wall is shown in **Figure 4.** The central component of the wall is the capillary **(C)** and in certain locations, associated connective tissue. On each side, where it faces the alveolus **(A),** a flat, squamous cell is interposed between the capillary and the air spaces. This is a pneumocyte type I cell. In some places, the type I cell is separated from the capillary endothelial cell by a single basal lamina shared by the two cells. This is the thin portion of the alveolar-capillary complex, readily seen in the upper part of the figure **(arrows).** Gas exchange occurs through the thin portion of the alveolar-capillary complex. Elsewhere, connective tissue is interposed between the pneumocyte type I cell and the endothelial cell of the capillary; each of these epithelial cells retains its own basal lamina.

A second cell type, the pneumocyte type II cell, or the septal cell **(SC),** also lines the alveolar air space. This cell typically displays a more rounded (rather than flattened) shape, and the nucleus is surrounded by a noticeable amount of cytoplasm, some of which may appear clear. The septal cell produces a surface active agent, different from that of the Clara cell, which also acts in permitting the lung to expand.

KEY

A, alveolus
C, capillary
CC, Clara cells
PsEp, pseudostratified squamous epithelium
SC, septal cell
SM, smooth muscle

arrows, Fig. 4, thin portion of alveolar-capillary complex
diamond, junction between pseudostratified columnar epithelium and Clara cells

PLATE 92

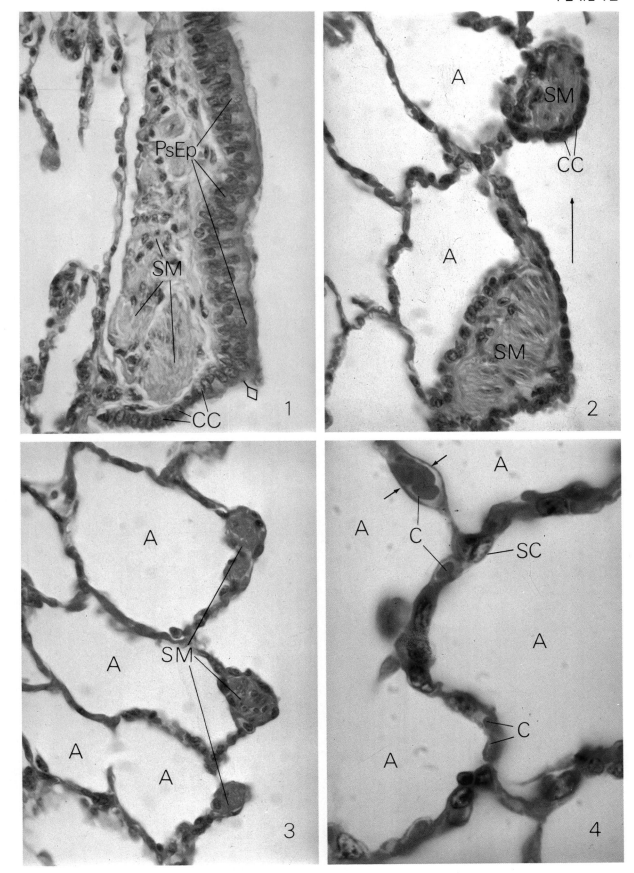

Urinary System

19

The urinary system consists of the two **kidneys,** the two **ureters,** the **urinary bladder,** and the **urethra.** The kidneys are highly vascular organs, receiving approximately 25 percent of cardiac output. They produce urine by a process that initially involves filtration of the blood. The urine, when formed, is conveyed by the ureters to the urinary bladder where it is stored until discharged via the urethra. Urine contains metabolic waste products, such as urea, uric acid, and creatinine, certain foreign substances or their breakdown products, electrolytes, and a variable amount of water. These urinary components reflect the functions of the kidneys in excretion, electrolyte balance, acid-base balance, and water balance. Kidney functions not reflected by urine production include the production of **renin,** a factor in blood pressure regulation; production of renal **erythropoietin,** a factor in the regulation of red blood cell formation; and the addition of hydroxyl groups to vitamin D.[1]

KIDNEYS

The kidneys are large, bean-shaped organs, located in the retroperitoneal tissue of the posterior abdominal cavity. On the upper pole of each kidney, embedded within the renal fascia, lies an adrenal gland. The medial border of the kidney is concave and contains a deep vertical fissure, called the **hilus,** through which the renal vessels and nerves pass and through which the expanded,

funnel-shaped origin of the ureter, called the **renal pelvis,** leaves. A section through the kidney shows the relationship of these structures as they lie just within the hilus of the kidney, in a space called the **renal sinus** (Fig. 19.1). Although not shown in the illustration, the space between and around these structures is filled largely with loose connective tissue and adipose tissue. The kidney surface is covered by a thin but tough connective tissue capsule. It passes inwardly at the hilus where it forms the connective tissue covering (Fig. 19.1) of the sinus and becomes continuous with the connective tissue forming the walls of the calyces and renal pelvis.

Cortex and Medulla

Examination of the cut face of a fresh hemisected kidney with the naked eye reveals that its substance can be divided into two distinct regions, an outer reddish brown-colored part, the **cortex,** and an inner much lighter colored part, the **medulla** (see Atlas section, Plate 93). The color seen in the cut surface of an unfixed kidney reflects the blood through the tissue. Approximately 90 to 95 percent of the blood passing through the kidney is in the cortex; 5 to 10 percent is in the medulla. The cortex consists of **renal corpuscles,** the straight and convoluted tubule segments of the kidney **nephron, collecting tubules,** and an extensive vascular supply. The nephron is the basic functional unit of the kidney and will be described later. The renal corpuscles are spherical structures, barely visible with the naked eye. They comprise the beginning segment of the nephron and contain a unique capillary network, called a **glomerulus.**

Examination of a section cut through the cortex at an angle perpendicular to the surface of the kidney reveals a series of vertical striations that

---

[1] Despite its name, vitamin D is actually a steroid prohormone. It is converted to the highly active 1,25 $(OH)_2$ vitamin D by successive metabolic steps that take place first in the liver and then in the kidney. This hormone plays an essential role in calcium balance. It is worthy of note that patients on prolonged renal dialysis, unless treated, often suffer severe disturbance of calcium homeostasis.

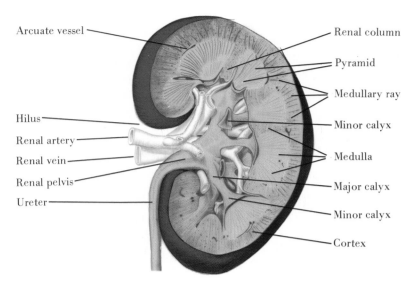

Figure 19.1. Diagram of a kidney seen from behind. Part of the kidney has been removed to show the internal structure. (Based on Braus H: *Anatomie der Menschen.* Berlin, Springer, 1924.)

appear to emanate from the medulla. These are the *medullary rays* (of Ferrein). The name reflects their appearance, since the striations seem to emanate as rays from the medulla. Each medullary ray represents an aggregation of the straight tubule component of the nephrons and associated collecting ducts. The regions between medullary rays contain the convoluted portion of the nephrons and the renal corpuscles. These areas are referred to as *cortical labyrinths.*

The medulla is comprised of the continuation of both the straight tubular segments of the nephrons and the collecting ducts, and a capillary network, the *vasa recta,* that parallel the various tubules and represent part of an important exchange system that ultimately determines the concentration of the urine. The tubules in the medulla, because of their arrangement and because of differences in length, form a number of conical structures called *pyramids.* Usually 8 to 12, but as many as 18 pyramids may occur in the human kidney. The bases of the pyramids face the cortex and the apices face the renal sinus. Each pyramid is divided into an outer zone (adjacent to the cortex) and an inner zone. The outer zone is further divided into an inner and outer strip. The zonation as well as the stripes are readily recognized in a sagittal section through the pyramid of a fresh specimen. They are a reflection of the location of distinct segments of the nephron at specific levels within the pyramid (see Figs. 19.1 and 19.2).

The caps of cortical tissue over the pyramid also extend peripherally around the lateral portion of the pyramid, forming the *renal columns* (of Bertin). Although comprised of the same components as the cortical tissue, the renal columns are regarded as part of the medulla. The apical portion of each pyramid, which is known as the *papilla,* projects into a *minor calyx,* a cup-shaped structure that represents an extension of the renal pelvis. The tip of the papilla, also known as the *area cribrosa* is perforated by the openings of the collecting tubules. The minor calices are branches of two or three *major calices* that are major divisions of renal pelvis (Fig. 19.1).

Kidney Lobes

Together, a pyramid, its overlying cortical tissue, and the neighboring tissue in the renal columns are referred to as a *lobe* of the kidney. In the developing fetal kidney, the lobar organization of the kidney is conspicuous. Each lobule is reflected as a convexity on the outer surface of the organ, but these convexities disappear after birth. The surface convexities that are typical of the fetal kidney may persist until the teenage years and in some cases in the adult as well. The lobes of the kidney are further subdivided into *lobules,* consisting of a central medullary ray and the surrounding cortical material (Fig. 19.2). Although the center, or axis, of a lobule is readily identified, the boundaries between adjacent lobules are not obviously demarcated from one another by connective tissue septa. The concept of the lobule has an important physiological basis, since the medullary rays con-

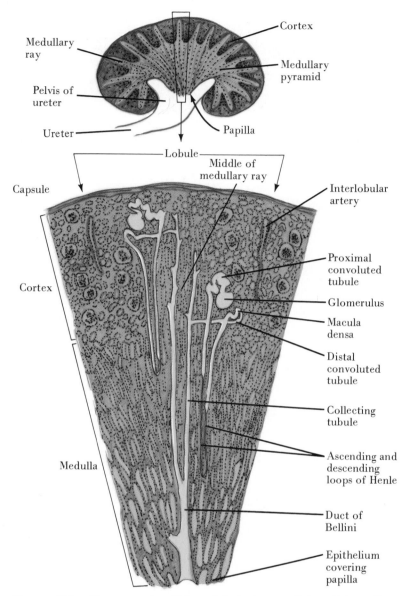

Figure 19.2. Diagram of a kidney lobule in a unilobar kidney. Two nephrons and their collecting tubules (yellow) have been drawn to show their relationship to the cortex and medulla. The **upper one,** depicting a cortical nephron, extends only a short distance into the medulla and possess a short thin segment in the loop of Henle. The juxtamedullary nephron has a long loop of Henle that includes a long thin segment that extends deep into the medulla. (Based on Ham AW, Cormack DH: *Histology,* 8th ed. Philadelphia, JB Lippincott, 1979.)

tain the collecting tubule for a group of nephrons (corresponding to a secretory unit) that drains into a common duct. Kidneys of some laboratory animals possess only one pyramid (see Fig. 19.2); these kidneys are classified as unilobar, in contrast to the multilobar kidney of the human.

Nephron

The functional unit of the kidney is the ***nephron*** (Fig. 19.3). It consists of a tuft of capillaries, called the ***glomerulus,*** and a ***uriniferous tubule.*** Each uriniferous tubule begins with what is often

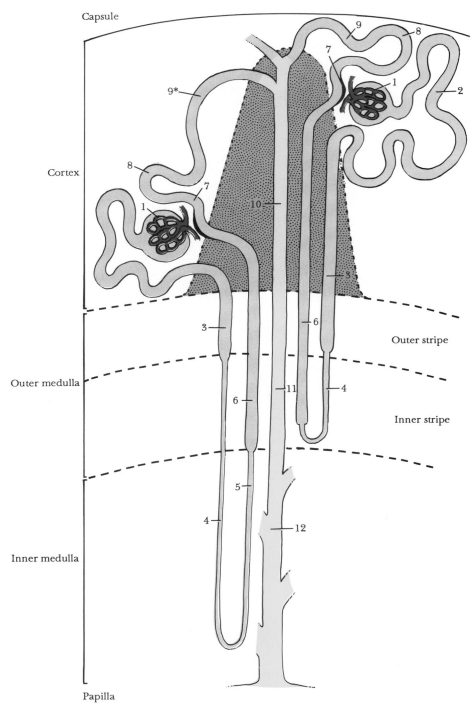

Capsule

Cortex

Outer stripe

Outer medulla

Inner stripe

Inner medulla

Papilla

Figure 19.3. Schematic diagram of a long-looped nephron **(left side)** and a short-looped nephron **(right side)** together with the associated collecting duct system. The relative position of the cortex, medulla, papilla, and capsule are indicated. The cone-shaped **dashed line** in the cortex represents a medullary ray. (Modified from Kriz W, Bankir L: A standard nomenclature for structures of the kidney. *Kid Internat* 33:1-7, 1988.) Key: **1** = renal corpuscle including the glomerulus (tuft of capillaries) and Bowman's capsule; **2** = proximal convoluted tubule; **3** = proximal straight tubule; **4** = descending thin limb; **5** = ascending thin; **6** = thick ascending limb (distal straight tubule); **7** = macula densa located in the final portion of the thick ascending limb; **8** = distal convoluted tubule; **9** = connecting tubule; **9*** = collecting tubule that forms an arcade; **10** = cortical collecting duct; **11** = outer medullary collecting duct; **12** = inner medullary collecting duct.

described as a double-layered cup, called *Bowman's capsule.* Within the cup is the glomerulus. Together, the glomerulus and Bowman's capsule constitute the *renal,* or *Malpighian, corpuscle.* Continuing from Bowman's capsule, the remaining segments of the uriniferous tubule are: the proximal thick segment (comprised of a *pars convoluta* and a *pars recta*); the thin segment; and the distal thick segment (comprised of a *pars recta,* a *macula densa,* and a *pars convoluta*).

The proximal thick segment begins as the *proximal convoluted tubule* (pars convoluta) at Bowman's capsule; it makes a short turn toward the cortex and then returns to its site of origin where most of its convolutions are located. It then enters the medullary ray and continues as the descending straight segment (pars recta) into the pyramid. Next, the *thin segment* descends farther toward the apex of the pyramid, but at some point before reaching the apex it makes a hairpin turn and returns toward the cortex. The distal thick segment ascends through the pyramid and medullary ray as the ascending straight segment (pars recta) to the vicinity of its renal corpuscle of origin. It leaves the medullary ray and makes contact, as the *macula densa,* with the vascular pole of the parent renal corpuscle. The distal thick segment becomes the distal convoluted tubule (pars convoluta) and then empties into a collecting tubule. The descending limb (pars recta) of the proximal thick segment, the thin segment and its hairpin turn, and the ascending limb (pars recta) of the distal thick segment are collectively called the *loop of Henle.* In some cases, the thin segment is extremely short and the hairpin turn may be made by the distal thick segment.

Two types of nephrons are identified, based, in part, on where the glomerulus is located (see Fig. 19.2). A nephron whose glomerulus is adjacent to the base of the pyramid is called *juxtamedullary;* other nephrons are called *cortical.* Juxtamedullary nephrons have long loops of Henle and long thin segments that extend well into the inner region of the pyramid. Cortical nephrons have short loops of Henle, extending only into the outer region of the pyramid. They are typical of the nephrons wherein the hairpin turn occurs in the distal thick segment.

The nephrons empty into collecting tubules. These drain into increasingly larger tubules that travel first in the medullary rays and then in the pyramid to its apex where a number of large collecting ducts, called *ducts of Bellini,* open into the calyx (Fig. 19.4). The area on the papilla that contains the openings of the large collecting ducts is called the *area cribrosa.* It should be noted that the arrangement of the nephrons and the collecting tubules accounts for the characteristic appearance of the cut surface of the kidney, as can be seen in Figure 19.2.

Renal (Malpighian) Corpuscle

The renal corpuscle (Fig. 19.5) is a filtration apparatus of the kidney, producing as much as 180 liters of plasma filtrate during a 24-hr period. The glomerular capillaries, which are the vascular part of the corpuscle, contain numerous fenestrations (Fig. 19.6). These fenestrations are slightly larger and somewhat more irregular in outline than fenestrations seen in other capillaries. Moreover, the diaphragm that spans the fenestrations in other capillaries is absent in many of the glomerular capillaries.

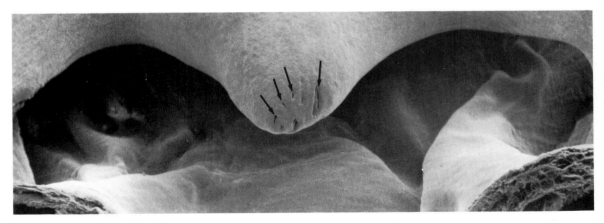

Figure 19.4. SEM of renal papilla and calyx, showing a conical structure, the apex of the renal papilla, projecting into a space, the renal calyx. The apex of the papilla contains openings **(arrows)** of the ducts of Bellini. These ducts deliver urine from the pyramids to the calyx. The surface of the apex of the papilla containing the openings is designated the area cribrosa. (C. C. Tisher, 1976.)

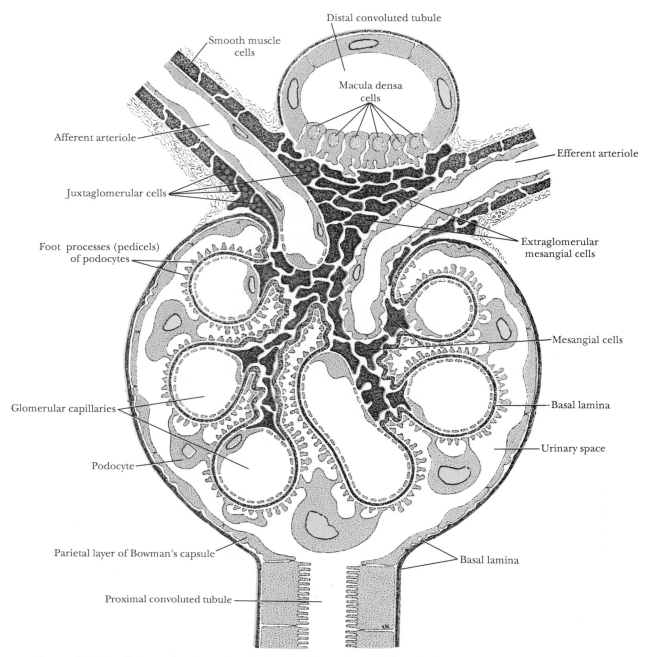

Figure 19.5(a). Schematic diagram of a renal glomerulus and the structures associated at the vascular pole **(top)** and urinary pole **(bottom)** (not drawn to scale). Mesangial cells are associated with the capillary endothelium and the glomerular basement membrane. The macula densa cells of the distal tubule are shown intimately associated with the juxtaglomerular and the extraglomerular mesangial cells. (Modified from Kriz W, Sakai T: In: Morphological aspects of glomerular function. *Proceedings of the Tenth International Congress of Nephrology,* London, 1987.)

The inner layer of Bowman's capsule, called the *visceral layer,* consists of modified epithelial cells designated as *podocytes.* They contain numerous processes, which, in turn, contain secondary processes, called *foot processes* or *pedicels.* The foot processes interdigitate with similar foot processes of neighboring podocytes (Fig. 19.7). The elongate spaces between them are called *filtration slits.* The foot processes contain numerous microfilaments that are considered to be instrumental in regulating the passage of substances through the filtration slits. An additional factor that influences the pas-

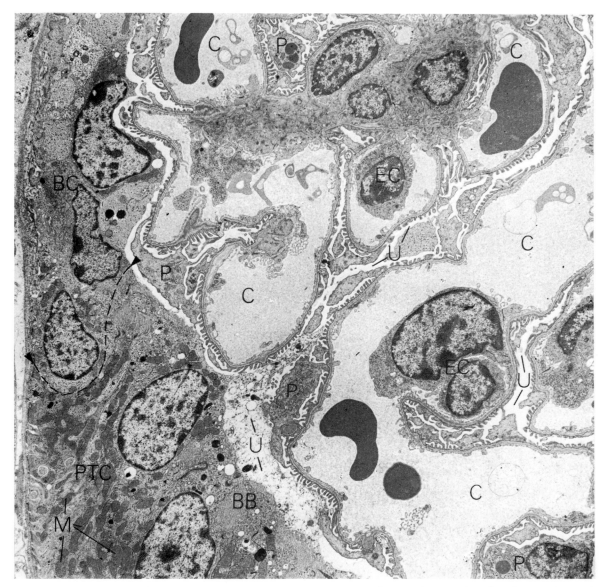

Figure 19.5(b). TEM of glomerulus in the region of the urinary pole. The nuclear and perinuclear regions of the endothelial cells (EC) that line the glomerular capillaries (C) bulge into the vascular lumen. On the outer surface of the capillaries are the podocytes (P). External to the podocytes is the urinary space (U). The Bowman's capsule (BC) is shown on the left; it is continuous at the **broken line (marked by arrowheads)** with the proximal tubule cell (PTC) of the tubule. Note the numerous mitochondria (M) in the base of these cells and the brush border (BB) at the apex projecting into the urinary space. The nuclei of three adjacent mesangial cells can be seen in the **upper right corner** of the electron micrograph. × 4700.

sage of substances through the filtration slits is the presence of a thin membrane similar to the diaphragm of capillary fenestrations. This membrane, the *filtration slit membrane,* spans the slits (Fig. 19.8).

The glomerular capillary endothelium and the podocytes constitute two of the three components of the filtration apparatus. The third component is the glomerular basement membrane

that occupies the space between the endothelium and podocytes. The basal lamina, which serves both the capillary endothelium and the podocytes, measures about 300 to 350 nm, in thickness.

The outer layer of Bowman's capsule, called the *parietal layer,* is a simple squamous epithelium. At the *uriniferous pole* of the renal corpuscle, it opens into the proximal convoluted tubule.

The space between the visceral and parietal

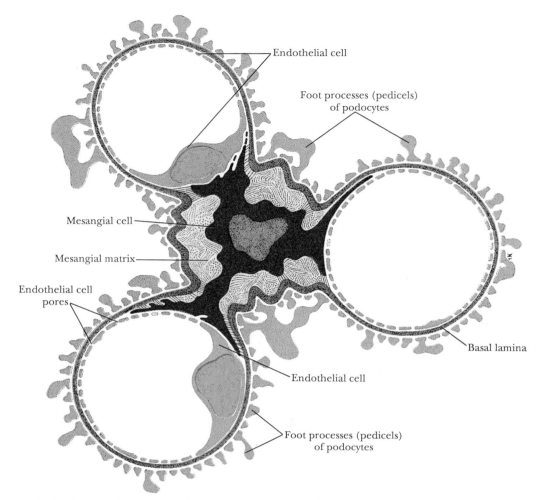

Figure 19.5(c).   Schematic diagram showing the relationship between the intraglomerular mesangial cells and the glomerular capillaries. The mesangial cell and its surrounding matrix are enclosed by the basal lamina of the glomerular capillaries. Note that they are in the same compartment as the endothelium and that they can be intimately associated with the basal lamina as well as the endothelial cells. (Modified from Sakai T, Kriz W: *Anat Embryol* 176373-386 1987.)

layers of Bowman's capsule is called the **urinary** or **Bowman's space** (see Fig. 19.5b). It is the receptacle for the plasma filtrate produced by the filtration apparatus of the renal corpuscle. The production of this plasma filtrate is the first step in the process of urine formation. Under normal conditions, the filtration barrier prevents cells and large molecules, such as proteins, from entering Bowman's space. The fact that albumin, though not a usual constituent, may sometimes be found in urine indicates that the size of albumin is close to the effective pore size of the filtration barrier. Despite the ability of the filtration barrier to restrict protein, several grams of protein do pass through the barrier each day. This protein is reabsorbed by endocytosis in the proximal convoluted tubule.

Urinalysis is an important part of the examination of patients who are thought to be suffering from renal disease. Part of this analysis includes the determination of the amount of protein excreted in the urine. The excretion of excessive amounts of protein, i.e., *proteinuria* (albuminuria), is an important diagnostic sign of renal disease. Normally, less than 150 mg of protein is excreted into the urine each day. Although excessive excretion of protein is almost always an indication of renal disease, it should be noted that extreme exercise, such as jogging, or severe dehydration may produce increased proteinuria in people without renal diseases.

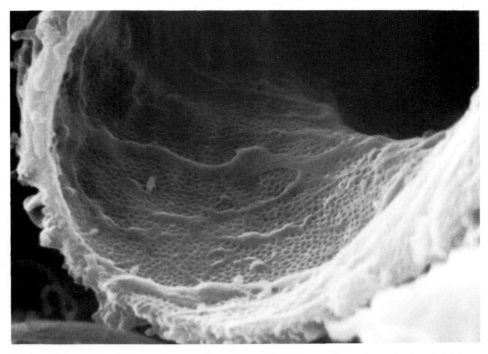

Figure 19.6. SEM of glomerular capillary. The wall of the capillary shows horizontal ridges formed by cytoplasm of the endothelial cell. Elsewhere, fenestrations are seen as numerous **dark oval** and **circular profiles.** (C. C. Tisher, 1976.)

The renal corpuscle contains an additional group of cells called *mesangial cells.* These cells and their surrounding matrix constitute the *mesangium,* which is separated from the capillary lumen by the endothelium and is most obvious at the vascular stalk of the glomerulus. Mesangial cells are positioned much the same as pericytes in that they are enclosed by the basal lamina of the glomerular capillaries (see Fig. 19.5a). The mesangial cells are not entirely confined to the renal corpuscle; some are located outside of the corpuscle along the vascular pole where they are also designated as *lacis cells* and form part of what is called the juxtaglomerular apparatus. Although the functions of mesangial cells are not fully known, experimental data shows that: (1) they are phagocytic and can remove trapped residues and aggregated proteins from the glomerular basal lamina keeping the glomerular filter free of debris and (2) they provide structural support at sites where the epithelial basement membrane is lacking. It has also been proposed that the mesangial cells, which have contractile ability, may function in the regulation of glomerular blood flow. Clinically, it has been observed that mesangial cells proliferate in certain kidney diseases.

Embryologically, the cells of the renal corpuscle and those cells intimately associated with it are derived from two basic cell types. One type, the smooth muscle-derived cells, include the juxtaglomerular cells and the extra- and intraglomerular mesangial cells. The second type, the epithelial-derived cells, include both layers of Bowman's capsule and the macula densa cells (see below) of the distal tubule.

Juxtaglomerular Apparatus

Lying directly adjacent to the afferent and efferent arterioles and to some extraglomerular mesangial cells at the vascular pole of the corpuscle is the terminal portion of the distal thick segment. It contains, as part of its wall, cells that collectively are referred to as the *macula densa.* When viewed with the light microscope the cells of the macula densa cells are distinctive in that they are narrower and usually taller than other distal tubule cells. The nuclei of these cells appear crowded, even to the extent that they may appear partially superimposed over one another—thus, the name macula densa. In this same region, the smooth muscle cells of the adjacent afferent arteriole (and sometimes the efferent arteriole) are modified in that their nuclei are spherical, as opposed to the typical elongate smooth muscle cell nucleus, and they contain secretory granules. These modified smooth muscle cells, referred to as *juxtaglomerular cells* (Fig. 19.5a), require special stains to reveal the

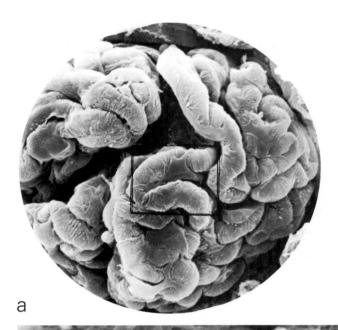

a

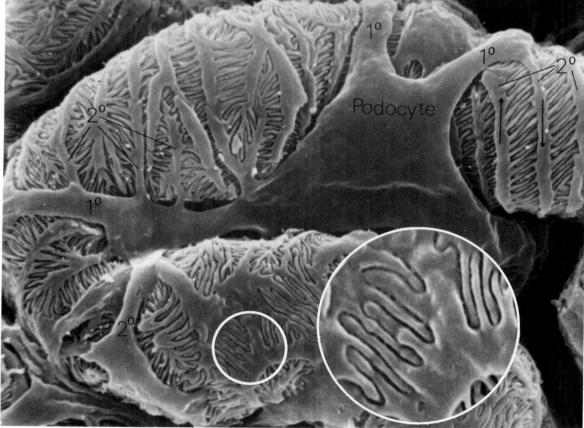

b

Figure 19.7(a). SEM of a glomerulus at low magnification. The parietal layer of Bowman's capsule has been removed revealing the tortuous course of the glomerular capillaries covered by podocytes within the renal corpuscle. × 700. **(b).** A higher magnification of the area in the rectangle in Figure 19.7a showing the epithelial podocytes (visceral layer of Bowman's capsule) covering the capillary. Note the podocyte and its processes embracing the capillary wall. The primary processes (1) of the podocyte give rise to secondary processes (2) and

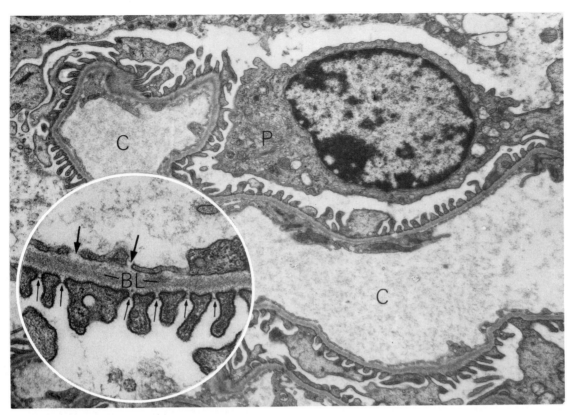

Figure 19.8. TEM of glomerular capillary (C) and adjacent podocyte (P). The pedicels of the podocytes rest on the basal lamina surrounding the capillary endothelium, and together the three components, the capillary endothelium, basal lamina, and podocytes, form a filtration apparatus. These are seen at higher magnification in the **inset. Large arrows** point to the fenestrations in the capillary; external to these is the basal lamina (Bl), and external to this are the pedicels of the podocytes. Note the slit membrane **(small arrows)** spanning the gap between adjacent pedicels.

granules in the light microscope. It has been demonstrated that the granules contain an aspartyl peptidase, known as ***renin.*** Renin is synthesized, stored, and released into the blood from the modified smooth muscle cells. In the blood, it serves to catalyze the cleavage of angiotensin I from angiotensinogen. A converting enzyme, in turn, transforms angiotensin I to the physiologically active form, angiotensin II. The latter is a potent vasoconstrictor that has a regulatory role in the control of renal and systemic vascular resistance. It

is also a regulator of salt balance by promoting aldosterone release from the adrenal cortex. The macula densa, the juxtaglomerular cells, and the extraglomerular mesangial cells constitute the ***juxtaglomerular apparatus.*** The unique intimate association of the cells in the juxtaglomerular apparatus has led to the concept that tubular fluid composition at the macula densa influences renin release from the juxtaglomerular cells. In fact, recent in vitro studies, utilizing microperfusion of dissected juxtaglomerulus apparatuses, have re-

these, in turn, give rise to the pedicels. The space between the interdigitating pedicels creates the slit pores. The area in the **inset** (enlarged from the area indicated by the **black circle**) reveals the slit pores at higher magnification. An interesting feature is that alternating pedicels belong to the secondary process of one cell; the intervening pedicels belong to the process of another cell. For example, the **two arrows on the right** of the micrograph are aligned on secondary processes; the **arrow pointing down** is on a process of the podocyte visible from the perspective shown whereas the process with the **arrow pointing up** is from another podocyte (which is not visible from the perspective shown here.) Note how each secondary process provides pedicels, which then interdigitate with the opposing pedicel of the other cell's secondary process. × 4000 (**inset,** × 6000).

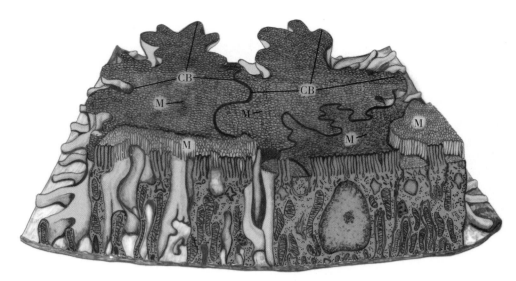

Figure 19.9. Diagram showing both sectioned faces and three-dimensional aspects of proximal convoluted tubule cells. The basolateral interdigitations are numerous; some of the interdigitating processes extend the full height of the cell. The processes are long in the basal region and create an elaborate extracellular compartment adjacent to the basal lamina (see Fig. 19.10). Apically, the microvilli (M) constitute a brush border. In some locations, the microvilli have been omitted, thereby revealing the convoluted character of the apical cell boundary (CB). (Based on Bulger R: *Am J Anat* 116:237, 1965.)

vealed that a fall in NaCl concentration serves as a local tubular signal for stimulation of renin secretion. It would appear, as previously postulated, that the cells of the macula densa sense changes in NaCl concentration and, in turn, mediate renin secretion by the juxtaglomerular cells.

Kidney Tubules

As the glomerular filtrate passes through the uriniferous and collecting tubules of the kidneys, it undergoes the following changes: (1) many of the substances within the filtrate are reabsorbed, some partially (for example, sodium) and some completely (for example, glucose); (2) certain substances (for example, creatinine) are added to the filtrate and, thus, to the urine by secretory activity of the tubule cells; (3) the volume of the filtrate is reduced substantially; and (4) the urine is made hypertonic. The long loops of Henle and collecting tubules that pass parallel to similarly arranged blood vessels, serve as the basis for the countercurrent multiplier mechanism that is instrumental in concentrating the urine and thereby making it hypertonic.

Proximal thick segment. The two major parts of the proximal thick segment have already been identified as the proximal convoluted tubule and the straight portion that is the first part of the descending limb of Henle.

The proximal thick segment, also called the proximal tubule, is made up of large, simple cuboidal epithelial cells. Numerous closely packed, tall microvilli (about 1.0 to 1.3 μm) on the apical surface of the cells constitute the **brush border,** a structure evident with the light microscope. The lateral surfaces of proximal tubule cells interdigitate extensively as illustrated in Figure 19.9. The interdigitations are even more extensive in the basal region of the epithelial layer, thereby forming a tortuous basal and lateral extracellular space (Fig. 19.10). The basolateral extracellular space is separated from the tubular lumen by apically placed junctional complexes, long recognized with the light microscope as the **terminal bar apparatus.** The space is important in sodium and water transport.[2] Large elongate mitochondria adjacent to the plasma membrane provide energy for this work. The mitochondria are oriented at right angles to the base of the cell (Fig. 19.11) and, in the pars convoluta, they tend to give the cell the appearance of having basal striations, a characteristic that is evident with the light microscope.

_____

[2] Sodium and water enter the proximal tubule cell by diffusion through the apical plasma membrane. The sodium is then pumped out of the cell, across the plasma membrane into the basolateral extracellular space, and water follows osmotically. Thus, as a consequence of active sodium transport, as much as 70 percent of the fluid is reabsorbed from the lumen of the proximal convoluted tubule.

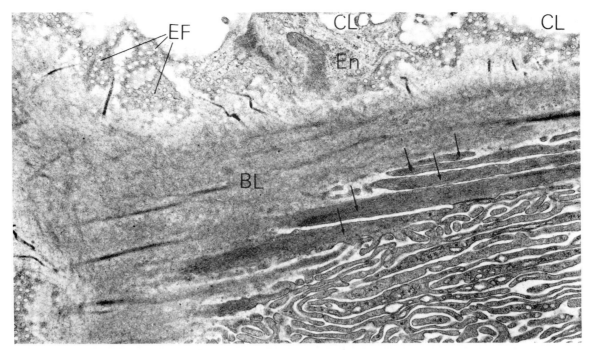

Figure 19.10. Electron micrograph (EM) of a section that is almost tangential to the base of a proximal convoluted tubule cell, and the subjacent basal lamina and capillary. In the upper part of the micrograph is the capillary lumen (CL) bounded by the capillary endothelium (En). Characteristically, the endothelium possesses numerous fenestrations (EF) and, in this plane of section, the fenestrations are seen in face view, displaying circular profiles. The basal lamina (BL) appears as a broad band of homogeneous material below that **(lower right)** are the interdigitating basal processes of the proximal tubule cells. The long, straight processes contain longitudinally oriented microfilaments **(arrows)**. In this plane of section, the basal extracellular space appears as a maze between the cellular processes. × 15,000.

At the very base of the cell, that is, at the bottom of the interdigitating processes, bundles of 6-nm microfilaments are present (see **arrows,** Figs. 19.10 and 19.11). It has been suggested that they play a role in facilitating the movement of fluid from the basolateral extracellular space toward the adjacent peritubular capillary.

Present at the apical surface of the cells are numerous pinocytotic vesicles. These pinch off from the plasma membrane between the base of the microvilli (Fig. 19.11). The pinocytotic vesicles coalesce to form larger vesicles and together form a functional link with lysosomes of the tubule cell. The pinocytotic vesicles and lysosomes are active in the endocytosis and disposal, respectively, of protein from the tubular lumen.

With the light microscope, the cytoplasm of the proximal tubule cells stains with eosin. As already indicated, the basal striations are pronounced only in the convoluted portion because in the straight portion the mitochondria are smaller and not as concentrated in the basal part of the cell. The interdigitations of the lateral surfaces of the cells obscure the boundaries of the cells so that they are not evident with the light microscope. When adequately preserved, the brush border serves to distinguish proximal tubule cells clearly from other kidney tubule cells.

Thin Segment. The thin segment in cortical nephrons is short or sometimes absent. These nephrons possess relatively short loops of Henle and the thin segment is in the descending portion of the loop. In juxtamedullary nephrons, the thin segment is substantially longer. It begins in the descending portion of the loop, makes the hairpin turn, and continues as the first part of the ascending limb.

In the 1960s, electron microscopists described the thin segment as consisting of a simple squamous epithelium, in which at least two structurally distinct types of cells are recognizable in different regions of the thin segment. The chief ultrastructural difference between the two types of epithelium relates to the association of the adjacent cells. Complex interdigitations between adjacent cells were seen in thin descending limb and a more simple epithelium was observed in the more distal portion. In subsequent studies of several other

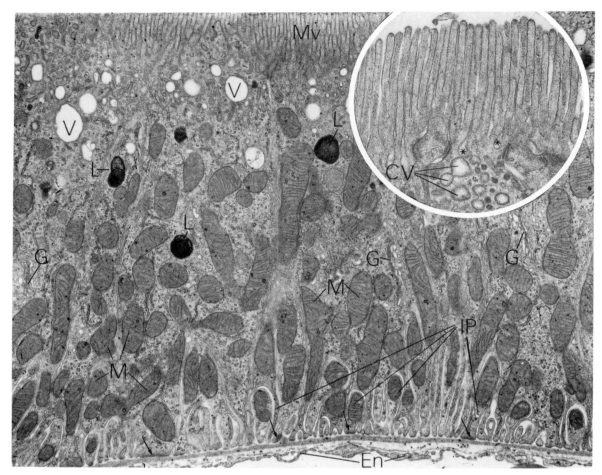

Figure 19.11. EM of a proximal tubule cell. The apical surface of the cell shows numerous microvilli (Mv) that collectively are recognized as the brush border in the light microscope. Numerous vesicles (V) are evident in the apical cytoplasm. These form by fusion of smaller vesicles (CV, inset) that pinch off from the plasma membrane **(asterisks)** at the base of the microvilli **(inset)**. Also present in the apical and midregion of the cell are lysosomes (L) and Golgi profiles (G). The nucleus has not been included in the plane of section. Many mitochondria longitudinally oriented (M) are seen within the interdigitating processes (IP) directly adjacent to the infolded plasma membrane. The mitochondria (M) responsible for the appearance of the basal striations seen in the light microscope, particularly if the extracellular space is enlarged. In the base of the foot processes there is a dense material **(arrows)** that represents bundles of cross-sectioned microfilaments (these are the same filaments as seen in longitudinal section in Fig. 19.10). The electron micrograph also reveals a small amount of connective tissue and the fenestrated endothelium (En) of an adjacent peritubular capillary. × 15,000.

species, four different types of epithelium have been identified. Although it is not known if the four types exist in man, the epithelium has been reported to be of a similar type.

Type I epithelium is found in the thin segment of the loop of Henle in short-looped nephrons; types I through IV, in sequential regions of the thin segment in long-looped nephrons (Fig. 19.12). Type I epithelium, found in the descending thin limb of short-looped nephrons, consists of a thin, simple epithelium. The cells have almost no interdigitations with neighboring cells

and have few organelles. Type II epithelium, found in the thin descending limb of long-looped nephrons located in the outer medulla, consists of taller epithelium. These cells possess more abundant organelles and have many small, blunt microvilli. The extent of lateral interdigitations with neighboring cells shows species variation. For example, in the rat, numerous, complex interdigitations are seen; in the rabbit, the cells do not interdigitate. Type III epithelium, found in the thin descending limb in the inner medulla, consists of a lower epithelium. The cells have simpler

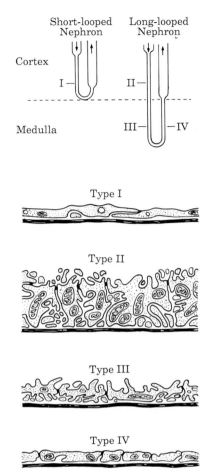

Short-looped Nephron   Long-looped Nephron

Cortex

Medulla

Type I

Type II

Type III

Type IV

Figure 19.12. Schematic diagrams of a short-looped nephron **(top, left side)**, a long-looped nephron **(top, right side)**, and four regions of the epithelium of the thin limb of the loop of Henle. The Roman numerals (I–IV) identify the various segments of the epithelium and the region where they are found in the thin limb of the loops. The diagrams of the epithelium do not include nuclear regions of the epithelial cells. See text for further explanation. (Modified from Madsen KM, Tisher CC: Physiologic anatomy of the kidney. *Kidney Hormones* 3:45–100, 1986.)

structure and have fewer microvilli than cells of the type II epithelium. The cells do not have lateral interdigitations. Type IV epithelium, found at the bend of long-looped nephrons and through the entire thin ascending limb, consists of a low, flattened epithelium without microvilli on the luminal surface. The cells possess few organelles but do demonstrate numerous, elaborate lateral interdigitations.

The functional significance of these differences is not yet clear, although it should be noted that the thin segment is part of the countercurrent exchange system that functions in concentrating the urine and these differences probably reflect specific roles in this process.

Distal Thick Segment. The three parts of the distal thick segment, also called the distal tubule, are the pars recta, the macula densa, and the pars convoluta. The macula densa has already been described. Cells constituting the pars recta and pars convoluta are essentially similar. They are large cuboidal epithelial cells. As in the case of proximal tubule cells, the distal tubule cells display elaborate lateral and basal interdigitations, an elaborate basolateral extracellular space exists between the cells, and terminal bars separate the space from the lumen of the tubule. Large, basal mitochondria (Fig. 19.13) account for the appearance of basal striations in the cells when viewed with the light microscope. The nucleus is located in the apical region and sometimes, especially in the pars recta, causes a bulge of the cell into the lumen. There is no brush border, but small apical microvilli are present in some regions of the segment. The cytoplasm of distal tubule cells stains lightly with eosin. Also to be noted is that, with the light microscope, the boundaries between distal tubule cells are not distinct.

Collecting Tubules. Collecting tubules begin in the cortical labyrinth and proceed to the medullary rays where they drain into larger collecting tubules. The collecting tubules of the medullary rays extend as straight tubules into the pyramid. As the tubules approach the apex of the pyramid, they converge and form larger collecting tubules called **ducts of Bellini.** Some collecting tubules continuing from juxtamedullary nephrons ascend in the cortical substance and then descend before merging with the **straight collecting tubules.** These initial segments, because of their course, are called **arched collecting tubules.**

The collecting tubules consist of simple cuboidal epithelium. The cells that make up the larger ducts, those in the inner part of the pyramid, are taller than those found in the outer part of the medulla and in the cortex. Two cell types are seen in the collecting ducts of the cortex: **light cells** or **collecting duct (CD) cells** and **dark cells** or **intercalated cells (IC).** CD cells possess microvilli on their apical surface and a single cilium. Larger ducts deep in the pyramid contain only light cells. The boundaries between the light cells of collecting ducts are readily seen with the light microscope. Intercalated cells have numerous short projections in the form of **lamellapodia.** These are easily identified with the scanning electron microsce (SEM) (Fig. 19.14), but may be mistaken for microvilli with the transmission electron microsce (TEM). The IC (or dark cells) have many mito-

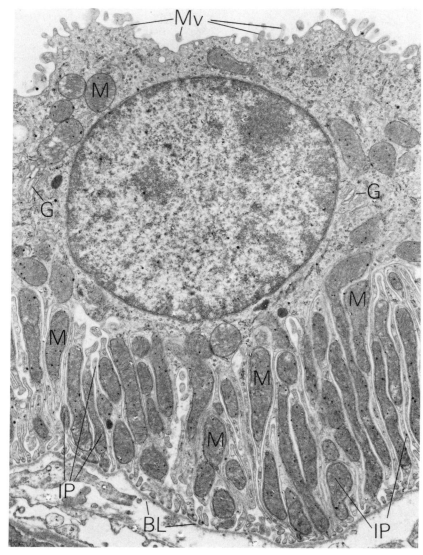

Figure 19.13. EM of a distal convoluted cell, longitudinal section. The apical surface of the cell displays some microvilli (Mv), but they are not sufficiently long or numerous to give the appearance of a brush border (compare with Fig. 19.11). The nucleus and Golgi profiles (G) are in the upper portion of the cell. Mitochondria (M) are chiefly in the basal region of the cell within the interdigitating processes (IP). As in the proximal tubule cell, the mitochondria account for the appearance of basal striations in the light microscope. Beneath the distal tubule cell is a basal lamina (BL). × 12,000.

chondria, a denser cytoplasm, apical vesicles, and basally located interdigitations with neighboring cells. IC cells are rarely found in the inner medullary segment. The CD cells gradually increase in height from low cuboidal in the outer part of the medulla to low columnar in the papillary ducts. The CD cells are arranged in a single layer with their nuclei in register at one level and their free surfaces bulging into the lumen of the collecting duct. The simple columnar epithelium lining the

ducts continues onto the surface of the papilla in the region of the cribrosa.

Interstitial Cells

In the kidney, connective tissue (called *interstitial tissue*) is found in the space outside of the basal laminae and surrounding the components of the nephrons, the blood, and lymphatic vessels. This tissue increases considerably in amount from

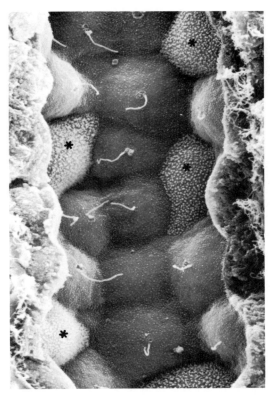

Figure 19.14. SEM of a collecting tubule showing dark cells **(asterisks)**, with numerous short lamellapodia or microridges on their surface, and light cells, each with a single cilium on its free surface along with small microvilli. [Note the terms "light" and "dark" refer to the staining character of sectioned cells. Here the density differences reflect charge characteristics of the coated surface of the specimen.] (Courtesy of C. C. Tisher, 1976.)

from lymphocytes or the monocyte-phagocyte series and function in the immune response.

In the medulla of the kidney, three types of interstitial cells, types I to III, have been described in studies utilizing the rat. The type I cell is considered to be the typical interstitial cell of the medulla and is the only interstitial cell type normally present in the inner region of the inner medulla. It is the most thoroughly studied interstitial cell type because it is thought to have an endocrine function. Type I cells, although highly pleomorphic, are stellate cells with their long axis oriented perpendicular to the long axis of the adjacent tubule and capillaries. Type I cells contain abundant rough endoplasmic reticulum (rER), a well-developed Golgi, lysosomes, and lipid inclusions or droplets that vary in relation to the diuretic state of the animal. The function of these cells is not known but they are thought to be involved in the urine-concentrating mechanism. It has also been suggested that the type I cells secrete a hormone, yet to be isolated, involved in the regulation of blood pressure. Type II cells are rounded, lymphocyte-like cells with sparse cytoplasm and without lipid droplets. They have abundant free ribosomes but a poorly developed endoplasmic reticulum. The function of the type II cells is not known but it has been speculated that they have phagocytic properties. Type III cells are pericytes that are associated with the descending vasa recta. Again, the function of the type III cells is not known, but it has been suggested that they are related to smooth muscle cells and have contractile properties.

Formation of Concentrated Urine

The plasma filtrate reabsorbed by the proximal tubule is essentially isotonic, that is, it is not concentrated by the proximal tubule cells. The production of a hypertonic urine is a function of the loop of Henle, the collecting tubules, and the adjacent parallel medullary blood vessels. Together, these constitute the *countercurrent multiplier and exchange system.* This mechanism is the subject of physiology texts, but it should be noted that, in principle, the system works by active transport of sodium and accompanying passive movement of water and chloride from the lumen of the nephron in the pars recta of the proximal tubule and active cotransport of sodium and chloride from the lumen of the nephron in the thick ascending limb of the loop of Henle. The ascending limb is highly impermeable to water and NaCl, therefore, active transport mechanisms are re-

the cortex (where it constitutes about 7 percent of the volume) to inner region of the medulla and papilla. Until it was recognized that the concentration of solutes in the intertubular spaces of the medulla had an important role in concentration of urine by influencing the resorption of water, the interstitial tissue was of limited research interest.

In the cortex of the kidney, two types of interstitial cells have been identified. The most common cell type resembles fibroblasts and is found between the basement membrane of the tubules and the adjacent peritubular capillaries. The less common and smaller second cell type resembles lymphocytes or mononuclear cells and contains lysosomes and phagocytic vacuoles but few lipid inclusions. Although the functions of these cells have not been firmly established, it is likely that the fibroblast-like cells produce collagen and glycosaminoglycans of the extracellular matrix of the interstitium. The small cells may be derived

quired to remove the sodium and chloride. Essentially, this active cotransport mechanism in the ascending limb of the loop of Henle results in a concentration of NaCL in the interstitium of the medulla. Because this limb of the loop is relatively impermeable to water, the water does not follow the sodium osmotically. This means that the fluid in the limb becomes more dilute (hypotonic) as it approaches the cortex. At the same time, the interstitium of the pyramid becomes very hypertonic, up to 1200 milliosmoles (mOsm) per liter in the apex of the pyramid.

The antidiuretic hormone (ADH) of the pituitary gland acts on the collecting tubule cells, making them permeable to water. In the presence of ADH, water passes from the collecting tubule to the interstitium, making the urine hypertonic. In the absence of ADH, the water fails to pass out of the collecting tubules and a dilute urine is produced. Insufficient production of ADH by the pituitary gland leads to the production of copious amounts of dilute urine, a condition known as *diabetes insipidus.* Another hormone, aldosterone, a product of the adrenal gland, acts on the renal tubules to stimulate sodium reabsorption and potassium secretion.

Blood Supply

Each kidney receives a large branch from the abdominal aorta called the *renal artery.* The artery branches within the renal sinus and sends *interlobar* branches into the substance of the kidney (Fig. 19.15). The interlobar arteries travel between the pyramids as far as the cortex and then turn to follow a course along the base of the pyramid. In this location, that is, between the base of the pyramid and the cortex, the artery is designated as an *arcuate artery. Interlobular arteries* branch from the arcuate arteries and travel through the cortex toward the capsule. Although the boundaries between lobules are not distinct, it should be noted that the interlobular arteries, when included in the section, are usually located at some midpoint between adjacent medullary rays, travelling in the cortical labyrinth. As they traverse the cortex toward the capsule, the interlobular arteries give off branches, the *afferent arterioles,* with one distributed to each glomerulus. A single afferent arteriole may spring directly from the interlobular artery, or a common stem from the interlobular artery may branch to form several afferent arterioles. (The common stem, having left the interlobular location to enter the lobule, is properly called an *intralobular artery*). Some interlobular arteries terminate near the periphery of the cor-

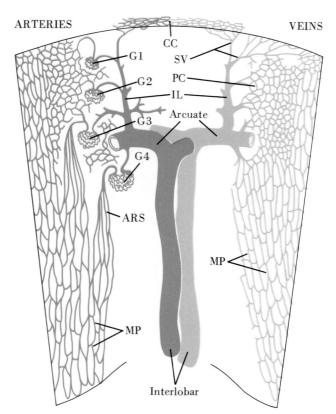

Figure 19.15. Schematic diagram of renal blood supply. Renal arteries give rise to interlobar arteries that branch into arcuate arteries at the border between medulla and cortex. Interlobular arteries (IL) branch from the arcuate arteries and travel toward the renal capsule, giving off afferent arterioles to the glomeruli (G). Glomeruli in the outer part of the cortex (G1, G2) send efferent arterioles to the peritubular capillaries (PC) that surround the tubules in the cortex; glomeruli near the medulla (G3, G4), the juxtamedullary glomeruli, empty almost entirely into the medullary plexus (MP) of capillaries via the arteriolae rectae spuriae (ARS). Blood returns from the capillaries via veins that enter the interlobular (or arcuate) veins. Stellate veins near the capsule drain both the capsular capillaries (CC) as well as peritubular capillaries. (Based on Morrison DM: *Am J Anat* 37:53, 1926.)

tex, whereas others enter the kidney capsule for its supply.

Afferent arterioles give rise to the glomerular tuft of capillaries. The glomerular capillaries reunite to form an *efferent arteriole* that, in turn, gives rise to a second network of capillaries, the *peritubular capillaries.* The arrangement of these capillaries differs according to whether they spring from cortical or juxtamedullary glomeruli. Efferent arterioles from cortical glomeruli lead into a peritubular capillary network that surrounds the local uriniferous tubules (see G1 and G2, Fig. 19.15). Efferent arterioles from juxtamedullary glomeruli descend into the medulla alongside the loop of Henle; they break up into smaller vessels that continue toward the apex of the pyramid but make hairpin turns at various levels to return, again as straight vessels, toward the base of the pyramid (see G3 and G4, Fig. 19.15). The terms used to describe these vascular patterns are not always consistent, but the following apply to the medullary circulation. *Arteriolae rectae spuriae* is the name given to the arterial vessels from the juxtamedullary glomeruli that descends into the medulla. *(Arteriolae rectae verae* is a term given to arterioles that spring directly from the arcuate arteries, bypassing juxtamedullary glomeruli. These connections have been described in experimentally treated animals and in diseased kidneys. Their presence in the normal kidney is questioned.) *Vasa recta* is the term given to the straight vessels somewhat larger than capillaries that continue from the arteriolae rectae spuriae. The descending limb of the vasa recta forms the *arterial limb;* the ascending limb of the vasa recta forms the *venous limb.*

The venous return from the peritubular capillary networks follows the reverse routes (Fig. 19.15): (1) peritubular cortical capillaries to interlobular veins to arcuate veins to interlobar veins to the renal vein; (2) medullary vascular network to arcuate veins, and so forth; (3) peritubular capillaries near the kidney surface and capillaries from the capsule to veins called *stellate veins* to interlobular veins, and so forth.

Lymphatic Vessels

The kidneys contain lymphatic vessels, but they are not usually evident in routine histological preparations. However, they can be displayed by experimental methods. Such methods show that two major networks of lymphatic vessels exist. One network is located in the outer regions of the kidney substance and drains into larger lymphatic vessels in the capsule. The second network is more deeply located and drains into lymphatic vessels in the sinus of the kidneys. Anastomoses exist between the two networks.

Nerves

The kidney receives nerve fibers from the sympathetic network of the abdominal cavity. While the details of renal innervation have not yet been established, it is known that experimental stimulation of the sympathetic nerves diverts renal circulation primarily through the medulla and causes blanching of the kidney cortex. Whereas this diversion of cortical blood is experimental, some cortical blanching does occur during the sympathetic stimulation that occurs in day-to-day

stress. The kidneys also contain afferent nerve fibers and possibly parasympathetic fibers.

EXCRETORY PASSAGES

The excretory passages for the urine for each kidney are the calyces, major and minor, the renal pelvis, the ureter, the urinary bladder (where the urine is temporarily stored), and the urethra. All of these except the urethra have the same general structure namely, an adventitia (or, in some regions, a serosa), a muscularis, and a mucosa.

Ureter

The ureters conduct urine from the renal pelvis to the urinary bladder. They serve not only as a route for the urine, but also contribute to its flow by means of their regular peristaltic contractions. The ureter enters the bladder obliquely so that contraction of the bladder to expel urine tends to close off the ureteral openings and force it out through the urethra.

The muscle of the ureter and in the other urinary excretory passages is smooth. It is arranged in bundles and these are generally disposed as an inner longitudinal layer, a circularly arranged middle layer, and an outer longitudinal layer.

The renal pelvis is partly inside the kidney and partly outside. In the unilobar kidney, it collects urine directly from the collecting ducts that open at the apex of the pyramid. In multilobar kidneys, the pelvis connects to tributaries, the major calyces, and by these to subtributaries, the minor calyces, which collect the urine from the pyramids.

Urinary Bladder

The urinary bladder is situated in the pelvic region of the abdominopelvic cavity. It contains three openings, two for the ureters and one for the urethra. The triangular region between these three openings, the *trigone,* is relatively smooth and constant, whereas the remainder of the bladder wall is thick when the bladder is empty and thinner when the bladder is distended. The arrangement of muscle layers in the muscularis is usually more difficult to ascertain than in the ureter. Muscle fibers around the urethral opening form an *internal sphincter* for this aperture.

On its superior aspect, the bladder is covered by peritoneum, and thus, this part of the bladder wall shows a serosa. Elsewhere, the outer layer of the urinary bladder consists of an adventitia. This adventitia, as well as that of other excretory passages (excluding the urethra), consists of fibroelastic connective tissue. In addition to afferent nerve supply, the urinary bladder receives both the sympathetic and parasympathetic innervation, and autonomic ganglia cells are present in the bladder adventitia.

Transitional epithelium. The mucosa of the calyces, ureters, and urinary bladder consist of a lamina propria of loose connective tissue and transitional epithelium (Fig. 19.16). Transitional epithelium displays two unique features. It forms an osmotic barrier between the hypertonic urine and the tissue fluids, and its cells possess a large reserve of surface membrane that is brought into position when the bladder is distended. Structurally, the special feature of transitional epithelium is the

presence of modified areas of plasma membrane designated as *plaques* (Fig. 19.17). These plaques, measuring about 12 nm, are thicker than normal membrane. They appear to be relatively rigid, and with special negative staining procedures for viewing with the TEM, they are seen to consist of hexagonal subunits. When the bladder is empty, the plaques fold inward, occupying space in the superficial reaches of the cell; when the bladder is distended, the plaques are returned to a surface position (Fig. 19.18). Filaments joined to the undersurface of the plaque are believed to prevent the undue stretching of the plaques in the distended bladder and participate in their infolding in the empty bladder. In thin sections (Fig. 19.17),

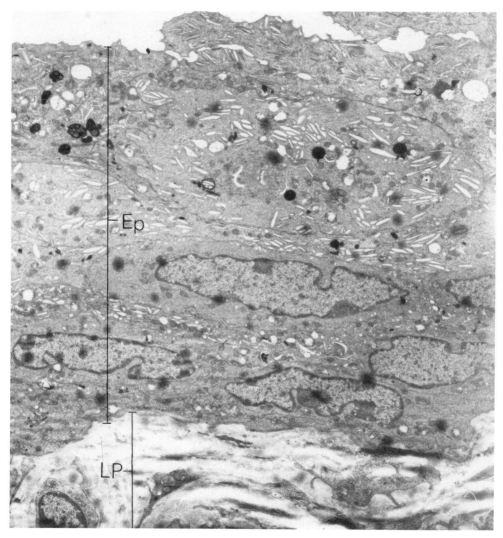

Figure 19.16. TEM of epithelial cells of the urinary bladder. The mucous membrane of the urinary bladder consists of transitional epithelium (Ep) with an underlying lamina propria (LP). The surface cells of transitional epithelium are large; the plasma membrane facing the lumen of the bladder possesses unique areas, designated plaques, seen at higher magnification in Figure 19.17. × 5000.

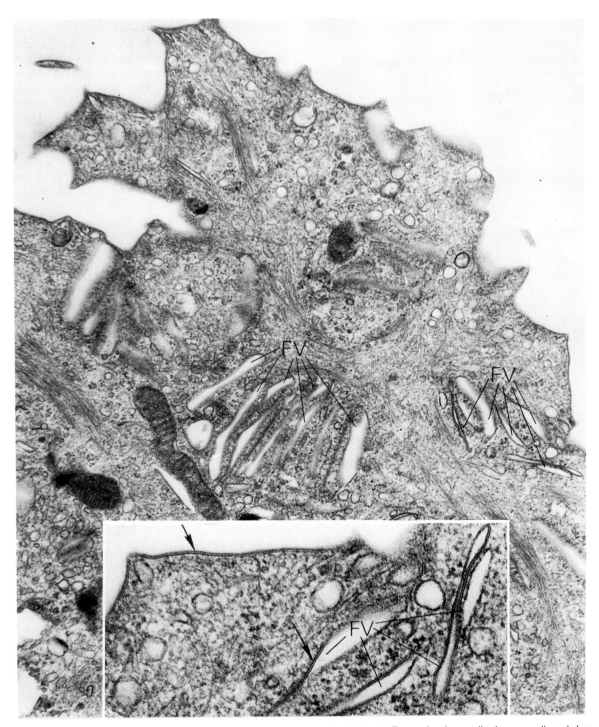

Figure 19.17. TEM of the apical region of a transitional epithelial cell. The cytoplasm displays small vesicles, filaments, and mitochondria, but the most distinctive feature of the cell is its fusiform-shaped vesicles (FV). At higher magnifications **(inset)**, the membrane forming the vesicles is seen to be similar to the plasma membrane of the cell surface **(arrows)**. Both of these are thickened and give the impression of possessing a degree of rigidity greater than that of plasma membrane in other locations. The thickened plasma membrane represents a sectioned view of a surface plaque. The fusiform vesicles are formed by the infolding of the plaques in the relaxed urinary bladder. × 27,000 **(inset** × 60,000).

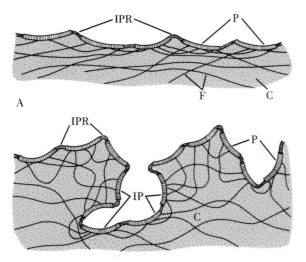

Figure 19.18. Diagrams of luminal surface of transitional epithelial cells in distended (A) and relaxed (B) bladder. The plasma membrane is thickened in regions to form plaques (P). The interplaque regions (IPR) consist of membrane that is not thickened. In the relaxed bladder, the plaques are invaginated into the cell and, although they retain their continuity with the surface, the invaginated plaques (IP) typically appear as isolated fusiform vesicles in electron micrographs. Filaments (F) attached to the undersurface of the plaques may prevent undue stretching in the distended bladder. (Modified from Staehelin LA, et al: *J Cell Biol* 53:73, 1972).

the infolded plaques appear as fusiform vesicles, their connections to the surface are usually not included in the plane of the section, thus the elongate vesicle-like appearance.

Urethra

The male urethra is divided into three parts: prostatic, membranous, and penile. The prostatic portion of the urethra passes through the prostate gland, and numerous ducts from the gland open into this part of the urethra (see also Chapter 21). On its posterior wall, there is a rounded elevation, the **seminal colliculus.** This is a small cul-de-sac, a vestige of the fused müllerian (paramesonephric) ducts. On its summit, the colliculus has an opening for the prostatic utricle and on either side are the openings of the ejaculatory ducts. The prostatic urethra is lined by transitional epithelium.

The membranous portion of the urethra is short; it penetrates the urogenital diaphragm. The latter contains striated muscle that serves as the **external sphincter** of the urethra. (The smooth muscle in the bladder wall surrounding the origin of the urethra serves as the **internal urethral sphincter).** The membranous portion of the urethra is lined by pseudostratified columnar epithelium.

The penile portion of the urethra is the longest portion. It extends through the corpus spongiosum of the penis. It is lined mostly with pseudostratified columnar epithelium, but near its opening the epithelium becomes stratified squamous. At its proximal end, two ducts of the bulbourethral glands open into the urethra; along its length mucus-secreting glands (of Littre) open into the urethra.

The female urethra is short, measuring from 3 to 5 cm in length. It is lined partly with pseudostratified columnar epithelium and partly with stratified squamous epithelium. The female urethra also penetrates the urogenital diaphragm and the striated muscle of this structure constitutes the external urethral sphincter. Smooth muscle fibers, chiefly around the origin of the urethra from the bladder, constitute the internal urethral sphincter.

ATLAS PLATES

93–98

PLATE 93. Kidney I

The kidney is a flattened, bean-shaped structure with a hilus on its medial border. Blood vessels, nerves, and lymphatic vessels enter or leave the kidney through the hilus; in addition, the funnel-shaped pelvis of the ureter leaves the kidney at the hilus. A section through the hilus is shown in **Figure 1.** The hilar region of the kidney is below and the convex lateral border is above. The outer part of the kidney (except at the hilus) has a reddish brown appearance; this is the cortex. It is easily distinguished from the inner portion, the medulla, which is further divided into an outer portion **(OM),** identified here by the presence of straight blood vessels, the vasa recta **(VR),** and an inner portion **(IM),** which has a light appearance. The medulla consists of pyramidal structures, the pyramids, which have their base facing the cortex and their apex in the form of a papilla **(P)** facing the hilar region of the kidney. The pyramids are separated, sometimes only partially as in **Figure 1,** by cortical material that is designated the renal columns **(RC).** Also to be noted is that the two pyramids depicted in the illustration share the same papilla. Most of the pyramid belonging to the other papilla, on the left, has not been included in the plane of the section. The papillae are free tips of the pyramids that project into the first of a series of large collecting vessels, the minor calyces **(MC);** the inner surface of the calyx is white. (Minor calyces drain into major calyces and, in turn, these open into the pelvis, which funnels into the ureter.)

An interesting feature of the kidney section shown in **Figure 1** is that the blood has been retained in many of the vessels, thereby allowing for a visualization of several renal vessels in their geographical location. Among the vessels that can be identified in the cut face of the kidney shown in **Figure 1** are the interlobular vessels **(IV)** within the cortex; the arcuate veins **(AV)** at the base of the

pyramids; and, in the medulla, the vessels going to and from the capillary network of the pyramid. The latter vessels, both arterioles and venules, are relatively straight and are designated collectively as the vasa rectae **(VR).**

A histological section including the cortex and part of the medulla is shown in **Figure 2.** Located at the boundary between the two (partly marked by the **dashed line**) are numerous profiles of arcuate arteries **(AA)** and arcuate veins **(AV).** The most distinctive feature of the renal cortex, regardless of the plane of section, are the renal corpuscles **(RC).** These are spherical structures comprised of the glomerulus surrounded by the Bowman's capsule. Also seen in the cortex are groups of tubules that are more or less straight and disposed in a radial directions from the base of the medulla **(arrows);** these are the medullary rays. In contrast, the medulla presents profiles of tubular structures that are arranged as gentle curves in the outer part of the medulla, turning slightly to become straight in the inner part of the medulla. The disposition of the tubules (and blood vessels) gives the cut face of the pyramid a slightly striated appearance that is also evident in the gross specimen **(Figure 1).**

PLATE 93

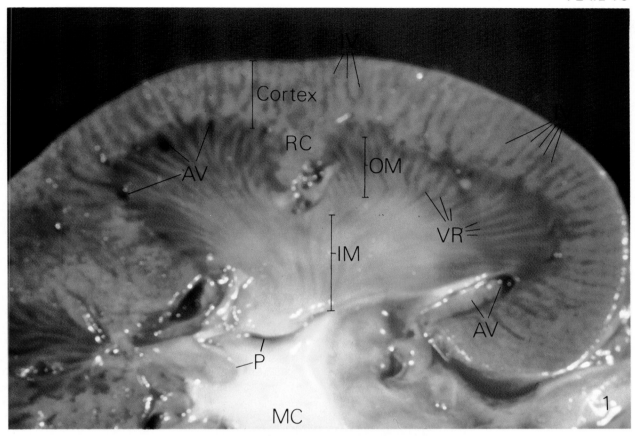

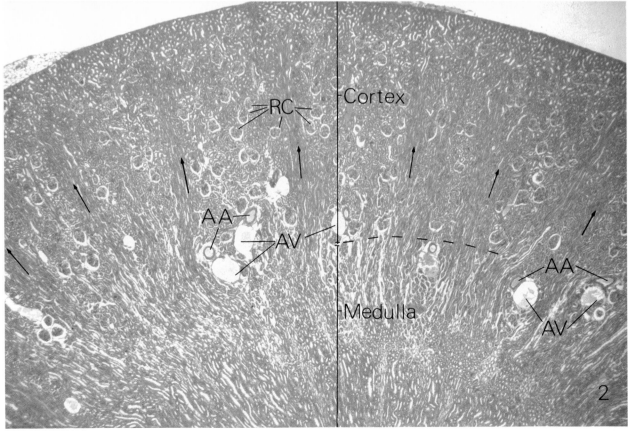

PLATE 94. Kidney II

The functional unit of the kidney is the nephron. It is made up of the following parts: the renal corpuscle (consisting of a glomerulus and Bowman's capsule) and the renal tubule, which itself consists of three major segments: the proximal thick segment (proximal convoluted tubule and the descending limb of Henle's loop); the thin segment; and the distal thick segment (ascending limb of Henle's loop, macula densa, and distal convoluted tubule). Nephrons empty into collecting ducts that drain into progressively slightly larger ducts that ultimately pass from the cortex into the pyramid, where they open at the papilla into a calyx. The collecting ducts opening at the papilla are called ducts of Bellini.

The renal cortex can be divided into regions referred to as the cortical labyrinth (CL) and the medullary rays (MR) (Fig. 1). The cortical labyrinth contains the renal corpuscles (RC), which appear as relatively large spherical structures. Surrounding each renal corpuscle are the proximal and distal convoluted tubules. They are also part of the cortical labyrinth. The convoluted tubules, particularly the proximal, because of their tortuosity, present a variety of profiles, most of which are oval or circular; but others, more elongate, are in the form of J, C, or even S shapes. The medullary rays are comprised of groups of straight tubules oriented in the same direction and appear to radiate from the base of the pyramid. When the medullary rays are cut longitudinally, as they are in **Figure 1,** the tubules present elongated profiles. The medullary rays contain proximal thick segments (descending limb of Henle's loop), distal thick segments (ascending limbs of Henle's loop), and collecting tubules.

At a somewhat higher magnification of the renal cortex **(Fig. 2),** but cut in a plane at a right angle to the section in **Figure 1,** is another profile of the renal cortex. The peripheral part of the micrograph shows the cortical labyrinth in which the tubules display chiefly round and oval profiles but also some that are more elongate and curved. The appearance is the same as the cortical labyrinth areas of **Figure 1.** (A renal corpuscle **(RC)** is also present in the cortical labyrinth). In contrast, the profiles presented by the tubules of the medullary ray in **Figure 2** are quite different from those seen in **Figure 1.** All of the tubules bounded by the **dashed line** belong to the medullary ray **(MR)** and they are all cut in cross-section.

A general survey of the tubules within the medullary ray reveals that several distinct types can be recognized based on the size of the tubule, shape of the lumen, and size of the tubule cells. These features as well as those of the cortical labyrinth will be considered in the following plate.

PLATE 94

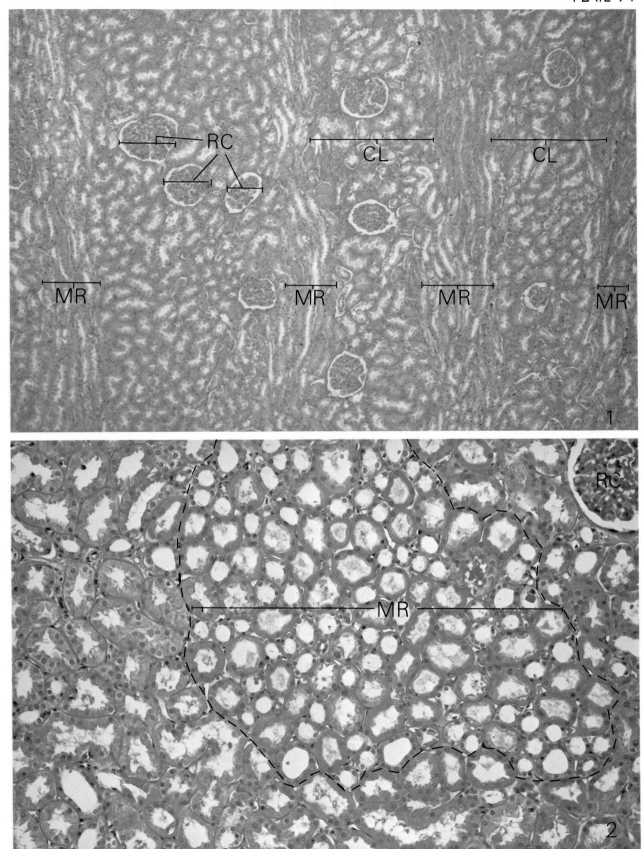

PLATE 95. Kidney III

Proximal and distal convoluted tubules display features that allow for their identification in H & E-stained paraffin sections. **(1)** The proximal convoluted tubule is more than twice as long and more tortuous than the distal convoluted tubule; thus, the majority of the tubular profiles in the cortical labyrinth will be proximal. In **Figure 1,** an area of cortical labyrinth, there are six distal convoluted **(DC)** tubule profiles (unlabeled). **(2)** The proximal tubules have a slightly larger outside diameter than distal tubules. **(3)** Proximal tubules have a brush border, whereas the distal tubules have a cleaner, sharper luminal surface. **(4)** The lumen of the proximal tubules is often star-shaped; this is not the case with distal tubules. **(5)** Typically fewer nuclei appear in a cross section of a proximal tubule than in an equivalent segment of a distal tubule.

Most of the above points can also be utilized in distinguishing the straight portions of the proximal and distal thick segments in the medullary rays. There are, however, certain differences. The medullary rays consist of tubules that are straight and parallel. Thus, instead of the occasional U, J, or S shapes seen in the cortical labyrinth, the proximal and distal thick segments within the medullary rays all display essentially the same profiles, be they rounded or elongate. For example, in **Figure 2** they are all rounded except for a proximal convoluted tubule (PC) included in the lower right corner of the figure (it belongs to the adjacent cortical labyrinth). Secondly, the number of proximal (P) and distal (D) tubular profiles are about equal in the medullary ray, as is shown by the labeling of each tubule in **Figure 2.** Note that, in contrast to the distal tubules, the proximal tubules display a brush border, they have a larger outside diameter, and many display a star-shaped lumen. The medullary ray also contains collecting tubules (CT). They will be considered in the next plate.

The renal corpuscle appears as a spherical structure whose periphery is comprised of a thin capsule that encloses a narrow clear-appearing space, the urinary space **(asterisks),** and a capillary tuft or glomerulus that appears as a large cellular mass **(Figs. 3 and 4).** The capsule of the renal corpuscle, known as Bowman's capsule, actually has two parts: a parietal layer, which is marked **(BC),** and a visceral layer. The parietal layer consists of simple squamous epithelial cells. The vis-

KEY

A, arteriole
BC, Bowman's capsule (parietal layer)
CT, collecting tubule
D, distal thick segment (straight portion)
DC, distal convoluted tubule
MD, macula densa
P, proximal thick segment (straight portion)

PC, proximal convoluted tubule
Pod, podocytes (visceral layer of Bowman's capsule)
asterisks, urinary space
double-headed arrow, blood vessel at vascular pole of renal corpuscle (Fig. 4).

Fig. 1, × 240
Fig. 2, × 240
Fig. 3, × 360
Fig. 4, × 360 (all human).

ceral layer consists of cells, called podocytes **(Pod),** which lie on the outer surface of the glomerular capillary. Except where they clearly line the urinary space as the labeled cells do in **Figure 3,** podocytes may be difficult to distinguish from the capillary endothelial cells. To complicate matters, the mesangial cells are also a component of the glomerulus. In general, nuclei of podocytes are larger and stain less intensely than the endothelial and mesangial cells.

A distal **(DC)** and two proximal **(PC)** convoluted tubules are marked in **Figure 3.** The cells of the distal tubule are more crowded on one side, as is also the case in the adjacent distal tubule. These crowded cells constitute the macula densa **(MD)** of the distal thick segment. The macula densa is adjacent to the afferent arteriole.

In **Figure 4,** both the vascular pole and the urinary pole of the renal corpuscle are evident. The vascular pole is characterized by the presence of arterioles **(A),** one of which is entering or leaving **(double-headed arrow)** the corpuscle. The afferent arteriole possesses modified smooth muscle cells with granules, the juxtaglomerular cells (not evident in **Fig. 4).** At the urinary pole, the parietal layer of Bowman's capsule is continuous with the beginning of the proximal convoluted tubule (PC). Here the urinary space of the renal corpuscle continues into the lumen of the proximal tubule, and the lining cells change from simple squamous to simple cuboidal or low columnar with a brush border.

PLATE 95

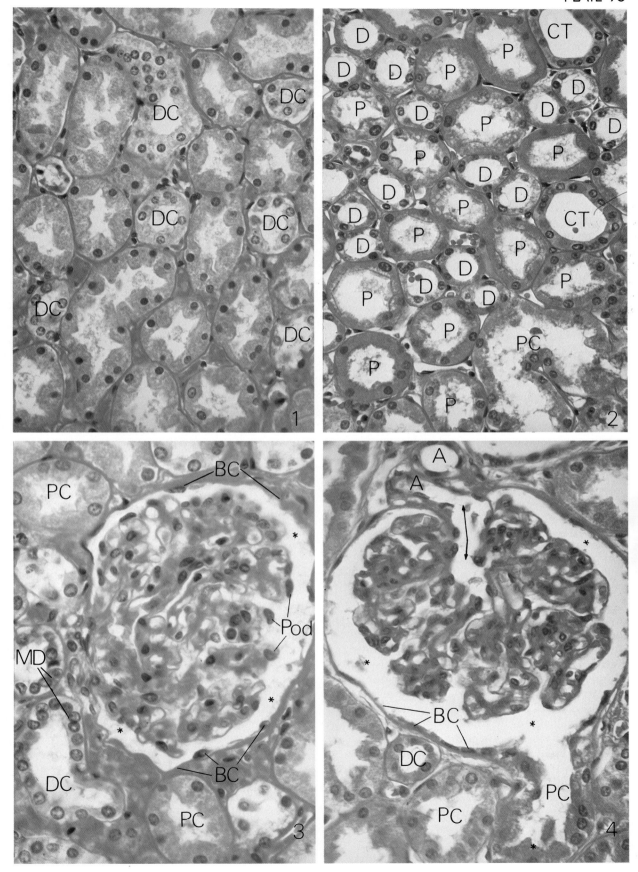

PLATE 96. Kidney IV

A section through the outer portion of the medulla is shown in **Figure 1.** This region contains proximal and distal thick segments, thin segments, and collecting tubules. All of the tubules are parallel and all are cut in cross-section; thus, they present circular profiles. The proximal **(P)** thick segments display typical star-shaped lumens and a brush border (or the fragmented apical cell surface from which the brush border has been partially broken). These tubules have outside diameters that are generally larger than those of the distal tubules **(D).** As mentioned previously, and as noted in **Figure 1,** the distal tubules display a larger number of nuclei than do comparable segments of proximal tubule cells. Also, it should again be noted that the lumen of the distal tubule is more rounded and the apical surface of the cells is sharper. The collecting tubules **(CT)** have outer diameters that are about the same as those of the proximal tubules and larger than those of distal tubules. The cells forming the collecting tubules are cuboidal and smaller than those of proximal tubules; thus, they also display a relatively large number of nuclei than comparable segments of proximal tubule cells. Count them! Finally, boundaries between the cells which constitute the collecting tubules are usually evident **(asterisks),** and this serve as one of the most dependable features for the identification of collecting tubules.

The thin segments **(T)** have the thinnest walls of all renal tubules seen in the medulla. They are formed by a low cuboidal or simple squamous epithelium, as seen in **Figure 1,** and the lumens are relatively large. Occasionally a section includes the region of transition from a thick to a thin segment and can be recognized even in a cross-section through the tubule. One such junction is evident in **Figure 1** (the tubule with **two arrows** in the lumen). On one side, the tubule cell **(arrow pointing to left)** is characteristic of the proximal segment, and it possesses a distinctive brush border; the other side of the tubule **(arrow pointing to right)** is comprised of low cuboidal cells that resemble the cells forming the thin segments. In addition to the renal and collecting tubules, there are many other small tubular structures in **Figure 1.** Thin-walled and lined by endothelium, they are small blood vessels. These vessels (along with the loops of Henle and collecting tubules) play an important role in the countercurrent mechanism that concentrates urine in the pyramids.

Figure 2 shows a renal pyramid at low magnification. The pyramid is a conical structure com-

KEY

AV, arcuate vessels
CT, collecting tubules
D, distal thick segment
P, proximal thick segment
RC, renal corpuscle
SCEp, simple columnar epithelium
T, thin segment
TEp, transitional epithelium
arrow pointing to left, proximal tubule cell (Fig. 1)

arrow pointing to right, thin segment cell (Fig. 1)
arrowhead, location of apex of pyramid
asterisks, boundaries between cells of collecting tubule
diamonds, boundary between transitional and columnar epithelium

Fig. 1, human, × 240   **Fig. 2,** human, × 20.

prised principally of medullary straight tubules, ducts, and the straight blood vessels (vasa recta). The **dashed line** at the left of the micrograph is placed at the junction between cortex and medulla; thus, it marks the base of the pyramid. Note the arcuate vessels **(AR)** that lie at the boundary of cortex and medulla. They define the boundary line. The few renal corpuscles **(RC),** upper left, belong to the medulla they are referred to as juxtamedullary corpuscles.

The pyramid is somewhat distorted in this specimen as evidenced by regions of longitudinally sectioned tubules, lower left, and cross- and oblique-sectioned tubules in other regions. In effect, part of the pyramid was bent, thus the change in the plane of section of the tubules.

The apical portion of the pyramid, known as the renal papilla, is lodged in a cup or funnel-like structure referred to as the calyx. It collects the urine that leaves the tip of the papilla from the papillary ducts (of Bellini). (The actual tip of the papilla is not seen within the plane of section, nor are the openings of the ducts at this low magnification.) The surface of the papilla that faces the lumen of the calyx is simple columnar or cuboidal epithelium **(SCEp).** (In places, this epithelium has separated from the surface of the papilla and appears as a thin strand of tissue.) The calyx is lined by transitional epithelium **(TEp).** Although not evident in the low magnification shown here, the boundary between the columnar epithelium covering the papilla and the transitional epithelium covering the inner surface of the calyx is marked by the **diamonds.**

PLATE 96

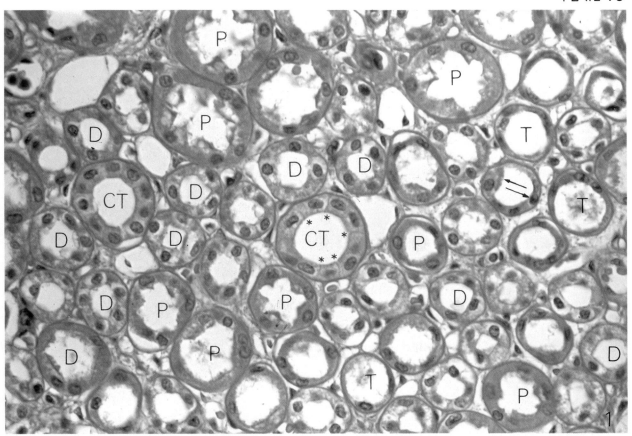

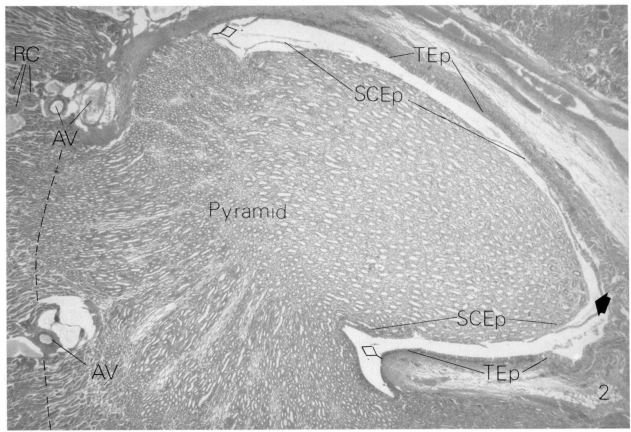

PLATE 97. Ureter

The ureters are paired tubular structures that convey urine from the kidneys to the urinary bladder. They not only serve as a route to the bladder but they contribute to the flow of urine by means of their regular peristaltic activity.

As shown in **Figure 1,** the adjacent low-power orientation micrograph, the wall of the ureter consists of a mucosa **(Muc)**, a muscularis **(Mus),** and an adventitia **(Adv).** It should be noted that the ureters are located behind the peritoneum of the abdominal cavity in their course to the bladder. Thus, a serosa **(Ser)** may be found covering a portion of the circumference of the tube. Also, due to contraction of smooth muscle of the muscularis, the lumenal surface is characteristically folded, thus creating a star-shaped lumen.

The wall of the ureter is examined at higher magnification in **Figure 2.** One can immediately recognize the thick epithelial lining, which appears distinct and sharply delineated from the remainder of the wall. This is the transitional epithelium **(Ep).** The remainder of the wall is made up of connective tissue **(CT)** and smooth muscle. The latter can be recognized as the darker-staining layer. The section also shows some adipose tissue **(AT),** a component of the adventitia.

The transitional epithelium and its supporting connective tissue constitute the mucosa **(Muc).** A distinct submucosa is not present, although the term is sometimes applied to the connective tissue that is closest to the muscle.

The muscularis **(Mus)** is arranged as an inner longitudinal layer **[SM(l)],** a middle circular layer **[SM(c)],** and an outer longitudinal layer **[SM(l)].** However, the outer longitudinal layer is present only at the lower end of the ureter. In a cross-section through the ureter, the inner and outer smooth muscle layers are cut in cross-section, whereas the circular middle layer of muscle cells is cut longitudinally. This is as they appear in **Figure 2. Figure 3** shows the inner longitudinal smooth muscle layer **[SM(l)]** at higher magnification. Note that the nuclei appear as round profiles, indicating that the muscle cells have been cross-sectioned.

Figure 3 also shows the transitional epithelium to advantage. The surface cells are characteristically the largest and some are binucleate **(arrow).** The basal cells are the smallest and, typically, the nuclei appear crowded due to the minimal cytoplasm of each cell. The intermediate cells appear to consist of several layers and are comprised of cells larger in size than the basal cells but smaller than the surface cells.

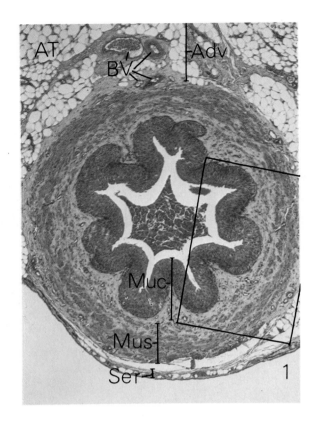

KEY	
A, artery	**Mus,** muscularis
Adv, adventitia	**Ser,** serosa
AT, adipose tissue	**SM(c),** circular layer of
BV, blood vessels	smooth muscle
CT, connective tissue	**SM(l),** longitudinal layer
Ep, transitional	of smooth muscle
epithelium	**arrow, Fig. 3,** binucleate
Muc, mucosa	surface cell
Fig. 1, × 35	**Fig. 3,** × 400.
Fig. 2, × 160	All monkey.

PLATE 97

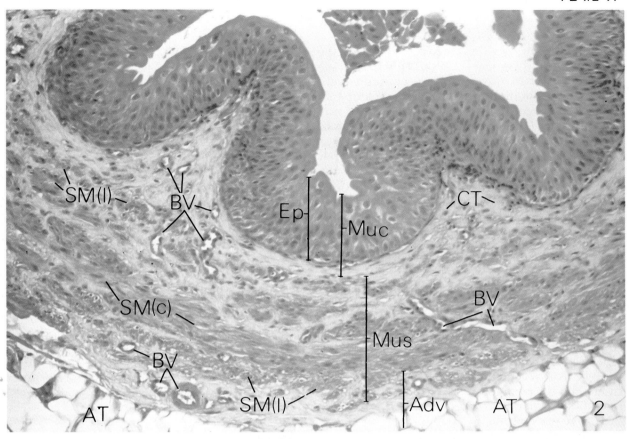

SM(l) BV Ep Muc CT
SM(c) Mus
BV BV
AT SM(l) Adv AT **2**

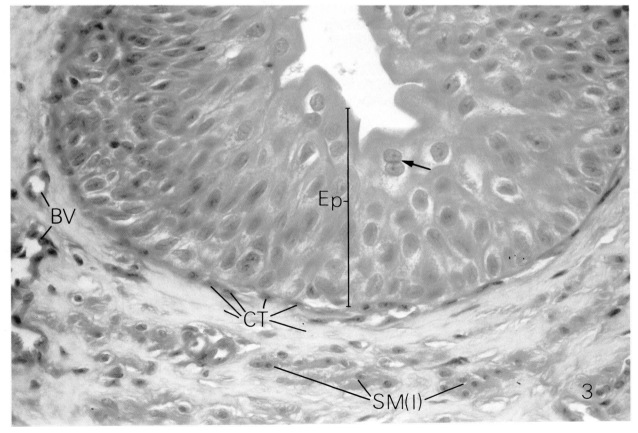

BV Ep CT SM(l) **3**

PLATE 98. Urinary Bladder

The urinary bladder receives urine from the two ureters and stores it until it is discharged via the urethra. Its structure reflects these functions. It possesses a lining of transitional epithelium that adapts to changes in bladder volume, and the wall contains bundles of smooth muscle that functions in the discharge of urine.

The full thickness of the urinary bladder is illustrated in **Figure 1.** It shows the mucosa (**Muc**), the muscularis (**Mus**), and the serosa (**S**). The mucosa consists of transitional epithelium (**Ep**) and its supporting connective tissue (**CT**). A distinct submucosa is not present, although, as with the ureter, the connective tissue closest to the muscle is sometimes referred to as a submucosa. The muscularis consists of smooth muscle which, like that of the ureter, is arranged in three layers: an inner longitudinal [**SM(L)**], middle circular [**SM(C)**], and outer longitudinal [**SM(L)**]. The smooth muscle in this preparation stains more in intensely than the connective tissue. On the basis of organization, the bundles of smooth muscle cells can be recognized because they are surrounded by connective tissue (**CT**). This relationship is especially evident when the smooth muscle is cut obliquely or in cross-section. When the smooth muscle is cut longitudinally, the relationship is less evident, but then the elongated profiles of the smooth muscle cell nuclei serve as a diagnostic feature. Another extremely useful criterion for distinguishing smooth muscle from connective tissue in **Figure 1** is that the number of nuclei in a given area of smooth muscle (**white circle**) is greater than the number of nuclei in a comparable area of connective tissue (**black circle**).

A serosa is present on the upper surface of the bladder; it consists of a layer of simple squamous epithelium (mesothelium) that rests on a small amount of supporting connective tissue. Else-

KEY

CT, connective tissue
Ep, epithelium
Lym, lymphocytes
Muc, mucosa
Mus, muscularis
S, serosa

SM(C), circular layer of
   smooth muscle
SM(L), longitudinal layer
   of smooth muscle
arrows, binucleate cells

Fig. 1, × 65
Fig. 2, × 160

Fig. 3, × 640.
All monkey.

where, the outer layer of the wall consists of a fibrous adventitia.

The **rectangle** in **Figure 1** and in **Figure 2** indicates areas that are shown at higher magnification in **Figures 2 and 3,** respectively, to demonstrate the transitional epithelium. In the contracted state, the epithelium (Ep) is characterized by the presence of dome-shaped cells at the free surface and large numbers of pear-shaped cells immediately under the surface cells. The cells at the surface are large and sometimes have two nuclei (**arrows**). The deeper cells, on the other hand, are smaller. Because of the absence of connective tissue papillae, the epithelial-connective tissue junction is rather even. An aggregation of lymphocytes (**Lym**) is immediately under the epithelial surface. This is not an unusual observation.

The thickness of the transitional epithelium depends on the degree of bladder (or ureteral) distention. In the empty ureter or bladder, it appears to be about five cells deep. However, when they are distended, it appears to have a thickness of only three cells, a basal layer, an intermediate cell layer, and a surface cell layer.

PLATE 98

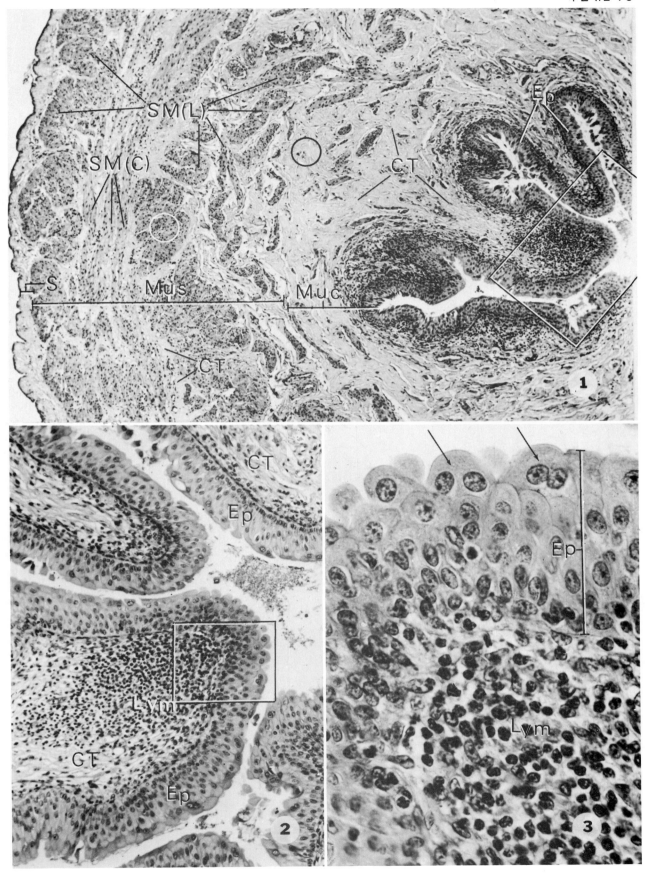

Endocrine Organs

20

In multicellular organisms, intercellular communication is necessary to maintain homeostasis (physiological balance or equilibrium), to coordinate normal growth and development, to adapt to internal and external environmental stress, and to contribute to the processes of sexual reproduction. Two communication systems—the nervous system and the endocrine system—have evolved to satisfy this need. These two systems are closely interrelated and may overlap in their function as they coordinate the activities of various cellular systems. The interaction of the nervous and endocrine systems is coordinated at the hypothalamus, which is one of the major controlling centers for the autonomic nervous system.

The nervous system communicates through neural impulse transmission and the local release of neurotransmitters in the immediate vicinity of the target cell. In general, the nervous system induces a rapid and localized response. The endocrine system communicates through the release of **hormones,** secretory products that pass into the circulatory system and are transported to target cells. It induces a slower and less localized response as specific target cells, tissues, or organs respond to an individual hormone. Each hormone elicits a response from cells that possess receptors for that specific hormone. Classically, endocrine glands have been defined as being ductless glands, because they release their secretory products directly into the blood or lymph. In contrast, exocrine glands have ducts to convey their secretory products.

Over 50 hormones have been identified as products of the cells of the endocrine system. Chemically, these hormones can be divided into three classes: steroid hormones, protein (peptide) hormones, and amino acid analogues and derivatives.

Steroid hormones (for example, testosterone and estradiol) are produced by cells that originate from embryonic mesodermal tissue. Glands that secrete steroid hormones include the ovaries, testes, and adrenal cortex.

Protein hormones (for example, insulin and prolactin) are produced by cells that most likely originate from endodermal tissue of the gastrointestinal tract with the exception of the adenohypophysis, which originates from ectodermal tissue of the oral cavity. Glands that secrete peptide hormones include the hypophysis (or pituitary), thyroid, parathyroid, and pancreas. Peptide hormones are also secreted by scattered endocrine cells present in the epithelial lining of the gastrointestinal tract and lungs.

Amino acid analogues and derivatives (for example, norepinephrine, epinephrine, and thyroxine) are structurally simple substances. Glands that secrete these hormones include the thyroid and adrenal medulla. Chemically, norepinephrine and epinephrine are classified as catecholamines. Norepinephrine is also the neurotransmitter found in most of the postganglionic sympathetic nerve fibers.

The components of the endocrine system vary greatly in their organization and include: (1) the discrete endocrine glands—hypophysis, thyroid, parathyroid, adrenal, and pineal; (2) the endocrine component of glands with both exocrine and endocrine function—kidney, pancreas, gonads, and placenta (a unique transitory form of this type of gland); and (3) scattered cells with endocrine function, known as the **diffuse neuroendocrine system.**

This chapter will deal primarily with a description of the discrete endocrine glands. A common structural feature of these glands is an exceptionally rich blood supply, the bloodstream providing the route not only for the supply of metabolites

---

DIFFUSE NEUROENDOCRINE SYSTEM

The diffuse neuroendocrine system is composed of hormone-secreting cells that synthesize structurally related peptides and active amines. These products act as hormones or neurotransmitters. Histochemical and cytochemical studies have revealed that these cells demonstrate the presence of common enzyme systems involved in amine handling and the production of their common secretory peptides. The cells are identified as APUD (amine precursor uptake and decarboxylation) cells. The APUD cells may act upon contiguous or nearby cells (paracrine) or upon distant cells (endocrine). APUD cells are present in the hypothalamus, adenohypophysis, pineal, parathyroids, thyroid, adrenals, placenta, pancreas, stomach, intestine, lungs, urogenital tract, skin, carotid body, and sympathetic ganglia. Early in embryonic de-velopment the APUD cells are programmed for their neuroendocrine function. Clinically, the common neuroendocrine programming of the APUD cells has been suggested to explain the excessive production of a hormone by endocrine cells that are not normally the source of that hormone. Symptoms of cancers are often associated with the production of excessive amounts of peptide hormones in tissues that do not normally produce significant amounts of hormones. Although APUD cells in neoplastic tissue may be the source of the ectopic hormones, the mechanism by which genes are expressed in these cells is not known. APUD cells are found in many tumors including oat cell carcinoma of the lung, thymomas, and carcinoid tumors.

---

from which the hormones are synthesized, but also for the transport of the released hormones. Descriptions of the endocrine components of glands and cells with endocrine function are included in the chapters on the digestive, respiratory, urinary, and reproductive systems. Th endocrine cells of the gastrointestinal tract and pancreas, referred to as the gastroenteropancreatic (GEP) system (see page 436), collectively represent the largest endocrine gland in the body. It should also be noted that endocrine cells of the gastrointestinal tract may influence the activity of adjacent epithelial cells via the local diffusion of a peptide to its target cells through the extracellular space (*paracrine* control). By definition, *endocrine* control involves the circulatory system to transport the hormone.

HYPOPHYSIS (PITUITARY GLAND)

The hypophysis, or pituitary gland, is a compound endocrine gland suspended from the hypothalamus and located in the sella turcica, a depression in the bony floor of the cranial cavity. A short stalk, the *infundibulum,* attaches the pituitary to the hypothalamus. This small gland, which is about the size of a pea, is often referred to as the "master gland" because it produces several hormones that influence the activity of other endocrine glands.

The hypophysis may be divided into a glandular portion, the *adenohypophysis,* and a neural portion, the *neurohypophysis.* The embryological development of the hypophysis explains the presence of these two distinct tissue types. The adenohypophysis is derived from an outpocketing (called Rathke's pouch) of the ectoderm of the primitive oral cavity; the neurohypophysis, from an outpocketing of the neuroectoderm of the primitive brain (specifically, the diencephalon) (Fig. 20.1).

The adenohypophysis is further divided into a **pars distalis,** which comprises the bulk of the adenohypophysis, a **pars tuberalis,** and a **pars intermedia.** The neurohypophysis is divided into a **pars nervosa** and the infundibulum. The latter forms the stalk of the hypophysis. Additionally, the pars distalis and pars tuberalis are considered to be the **anterior lobe** of the gland, and the pars nervosa and pars intermedia are called the **posterior lobe.**

Blood Supply

A knowledge of the unusual blood supply of the hypophysis is essential in understanding its activities. The hypophysis is supplied by two sets of vessels (Fig. 20.2): several *superior hypophyseal arteries* and a pair of *inferior hypophyseal arteries.* The inferior hypophyseal arteries primarily supply the pars nervosa, although some branches anastomose with branches of the superior hypophyseal arteries to supply the lower part of the infundibulum. The superior hypophyseal arteries supply the median eminence, the upper part of the infundibulum, and the lower part of the infundibulum (through the connection with the inferior hypophyseal arteries). It should be noted that both the superior and inferior hypophyseal arteries supply the neurohypophysis. In contrast, most of the anterior lobe of the hypophysis has no direct arterial supply.

The arteries that supply the median eminence and the infundibulum end in capillary plexuses

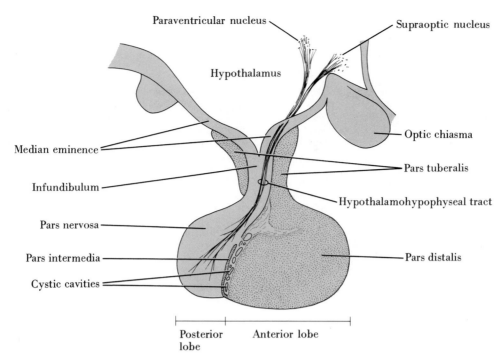

Figure 20.1. Drawing of a section through the human pituitary and related regions of the hypothalamus. The adenohypophysis consists of the pars distalis, pars tuberalis, and pars intermedia; the neurohypophysis consists of the infundibulum and pars nervosa. (Based on Junqueira LC, Carneiro J: *Basic Histology,* 3rd ed. Los Altos, CA, Lange, 1980.)

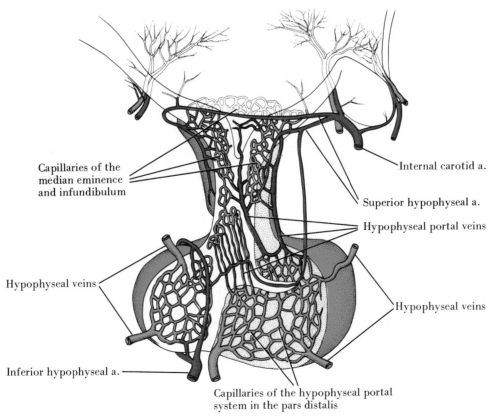

Figure 20.2. Diagram of the blood supply to the pituitary. The hypophyseal portal veins are indicated. The hypophyseal portal veins begin in the capillary beds of the median eminence and infundibulum and end in the capillaries of the pars distalis. (Based on Junqueira LC, Carneiro J: *Basic Histology,* 3rd ed. Los Altos, CA, Lange, 1980.)

HORMONAL REGULATING FACTORS

The release of hormones from the adeno-hypophysis is regulated by the hypothalamus through the release of **hypothalamic regulating factors** (hormones) into the hypophyseal portal veins. These hypothalamic regulating factors can stimulate secretion (**releasing factors**) or inhibit it (**inhibitory factors**). The regulating factors are produced in the cells of the hypothalamus in response to circulating levels of hormones. Thus, the cells of the adenohypophysis can be selectively inhibited or stimulated. A simple negative feedback system controls the synthesis and discharge of the releasing factors. Consider the production of thyroid hormones (Fig. 20.3). If blood levels of thyroid hormones are high, thyrotropin-releasing factor

(TRF) is not produced or released. If blood levels of thyroid hormones are low, the hypothalamus discharges TRF into the hypophyseal portal vein. This stimulates specific cells within the adenohypophysis to produce thyroid-stimulating hormone (TSH), or thyrotropin, which, in turn, stimulates the thyroid to produce and release more thyroid hormone. As the thyroid hormone level rises, the negative feedback system stops the hypothalamus from discharging TRF. Most of the tropic hormones produced by the adenohypophysis are regulated by releasing factors. Prolactin production is regulated by an inhibitory factor, that is, prolactin secretion is tonically inhibited by the release of prolactin-inhibiting factor (PIF) by the hypothalamus.

(primary capillary plexuses). These areas are drained by portal veins, known as the *hypophyseal portal veins.* The veins pass to the pars distalis and end in a secondary capillary plexus. This system of vessels provides a route for neurosecretory substances released from hypothalamic nerve endings in the median eminence and infundibular stem to pass to cells in the pars distalis. Evidence suggests

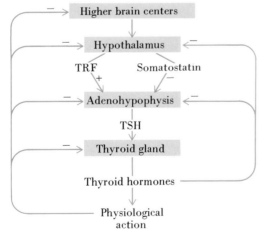

Figure 20.3. Hypothalamic-adenohypophysis-thyroid interaction. Production of thyroid hormones is regulated through a negative feedback system. Both the thyroid hormones and the physiological actions that they induce, such as an increase in the metabolic rate, can feedback on the system and inhibit further release of thyroid hormones. Such inhibition may occur at the level of the thyroid gland, adenohypophysis, hypothalamus, or higher brain centers. The system is activated in response to low thyroid hormone levels or in response to metabolic needs.

that blood flow may be reversed within hypophyseal portal veins, thus establishing a vascular route for feedback between the various endocrine components and the brain.

Electron microscopic studies have established that the capillaries of both the anterior and posterior lobes of the hypophysis are fenestrated. This feature presumably allows passage of the neurosecretory substances. The venous blood leaving the hypophysis carries the hormones to target cells in various parts of the body.

Adenohypophysis

The adenohypophysis synthesizes and releases several hormones in response to signals from the hypothalamus (Table 20.1). Most of the hormones are called *tropic hormones* because they influence the activity of cells in other target glands and tissues. Although a description of the complex metabolic effects of these hormones is beyond the scope of this chapter, general effects are indicated in the table to aid in correlating structure and function.

Cell Types. Earlier histologists distinguished various cell types within the adenohypophysis on the basis of staining properties of cells exposed to mixtures of acidic and basic dyes (Fig. 20.4). It is important to note that the identification of cells as *basophilic* or *acidophilic* refers to the binding affinity of the specific granules in the cells and *not* to the binding affinity of cytoplasmic ribonucleoproteins or other cytoplasmic constituents. Based on these binding affinities two general classes of cells were identified: (1) *chromophobes,* which show little affinity for the dyes and (2) *chromophils,* which stain strongly. The chromophilic cells that

TABLE 20.1. Hormones of the Adenohypophysis

HORMONE[a]	SOURCE (CELL TYPE)		FUNCTIONS[b]
	GENERAL	SPECIFIC	
Adrenocorticotropic hormone (ACTH), or adrenocorticotropin, or corticotropin	Basophil	Adrenocortico-lipotrop (or ACTH/LPH cell)	Stimulates production of glucocorticoids by cells of the adrenal cortex
Lipotropic hormone (LPH), or lipotropin	Basophil	Adrenocortico-lipotrop	Unknown in the human
Thyroid-stimulating hormone (TSH), or thyrotropin	Basophil	Thyrotrop	Stimulates production of thyroid hormones
Follicle-stimulating hormone (FSH)	Basophil	Gonadotrop	In females, stimulates growth of the ovarian follicles; in males, activates spermatogenesis
Luteinizing hormone (LH); or luteotropin (LH) in the female, also known as interstitial cell-stimulating hormone (ICSH) in the male	Basophil	Gonadotrop	In females, essential for ovulation, formation of the corpus luteum, and stimulation of steroid hormone production by the follicle and corpus luteum; in males, stimulates interstitial (Leydig) cells in the testes to produce androgens (particularly testosterone)
Growth hormone (GH)	Acidophil	Somatotrop	Stimulates body growth, particularly growth of long bones
Prolactin (PR), or lactogenic hormone (LTH)	Acidophil	Lactotrop (or mammatrop)	Promotes mammary gland development and lactation

[a] All hormones listed are peptide hormones.
[b] The purpose of this list is to orient the student in terms of basic function and, therefore, only major functions are given.

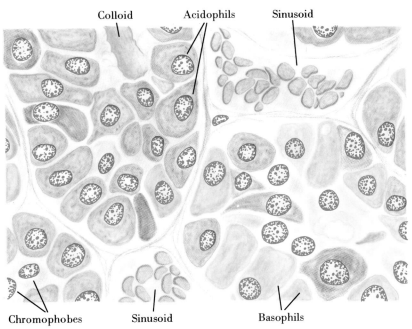

Figure 20.4. Drawing of cells within the human adenohypophysis. The drawing is of a histological section stained with aldehyde fuchsin-fast green-orange G. Acidophils appear orange; basophils, blue. Chromophobes appear lightly stained. The cords of cells are surrounded by a thin layer of connective tissue and sinusoids. (Based on *Bailey's Textbook of Histology,* 18th ed. Baltimore, Williams & Wilkins, 1984.)

567

bound acidic dyes were classed as *acidophils;* those that bound basic dyes, as *basophils.*

With recent advances in immunocytochemistry, it has been possible to identify the cells on the basis of the hormones they contain. The cell types identified on the basis of staining properties and immunolabeling are indicated for the adenohypophyseal hormones listed in Table 20.1. Immunolabeling studies have demonstrated that in two cases a single cell type produces more than one hormone: the adrenocorticolipotrops produce both adrenocorticotropic hormone (ACTH) and LPH and gonadotrops produce both lipotropic hormone (LH) and follicle-stimulating hormone (FSH).

The *pars distalis* constitutes about 75 percent of the hypophysis. It contains cells arranged in cords adjacent to large-bore, thin-walled, fenestrated capillaries. Although relatively little connective tissue is present among the cords of cells, the anterior lobe is surrounded by a dense connective capsule.

At least five distinct cell types have been identified within the pars distalis, based on immunocytochemical studies (Table 20.1): (1) somatotropic cells (acidophils), which secrete growth hormone (GH); (2) lactotropic cells (acidophils), which secrete prolactin; (3) gonadotropic cells (basophils), which secrete both LH and FSH, increase in number at puberty, and demonstrate subtle changes in women during the menstrual cycle; (4) thyrotropic cells (basophils), which secrete thyroid-stimulating hormone (TSH); and (5) adenocorticolipotropic cells (basophils), which secrete both ACTH and LPH. The chromophobes are considered to be reserve or transitory cells.

The *somatotrops* are the most common type of acidophilic cells. They are small, rounded cells with highly refractile granules that stain immunocytochemically for GH. They are most numerous in the posterolateral aspect of the pars distalis. The *lactotrops* are highly variable acidophilic cells that are scattered and wedged between adjacent cells in the cords. These cells undergo hypertrophy during lactation. At this time, they contain large secretion granules (approximately 600 nm in diameter).

The most common type of basophilic cells are *adrenocorticolipotrops.* They are usually round or oval cells whose granules are intensely periodic acid-Schiff (PAS)-positive and stain immunochemically for ACTH and LPH. These cells are most common in the anteromedian aspect of the pars distalis. The *thyrotrops* are large, irregularly shaped basophilic cells confined to the anteromedial aspect of the pars distalis. The granules of these cells stain intensely with aldehyde thionine. The *gonadotrops* are small basophilic cells that are most common in the posterolateral aspect of the pars distalis. The granules, which stain with aldehyde thionine and PAS, stain immunocytochemically for LH and FSH.

Ultrastructurally, the various acidophils and basophils demonstrate the presence of a moderately well-developed endoplasmic reticulum and Golgi complexes as well as secretion granules. Although the differences in the sizes of the secretion granules have been suggested as a criterion for distinguishing the various cell types, the overlap in granule size is so great that definitive identification requires immunocytochemical staining.

The *pars intermedia* demonstrates considerable species variation in its structure. In the human, it is located just posterior to a cleft or series of small cystic cavities that represent the residual lumen of Rathke's pouch. It contains basophilic and chromophobic cells (Fig. 20.5). These cells,

Figure 20.5. Drawing of a section through the pars intermedia of an adult human pituitary gland. Cords of basophilic (darkly staining) and chromophobic (lightly staining) cells grow into the neural lobe. Vesicles filled with colloid (black) are present within some of the cords of cells. (Based on *Bailey's Textbook of Histology,* 18th ed. Baltimore, Williams & Wilkins, 1984.)

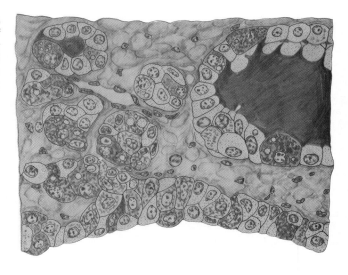

possessing cilia, commonly line the cysts that are filled with colloidal material. Extension of the basophilic cells into the pars nervosa is also seen in the human.

The function of the cells of the pars intermedia in the human remains unclear. In amphibians, the basophilic cells produce melanocyte-stimulating hormone (MSH) that stimulates pigment production in melanocytes. In humans, MSH does not appear to be a distinct hormone, but it is probably a product of LPH cleavage. Therefore, these basophilic cells are most likely adrenocorticolipotrops.

The *pars tuberalis* forms a sleeve around the infundibular stem (Fig. 20.1), which is about 25 to 60 μm thick. It is a highly vascular structure with cords or clusters of chromophilic and chromophobic cells associated with blood vessels, which include veins of the hypophyseal portal system. Nests of squamous cells and small follicles lined with cuboidal cells are scattered in the pars tuberalis. Gonadotrops are the most common functional cells present in this region.

Neurohypophysis

The cells of the neurohypophysis produce two peptide hormones: *oxytocin* and *antidiuretic hormone* (ADH), or *vasopressin.* The release of these substances into the systemic circulation is regulated by the hypothalamus and higher brain levels. General functions of the hormones are listed in Table 20.2. It should be noted that even though oxytocin does stimulate smooth muscle contraction in the pregnant uterus, this may not be a normal physio-

logical function of the hormone. ADH basically affects the permeability of the distal convoluted tubules and collecting ducts of the kidney and thus controls water absorption from these ducts. Individuals producing low levels of ADH (diabetes insipidus) excrete large amounts of dilute urine and suffer from extreme thirst.

The neurohypophysis consists of the posterior lobe, the infundibular stem, and the median eminence. It contains *pituicytes* and *axonal processes* of unmyelinated nerve fibers whose cell bodies are located in the paraventricular and supraoptic nuclei of the hypothalamus. The axonal processes (approximately 100,000) converge at the median eminence forming a bundle of fibers known as the *hypothalamohypophyseal tract* and pass through the infundibular stem to reach the pars nervosa (see Fig. 20.1). These nerve fibers are unusual in that they do not end on other neurons or effector cells, but end blindly close to vessels of the rich capillary plexus of the pars nervosa (Fig. 20.6). As was noted earlier, the capillaries of the hypophysis are fenestrated. The circular fenestrations in the attenuated endothelium are closed by thin diaphragms.

The terminal portions of axonal processes are expanded and commonly contain numerous secretory granules (100 to 300 nm in diameter), known as *Herring bodies* (Fig. 20.7). The neurosecretory substances contained in these granules are believed to be synthesized in the cell bodies and then transported through the axons to the nerve terminals where they are released in response to hypothalamic nerve impulses. The released hormonal substances transverse the perivascular space, enter

TABLE 20.2. Hormones of the Neurohypophysis

HORMONE[a]	SOURCE	FUNCTION
Oxytocin	Cell bodies of neurons located in the supraoptic and paraventricular nuclei of the hypothalamus[b]	Stimulates activity of the contractile cells around the ducts of the mammary glands to eject milk from the glands; stimulates contraction of smooth muscle cells in the pregnant uterus
Antidiuretic hormone (ADH) or vasopressin	Cell bodies of neurons located in the supraoptic and paraventricular nuclei of the hypothalamus[b]	Decreases urine volume by causing the kidneys to remove water from newly formed urine; decreases the rate of perspiration in response to dehydration; causes rise in blood pressure by stimulating contractions of smooth muscle cells in the wall of arterioles

[a] Oxytocin and ADH are peptide hormones.
[b] Immunocytochemical studies indicate that oxytocin and ADH are produced by separate sets of neurons within the supraoptic and paraventricular nuclei of the hypothalamus. Biochemical studies have demonstrated that the supraoptic nucleus contains equal amounts of both hormones, whereas the paraventricular nucleus contains more oxytocin than ADH, but less than the amount found in the supraoptic nucleus.

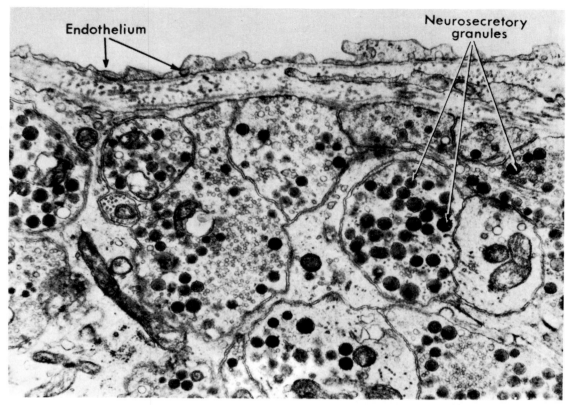

Figure 20.6. Electron micrograph of rat neurohypophysis. Neurosecretory granules and small vesicles are present in the terminal portions of axonal processes of the fibers of the hypothalamo-hypophyseal tract. Capillaries with fenestrated endothelium are present in close proximity to the nerve endings. × 22,000. (Courtesy of P. Orkland and S. L. Palay.)

the fenestrated capillaries, and are distributed to target organs, tissues, and cells via the systemic circulation. It should be noted that the neurohypophyseal hormones (ADH and oxytocin) are bound to a carrier protein, called *neurophysin,* during the axonal transport and storage in the pars nervosa. This hormone-neurophysin complex constitutes the bulk of the Herring bodies. The hormones are freed from the neurophysin when they are released from the nerve terminals.

The *pituicytes* resemble the neuroglial cells found in the central nervous system, except that the pituicytes may contain pigment granules. The nuclei of the pituicytes are round or oval, and the cytoplasm is drawn into processes that are often associated with the axonal processes and terminal expansion of the nerve fibers, but it is unknown if the pituicytes have metabolic activities associated with hormone secretion.

PINEAL GLAND

The pineal gland, or pineal body, is now usually considered an endocrine gland, but its functions in humans are unknown. In animal studies it has been shown to contain a number of neurotransmitters, including norepinephrine, dopamine, serotonin, histamine, and melatonin, and the hypothalamic peptides, somatostatin and thyrotropin releasing factor (TRF). Of all these biologically active substances, only melatonin has been shown to be released into the blood and can be considered a true hormone (Table 20.3). This substance appears to inhibit the steroidogenic activity of the gonads. Clinically, it is important to note that diseases of the pineal, which are rare, are often associated with abnormal gonadal function. Children with tumors that destroy the pineal parenchyma demonstrate precocious (or early onset of) puberty.

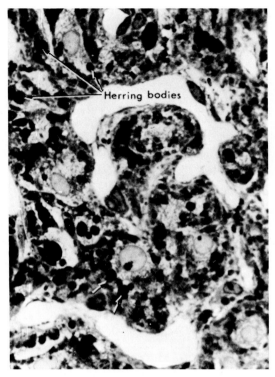

Herring bodies

Figure 20.7. Photomicrograph of rat neurohypophysis. **Arrows** indicate dark rounded masses called Herring bodies that are present in nerve endings adjacent to the capillaries. × 950. (Courtesy of P. Orkland and S. L. Palay.)

Structure

In the human adult, the pineal gland is a flattened, cone-shaped structure, measuring 5 to 8 mm in height and 3 to 5 mm in diameter and weighing 100 to 180 mg (Fig. 20.8). It is embryologically derived from the neuroectoderm of the diencephalic roof. Except at the attachment of the pineal gland to the roof of the third ventricle, pia mater covers its surface and forms a capsule from which connective tissue septa containing blood vessels and nerves penetrate into the gland dividing it into poorly defined lobules.

The pineal gland consists of two basic cell types: *pinealocytes,* which are in the majority and are arranged in clumps or cords within the lobules, and *glial cells* (*interstitial cells*). The most characteristic feature of the pinealocyte is the presence of a large, deeply infolded or lobulated nucleus with one or more prominent nucleoli. The cytoplasm often contains lipid droplets. At the ultrastructural level, typical cytoplasmic organelles are seen. The most distinctive features of the cell are the presence of dense-cored, membrane-bound granules (particularly in the cytoplasmic processes) and large numbers of microtubules arranged in parallel bundles within the cytoplasmic processes. Special silver impregnation techniques are required to demonstrate the extent of the cytoplasmic processes that radiate out from the cell body and have an expanded terminal portion. These terminal club-like endings, which are associated with blood capillaries, contain relatively few granules or vesicles, indicating that the cells may not store much secretory product.

Small numbers of glial cells, about 5 percent of the cells in the gland, are present in the perivascular areas and surrounding the clumps or cords of pinealocytes. The glial cells have small, often elongate nuclei that stain more intensely than those of the pinealocytes. Cytoplasmic processes containing numerous filaments (5 to 6 nm in diameter) extend from the glial cells, giving them the appearance of astrocytes.

In addition to the pinealocytes and glial cells, the human pineal gland contains calcified concretions, known as *corpora arenacea,* or *brain sand,* which form in the organic matrix of the substance secreted by the pinealocytes (Fig. 20.9). These concretions, consisting of calcium phosphates and carbonates, have an irregular shape and a lamellar appearance when seen in sectioned specimens. The concretions begin to form early in childhood and increase in number with age. They are easily

TABLE 20.3. Hormones of the Pineal Gland

HORMONE[a]	SOURCE	FUNCTION
Melatonin	Pinealocytes	Function obscure in humans; in other mammals, slows steroid secretion by the ovaries; may function in regulating endocrine activity of the gonads, particularly as related to the menstrual cycle

[a] Melatonin is an indolamine.

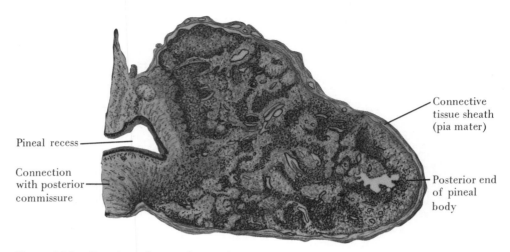

Figure 20.8. Drawing of a median section through the pineal gland of a newborn child. The blood vessels are empty. × 25. (After Schaffer in Bloom W, Fawcett DW (eds): *A Textbook of Histology,* 10th ed. Philadelphia, WB Saunders, 1975.)

identified on radiographic and CT scan films, providing a helpful landmark for identifying the location of the pineal gland. The concretions do not appear to interfere with normal functioning of the gland.

Innervation and Function

The pineal gland is innervated by postganglionic sympathetic nerves that arise in the superior cervical ganglia. The sympathetic inflow is regulated by the relay (through the hypothalamus and spinal cord) of impulses that originate in the retinal neurons. Therefore, the gland's activity is influenced by changes in the external lighting, that is, by periods of light and darkness. Light entering the eye stimulates neurons to transmit impulses to the pineal gland that inhibit the secretion of melatonin. Nighttime levels of the hormone are 10 times higher than daytime levels. It is currently

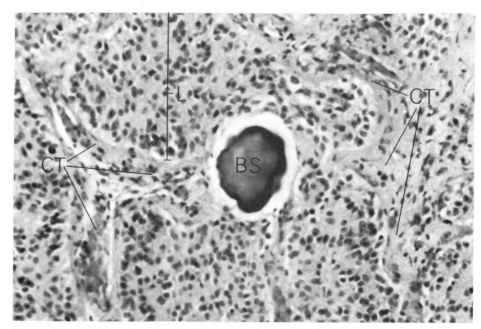

Figure 20.9. Photomicrograph of human pineal gland. A characteristic concretion called brain sand (BS), or corpora arenacea, can be seen. Lobules (L) of the gland are surrounded by connective tissue (CT). × 250. (Courtesy of M. H. Ross)

believed that the pineal gland, through the secretion of melatonin, influences the gonads in response to light, modulating their daily physiological activity (circadian rhythm). In animals who demonstrate seasonal or annual changes (circannual rhythms) in their reproductive function, the pineal gland may respond to changes in the length of the light-dark cycle.

Nerve endings of the postganglionic sympathetic fibers are associated with the pinealocytes, influencing their secretory activity, and with smooth muscle cells of the blood vessels, regulating blood flow through the gland. The structure of the blood vessels remains obscure in the human. Studies of human fetal pineal glands have demonstrated the presence of tight junctions between the endothelial cells. Furthermore, unlike other endocrine glands, fenestrations have not been reported within the endothelial cells of the blood capillaries. Such fenestrations have been reported in other species, and rat studies utilizing dyes injected into the bloodstream have demonstrated diffusion of the dyes into the pineal gland. It is important to remember that the brain tissue in general is isolated from the blood (blood-brain barrier). Although the absence of such a barrier has been demonstrated in the case of the rat pineal, current evidence suggests that a barrier is present in the human pineal gland.

THYROID GLAND

The thyroid gland is a bilobed structure located in the neck. A narrow central portion, the *isthmus,* crosses anterior to the trachea and connects two lateral lobes. An additional *pyramidal lobe* commonly extends superiorly from the isthmus. The thyroid weighs about 40 g.

Embryologically, the thyroid is of endodermal origin, arising from a median downward growth in the floor of the pharyngeal gut near the base of the tongue. The parafollicular cells (see below) are derived from neural crest cells that migrate into the ultimobranchial bodies of the fourth pharyngeal pouches. The thyroid gland, which begins functioning at about the 10th week of fetal life, plays an essential role in regulating tissue metabolism and general growth and development (Table 20.4). Deficiencies in the thyroid hormones during fetal development result in irreversible damage including the development of fewer and smaller neurons, defective myelination, stunted body growth, and mental retardation.

Body Supply and Nerves

The thyroid gland receives its blood supply primarily through the superior and inferior thyroid arteries. These unusually large vessels, which have numerous anastomoses, provide the gland with a rich blood supply. The veins of the gland form a venous plexus, associated with the capsule of the gland. Unusually extensive blood and lymphatic capillary plexuses surround the parenchymal tissue within the gland. As is typical of most endocrine tissue, the endothelium of the blood capillaries is fenestrated. In the thyroid, the lymphatic capillaries provide an important route for conveying the hormones from the gland.

TABLE 20.4. Hormones of the Thyroid Gland

HORMONE[a]	SOURCE	FUNCTION
Tetraiodothyronine (T_4) or thyroxine Triiodothyronine (T_3)	Principal cells	Calorigenic effect—regulates tissue metabolism (increases rate of carbohydrate utilization, protein synthesis and degradation, and fat synthesis and degradation); influences body and tissue growth and development of the nervous system in the fetus and young child[b]; increases absorption of carbohydrates from the intestine
Thyrocalcitonin	Parafollicular cells	Lowers blood calcium level by inhibiting bone resorption and stimulating adsorption of calcium by the bones

[a] T_3 and T_4 are iodinated tyrosine derivatives (T_3 acts more rapidly and is more potent): thyrocalcitonin is a peptide hormone.
[b] Deficiency of T_3 and T_4 during development results in fewer and smaller neurons, defective myelination, and mental retardation.

Most of the nerve fibers entering the thyroid with the larger branches of the thyroid arteries are postganglionic sympathetic fibers from the superior, middle, and inferior cervical (sympathetic) ganglia. These nerves are believed to function primarily in regulating blood flow in the gland, but some evidence suggests that the sympathetic fibers may stimulate secretion of thyroid hormones.

Structure

The thyroid is surrounded by a thin, connective tissue capsule from which septa extend into the gland, dividing it into irregular lobes and lobules. The parenchymal cells are organized in spherical or short, blind ending cylindrical masses called *follicles.* The follicles are cyst-like structures consisting of a single layer of epithelial cells surrounding a central mass of gelatinous colloidal material (Fig. 20.10). In humans, the follicles vary in size from 0.02 to 0.9 mm in diameter.

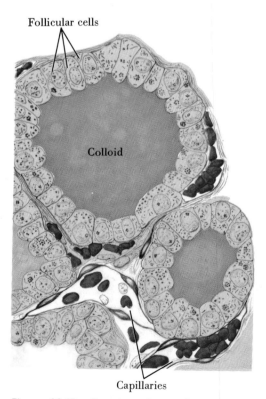

Follicular cells

Colloid

Capillaries

Figure 20.10. Drawing of a section through follicles of a human thyroid gland. Follicles consist of a single layer of epithelial cells surrounding a central mass of colloidal material. (Based on Bensley RR: In Bloom W, Fawcett DW (eds): *A Textbook of Histology,* 10th ed. Philadelphia, WB Saunders, 1975.)

Rich blood and lymphatic capillary plexuses are present in the connective tissue that separates the follicles.

The follicular epithelial cells, which rest on a very thin basal lamina, vary in height from cuboidal to squamous. The height of the epithelium is indicative of the functional activity; the squamous follicular cells are referred to as "resting." Two cell types identified in the follicles are *principal* or *follicular cells* and *parafollicular* or *C cells.* The luminal colloid stains with both basic and acidic dyes and is PAS-positive. The colloid consists of proteolytic enzymes, mucoproteins, and a glycoprotein called *thyroglobulin,* which is the storage form of the thyroid hormone. It should be noted that the thyroid is unique among the endocrine glands in its ability to store its secretory product.

Principal Cells. The activities of the *principal cells* include the synthesis of thyroglobulin, iodination, and storage of thyroglobulin within the follicular lumen, resorption and hydrolysis of thyroglobulin, and release of the thyroid hormones into the blood and lymphatic capillaries.

Most of the follicular epithelial cells are *principal cells* resting on the basal lamina with their apices directed inward toward the follicular cavity. The principal cells vary in height from columnar to squamous. Their nuclei are spherical and contain one or more prominent nucleoli. With the light microscope a supranuclear Golgi complex, lipid droplets, and PAS-positive droplets can be identified in the basophilic cytoplasm. Ultrastructural studies of the active cuboidal or columnar cells reveal the presence of organelles commonly associated with both secretory and absorptive cells as shown schematically in Figure 20.12: (1) typical junctional complexes at the apical end of the lateral plasma membrane; (2) short microvilli on the apical surface of the cells; (3) numerous profiles of rough endoplasmic reticulum in the basal region; (4) a well-developed, supranuclear Golgi complex; (5) numerous small vesicles in the apical cytoplasm, which are morphologically similar to vesicles associated with the Golgi; (6) abundant lysosomes and multivesicular bodies; and (7) membrane-limited vesicles, identified as *colloidal resorption droplets,* in the apical region.

Parafollicular Cells. The *parafollicular cells* (Fig. 20.11) may be present in the follicular epithelium or scattered in the connective tissue between the follicles. When present in the follicle, they are located near the basal lamina and do not extend to the follicular lumen. Ultrastructurally, the most characteristic feature of these cells is the presence of numerous, dense, membrane-bound secretory granules measuring 0.1 to 0.5 μm in diameter.

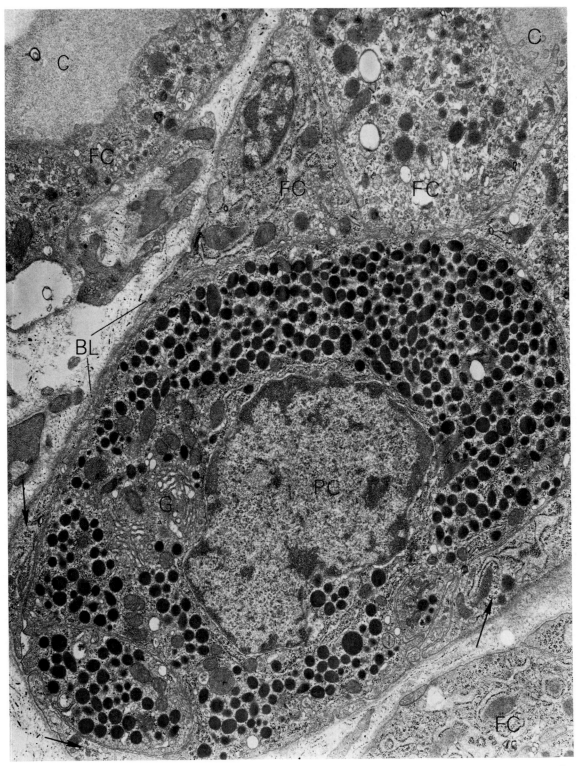

Figure 20.11. Electron micrograph of a parafollicular cell. Cytoplasmic processes of follicular cells (**arrows**) partially surround the parafollicular cell, which contains numerous electron-dense granules and a prominent Golgi complex (G). Basal lamina (BL) is associated with the follicular cells (FC). The central mass of colloidal material (C) in two adjacent follicles can be seen in the upper portion of the micrograph. × 12,000 (Courtesy of E. Nunez).

Thyroid Hormones

The synthesis, storage, and secretion of the thyroid hormones involves a number of functional events that can be correlated with the structure of the principal cells (Fig. 20.12).

1. Synthesis of thyroglobulin: The polypeptide component is synthesized in the granular endoplasmic reticulum and carried to the Golgi complex where it is conjugated with the carbohydrate moiety.
2. Release of noniodinated thyroglobulin into the follicular lumen.
3. Iodination of the thyroglobulin: Iodide is oxidized to iodine by thyroperoxidase, also produced by the principal cells and then released into the follicular lumen. (The principal cells have the capacity to concentrate iodides 30 to 40 times the serum level.) Iodination of some of

the tyrosine residues within the thyroglobulin then rapidly occurs at the microvillous membrane.

4. Storage of the iodinated thyroglobulin: Most, if not all, thyroid hormones produced by principal cells reside at least briefly in the follicular lumen. (Studies indicate that thyroglobulin may be stored for a period of 10 months or more.)
5. Endocytosis of the iodinated thyroglobulin by the principal cells: In response to secretory stimulus, the principal cells take up thyroglobulin from the central colloid material of the follicle through receptor-mediated endocytosis (see Chapter 2).
6. Hydrolysis of the thyroglobulin: Lysosomal vesicles produced by the Golgi apparatus fuse with the endocytic vesicles. Hydrolysis of the thyroglobulin by proteases from the lysosome results in the breakdown of the molecule into its constituent amino acids, carbohydrates, and the

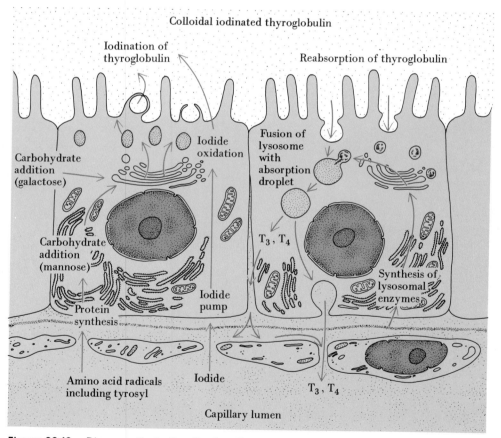

Figure 20.12. Diagram illustrating the functional architecture of the thyroid follicular cells. **Arrows** indicate the general metabolic pathways. The synthesis, secretion, and iodination of thyroglobulin are shown in the cell on the left. Colloidal iodinated thyroglobulin is stored in the follicular lumen. The cell on the right shows the endocytosis and hydrolysis of the thyroglobulin and the release of the active thyroid hormones into the capillaries. (Modified from Junqueira LC, Carneiro J: *Basic Histology*, 3rd ed. Los Altos, CA, Lange, 1980.)

thyroid hormones *triiodothyronine (T_3)* and *tetraiodothyronine (T_4)*, or *thyroxine.*

7. Release of T_3 and T_4 into the lymphatic and blood capillaries: T_4 and T_3 (in a ratio of 20:1) move through the basal plasma membrane and enter lymphatic and blood capillaries.

As T_3 and T_4 are released into the capillaries, most of the molecules are immediately bound to specific plasma proteins. Only the unbound (free) fractions of these hormones are metabolically active. The free hormone also functions in the feedback system that regulates the secretory activity of the thyroid.

The release of the thyroid hormones T_3 and T_4 is regulated by a simple feedback system. The secretion of thyroid hormones is controlled by the release of thyroid-simulating hormone (TSH), or thyrotropin, from the adenohypophysis into the bloodstream. The TSH stimulates the principal cells of the thyroid to release T_3 and T_4. Low levels of free T_3 and T_4 initiate the release of thyrotropin-releasing factor (TRF) from the hypothalamus, and, in turn, TRF stimulates thyrotropic cells in the adenohypophysis to secrete TSH. High serum levels of free T_3 and T_4 inhibit the synthesis and release of TSH. Somatostatin, which is also released from the hypothalamus, functions as an antagonist to TRF, inhibiting TSH release (Fig. 20.3).

Thyrocalcitonin is a physiological antagonist to parathyroid hormone. These two hormones presumably act in concert to maintain the normal concentration of calcium in the serum and the extracellular fluids. Thyrocalcitonin appears to lower blood calcium levels by inhibiting bone resorption and accelerating adsorption of calcium to bones. Clinically, thyrocalcitonin is used to treat patients with hypercalcemia. However, the actual importance of thyrocalcitonin in maintaining calcium homeostasis in the human has not been established. No clinical diseases have been associated with thyrocalcitonin deficiency.

The release of thyrocalcitonin from the parafollicular cells appears to be regulated by blood calcium levels; high levels of calcium stimulate secretion, while low levels inhibit it.

PARATHYROID GLANDS

The parathyroid glands, named because of their association with the thyroid gland, are usually found embedded in the connective tissue capsule on the posterior surface of the thyroid. In the human usually two pairs of small, yellowish-brown, oval structures are present. They typically measure about 6 mm in length, 3 to 4 mm in width, and 1 to 2 mm in thickness. They are identified by their location as **superior** and **inferior parathyroid glands.** In some individuals (estimates on the frequency vary from 2 to 10 percent), additional glands are associated with the thymus.

Embryologically, the inferior parathyroid glands and the thymus are derived from the third branchial pouch and the superior glands from the fourth branchial pouch. Both the inferior parathyroids and the thymus migrate caudally during development. Normally, the inferior parathyroids separate from the thymus and come to lie below the superior parathyroids. Failure of these structures to separate results in the atypical association of the parathyroids with the thymus in the adult.

The parathyroids function in the regulation of blood ion levels, especially calcium and phosphate. These glands are essential for life. Therefore, care must be taken during thyroidectomy to avoid removing the parathyroids. If the glands are removed, death will ensue as muscles, including the laryngeal and other respiratory muscles, go into tetanic contraction as the blood calcium level falls.

Blood Supply and Innervation

The parathyroids receive their blood supply from the inferior thyroid arteries or anastomoses between the superior and inferior thyroid arteries. The parenchyma of the gland is surrounded by rich blood and lymphatic capillary plexuses. Fenestrations are present in the endothelial cells of the blood capillary plexus.

The autonomic nerve fibers present in the gland appear to be involved in the regulation of blood flow and are not secretomotor in function.

Structure

Each glandular mass is surrounded by a thin, connective tissue capsule from which septa extend into the gland, dividing it into poorly defined lobules and separating the densely packed parenchymal cells into anastomosing cords. The extent of the connective tissue becomes more obvious in the adult as the number of fat cells increases with age. Their number increases dramatically at puberty and continues to increase throughout life. In the elderly adult, 60 to 70 percent of the glandular mass may be occupied by fat cells. The septa provide a route of access for the blood and lymphatic vessels and nerves.

Two basic cell types are identified in the glandular epithelium (Fig. 20.13): *principal* or

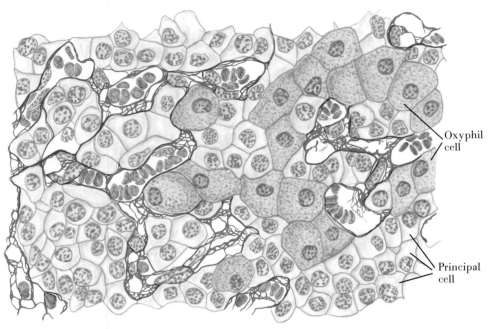

Oxyphil
cell

Principal
cell

Figure 20.13. Drawing of cells within the human parathyroid gland. Principal cells are small and often vacuolated. The oxyphilic cells are much larger and contain fine granules. (Modified from Bloom W, Fawcett DW (eds): *A Textbook of Histology,* 10th ed. Philadelphia, WB Saunders, 1975.)

chief cells and *oxyphil cells.* Some investigators identify a third, transitional cell type that is intermediate in structure between the two, however, the features associated with these cells may result from poor fixation of the tissue.

The *principal cells* are the most common parenchymal cell in the parathyroid. They are small, polygonal cells, measuring about 7 to 10 μm in diameter. They have a centrally located, vesicular nucleus and a pale-staining, slightly acidophilic cytoplasm. Lipofuscin granules, large accumulations of glycogen, lipid droplets, and small, dense membrane-limited granules (presumably containing the storage form of parathyroid hormone) are seen in addition to the typical cytoplasmic organelles.

The *oxyphil cells* constitute a minor portion of the parenchymal cells. They are distinctly larger than the principal cells and have intensely eosinophilic cytoplasm. Their nuclei are often smaller and more heterochromatic than those of the principal cells. Ultrastructural studies have revealed that the eosinophilic staining of the cytoplasm is due to the presence of numerous large mitochondria. Morphologically, the cells are further characterized by limited amounts of endoplasmic reticulum, a small Golgi complex, and the absence of secretory granules.

Function

The parathyroids produce *parathyroid hormone (PTH)* or *parathormone* (Table 20.5). This hormone is essential in maintaining normal blood calcium levels. The secretion of PTH is regulated by the serum calcium level. Through a simple feedback system, low levels of serum calcium stimulate secretion of PTH; high levels of serum calcium inhibit its secretion. Although the principal cells are believed to be the primary source of PTH, some evidence suggests that the oxyphil cells may also produce this hormone.

ADRENAL GLANDS

In the human, the *adrenal* or *suprarenal glands* are a pair of flattened, triangular bodies located adjacent to the superior pole of each kidney. They measure approximately 5 × 3 × 1 cm and have a combined weight of about 10 to 15 g. Each gland is enclosed in a thick, connective tissue capsule.

The glands are composed of two distinct parts, a central *medulla* and an outer *cortex,* which differ in their origin, function, and structure. In the adult, the medulla represents about 10 percent of the total weight of the adrenal gland. The paren-

TABLE 20.5. Hormones of the Parathyroid Glands

HORMONE[a]	SOURCE	FUNCTION
Parathyroid hormone (PTH) or parathormone	Principal, or chief, cells[b]	Increases blood calcium level in three ways: (1) promotes calcium release from bone (increases relative number of osteoclasts); (2) stimulates calcium resorption by tubular cells of kidney, while inhibiting phosphate resorption; (3) causes formation of 1,25-dihydroxycholecalciferol in the kidneys (hormone that promotes absorption of calcium by the intestinal epithelial cells)

[a] PTH is a peptide hormone.
[b] Some evidence suggests that oxyphilic cells, which first appear in the parathyroid gland at about 4 to 7 years of age and increase in number after puberty, may also produce PTH.

chymal cells of the medulla are embryologically derived from neural crest cells. The hormones produced by the secretory cells of the medulla, the **chromaffin cells,** influence the activity of glandular epithelium, cardiac muscle, and the smooth muscle located in the walls of blood vessels and viscera. Most of the parenchymal cells of the adrenal cortex are under partial control of the adenohypophysis and function in regulating metabolism and maintaining normal electrolyte balance (Table 20.6).

Blood Supply, Lymphatic Drainage, and Innervation

The suprarenals are highly vascular glands, receiving blood via three groups of arteries, the superior, middle, and inferior suprarenal arteries, arising from the inferior phrenic artery, aorta, and renal artery, respectively. The suprarenal arteries usually branch before entering the capsule and form an extensive arterial plexus over the surface of the gland. Branches from these capsular arteries enter the gland. Two sets of vessels—*cortical* and *medullary arterioles*—supply the parenchyma of the adrenal (Fig. 20.14 and 20.15). Most branches of the capsular arteries, specifically the *cortical arterioles,* contribute to a subcapsular plexus that gives rise to numerous anastomosing *cortical sinusoids* that distribute blood to the cells of the cortex. The sinusoids are lined by fenestrated endothelial

cells. At the junction between the medulla and cortex the sinusoids merge and communicate with the vascular beds in the medulla. In addition, medullary arterioles pass through the cortex to supply the medulla directly. Thus, the medullary capillary bed, which is also lined by a fenestrated endothelium, receives its blood supply by two routes. This system allows hormones produced by the cortical cells to influence the activity of the medullary cells.

The cortex of the adrenal does not have a separate venous drainage. Blood from the capillary plexuses of both the cortex and medulla enters medullary veins that join a single suprarenal vein. In humans, medullary veins are unusual in that there are conspicuous bundles of longitudinally oriented smooth muscle fibers surrounding them.

Lymphatic vessels are present in the capsule and the connective tissue around the larger blood vessels in the gland. No lymphatic vessels are present in association with the parenchyma of the gland.

An unusually large number of autonomic nerve fibers are present in the adrenals. Most of the fibers are myelinated (preganglionic) sympathetic fibers that pass to the medulla and end on parenchymal cells located there. The sympathetic fibers convey impulses that stimulate the cells to secrete epinephrine. The autonomic fibers located in the cortex are primarily associated with the blood vessels, controlling vasodilation and vaso-

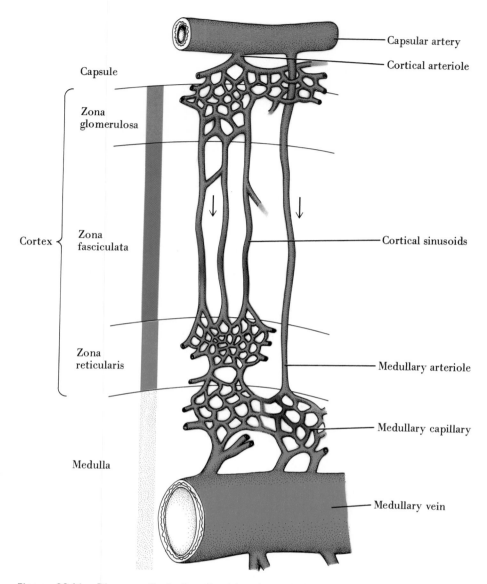

Figure 20.14. Diagram illustrating the blood supply to the human adrenal gland. The region of the capsule, the zones within the cortex, and the medulla are indicated. (Modified from *Gray's Anatomy*, 36th British ed.)

constriction. Secretory activity of most of the cortical parenchymal cells is stimulated by ACTH from the adenohypophysis.

Adrenal Cortex

The adrenal cortex is invested externally by a connective tissue capsule from which septa, or trabeculae, extend into the cortex. Blood vessels, nerves, lymphatics, and smooth muscle fibers are present in the trabeculae. The adrenal cortex is subdivided into three concentric layers (Fig. 20.15): (1) the *zona glomerulosa,* a thin, outer layer

adjacent to the capsule; (2) the *zona fasciculata,* a thick, middle layer; and (3) the *zona reticularis,* a thin, inner layer adjacent to the medulla. The parenchymal cells of the cortex are arranged in clusters or cords that are separated by blood capillaries and sinusoids. Morphologically, the transition from one layer to the next is gradual.

The *zona glomerulosa* consists of small columnar or pyramidal cells arranged in rounded clusters and curved columns that are continuous with the cords of cells in the zona fasciculata. In the human, the zona glomerulosa may be absent in areas of the cortex. The cells have intensely stain-

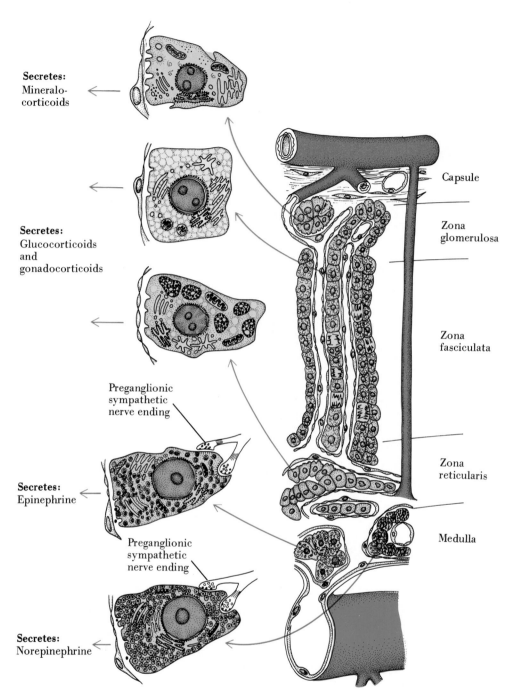

Secretes:
Mineralo-
corticoids

Secretes:
Glucocorticoids
and
gonadocorticoids

Preganglionic
sympathetic
nerve ending

Secretes:
Epinephrine

Preganglionic
sympathetic
nerve ending

Secretes:
Norepinephrine

Capsule

Zona
glomerulosa

Zona
fasciculata

Zona
reticularis

Medulla

Figure 20.15. Diagram illustrating the organization of the cells within the adrenal gland and their relationship to the blood vessels. Refer to Figure 20.14 for identification of the blood vessels. The ultrastructural features of the basic cell types and a brief description of their function are included. (Modified from *Gray's Anatomy*, 36th British ed.)

TABLE 20.6. Hormones of the Adrenal Glands

HORMONE[a]	SOURCE	FUNCTION
ADRENAL CORTEX		
Mineralocorticoids (95% of mineralocorticoid activity in aldosterone)	Parenchymal cells of the zona glomerulosa	Aid in controlling electrolyte homeostasis (act on distal tubule cells of kidney to increase sodium resorption and decrease potassium resorption); function in maintaining the osmotic balance in the urine and in preventing serum acidosis
Glucocorticoids (hydrocortisone, corticosterone, and cortisone; 95% of glucocorticoid activity in hydrocortisone)	Parenchymal cells of the zona fasciculata (and to a lesser extent of the zona reticularis)	Promote normal metabolism, in particular, affect carbohydrate metabolism (increase rate of amino acid transport to liver, promote removal of protein from skeletal muscle and its transport to the liver, reduce rate of glucose metabolism by cells and stimulate glycogen synthesis by liver, stimulate mobilization of fats from storage deposits for energy utilization); provide resistance to stress; suppress inflammatory response and some alllergic reactions
Gonadocorticoids (sex steroids)	Parenchymal cells of the zona reticularis (and to a lesser extent of the zona fasciculata)	Amount usually so small that it is insignificant (for specific functions, see chapters on male and female reproductive systems)
ADRENAL MEDULLA		
Norepinephrine and epinephrine (in human, 80% epinephrine)	Chromaffin cells	Sympathomimetic (produce effects similar to those induced by the sympathetic division of the autonomic nervous system)[b]: increase heart rate, increase blood pressure, reduce blood flow to viscera and skin; stimulate conversion of glycogen to glucose; increase sweating; induce dilation of bronchioles; increase rate of respiration; decrease digestion; decrease enzyme production by digestive system glands; decrease urine production

[a] Mineralocorticoids, glucocorticoids, and gonadocorticoids are steroid hormones (cholesterol derivatives); epinephrine and norepinephrine are catecholamines (amino acid derivatives).
[b] The catecholamines influence the activity of glandular epithelium, cardiac muscle, or smooth muscle located in the walls of blood vessels or viscera.

ing, spherical nuclei and a relatively small amount of cytoplasm containing a few lipid droplets, small amounts of basophilic material, and abundant smooth endoplasmic reticulum (sER). The Golgi complex is present on the side of nuclei adjacent to the blood vessels.

The *zona fasciculata* consists of large, polyhedral cells arranged in parallel columns or cords usually one or two cells thick. The columns are separated by the sinusoids. The cells of the zona fasciculata have a lightly staining, spherical nucleus; binucleate cells are common in this zone. Present in the generally acidophilic cytoplasm are numerous lipid droplets containing neutral fats, fatty acids, cholesterol, and phospholipids. These substances represent precursors for the steroid hormones produced by the cells. The lipid is extracted during typical histological procedures, thus giving the cells a vacuolated or spongy appearance. Ultrastructurally, features associated with steroid-secreting cells are observed, including abundant sER, mitochondria with tubular cristae, large numbers of lipid droplets, a well-developed

Golgi complex, and profiles of granular endoplasmic reticulum (Fig. 20.16).

The **zona reticularis** consists of rounded cells arranged in branching and anastomosing cords or columns. Compared to the cells of the zona fasciculata, the cells are smaller, the nuclei of the cells are more deeply stained, and the cytoplasm contains

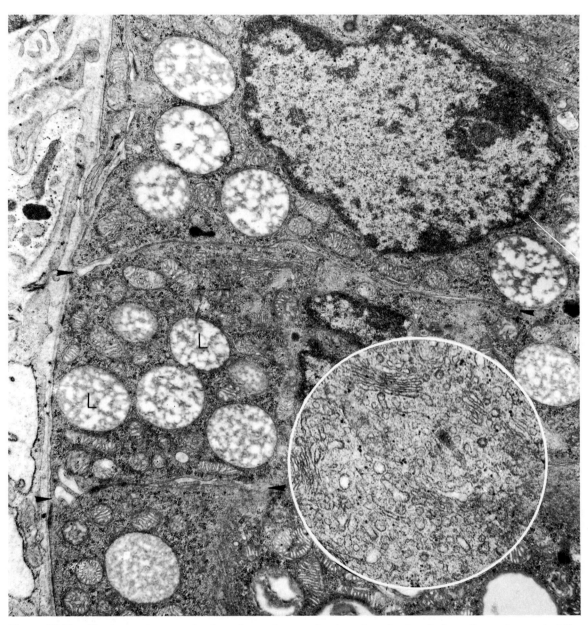

Figure 20.16. Electron micrograph of portions of several adrenal cortical cells from the outer part of the zona fasciculata. The boundary between adjacent cells of the cord is indicated by the **arrowheads**. Lipid droplets (L) are numerous (the lipid has been partially extracted), as are the mitochondria. A higher magnification of an area in the cell at the top of the micrograph (**inset**) reveals the extensive smooth endoplasmic reticulum characteristic of steroid-secreting cells. A portion of the Golgi is also evident. × 15,000 (**inset**, × 40,000).

Chromaffin cells (named because they react with chromate salts) of the adrenal medulla are a part of the APUD system of cells. The chromaffin reaction is thought to involve oxidation and polymerization of the catecholamines contained within the secretory granules of the cells. Classically, chromaffin cells have been defined as being derived from neuroectoderm, innervated by preganglionic sympathetic nerve fibers, and capable of synthesizing and secreting catecholamines. Chromaffin cells are found in the adrenal medulla, in paravertebral and prevertebral sympathetic ganglia, and in various other locations. Those scattered groups of chromaffin cells located among or near the components of the autonomic nervous system are referred to as *paraganglia*.

relatively few lipid droplets. In the zona reticularis, light- and dark-staining cells can be identified. The dark cells have more intensely staining nuclei and lipofuscin granules in their cytoplasm. The physiological significance of the two cell types is unknown. Ultrastructurally, the cells demonstrate features seen in other cortical parenchymal cells including abundant sER.

Adrenal Medulla

The central portion of the adrenal gland, the *medulla,* is composed of endocrine parenchymal cells (called *chromaffin cells*), connective tissue, and numerous blood vessels and nerves. The parenchymal cells are organized in short, interconnecting cords surrounded by blood vessels.

Chromaffin cells of the adrenal medulla are relatively large, rounded cells. Histochemical studies have demonstrated that two cell types are present; one contains norepinephrine, the other epinephrine. Ultrastructurally, the cells are characterized by the presence of numerous membrane-bound granules measuring 100 to 300 nm in diameter. On the basis of the staining of the granules, two populations of cells can also be identified (see Fig. 20.17). One population of cells, containing granules with very dense cores, secretes norepinephrine; the other population of cells, containing homogeneous and less densely staining granules, secretes epinephrine. Other ultrastructural features of both cell populations include relatively abundant granular endoplasmic reticulum and a well-developed Golgi complex.

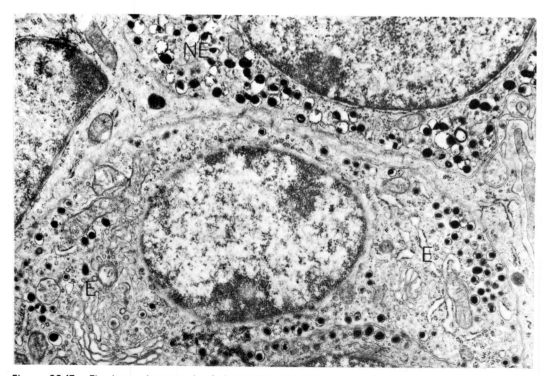

Figure 20.17. Electron micrograph of chromaffin cells in the mouse adrenal medulla. Two types of medullary cells are present. The norepinephrine-secreting cells (NE) contain granules with very dense cores; the epinephrine-secreting cells (E) contain less intensely staining granules. × 15,000.

From studies utilizing the techniques of cell fractionation and density gradient centrifugation to isolate the secretory granules from the cells of the adrenal medulla, it has been shown that the granules contain large amounts of a soluble protein called **chromogranin,** in addition to hormone. It is not clearly understood how the low molecular weight catecholamines are reatined in the substance of the granules. It appears that the uptake of catecholamine by the granules occurs through an active transport mechanism involving a magnesium-activated ATPase in the limiting membrane of the granule. Drugs, such as reserpine, which cause depletion of catecholamines from the granules may inhibit the active transport mechanism. The contents of the granules including the hormone and chromogranin is released by exocytosis.

Functions

The parenchymal cells of the adrenal cortex secrete a variety of hormones collectively referred to as **corticosteroids** (Table 20.6). The parenchymal cells of the zona glomerulosa secrete a class of steroid hormones called **mineralocorticoids,** which function in maintaining normal electrolyte balance. **Aldosterone** is the most potent mineralocorticoid and accounts for approximately 95 percent of the activity of this class. The parenchymal cells of the zona fasciculata (and, to a lesser extent, those of the zona reticularis) secrete a class of steroid hormones called **glucocorticoids,** which influence carbohydrate metabolism. **Hydrocortisone,** or cortisol, is the most important member of this class and accounts for most of the glucocorticoid activity. Studies indicate that small amounts of **gonadocorticoids,** or **sex steroids,** primarily andorgens, are secreted by the parenchymal cells of the zona reticularis and to a lesser extent by those of the zona fasciculata.

The secretory activity of the cortical parenchymal cells of the inner two layers (zona fasciculata and zona reticularis) is regulated by the adenohypophysis through the secretion of ACTH. ACTH stimulates secretion and release of corticosteroids, promotes growth of the adrenal cortex, and increases blood flow through the adrenal gland. The release of ACTH is regulated by a feedback system that involves the adenohypophysis, the hypothalamus, and higher brain centers (Fig. 20.18). The hypothalamus produces corticotropin-releasing factor (CRF) that stimulates cells in the adenohypophysis to release ACTH. The circulating levels of corticosteroids influence the release of both CRF and ACTH. High plasma

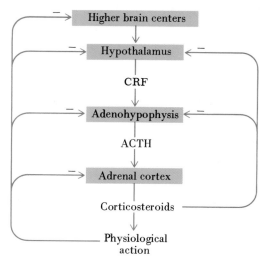

Figure 20.18. Diagram illustrating the neuroendocrine control of the adrenal cortex. Both the corticosteroids themselves and the physiological effects that they induce can inhibit further release of corticosteroids through negative feedback. As is indicated, inhibition may occur at a number of levels. The system is activated in response to low levels of hormone or in response to metabolic needs (stress).

levels of corticosteroids inhibit CRF and ACTH release. Low levels of corticosteroids trigger the hypothalamus to release CRF), which causes the adenohypophysis to release ACTH. Target cells within the adrenal cortex respond to the ACTH and release additional corticosteroids.

Aldosterone secretion by the cells of the **zona glomerulosa** is regulated by the **renin-angiotensin** system and plasma levels of sodium and potassium. ACTH has little or no direct effect on the secretion of aldosterone. The renin-angiotensin system is believed to be the major control system involved in aldosterone release. Stimulation of aldosterone secretion is believed to involve the following events.

Dehydration or sodium deficiency
↓
Decrease in blood volume
↓
Decrease in blood pressure
↓
Stimulation of juxtaglomerular cells in the kidney
↓
Release of renin into blood
↓
Conversion of plasma angiotensin to angiotensin I
↓

Conversion of angiotensin I to angiotensin II (in the lungs)
↓
Stimulation of parenchymal cells of the zona glomerulosa
↓
Release of aldosterone
↓
Retention of sodium (and water) through the activation of the distal tubule cells of the kidneys
↓
Increase in blood volume
↓
Increase in blood pressure
↓
Inhibition of renin release by juxtaglomerular cells

The parenchymal cells of the adrenal medulla secrete catecholamines (primarily epinephrine and smaller amounts of norepinephrine). These substances produce effects similar to those induced by the sympathetic division of the autonomic nervous system. The release of the catecholamines by the chromaffin cells of the adrenal medulla is initiated by impulses conveyed in the preganglionic sympathetic fibers that end on the chromaffin cells. In response to these signals the chromaffin cells release the catecholamines into the adjacent blood vessels.

ATLAS PLATES

99–105

PLATE 99. Pituitary Gland I

The pituitary gland, or hypophysis cerebri, is located in a small bony fossa in the floor of the cranial cavity. It is connected by a stalk to the base of the brain. Although it is joined to the brain, only part of the pituitary gland develops from the neural ectoderm; this is referred to as the neurohypophysis. The larger part of the pituitary gland develops from the oral ectoderm; this part is called the adenohypophysis. The adenohypophysis develops as a diverticulum of the buccal epithelium, called Rathke's pouch. In the fully developed gland, the lumen of Rathke's pouch may be retained as a vestigial cleft.

Both the adenohypophysis and the neurohypophysis are further subdivided as follows:

Adenohypophysis
   (a) pars distalis (anterior lobe)
   (b) pars tuberalis
   (c) pars intermedia

Neurohypophysis   (posterior lobe)

   (a) pars nervosa
   (b) infundibulum (infundibular stem and median eminence of tuber cinereum).

These parts are shown in a sagittal section of the pituitary gland in the accompanying figure. The neurohypophysis is marked by the **broken lines.** The pars nervosa is the expanded portion which is continuous with the infundibulum (**I**). The pars tuberalis (**PT**) is located around the infundibular stem. The pars intermedia (**PI**) is between the pars distalis and the pars nervosa. It borders a small cleft (**C**) that constitutes the remains of the lumen of Rathke's pouch. The pars distalis is the largest part of the pituitary gland. It contains a variety of cell types, some of which are more numerous in one region, some in another. This accounts for the difference in staining (light and dark areas) that is to be seen throughout the pars distalis.

The parts of the pituitary gland can be identified largely on the basis of their location and relation to each other. For example, the pars nervosa can be identified readily if it is continuous

KEY

C, vestigial cleft of   **PI,** pars intermedia
   Rathke's pouch   **PT,** pars tuberalis
I, infundibulum

Fig., monkey,
   × 40

with a stem or stalk of essentially the same kind of material. The pars intermedia is in an intermediate location and in relation to the vestigial cleft; however, the cleft may not be evident and the pars intermedia may be more extensive (in this specimen it continues along the surface of the gland).

Upon considering the cell types at higher magnification (Atlas section, Plate 100), one comes to realize that these 100 also serve as a major indication as to the part of the gland that is being examined.

The blood supply to the pars distalis of the pituitary gland is unique and requires special mention in that it is supplied by two sets of vessels. Capillaries at the outer layer of the pars distalis receive blood from arteries in the usual manner, but most of the capillary plexuses receive blood via the hypophyseal portal system. The latter originates in capillaries located in the median eminence and infundibulum (see Fig. 20.2). They then drain into a venous network that flows to the pars distalis where they empty into a second capillary network. This system serves as a route whereby releasing factors (hormones) from the hypothalamus are conveyed to the pars distalis. There is reported to be a specific releasing factor for each of the anterior pituitary hormones. The releasing factors cause the release, or discharge, of the specific pituitary hormones, and in this way, the hypothalamus regulates the secretory activity of the pars distalis.

PLATE 99

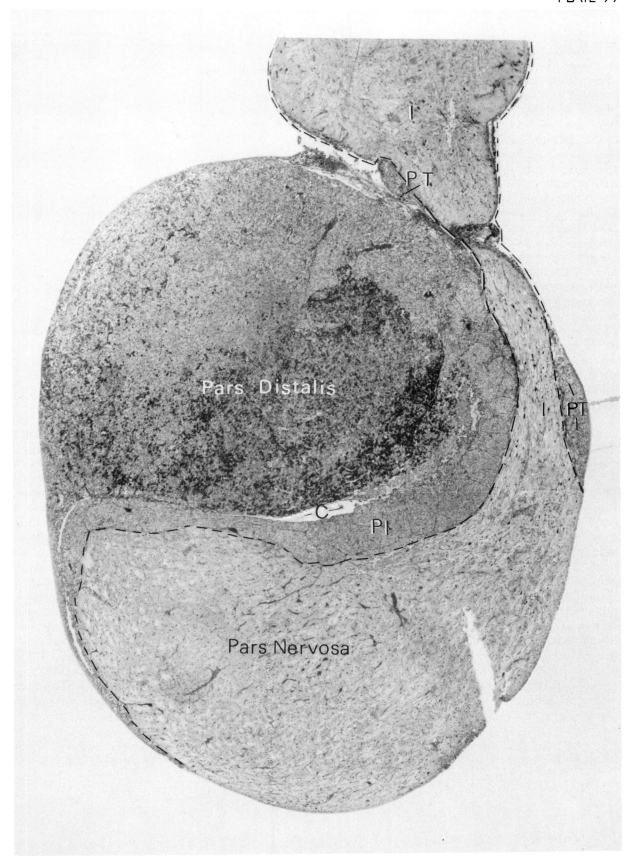

PLATE 100. Pituitary Gland II

The parenchyma of the pars distalis consists of two general cell types, chromophobes and chromophils. Chromophobes stain poorly; chromophils stain well. Chromophils are further subdivided into acidophils and basophils. Basophils stain with basic dyes or hematoxylin, whereas the cytoplasm of the acidophil stains with acid dyes such as eosin. Also, the cytoplasm of basophils stains with the PAS reaction due to the glycoprotein in the secretory granules.

A region of the pars distalis that shows a large number of basophils is illustrated in **Figure 1.** The field also contains acidophils, chromophobes, and stromal elements. The basophils (**B**) can be distinguished from acidophils (**A**) because the basophils are slightly larger and the cytoplasm of the acidophils stains with eosin. Both of these cell types can be distinguished from the chromophobes (**C**), which contain only a small amount of poorly staining cytoplasm. The parenchymal components of the pars distalis are arranged as cords of cells. These are separated by a delicate connective tissue stroma which contain capillaries. The elongated nuclei (**arrows**) belong either to cells of the connective tissue stroma or to the endothelial cells.

A region of pars distalis predominating in acidophils is shown in **Figure 2.** Eosinophilic cytoplasm can be seen in each cell. In contrast, the nuclei of chromophobes (**C**) are surrounded by a small amount of poorly staining cytoplasm. Acidophils can be further subdivided into two groups on the basis of special cytochemical and ultrastructural features. One group, called somatotrops, produces the growth hormone (somatotropic hormone, STH); the other group of acidophils, called mammotrops, or luteotrops, produce the lactogenic hormone (luteotropic hormone, LTH). The groups of basophils can also be distinguished with the electron microscope and/or with special cytochemical procedures. One group produces the thyroid-stimulating hormone, TSH; the other produces the gonadotropic hormones, FSH and LH. Chromophobes are also a heterogeneous group of cells. Many are considered to be depleted acidophils or basophils, however, one group of chromophobes is considered to produce the hormone ACTH.

The pars tuberalis (**Fig. 3**) surrounds the infundibular stem. It consists of small acidophil

and basophil cells. Frequently, these are arranged as small vesicles (**V**) that contain colloid. Its function is not known.

The pars intermedia (**PI**) varies in size in different mammals (**Fig. 4**). It is relatively small in the human. It consists of cords of cells that resemble basophils, except that they are smaller. They sometimes form colloid-filled vesicles. Cells from the pars intermedia are occasionally seen in the pars nervosa (**PN**). The function of the pars intermedia in man is not clear. Studies with frogs indicate that a hormone from the intermedia, called the melanocyte-stimulating hormone (MSH), brings about a darkening of the skin.

The neurohypophysis (**Fig. 5**) contains cells called pituicytes and nonmyelinated nerve fibers from the supraoptic and paraventricular nuclei of the hypothalamus. The pituicytes are comparable to neuroglial cells of the central nervous system. The nuclei of the cells are round or oval; the cytoplasm extends from the nuclear region of the cell as long processes. In H&E preparations, the cytoplasm of the pituicytes cannot be distinguished from the nonmyelinated nerve fibers. The hormones of the neurohypophysis, oxytocin and antidiuretic hormone ADH (also called vasopressin because of its action on vascular smooth muscle), are formed in the hypothalamic nuclei and pass via the fibers of the hypothalamo-hypophyseal tract to the neurohypophysis where they are stored in the expanded terminal protions of the nerve fibers. In histological sections, the stored neurosecretory material appears as the Herring bodies (**HB**).

PLATE 100

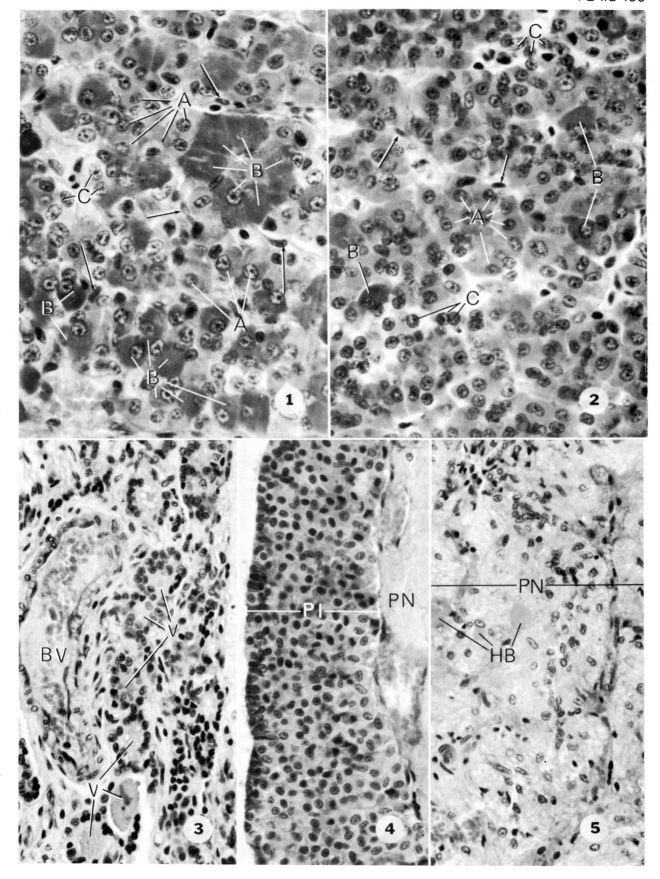

PLATE 101. Pineal Gland

The *pineal gland* (*pineal body, epiphysis cerebri*) is located in the brain above the superior colliculi. It develops from neuroectoderm, but in the adult it bears little resemblance to nerve tissue.

The pineal gland is surrounded by a capsule **(Cap),** except at its stalk. The capsule is formed by the *pia mater.* Trabeculae extend from the capsule into the substance of the gland and divide it into lobules **(Fig. 1).** The lobules **(L)** appear as the indistinct groups of cells surrounded by connective tissue **(CT).** The adult pineal body contains calcareous deposits **(BS)** that are regularly found in histological sections. They are called *brain sand* or *corpora arenacea.* When viewed with higher magnification they can be seen to possess a lamellated structure.

Two cell types have been described within the pineal gland: parenchymal cells and glial cells. The full extent of these cells cannot be appreciated without the application of special methods. These would show that the glial cells and the parenchymal cells have processes and that the processes of the parenchymal cells are expanded at their periphery. The parenchymal cells are more numerous. In an H&E preparation, the nuclei of the parenchymal cells are pale staining and somewhat vesicular. The nuclei of the glial cells, on the other hand, are smaller and stain more intensely. In **Figure 2,** two nuclear types can be seen. The more numerous nuclei are the larger ones; they stain less intensely and are somewhat vesiculated; they belong to parenchymal cells **(PC).** The less numerous nuclei are the smaller ones; they stain more intensely and belong to glial cells **(GC).**

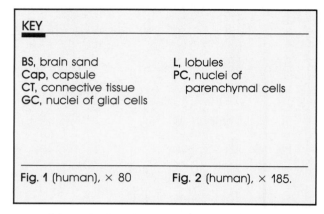

KEY

BS, brain sand
Cap, capsule
CT, connective tissue
GC, nuclei of glial cells

L, lobules
PC, nuclei of
   parenchymal cells

Fig. 1 (human), × 80   **Fig. 2** (human), × 185.

Although the physiology of the pineal gland is not well understood, the secretions of the gland evidently have an antigonadal effect. For example, hypogenitalism has been reported in pineal tumors that consist chiefly of parenchymal cells, whereas, sexual precocity is associated with nonparenchymal tumors (presumably in these the parenchymal cells have been destroyed). In addition, numerous experiments with laboratory animals indicate that the pineal gland has a neuroendocrine function whereby the pineal gland serves as an intermediary that relates endocrine function (particularly gonadal function) to cycles of light and dark. The external photic stimuli reach the pineal gland via optical pathways that connect with the superior cervical ganglion. In turn, the superior cervical ganglion sends postganglionic nerve fibers to the pineal gland. The extent to which these findings with laboratory animals apply to man is not yet clear.

PLATE 101

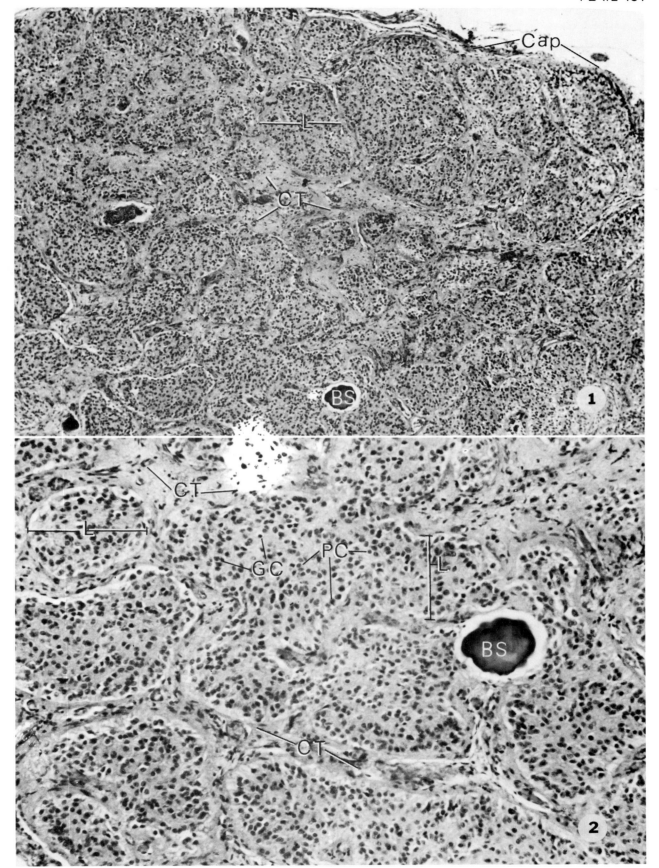

PLATE 102. Parathyroid and Thyroid Glands

The parathyroid glands are usually four in number. Each is surrounded by a capsule and lies on or is partially embedded in the thyroid gland. Connective tissue trabeculae extend from the capsule into the substance of the gland and, as seen in **Figure 1,** associated with the trabeculae are the larger blood vessels **(BV)** and, occasionally, adipose cells **(A).** The parenchyma of the parathyroid glands appears as cords or sheets of cells separated by capillaries and delicate connective tissue septa.

Two parenchymal cell types can be distinguished in routine H&E sections: chief cells (principal cells) and oxyphil cells **(Fig. 1).** The chief cells **(CC)** are more numerous. They contain a spherical nucleus surrounded by a small amount of cytoplasm. Oxyphil cells **(OC)** are less numerous. They contain a spherical nucleus surrounded by a small amount of cytoplasm. Also, oxyphil cells are conspicuously larger than chief cells but have a slightly smaller and more intensely staining nucleus. Their cytoplasm stains with eosin and the boundaries between the cells are usually well marked. Moreover, the oxyphils are arranged in groups of variable size that appear scattered about in a much larger field of chief cells. Even with low magnification it is often possible to identify clusters of oxyphil cells because a unit area contains fewer nuclei than a comparable unit area of chief cells, as is clearly evident in **Figure 1.** Oxyphil cells appear during the end of the first decade of life and become more numerous around puberty. A further increase may be seen in older individuals.

In addition to the chief and oxyphil cells, which are easy to identify, there may be other cells intermediate between these two and more difficult to identify. The significance of these intermediate cell types is not clear at present. Recent observations with the electron microscope verify the presence of cells that appear to be transitional between chief and oxyphil cells. This finding tends to support the concept that chief and oxyphil cells represent two functional variations of the same cell.

The parathyroid glands elaborate a hormone that influences calcium and bone metabolism. Injection of parathyroid hormone into laboratory animals results in the release of calcium from bone by the action of osteocytes (osteocytic osteolysis) and osteoclasts (osteoclasia). Removal of parathyroid glands results in a rapid drop in blood calcium levels.

The thyroid gland is located in the neck in close relation to the upper part of the trachea and the lower part of the larynx. It consists of two lateral lobes that are joined by a narrow isthmus. The functional unit of the thyroid gland is the follicle, which consists of a single layer of cuboidal or low columnar epithelium surrounding a colloid-filled space. A rich capillary network is present in the connective tissue that separates the follicles. The connective tissue also contains lymphatic capillaries.

A histological section of the thyroid gland is shown in **Figure 2.** The follicles **(F)** vary somewhat in size and shape, and they appear closely packed. The homogeneous mass in the center of each follicle is the colloid. The thyroid cells appear to form a ring around the colloid. Although the individual cells are difficult to distinguish at this magnification, the nuclei of the cells serve as an indication of their location and arrangement.

Large groups of cells are seen in association with some follicles. Where the nuclei are of the same size and staining characteristics, one can conclude that, in these sites, the section includes the wall of the follicle **(arrows)** in a tangential manner without including the lumen.

KEY

A, adipose cells
BV, blood vessels
CC, chief cells
CT, connective tissue
F, follicles

OC, oxyphil cells
arrows, tangential section of follicle wall
asterisks, shrinkage artifact

| **Fig. 1,** human, × 320 | **Fig. 2,** human, × 200 |

PLATE 102

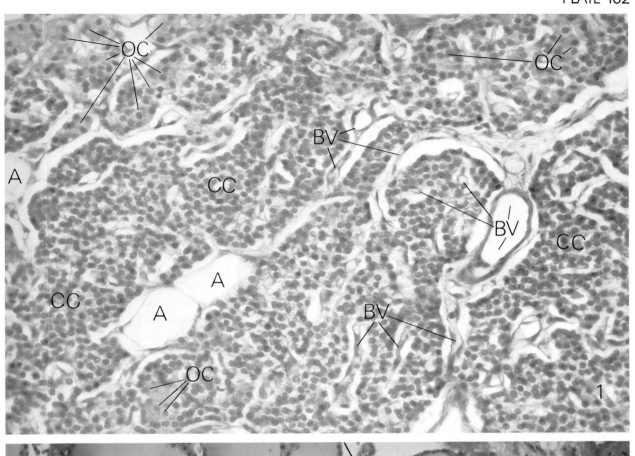

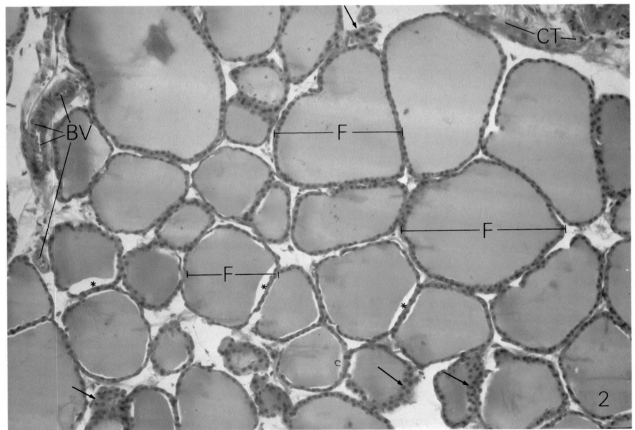

PLATE 103. Thyroid Follicle Cells, Light and Electron Microscopy

The **circular inset** shows parts of three thyroid follicles. The colloid is generally homogeneous in each, although different follicles show different degrees of staining. In one, the colloid has separated from the cells **(asterisk);** this is an artifactual separation. The thyroid follicular cells are cuboidal. They are the major glandular cell type of the thyroid gland: they synthesize thyroglobulin and secrete it into the follicle; later, the cells remove the colloid from the follicle by endocytosis, degrade the thyroglobulin of the colloid, and discharge the products into the underlying blood vessels. Another glandular cell type is also found in the thyroid gland, namely, the parafollicular cell. These cells may be present singly or in small groups. They produce calcitonin and they are also called C cells. The cell with the large amount of cytoplasm at the junction of the three follicles may be parafollicular cell. In many places adjacent follicles are extremely close to each other, separated only by a small amount of connective tissue in which there are capillaries **(arrows)** and sometimes nerves (see below). The electron micrograph shows portions of two adjacent follicles from a region roughly equivalent to one that is marked by the two **arrows.**

The most conspicuous organelles of the thyroid follicularcells are numerous profiles of rough-surfaced endoplasmic reticulum, Golgi profiles, and mitochondria. Less obvious are the small microvilli on their apical surface, lysosomes, small vesicles, and—when endocytosing colloid—large

apical pseudopods extending into the colloid. Because such apical pseudopods are not seen within the colloid, it is considered that these cells are not actively engaged in removal of colloid. The main point of the electron micrograph is to show the minimal space between follicles. At its narrowest point, the space contains a bundle of nonmyelinated nerve fibers **(NF)** and a thin cellular process of a fibroblast. Also to be noted in the electron micrograph are the capillaries in proximity to the follicle cells in the upper and lower part of the micrograph. The capillary endothelium **(En)** is extremely thin; the endothelium is fenestrated, and the electron micrograph shows very little perinuclear cytoplasm. There are red blood cells **(RBC)** within the capillaries.

PLATE 103

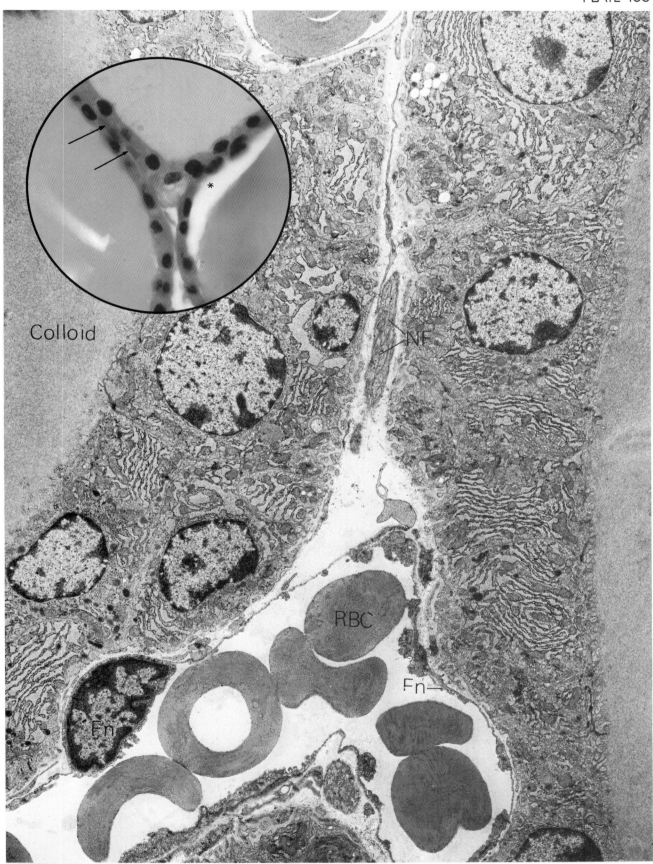

Colloid

NF

RBC

En

En

*

PLATE 104. Adrenal Gland I

There are two adrenal glands, one situated at the upper pole of each kidney. An adrenal gland is a composite of two distinct structural and functional components: the cortex and the medulla. The cortex develops from mesoderm, the medulla from ectoderm.

A section through the entire thickness of an adrenal gland is shown in **Figure 1.** Several histological features are readily evident in this low-power micrograph. The outer part of the gland, the cortex, has a distinctly different appearance, both in structural organization and staining characteristics, from the inner portion, the medulla. Very large blood vessels **(V)** are typically found in the medulla. These are veins that drain both the cortex and medulla. A capsule **(Cap)** surrounds the gland and from it delicate trabeculae extend into the substance of the gland **(Figs. 1 and 2).**

The cortex is divided into three parts according to the type and arrangement of cells. These are designated as the zona glomerulosa, the zona fasciculata, and the zona reticularis.

The zona glomerulosa **(ZG)** is located at the outer part of the cortex, immediately under the capsule **(Fig. 2).** The parenchyma of this zone consists of small cells that appear as arching cords or as oval groups. The nuclei of the parenchymal cells are spherical and the cells possess a small amount of lightly staining cytoplasm. Because of the small amount of cytoplasm, the nuclei in this zone appear relatively crowded. Between the cords of cells are elongated nuclei **(arrows, Figs. 2 and 3)** that belong either to cells of the delicate connective tissue stroma or to the endothelial cells of the capillaries that course between the cell cords.

The zona fasciculata consists of radially oriented cords and sheets of cells, usually two cells in width. It can be divided into two parts, an outer and an inner, based on the appearance of the cells in routine H&E preparations. The outer part of the zona fasciculata **(ZF)** is shown where it begins just beneath the zona glomerulosa in **Figure 2.** A deeper portion of the zona fasciculata is shown in

KEY	
Cap, capsule	**arrows,** nuclei of
V, vein of medulla	endothelial cells or of
ZF, zona fasciculata	connective tissue cells
ZG, zona glomerulosa	**asterisk,** binucleate cell
Fig. 1, monkey, × 30	**Figs. 2 and 3,** monkey, × 400

Figure 3. The nuclei of these cells are about the same size or slightly larger than those of the zona glomerulosa; however, there is more cytoplasm and the nuclei consequently are more distant from one another than those of the zona glomerulosa. Occasionally, binucleate cells **(asterisk)** are seen in the zona fasciculata. These may be difficult to recognize because the cell boundaries are not always conspicuous. The cells of the outer part of the zona fasciculata contain a considerably greater amount of lipid than the cells in the other parts of the cortex. During the preparation of routine H&E specimens, the lipid is lost, and the cytoplasm then has a noticeably foamy or spongy appearance.

The zones of the adrenal cortex are not only morphologically distinct, but the zones also reflect a functional specialization. The zona glomerulosa secretes the mineralocorticoids (aldosterone and deoxycorticosterone). On the other hand, the zona fasciculata secretes the glucocorticoids (cortisol, cortisone and corticosterone), and the zona reticularis is active in the production of adrenal androgens. The zona fasciculata has also been found to secrete adrenal androgens. There is yet another functional distinction in that the inner two zones of the adrenal cortex are regulated by ACTH whereas the zona glomerulosa is not.

PLATE 104

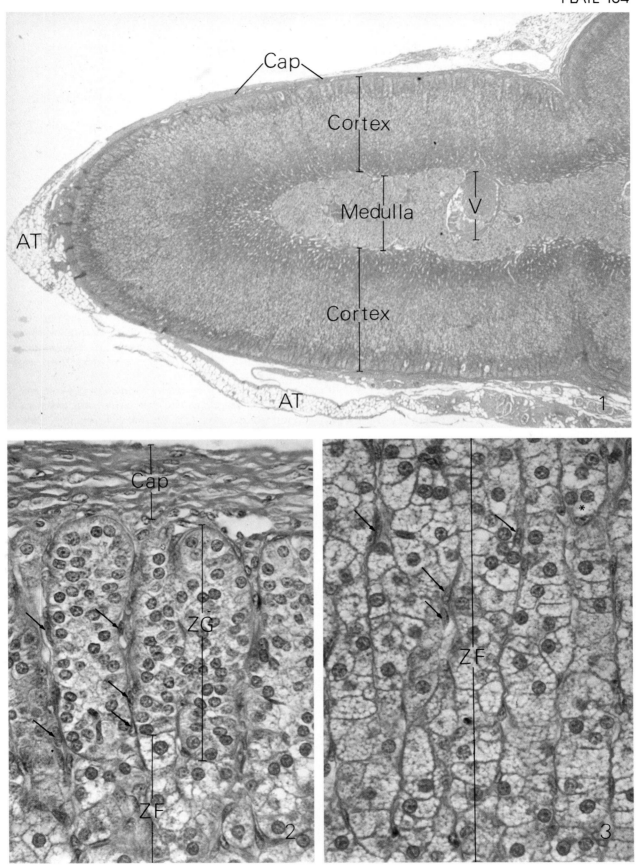

PLATE 105. Adrenal Gland II

The junction between the outer and inner parts of the zona fasciculata, as well as the junction between the inner portion of the zona fasciculata and the zona reticularis, are shown in **Figure 1.** The outer part of the zona fasciculata, as described in the previous plate, consists of cells whose cytoplasm has a spongy appearance [**ZF(S)**]. It constitutes the bulk of the fascicular zone. The inner part of the zona fasciculata consists of slightly smaller cells [**ZF(C)**]. The cytoplasm of these cells appears more compact than that of the cells in the outer part due the considerably reduced amount of lipid droplets. Throughout the entire zona fasciculata the cells appear as cords and between the cords one can see the elongated nuclei (**arrows**) that belong either to cells of the delicate connective tissue stroma or to endothelial cells.

The zona reticularis (**ZR**) is shown in the lower portion of **Figure 1.** This is the deepest part of the cortex, immediately adjacent to the medulla. It consists of interconnecting, irregular cords and sheets of relatively small cells. The cords and sheets are narrower than those of the other parts of the cortex; in many places they are only one cell wide. Between the cords of cells are the capillaries that, in this zone, frequently appear dilated as compared to the collapsed appearance of the capillaries of the zona glomerulosa and outer fasciculata. As in the other parts of the gland, the elongated nuclei (**arrows**) belong to the endothelial cells or to cells of the connective tissue stroma.

In mammals, the adrenal medulla is in the center of the gland, surrounded by the cortex. It consist of large cells (**Fig. 2**) that are organized in ovoid groups or as short interconnecting cords. The cytoplasm of neighboring cells may stain with different intensity. These cells color when treated

---

KEY

GC, ganglion cells
ZF(C), zona fasciculata, compact cells
ZF(S), zona fasciculata, spongy cells

ZR, zona reticularis
arrows, nuclei of endothelial cells or of connective tissue cells
asterisk, binucleate cell

Figs. 1 and 2, monkey, × 400

---

with chromate reagents and, for this reason, they are sometimes called chromaffin cells. Elongated nuclei (**arrows**) of vascular or connective tissue cells can be seen in the delicate stroma that separates the groups of parenchymal cells. Ganglion cells (**GC**) are occasionally seen in sections of the adrenal medulla.

The cells of the adrenal medulla develop from the same source as the postganglionic cells of the sympathetic nervous system. They are directly innervated by preganglionic cells of the sympathetic system and may be regarded as modified postganglionic cells that are specialized to secrete. These cells produce epinephrine and norepinephrine.

The adrenal medulla receives its blood supply via two routes. It is supplied by arterioles that pass through the cortex and it is supplied by capillaries that continue from the cortex. This means that some of the blood reaching the medulla contains cortical secretion.

PLATE 105

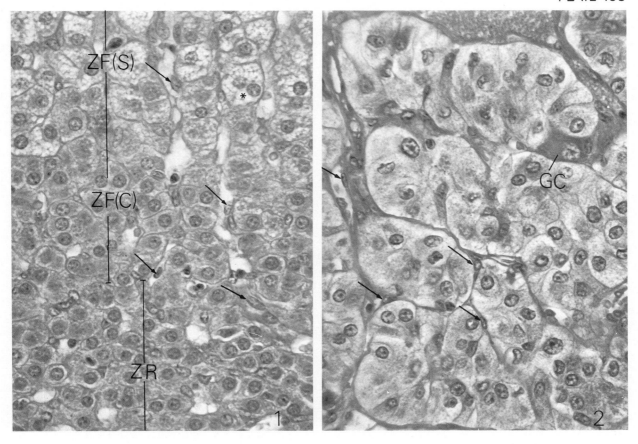

Male Reproductive System

21

The male reproductive system consists of the testes, epididymides and genital ducts, accessory reproductive glands, and penis (Fig. 21.1). The genital duct system includes the tubuli recti and rete testis, which lie within the testis; and the ductuli efferentes, ductus epididymidis, and ductus deferens, which constitute the ducts lying outside of the testis. The accessory glands include the seminal vesicles, prostate, and bulbourethral glands.

Included in this chapter is a brief description of mitosis and meiosis. A basic understanding of these processes is essential in understanding the proliferation of the germ cells and the production of the gametes in both the male and the female reproductive systems.

TESTIS

The testes have two interrelated functions: the production of gametes *(gametogenesis)* and the production of steroids *(steroidogenesis)*. In the male, the production of gametes, the *spermatozoa,* is referred to as *spermatogenesis.* A suspending medium secreted by the testis and other parts of the duct system provides a medium essential for the transport, maintenance, and further maturation of the sperm. Steroid hormones, primarily testosterone, function in the regulation of the development of the spermatozoa and the growth, development, and maintenance of the accessory reproductive glands. These hormones also influence the development of secondary sex characteristics and, to some extent, sexual behavior.

Each testis is covered on the anterolateral surface by a serous membrane called the visceral layer of the *tunica vaginalis* (Figs. 21.1 and 21.2). The tunica vaginalis is actually a closed serous cavity with an outer parietal layer and a visceral layer contacting the surface of each testis. (The testes develop in the abdominal cavity and then descend into the scrotum during fetal development. They carry with them an outpocketing of the peritoneum that becomes the tunica vaginalis.) Blood and lymphatic vessels and nerves enter the testis along its posterior surface, which is not covered by the tunica vaginalis. The epididymis, which lies along the lateral part of the posterior aspect of the testis, is only partially covered with the serous membrane.

Enclosing the seminiferous tubules of each testis is a thick fibrous capsule, the *tunica albuginea* (Fig. 21.2). The tunica vaginalis is applied to the external surface of this layer. Along the posterior border of the testis, the tunica albuginea projects into its interior, forming the *mediastinum testis.* Ducts, nerves, and testicular vessels exit and enter the testis through the mediastinum. Numerous thin fibrous septa extend from the tunica albuginea to the mediastinum. The septa divide the testis into 200 to 300 pyramidal lobules. Each lobule contains one to four highly convoluted seminiferous tubules, which produce the spermatozoa. Small blood vessels and lymphatic channels, as well as the *interstitial* or *Leydig cells* lie between the tubules (Fig. 21.3). These are endocrine cells that produce steroid hormones, including testosterone.

Macrophages are also present, but other connective tissue cells including typical fibroblasts are normally absent.

In humans, each testis contains 400 to 600 seminiferous tubules which measure about 150 to 250 μm in diameter and 30 to 80 cm in length. The combined length of the tubules in each testis is about 250 m. The seminiferous tubules usually

603

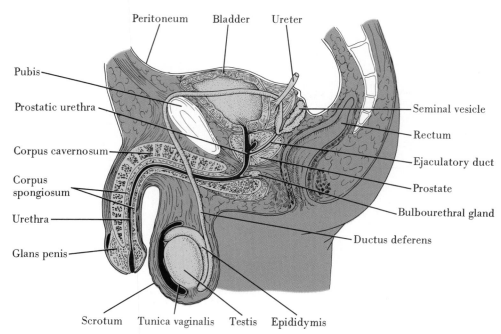

Figure 21.1. Schematic diagram demonstrating the components of the male reproductive system. Midline structures are depicted in sagittal section: bilateral structures including the testis, epididymis, vas deferns, and seminal vesicle are shown intact. (After Turner CD: In Bloom W, Fawcett DW (eds): *A Textbook of Histology*, 10th ed. Philadelphia, WB Saunders, 1975.)

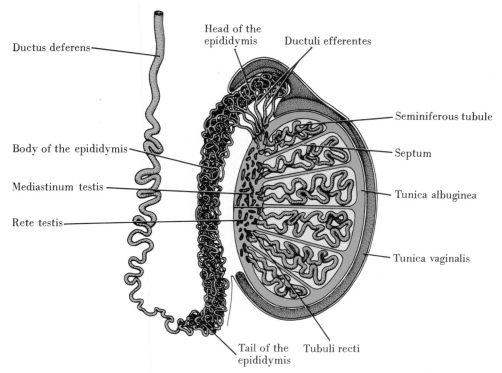

Figure 21.2. Schematic diagram of a longitudinal section through the human testis. The genital duct system, which includes the tubuli recti, rete testis, ductuli efferentes, ductus epididymidis, and ductus deferens, is also shown. (Modified from M. Dym, 1977.)

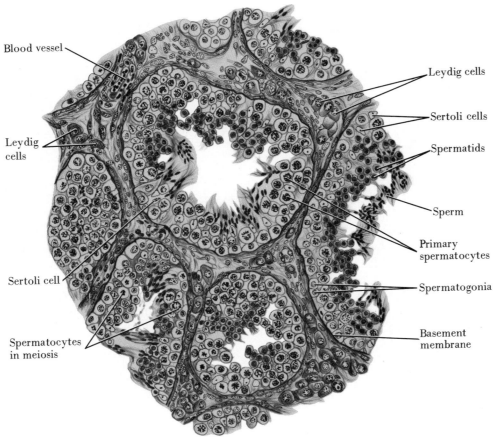

Figure 21.3. Drawing of a section of human testis. Several seminiferous tubules containing Sertoli and spermatogenic cells are shown. Leydig cells are seen in the interstitial tissue filling the interstices between the adjacent seminiferous tubules. (After Maximow AA: In Bloom W, Fawcett DW (eds): *A Textbook of Histology,* 10th ed. Philadelphia, WB Saunders, 1975.)

form an anastomic loop. Near the apex of the lobule the seminiferous tubules open into the *tubuli recti* (see Fig. 21.2), which form the first segment of the genital duct system. These ducts are continuous with the *rete testis,* a system of epithelial-lined spaces in the mediastinum.

Seminiferous Tubule

Boundary Tissue or Lamina Propria. The seminiferous tubules are surrounded by an outer layer of adventitial cells and associated connective tissue, the *lamina propria,* and a well-defined basement membrane (Figs. 21.3 and 21.4). The basement membrane lies adjacent to the seminiferous epithelium, separating it from the lamina propria.

The organization of the lamina propria demonstrates considerable species variation. In the common laboratory rodents, it consists of a single layer of flattened epithelioid cells, called *myoid cells*

or *peritubular contractile cells.* These contractile cells are in close apposition with one another at their margins and, thus, form a contiguous sheath around the epithelium. In humans and other primates, the contractile cells are not in close apposition, rather they are organized into three to five layers. At the ultrastructural level, the cells demonstrate features associated with smooth muscle cells, including the presence of large numbers of actin filaments. These cells demonstrate rhythmic contractions that assist in the movement of spermatozoa and testicular fluid through the seminiferous tubules and into the genital duct system. Thickening of the lamina propria normally occurs with aging and reduction of the size of the seminiferous tubules, but it has also been associated with many cases of infertility in the human male.

Seminiferous Epithelium. The *seminiferous epithelium* is a complex stratified epithelium composed of two basic cell types: *Sertoli cells* and

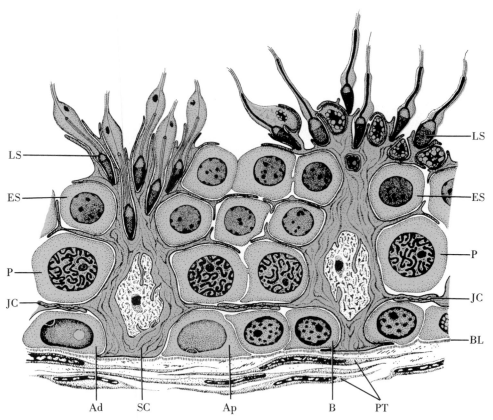

Figure 21.4. Schematic drawing of human seminiferous epithelium. The relationship of the Sertoli cells (SC) to the spermatogenic cells is indicated. The seminiferous epithelium rests on a basal lamina (BL), and a layer of peritubular cells (PT) surrounds the seminiferous tubule. Pale type A spermatogonium (Ap), dark type A spermatogonium (Ad), and type B spermatogonium are located in the basal compartment of the seminiferous epithelium below the junctional complex (JC) between adjacent Sertoli cells: pachytene primary spermatocytes (P), early spermatids (ES), and late spermatids (LS), with partitioning residual cytoplasm that becomes the residual body, are seen in the adluminal compartment above the junctional complex. (Redrawn from Y. Clermont, 1963).

spermatogenic cells (see Fig. 21.4). The *Sertoli cells* are a nonproliferating population composed of a single cell type. Each Sertoli cell extends from the basement membrane to the lumen of the seminiferous tubule. The *spermatogenic cells* are a proliferating population composed of cells at various phases of a complex differentiative process. For descriptive purposes, spermatogenesis can be divided into three distinct phases: (1) the spermatogonial phase; (2) the spermatocyte phase or meiosis; and (3) the spermatid phase or spermiogenesis. The most immature cells are located near the basement membrane. As the cells proliferate and undergo differentiation, they move toward the lumen of the seminiferous tubule. Usually four or five concentric layers of cells, representing generations of cells at various phases in their development, can be identified within the seminiferous epithelium. These morphologically distinct sper-

matogenic cells are at one of the three basic phases in the development and are identified as *spermatogonia, spermatocytes,* or *spermatids* (early or late). *Spermatogonia,* derived from stem cells, undergo a series of mitotic divisions during which they undergo limited morphological differentiation. The final division of these spermatogonia produces *spermatocytes,* which divide meiotically and produce *spermatids.* These haploid cells undergo dramatic morphological differentiation, referred to as *spermiogenesis,* as they are transformed into spermatozoa. (The morphology of the spermatogenic cells will be described in the section on spermatogenesis.)

Sertoli Cell

Structural Features. The Sertoli cells are columnar cells with complex apical and lateral processes that surround the adjacent spermatogenic cells and fill the spaces between them. However, the complex, elaborate configuration of the Sertoli cells cannot be seen distinctly in routine hematoxylin and eosin (H&E) preparation. The Sertoli cells give structural organization to the tubules as they extend through the full thickness of the seminiferous epithelium.

The Sertoli cell nucleus, containing finely dispersed chromatin, is generally ovoid or triangular in shape and may have one or more deep infoldings. Its shape and location vary. The shape may be flattened, lying in the basal portion of the cell near and parallel to the basement membrane, or it may be triangular or ovoid, lying near or some distance from the basement membrane. In some species, the Sertoli cell nucleus contains a unique tripartite structure that consists of an RNA-containing nucleolus flanked by a pair of DNA-containing bodies called *karyosomes.*

With the light microscope, the extent and morphology of the apical and lateral processes are poorly defined. At the ultrastructural level, the limits of the cell can be identified and the cytoplasm is seen to contain abundant smooth and some granular endoplasmic reticulum, numerous spherical or elongated mitochondria, a well-developed Golgi complex, and varying numbers of microtubules, lysosomes, lipid droplets, vesicles, glycogen granules, and fine filaments (Figs. 21.5 and 21.6). A sheath of 7- to 9-nm filaments surrounds the nucleus and separates it from other organelles. In humans, the basal cytoplasm also contains characteristic *inclusion bodies of Charcot-Böttcher.* These slender, fusiform, crystalloid inclusions, measuring 10 to 25 μm in length and 1 μm in width, are often visible with the light microscope. At the ultrastructural level, they appear as rather poorly ordered parallel or converging, straight, dense filaments, 15 nm in diameter (Fig. 21.5). The chemical nature and function of these inclusions is unknown.

Junctional Complexes. Adjacent Sertoli cells are joined to one another by an unusual type of junction (Fig. 21.6). The Sertoli cell junctional complex is morphologically unique, not being found in other kinds of epithelia. A Sertoli-Sertoli junctional complex consists of: (1) an exceedingly tight junction composed of up to 50 or more parallel lines of fusion of the apposed membranes; (2) flattened cisternae of endoplasmic reticulum that parallel the plasma membrane in the region of the tight junction; and (3) hexagonally packed bundles of actin filaments that are interposed between the cisternae of endoplasmic reticulum and the plasma membrane (Fig. 21.7). The endo-

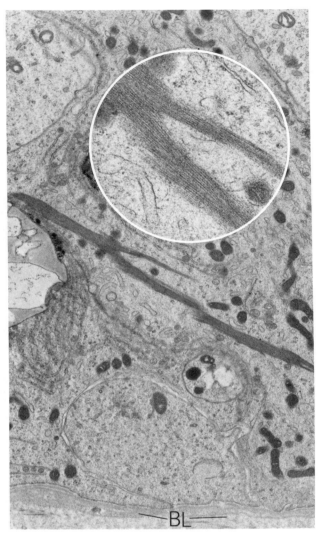

Figure 21.5. Electron micrograph of a human Sertoli cell. Characteristic crystalloid inclusion bodies of Charcot-Böttcher are present in the basal cytoplasm of the cell. The basal lamina (BL) is indicated for orientation. × 9000. The filaments of the crystalloid can be seen in the **inset.** × 27,000. (Courtesy of D. F. Cameron, 1984.)

plasmic reticulum associated with the junctional complex has ribosomes only on its cytoplasmic surface, which is directed away from the plasma membrane. A similar junctional complex also develops between Sertoli cells and spermatids. The Sertoli-spermatid junction is identical to the Sertoli-Sertoli junction except that there is no occluding junction between the two cells and there is no complementary specialization in the spermatid at the attachment site (see Fig. 21.7). It has been shown that the junctional complex at both sites is a strong adhesion device that holds the adjoining cells together.

Other types of junctions that have been de-

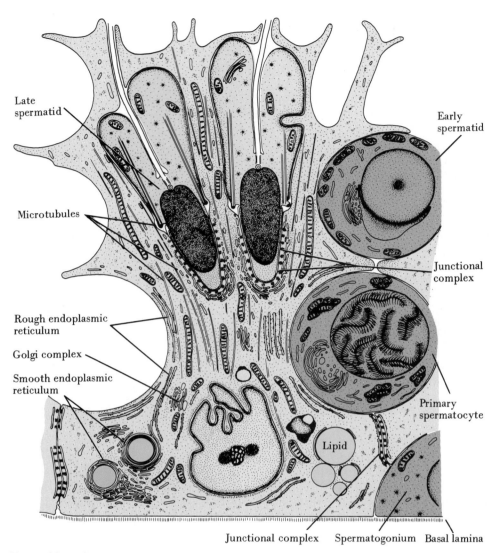

Figure 21.6. Schematic drawing of a Sertoli cell and adjacent spermatogenic cells. The ultrastructural features of the cells are illustrated. Junctional complexes between adjacent Sertoli cells and between the Sertoli cell and the late spermatids are illustrated. The late spermatids reside in recesses within the apical cytoplasm of the Sertoli cells. Lateral processes of the Sertoli cells extend over the surface of the spermatocytes and spermatids. (W. Bloom and D. W. Fawcett, 1975.)

scribed in Sertoli cells include gap junctions; hemidesmosomes, on the basal portion of the cell adjacent to the basal lamina; and desmosome-like complexes, between Sertoli cells and adjacent spermatogenic cells at early phases in their development.

Compartmentalization of the Seminiferous Epithelium. The Sertoli-Sertoli junctional complexes divide the seminiferous epithelium into two compartments: a ***basal compartment*** containing spermatogonia and young spermatocytes and an ***adluminal compartment*** containing later spermato-

cytes and spermatids (see Fig. 21.6). The compartmentalization of the seminiferous epithelium enables the Sertoli cells to establish microenvironments that allow the spermatogenic cells to proceed through meiosis and other differentiative events. The young spermatocytes, produced by the final mitotic division of the spermatogonia, must pass through the junctional complexes in order to enter the adluminal compartment. This process is not fully understood, but apparently occurs in a manner which maintains the integrity of the two compartments.

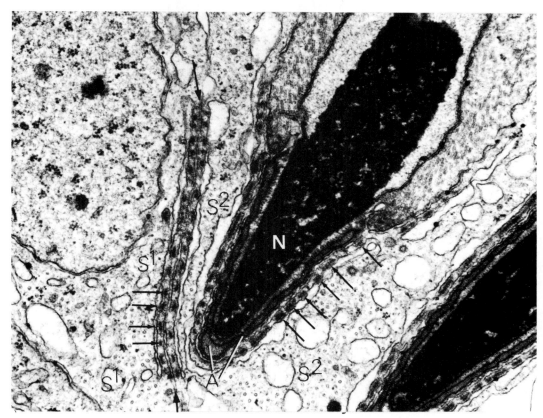

Figure 21.7. Electron micrograph demonstrating a Sertoli-Sertoli junctional complex and in close proximity a Sertoli-spermatid junctional specialization. Condensation and shaping of the spermatid nucleus (N) are well advanced. The acrosome (A) of the spermatid appears as a V-shaped profile, and in close association with it is the Sertoli cell junctional specialization characterized by bundles of microfilaments (**small arrows**) and the associated profile of endoplasmic reticulum, which resides immediately adjacent to the microfilament bundles. The Sertoli-Sertoli junction lies just to the left, joining one Sertoli cell (S^1) to the adjacent Sertoli cell (S^2). The **large arrows** indicate the limits of the junction. Note that the junction here reveals the same elements—the microfilament bundles (**small arrows**) and a profile of endoplasmic reticulum—as are seen in the Sertoli-spermatid junction. Not evident at this magnification is the tight junction that is associated with the Sertoli-Sertoli junctional complex. × 30,000.

Blood-Testis Barrier. Physiological and morphological studies have established that the Sertoli-Sertoli junctional complexes are the site of the *blood-testis barrier.* The concept of physiological barriers that separate tissues from blood-borne substances arose from studies conducted in the early 1900s. Investigators studying the distribution of intravenously injected dyes found that when some dyes were injected, most tissues were stained, but the brain, testes, and a few other tissues were not. (The concept of a blood-brain barrier arose from these early observations.)

The observation that the seminiferous tubules were not stained received little attention until the late 1960s when studies with a variety of dyes confirmed the earlier observations and further demonstrated that dyes were not excluded from the seminiferous tubules of prepubertal rats. Subsequent physiological studies on the penetration of substances into the seminiferous tubules and the composition of testicular fluids have clearly demonstrated a physiological compartmentalization of the testis. Striking differences have been found in the ionic, amino acid, carbohydrate, and protein composition of fluids collected from the lumens of seminiferous tubules and genital ducts versus blood plasma and testicular lymph. Of particular interest is the absence of many of the serum proteins and immunoglobulins from the fluids of the seminiferous tubules and genital ducts. Morphological studies utilizing electron-opaque markers of various sizes have demonstrated that the junctional complexes between adjacent Sertoli cells act as the barrier to the penetration of the markers.

Studies in the rat on the development of the testis at puberty have shown that the Sertoli junctional complexes are initially formed and establish the permeability barrier when the spermatogenic cells first pass through the early stages of the spermatocyte phase.

In terms of the immunological importance of the blood-testis barrier, two basic facts are well-established: (1) spermatozoa and spermatogenic cells possess molecules that are unique to this cell type and are recognized as "foreign" (not self) by the immune system; (2) spermatozoa are first produced at puberty long after the individual has become immunocompetent, that is, capable of recognizing foreign molecules and producing antibodies against them. Therefore, the blood-testis barrier serves an essential role in isolating the spermatogenic cells from the immune system. Failure of the spermatogenic cells and spermatozoa to remain so isolated results in the production of sperm-specific antibodies. Such an immune response is seen subsequent to vasectomy and in some cases of infertility. After vasectomy, sperm-specific antibodies are produced as the cells of the immune system are exposed to the spermatozoa that no longer remain isolated from the immune system within the reproductive tract. It has also been shown that in some cases of infertility, unrelated to vasectomy, sperm-specific antibodies are present in the semen.

Functions. The Sertoli cells obviously play an essential role in the development of the spermatogenic cells, however, many of the specific activities remain to be clarified. Many of the Sertoli cell functions are directly related to the compartmentalization of the seminiferous epithelium. As the Sertoli cells secrete fluids or restrict the movements of molecules, they establish microenvironments that are essential for the development and differentiation of the spermatogenic cells.

Functions ascribed to the Sertoli cells include:

1. Providing physical support for the spermatogenic cells
2. Mediating the movements across the seminiferous epithelium of steroids, metabolites, and nutrients utilized by the spermatogenic cells
3. Restricting the movements of extracellular molecules into the seminiferous epithelium through establishment of occluding (or tight) junctions between the adjacent Sertoli cells
4. Phagocytosing degenerating spermatogenic cells and the excess cytoplasm shed from the differentiating spermatids as the residual bodies

5. Secreting androgen-binding protein, which serves to concentrate testosterone within the seminiferous epithelium and the proximal part of the genital duct system
6. Secreting various stimulatory and inhibitory substances involved in the regulation of mitosis, meiosis, steroidogenic functions of the Leydig cells, and the release of gonadotropins from the pituitary
7. Controlling the movements of the spermatogenic cells within the seminiferous epithelium and the release of the spermatozoa into the lumen of the seminiferous tubule

Spermatogenic Cell and Spermatogenesis

Spermatogenesis is the developmental process through which the spermatogenic cells are transformed from the undifferentiated, diploid (*2n*) spermatogonia into highly specialized haploid (*n*) spermatozoa. As was explained earlier, each cell passes through three principal phases during its development: (1) the *spermatogonial phase,* or spermatocytogenesis; (2) the *meiotic phase,* or meiosis; and (3) the *spermatid phase,* or spermiogenesis.

The testes form during embryonic and fetal development. The interstitial cells arise from mesenchyme, the Sertoli cells from the germinal epithelium, and the spermatogonia from primordial germ cells. At birth, the seminiferous cords contain only two cell types—Sertoli cells and primordial germ cells (or gonocytes). During the prepubertal years, the cords form seminiferous tubules that become populated with spermatogonia, but development does not proceed beyond this phase. At puberty, the production of mature spermatozoa is initiated. By the age of 14 or 15 years, spermatozoa are produced at normal adult levels (50 to 150 million spermatozoa daily per testis). Although sperm production begins to decline at about age 45 years, it normally continues throughout life.

Spermatogonial Phase. The diploid spermatogonia, which reside in the basal compartment of the seminiferous epithelium, proliferate by mitotic divisions, giving rise to generation after generation of cells that will proceed through spermatogenesis. In order for this process to continue, the mitotic cells must also perpetuate themselves, providing a population of *stem cells.* Some of the stem cells, the "reserve" stem cells, rarely divide or have a very long cell-cycle time. If the spermatogenic cells are destroyed, induction of the mitotic activity of the reserve stem cells can re-establish the spermatogenic cell population.

Three morphologically distinct types of spermatogonia have been described in men: dark type A (Ad); pale type A (Ap); and type B (see Fig. 21.4). Type Ad spermatogonia serve as the reserve stem cells, occasionally dividing to produce type Ap spermatogonia, which, in turn, divide mitotically to produce type B cells. The three types of spermatogonia are rounded cells that show little difference in their size, measuring about 12 μm in diameter, or in the morphological characteristics of their pale-staining cytoplasm. The nuclei, measuring 6 to 7 μm in diameter, differ in their morphology and staining intensity. The nuclei of type Ad and Ap are usually slightly ovoid in shape and contain finely granular chromatin and one or two nucleoli attached to the nuclear envelope (Fig. 21.4). Type Ad spermatogonia can be distinguished from type Ap by the more intense staining of the nucleoplasm and the presence of the large, pale-staining nuclear vacuole. The nuclei of type B spermatogonia are spherical in shape, contain clumps of chromatin adjacent to the nuclear envelope, and have a single, centrally located nucleolus. Mitotic division of type B gives rise to the primary spermatocytes, marking the beginning of the meiotic phase.

MITOSIS AND MEIOSIS

At fertilization in the human, fusion of the haploid nuclei from the egg and a spermatozoon results in the formation of the zygote with 23 pairs of chromosomes (22 pairs of autosomes + XX in females and 22 pairs of autosomes + XY in males). Each chromosome pair contains one member of maternal origin and one of paternal origin. Subsequent growth of the multicellular organism with the exception of gametogenesis occurs through the process of mitotic cell divison.

The zygote and all the somatic cells derived from it are described as being diploid (2n) in chromosome number; the gametes, having only one member of each chromosome pair, are haploid (n). During gametogenesis, reduction in chromosome number to the haploid state (23 chromosomes in the human) occurs through the meiotic divisions. This reduction is necessary in order to maintain a constant number of chromosomes in the species.

Mitosis. Mitosis is a process of cell duplication, or replication, through which a cell gives rise to two daughter cells, each of which is genetically identical to the parent cell. (In its strict use, the term mitosis is used to describe the duplication and distribution of the chromosomes.) The process of cell division usually includes division of both the nucleus, *karyokinesis,* and the cytoplasm, *cytokinesis.* If cytokinesis does not follow karyokinesis, a binucleate cell is formed.

Four phases are defined in mitosis (Fig. 21.8).

1. *Prophase.* (Duplication of the DNA occurs in the interphase preceding this phase.) Prophase begins as chromosomes become visible. As the chromosomes continue to condense, each can be seen to consist of two strands, called *chromatids,* which are held together by the *centromere,* or *kilnetochore.* Other changes include disappearance of the nucleolus, replication of the centrioles, and disintegration of the nuclear envelope.

2. *Metaphase.* During metaphase the mitotic spindle, consisting of microtubules organized around the centrioles located at opposite poles of the cell, becomes organized and directs the movements of the chromosomes to the plane in the middle of the cell, the *equatorial,* or *metaphase, plate.*

3. *Anaphase.* During anaphase, the chromatids separate (these are then identified as the chromosomes of the forming cells) and are pulled to opposite poles of the cell by the microtubules of the spindle that are attached to the *centromeres.* Since the separating chromosomes contain identical copies of the duplicated DNA, the future daughter cells will be genetically identical, containing the same kind and number of chromosomes as the parent cell.

4. *Telophase.* During telophase, a nuclear envelope forms around the chromosomes at each pole, the chromosomes uncoil and become indistinct except at regions that remain condensed in the interphase nucleus, the nucleoli reappear, and the cytoplasm divides to form two daughter cells.

Meiosis. Meiosis is a process of cell division through which the diploid cells (2n), containing pairs of chromosomes, give rise to haploid cells (n), containing one member of each pair. During this process, the chromosomes pair and may exchange chromosome segments, thus altering the genetic composition of the chromosomes. This genetic exchange, called *crossing-over,* and the random assortment of each member of the chromosome pairs into haploid gametes gives rise to infinite genetic diversity.

The nuclear events of meiosis are essentially

the same in both the male and female, but the cytoplasmic events are markedly different. Figures 21.8 illustrates the key nuclear and cytoplasmic events of meiosis as they occur in spermatogenesis and oogenesis. The events of meiosis through metaphase I are essentially the same in both processes. Therefore, the figure illustrates the differences in the process as they diverge after metaphase I.

Cytoplasmic events. In the male, the meiotic division of a primary spermatocyte results in the formation of *four* structurally identical, but genetically unique, haploid spermatids, each with the capacity to differentiate into a spermatozoon. In contrast, in the female, the meiotic division of a primary oocyte results in the formation of *one* haploid ovun and *three* haploid polar bodies. The ovum receives the majority of the cytoplasm and becomes the functional gamete; the polar bodies receive very little cytoplasm and undergo degeneration.

It should be noted that during the mitotic and meiotic divisions of spermatogenesis (spermatogonia divide by mitotic division and spermatocytes divide by meiotic division), cytokinesis is incomplete, resulting in the cells being connected by intercellular bridges (Described below).

Nuclear events. During the interphase that precedes meiosis, the chromosomes duplicate themselves. The cells, containing twice the normal amount of DNA (tetraploid), then undergo a *reductional division* (or *meiosis I*) and an *equatorial division (or meiosisII)*. During meiosis I, the maternal and paternal chromosomes pair, exchange segments, and then separate from one another, establishing the haploid number of chromosomes and reducing the DNA to the diploid amount. In meiosis II, the chromatids separate from one another, maintaining the haploid number of chromosomes and reducing the DNA to the haploid amount.

Phases in the process of meiosis are similar to the phases of mitosis. *Prophase I* of meiosis I is an extended phase which is subdivided into five stages (see Fig. 21.8).

1. *Leptotene.* The chromosome becomes visible as thin strands.
2. *Zygotene.* Homologous chromosomes of maternal and paternal origin pair. This pairing involves the formation of a *synaptonemal complex,* a tripartite structure that brings the chromosomes into physical association so that crossing-over may occur (Fig. 21.9).
3. *Pachytene.* As the chromosomes condense, the individual chromatids become visible. Crossing-over occurs early in this phase.
4. *Diplotene.* The chromosomes condense further and *chiasmata,* or contracts between the chromatids, appear. The chiasmata indicate crossing-over may have occurred.
5. *Diakinesis.* The chromosomes reach their maximum thickness, the nucleolus disappears, and the nuclear envelope disintegrates.

Metaphase I is similar to metaphase of mitosis except that the paired chromosomes are aligned at the equatorial plate with one member on either side. *AnaphaseI* and *telophaseI* are similar to the same phases in mitosis except that the centromeres do not split and the paired chromatids, held by the centromere, remain together. The maternal and paternal members of each homologous pair, now containing exchanged segments, move to opposite poles. *Segregation,* or *random assortment,* occurs because the maternal and paternal chromosomes of each pair are randomly aligned on one side or the other of the metaphase plate. As mentioned above, this is an important contributor to genetic diversity. At the completion of meiosis I, or the reductional division, the cytoplasm divides. Each resulting daughter cell (a secondary *spermatocyte* or *oocyte*) is haploid, containing one member of each chromosome pair.

The cells quickly enter meiosis II, or the equatorial division, which is more like mitosis because the centromeres divide. The chromatids then separate at *anaphaseII* and pass to opposite poles of the cell. During meiosis II the cells pass through prophase II, metaphase II, anaphase II, and telophase II. These stages are essentially the same as those described in mitosis except that they involve a haploid set of chromosomes. *A feature that should be emphasized is that unlike the cells produced by mitosis, which are genetically identical to the parent cell, the cells produced by meiosis are genetically unique.*

Meiotic phase. A description of the chromosomal events associated with the meiotic phase is given in the special section on mitosis and meiosis (see above).

The early preleptotene spermatocytes initially reside in the basal compartment and resemble the spermatogonia in structure. They soon migrate away from the basal lamina and pass through the Sertoli-Sertoli junctional complex into the adluminal compartment. The spermatogenic cells increase in size and demonstrate distinctive nuclear morphology as they pass through the leptotene, zygotene, pachytene, and diplotene stages of the meiotic prophase. Cells late in the pachytene stage measure about 16 μm in diameter. Pachytene is the longest stage in the meiotic phase and lasts about

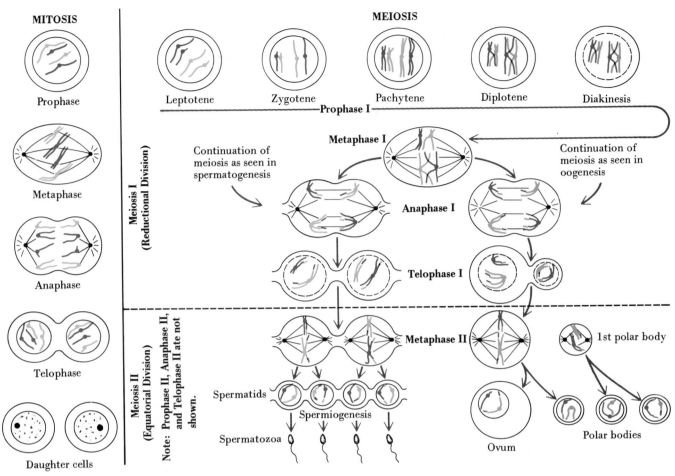

Figure 21.8. Comparison of mitosis and meiosis in an idealized cell having two pairs of chromosomes (2n). The chromosomes of maternal and paternal origin are depicted in red and blue, respectively. The mitotic division produces daughter cells that are genetically identical to the parental cell (2n). The meiotic division, which has two components, a reductional division and an equatorial division, produces a cell, which unlike the parental cell has only two chromosomes (n). In addition, during the chromosome pairing in prophase I of meiosis there is exchange of chromosome segments leading to further genetic diversity. It should be noted that in the human the first polar body does not divide. Division of the first polar body does occur in some species.

16 days in humans. The total duration of the meiotic phase is about 24 days. Secondary spermatocytes produced by the first meiotic division measure about 9 μm in diameter, but are infrequently seen because of the short duration (8 hr) of this stage. The secondary spermatocytes undergo equatorial division to form the spermatids.

Spermatid phase. Spermiogenesis refers to the differentiative process by which spermatids produced by the meiotic divisions are transformed into spermatozoa (Fig. 21.10). The major features of this transformation include: (1) formation of an acrosome; (2) development of a flagellum; (3) condensation of the chromatin, accompanied by changes in the shape and size of the nucleus;

and (4) loss of excess cytoplasm. These morphological changes are associated with the synthesis of numerous proteins unique to the spermatozoa.

The early spermatid is a round or polygonal cell with a spherical nucleus measuring about 6 μm in diameter and containing finely granular, pale-staining chromatin. Included among the typical cytoplasmic organelles are a prominent juxtanuclear Golgi complex, numerous mitochondria, a pair of centrioles, and an irregularly shaped basophilic mass called the chromatid body. During spermiogenesis, each of these structures undergoes marked changes.

One of the first changes observed in the developing spermatid is the appearance of dense,

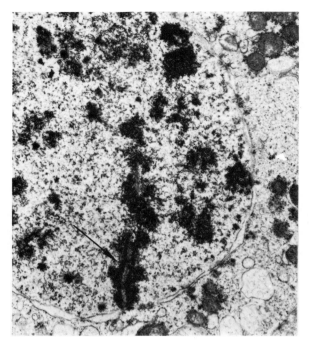

Figure 21.9. Electron micrograph of synaptonemal complex **(arrow)** in the nucleus of a pachytene primary spermatocyte. × 10,000.

PAS-positive granules in the Golgi complex, marking the beginning of the formation of the **acrosome.** As development continues membrane-limited granules, which are rich in carbohydrate, pinch off from the Golgi complex and then fuse, forming a single large **acrosomal vesicle** (see Fig. 21.10). As the acrosomal vesicle continues to enlarge by the fusion of additional granules produced by the Golgi, it becomes adherent to the nuclear envelope. The acrosome can be visualized as a membrane-limited sac that flattens and extends laterally over the anterior half of the round nucleus. The acrosome is present in all mammalian species, but its ultimate size and shape demonstrates tremendous species variation. The fully differentiated acrosome in humans has a relatively simple structure (Fig. 21.11). The acrosomal material is rich in carbohydrate and contains hydrolytic enzymes, including hyaluronidase, acrosin (an enzyme whose activity closely resembles that of trypsin), an acid phosphatase, and neuraminidase. These enzymes enable the mature spermatozoa to pass between the cells and penetrate the membranes that invest the egg.

As the acrosome is forming, paired centrioles, oriented perpendicular to one another, move to the opposite side of the cell near the plasma membrane. The distal centriole serves as a basal body directing the growth of an **axoneme,** consisting of a pair of central tubules surrounded by nine peripheral doublets. The axoneme serves as the central structural component in the flagellum (see Fig. 21.11). At about the time the acrosome reaches its most lateral extent and the nucleus begins to change in shape, the centrioles recede from the surface toward the nucleus. The proximal centriole becomes attached to a shallow groove on the caudal pole of the nucleus. At about this same time, cytoplasmic microtubules become organized into a circular band, the **manchette,** extending from the posterior margin of the acrosomal cap toward the caudal pole of the cell (see Fig. 21.10). The formation of the manchette is accompanied by: (1) the migration of the nucleus and overlying acrosome to a position adjacent to the plasma membrane; (2) the initial flattening and elongation of the nucleus; (3) the beginning of condensation of the chromatin; and (4) the initial elongation of spermatid that results from the displacement of the cytoplasm caudally.

As the flagellum develops, accessory structures are added to the basic axonemal complex including: (1) nine longitudinally oriented dense columns, the **outer dense fibers;** (2) the **connecting piece,** which unites the nucleus with the tail of the spermatozoon; and (3) the **fibrous sheath,** which is composed of two longitudinal columns and connecting ribs (see Fig. 21.11). As the flagellar membrane moves posteriorly along the flagellum, the manchette disappears and mitochondria migrate from the surrounding cytoplasm and become aligned in a helix around the proximal portion of the flagellum.

As was noted above, the condensation of the chromatin and changes in the shape of the nucleus begin at the time the manchette appears. Biochemical events involving changes in the histones and nuclear proteins associated with the nuclear DNA precede these morphological changes. As densely staining chromatin granules appear in the nucleus and increase in size, the nucleus becomes flattened and pyriform in shape. The substructure of chromatin is no longer visible as the chromatin condenses into the homogeneous, dense mass with occasional clear nuclear vacuoles (Fig. 21.11).

Spermiation. In the final stages of the maturation of the spermatid, the excess, **residual cytoplasm,** containing lipids and excess organelles, is partitioned off from the remainder of the spermatid. As the spermatozoon is released from the seminiferous epithelium, through the process

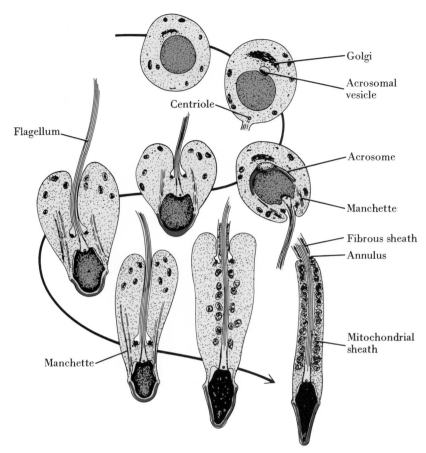

Figure 21.10. Schematic diagram of spermiogenesis in the human. The basic changes in the structure of the key organelles of the spermatid are illustrated (see text for detailed explanation). (Modified from M. Dym, 1977.)

known as **spermiation,** the excess cytoplasm is detached from the spermatozoon as a membrane-limited structure known as the **residual body** (of Reynaud). While it is known that the residual body is phagocytosed by the Sertoli cell (Fig. 21.4), recent evidence suggests that the process of degradation of the residual body is accomplished by a dual mechanism; initially by autophagic activity attributable to endogenous lysosomes in the residual body, and then phagocytosis of the partially degraded residual body by the Sertoli cell. Lipid droplets, which subsequently disappear from the apical Sertoli cell cytoplasm, are thought to be the last remnants of the digested residual body.

Spermatozoon. The differentiative events described above produce a structurally unique, motile cell capable of transporting its haploid complement of chromosomes to the egg. It carries with it the acrosomal enzymes required for its passage through the cells and membranes that invest the

egg and only those cellular components essential to provide the energy for its movement.

The mature spermatozoon in the human measures about 60 μm in length and is divided for descriptive purposes into a head, neck, and tail region (see Fig. 21.11). The head has a flattened pyriform shape and measures approximately 4 μm in length, 3 μm in width, and 1μm in thickness. The acrosomal cap covers the anterior two-thirds of the nucleus. The postacrosomal region of the head is of particular importance because it is this region of the sperm plasma membrane that fuses with the egg plasma membrane at fertilization. The condensed nucleus contains homogeneous, densely straining chromatin.

The neck is a short region containing the connecting piece composed of segmented columns and the proximal centriole.

The tail measures about 55 μm in length and is composed of a **middle piece, principal piece,** and

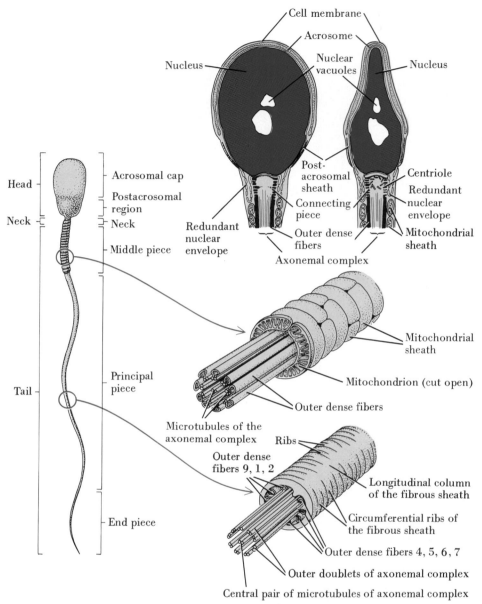

Figure 21.11. Diagram of a human spermatozoon. Regions of the spermatozoon are indicated on the left. Key ultrastructural features of the head (viewed in its major and minor diameters) and the middle piece and principal piece of the spermatozoon are illustrated on the right. (After Pederson and Fawcett, In Hafez ESE (ed): *Human Semen and Fertility Regulation in the Male*. St. Louis, CV Mosby, 1976.)

end piece. (Most of the details of the structure of the tail were described in the section on the spermatid phase of spermiogenesis and will not be repeated here.) The ***middle piece*** is about 5 to 9 μm in length and 1 μm in diameter. The core structure is the axoneme, which is surrounded by outer dense fibers and more externally by a sheath of helically arranged mitochondria. The ***principal piece*** is about 40 to 45 μm in length and is slightly narrower than the middle piece. The fibrous sheath, composed of two longitudinal columns and connecting ribs, is the characteristic component of this segment. The ***end piece*** is about 5 to 10 μm in length and contains only the axoneme and associated cytoplasm.

Intercellular bridges. Electron microscopic studies have revealed that the differentiating spermatogenic cells are interconnected by cytoplasmic bridges, the ***intercellular bridges.*** These bridges result from incomplete cytokinesis at the mitotic and meiotic divisions of the spermatogenic cells during the spermatogonial and meiotic phases of spermatogenesis (Fig. 21.12). The bridges measure about 2 to 3 μm in width and appear ultrastructurally to be reinforced by dense cytoplasmic material adjacent to membrane in the region of the bridges.

Studies of stem cell renewal suggest that as the stem cells divide, they produce either two separate daughter cells or two daughter cells connected by an intercellular bridge. Free cells continue to function as stem cells; interconnected cells are committed to proceed through spermatogenesis. At each subsequent division cytokinesis is incomplete, resulting in the formation of clones of interconnected cells, which remain connected throughout

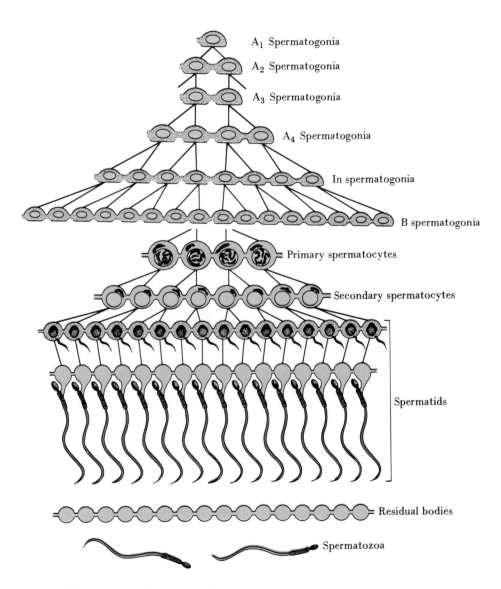

Figure 21.12. Schematic diagram illustrating the clonal nature of the various generations of spermatogenic cells. Cytoplasmic division is complete only in the primitive spermatogonia that serve as stem cells. All other spermatogenic cells remain connected by intercellular bridges as they undergo mitotic and meiotic division and differentiation of the spermatids. The cells separate as individual spermatozoa as they are released from the seminiferous epithelium. The residual bodies left within the seminiferous epithelium remain interconnected. (M. Dym and D. W. Fawcett, 1971.)

SPERMATOGENESIS IN THE RAT

Numerous biochemical, physiological, and morphological studies utilizing the rat as an animal model system have contributed greatly to our understanding of the events and control of spermatogenesis. Whereas a few aspects of spermatogenesis are unique in the human, the process in the rat is remarkably similar to that observed in all mammalian species that have been studied, including the primates. In the spermatogenic cycle of the rat shown in Figure 21.13, you can follow the successive changes an individual spermatogenic cell will undergo by starting with the A_1 cell located in the lower left-hand corner of the chart and following the path of differentiation indicated by the arrows. The most differentiated cell (shown in the top row, column VIII) is a spermatozoon that would be released from the seminiferous epithelium.

In the rat, six successive generations of spermatogonia (produced by augmentation divisions) with rather subtle morphological differences have been described as types A_1, A_2, A_3, A_4, In, and B. Type A_1 spermatogonia are produced by the mitotic division of the stem cells. (The superscript m indicates the time of a mitotic division.) The mitotic divisions give rise to the cells of the next generation. Type B spermatogonia divide to produce preleptotene primary spermatocytes (Pl). As the spermatogenic cells proceed through prophase of the first meiotic division, they pass through a series of morphologically distinct phases: preleptotene (Pl), leptotene (L), zygotene (Z), pachytene (P), diplotene (D), and diakinesis. The secondary spermatocytes (II) produced by the first meiotic (or reductional) division quickly complete the second meiotic (or equatorial) division and give rise to the haploid spermatid.

During spermiogenesis, the morphological transformation of the cells has been divided into a series of morphologically distinguishable *steps* indicated by arabic numerals in Figure 21.13. The primary criteria used to identify the steps are morphological alterations of the nucleus and acrosome. (The drawings of the cells, indicated in the chart, are based on observations of PAS-hematoxylin-stained preparations.)

CYCLE OF THE SEMINIFEROUS EPITHELIUM

The various generations of spermatogenic cells are not randomly distributed in the seminiferous epithelium, but are organized into well-defined cellular associations. This can be explained by examining Figure 21.13. Identify the spermatid at step 6 enclosed in the vertical column outlined in red. The vertical column indicates a cellular association. Spermatids at step 6 of spermiogenesis are always associated with types A_1 and B spermatogonia, pachytene spermatocytes, and step 18 spermatids. As the step 6 spermatids pass to the next step in their differentiation, step 7, all of the cells associated with it simultaneously pass to the next stage in their differentiation, that is, the cellular association enclosed in the vertical column outlined in blue. The vertical dashed lines in Figure 21.13 enclose 14 such distinct cellular associations identified in the rat. The cellular associations, indicated by roman numerals, are called *stages*. If the cellular association present in one portion of a rat seminiferous tubule was continually observed, one would see the cells passing successively through all 14 *stages* and then a repeat of the initial association would be observed. This series of changes between the appearances of the same cellular association is defined as the *cycle of the seminiferous epithelium*. The number of stages in the cycle of the seminiferous epithelium is constant for given species. In the human 6 stages have been defined (see Fig. 21.14); in the mouse and monkey, 12.

In all species, with the exception of the human, a particular cellular association occupies a relatively long segment along a seminiferous tubule. Therefore, a cross-section through a tubule typically includes only one type of cellular association (Fig. 21.15). The spermatogenic cells in a cross-section of a rat seminiferous tubule would consist of cells in 1 of the 14 cellular associations shown in Figure 21.13. This is *not* true of the human seminiferous tubule. Cellular associations occur in irregularly shaped areas along the tubule (see Fig. 21.15). Therefore, a cross-section through a tubule would reveal two or more distinct cellular associations.

Again with the exception of the human, the segments of seminiferous tubules containing the various cellular associations are organized in an orderly sequence along the seminiferous tubule (Fig. 21.16). The cellular associations in adjacent segments of a seminiferous tubule are always at the next higher or next lower stage of the cycle of the seminiferous epithelium. Thus, if one examines the cellular associations in the segments along the length of a seminiferous tubule, there is an orderly progression from one stage of the cycle to the next.

Autoradiographical studies, utilizing tritiated thymidine, which is incorporated into meiotically and mitotically dividing cells during the period of DNA synthesis (S phase of the cell cycle), have revealed that the cycle of the seminiferous epithelium is of a constant duration, lasting about 16 days in humans. It has been estimated that in humans it would require about 4.6 cycles (each of 16 days' duration), or approximately 74 days, for a spermatogonium produced by a stem cell to complete the process of spermatogenesis. It would then require about 12 days for the spermatozoa to pass through the epididymis. Therefore, if a drug is given that inhibits the initial phases of spermatogenesis, it would require approximately 86 days to recognize the effect of that compound.

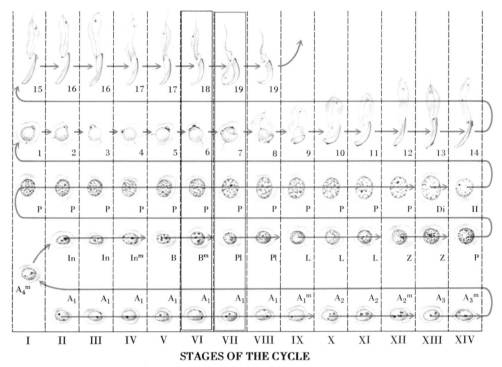

| I | II | III | IV | V | VI | VII | VIII | IX | X | XI | XII | XIII | XIV |

STAGES OF THE CYCLE

Figure 21.13. Schematic diagram depicting the spermatogenic cell associations of the 14 stages of the cycle of the seminiferous epithelium in the rat. Each numbered column **(roman numerals)** shows the spermatogenic cell types present in cellular associations found in cross-sections of seminiferous tubules. See the text for an explanation of the progression of the cells through the stages of the cycle. Steps in the development of the spermatids, numbered **1** to **19** and defined by changes in the structure of the nucleus and acrosome, are indicated with **arabic numerals.** Letters are used to identify spermatogonia and spermatocytes. A_1, A_2, A_3, and A_4, four generations of type a spermatogonia; In, intermediate spermatogonia; B, type B spermatogonia; Pl, preleptotene spermatocytes; L, leptotene spermatocytes; Z, zygotene spermatocytes; P, pachytene spermatocytes; Di, diplotene spermatocytes; II, secondary spermatocytes. The superscript m indicates mitotic division of the spermatogonia. (Modified from Dym M, Clermont Y: *Am J Anat* 128:265, 1970.)

their differentiation. At the time of sperm release the intercellular bridges remain as a component of the residual bodies, resulting in the release of unattached spermatozoa.

It has been proposed that the intercellular connections may function in synchronizing the development of the cells or in providing nutrients or genetic information essential for the development of the spermatogenic cells within the clone.

Interstitial Tissue

The space surrounding the seminiferous tubule is filled with *interstitial tissue;* it contains blood and lymphatic vessels forming peritubular plexuses, nerves, and loose connective tissue (see Fig. 21.3). In addition to its typical cellular elements, the connective tissue contains large, prominent *interstitial* or *Leydig cells.* In the adult human

testis, the interstitial tissue occupies about 35 percent of the total testicular volume, the Leydig cells about 12 percent.

The Leydig cells differentiate and secrete testosterone during the fetal period, promoting the development of the male reproductive tract. At about 4½ months of human fetal development, a period of gradual involution of the Leydig cells begins. The testis becomes essentially devoid of recognizable Leydig cells soon after birth. At puberty, in response to gonadotropic stimulation, the Leydig cells again develop and begin synthesizing and secreting androgens, primarily testosterone. It appears that the number of Leydig cells is constant and does not decline in the elderly.

The Leydig cells have a large, spherical nucleus containing a thin peripheral rim of heterochromatin and one or two prominent nucleoli. Binucleate cells are not uncommon. Numerous

Stage I

Stage II

Stage III

Stage IV

Stage V

Stage VI

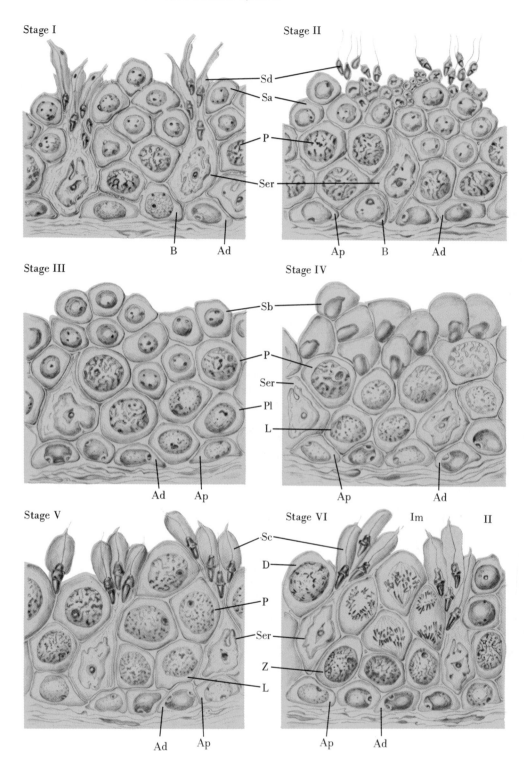

Figure 21.14. Schematic drawing of the six recognizable cell associations (or stages of the cycle of the human seminiferous epithelium). Ser, Sertoli cells; Ad, dark type A spermatogonia; Ap, pale type A spermatogonia; B, B type spermatogonia; Pl, preleptotene spermatocytes; L, leptotene spermatocytes; P, pachytene spermatocytes; D, diplotene spermatocytes; Im, primary spermatocytes in division; II, secondary spermatocytes; Sa, Sb, Sc, Sd, spermatids in various steps of differentiation; RB, residual bodies. (Based on Clermont Y: *Am J Anat* 112:50, 1963.)

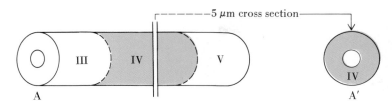

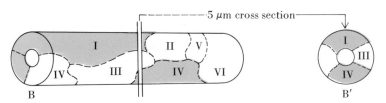

Figure 21.15. Schematic diagrams illustrating the difference in the organization of the seminiferous epithelium between most subhuman species **(A)** and man **(B)**. In subhuman species, a particular cellular association occupies a relatively long segment along the tubule. Therefore, in a typical cross-section only a single cellular association is observed (A'). In man, cellular associations occur in irregularly shaped areas along the tubule and, therefore, a cross-section typically shows two or more cellular associations (B'). (Modified from M. Dym, 1977.)

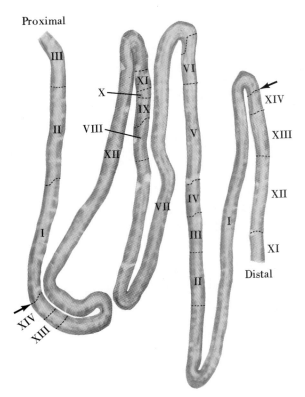

Figure 21.16. Drawing of a portion of an isolated seminiferous tubule from rat testis. The 14 cellular associations identified in the rat (see Fig. 21.13) are arranged in a linear array of segments along the length of the tubule. Stages are indicated by **roman numerals** on the segments. **Arrows** indicate the beginning and end of a series of segments including all stages of the cycle of the seminiferous epithelium in the rat. Proximal and distal ends of the isolated tubule are indicated. (After Perey B, Clermont Y, Leblond CP: *Am J Anat* 108:55, 1961.)

vacuoles, representing extracted lipid, are seen in typical light microscope preparations. At the ultrastructural level the most characteristic feature of the cells is the presence of abundant smooth endoplasmic reticulum (sER) (Fig. 21.17). Other ultrastructural features include gap junctions, numerous microvilli, scattered profiles of rough endoplasmic reticulum(rER) and a well-developed Golgi complex. The mitochondria vary in size and shape and may demonstrate either lamellar or tubular cristae. These ultrastructural features, particularly the presence of abundant sER, are also seen in other steroid-secreting cells, such as the cells of the adrenal cortex and the luteal and interstitial cells of the ovary.

The presence of cytoplasmic crystals, the *crystals of Reinke,* is a unique feature of human Leydig cells (Fig. 21.18). The crystals are not stained with common histological stains, but can be recognized as negative images in stained preparations. The crystals, composed of highly ordered 5-nm-thick filaments, may be 3 μm or more in thickness and up to 20 μm in length. Their functional significance is unknown.

The structure of the lymphatic vessels associated with the interstitial tissue demonstrates tremendous species variation. In rodents unusually large peritubular lymphatic vessels are present. In humans and other primates the lymphatics are of a more typical structure, but are quite extensive. The lymphatic vessels pass into the mediastinum of the testis and join, forming two or three vessels that will pass through the spermatic cord and convey lymph to para-aortic abdominal lymph nodes. This lymphatic drainage has important

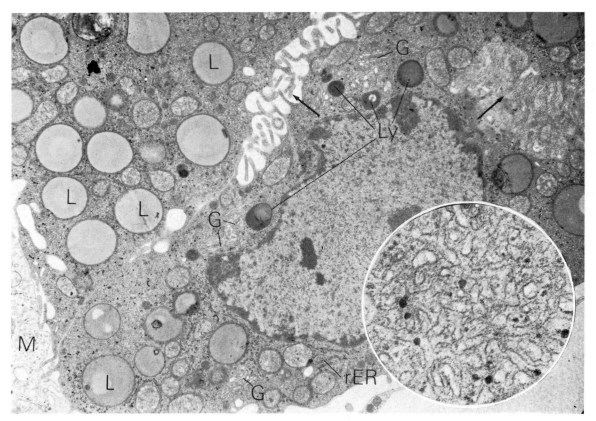

Figure 21.17. Electron micrograph of portions of several Leydig cells. The moderate electron density of the Leydig cell cytoplasm (compared with the lesser density of the small amount of cytoplasm of a macrophage (M) included in the micrograph) is due to the abundant smooth endoplasmic reticulum characteristic of Leydig cells. The **inset** shows at higher power the nature of the reticulum, particularly its close packing. The very dense particles represent glycogen. Other features characteristic of the Leydig cell seen in the lower-power micrograph are the numerous lipid droplets (L), the segmented profiles of the Golgi (G), and the presence of variable numbers of lysosomes (Ly). Occasional profiles of rough endoplasmic reticulum (rER) are also seen. Also note the presence of microvilli along portions of the cell surface **(arrows)**. × 10,000 (inset, × 60,000).

clinical implications because a malignant tumor of the testis, spreading by a lymphatic route, will metastasize to the para-aortic nodes. In contrast, a malignant tumor of the skin of the penis or scrotum will metastasize via the lymphatics into the inguinal lymph nodes. Involvement of the para-aortic nodes is more difficult to diagnose.

Hormonal Regulation of Spermatogenesis

The testis is a compound organ with both *exocrine* and *endocrine* functions. The exocrine function of the testis resides in the cells of the seminiferous epithelium that produce testicular fluids and spermatozoa. The endocrine function of the testis resides primarily in the Leydig cell population that synthesizes and secretes the principal circulating androgen, ***testosterone.*** Nearly all of the testosterone is produced by the testis; less than 5 percent is produced by the adrenal glands.

It has been estimated in humans that the total Leydig cell population produces about 7 mg of testosterone per day. As the testosterone leaves the Leydig cells, it may pass into blood or lymphatic capillaries or it may pass through the peritubular tissue and enter the seminiferous tubules. High local levels of testosterone within the testis (estimated to be as much as 200 times the circulating levels) are necessary for the proliferation and differentiation of the spermatogenic cells within the seminiferous epithelium. The lower peripheral level of testosterone influences (1) the differentiation of the central nervous system and the genital apparatus and duct system; (2) the growth and maintenance of secondary sexual characteristics

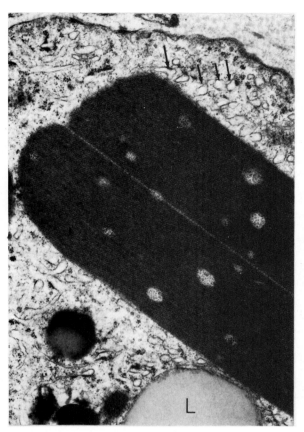

Figure 21.18. Electron micrograph of a Reinke crystal in the cytoplasm of a human Leydig cell. Smooth endoplasmic reticulum **(arrows)** and a lipid droplet (L) can be seen in the cytoplasm adjacent to the crystal. × 16,000. (Courtesy of Dr. D. F. Cameron, 1984.)

(such as growth of the beard, male distribution of pubic hair, and low-pitched voice); (3) the growth and maintenance of the accessory sex glands (seminal vesicles, prostate, and bulbourethral), genital duct system, and the external genitalia; (4) anabolic and general metabolic processes including skeletal growth, skeletal muscle growth, distribution of subcutaneous fat, and kidney function; and (5) behavior, including libido.

The steroidogenic and spermatogenic activities of the testis are modified or regulated by hormonal interaction among the hypothalamus, adenohypophysis, and the cells of the gonad—the Sertoli, spermatogenic, and Leydig cells (Fig. 21.19). The adenohypophysis produces three hormones involved in this process: luteinizing hormone (LH), which in the male is sometimes referred to as interstitial cell-stimulating hormone (ICSH); follicle-stimulating hormone (FSH); and

prolactin. In response to LH release by the adenohypophysis, the Leydig cells produce increasing amounts of androgenic steroids, particularly testosterone. Prolactin appears to have little effect by itself, but in combination with LH increases the steroidogenic activity of the Leydig cells. (Prolactin receptors are present on the plasma membrane of Leydig cells. Prolactin may also function in other reproductive tissues by causing an increase in the number of androgen receptors present in those tissues.)

FSH and testosterone stimulate the process of sperm production within the seminiferous epithelium. The Sertoli cells have been shown to be the primary target for FSH and androgens. Therefore, the Sertoli cells are considered to be the primary regulators of spermatogenesis, but the cellular mechanisms involved in this process remain poorly understood. It should be noted that some experimental evidence suggests that androgens may bind directly to spermatogenic cells.

The release of LH from the adenohypophysis is regulated by serum testosterone levels through a simple negative feedback system (see Fig. 21.19). This occurs either through a direct inhibitory action on the adenohypophysis or through inhibition of the secretion of gonadotropin-releasing factors by the hypothalamus. When testosterone is present in low concentrations, an LH-specific gonadotropin-releasing factor is secreted by the cells of the hypothalamus and LH is released by the adenohypophysis.

Three substances produced by the Sertoli cells are apparently involved in the hormonal regulation of male reproductive function. ***Androgen-binding protein*** (ABP) is a protein released from the Sertoli cells. It binds testosterone, thereby establishing a local environment in the seminiferous tubules and initial portion of the genital duct system, which is high in androgen content. ***Inhibin*** is a molecule that reportedly functions in the regulation of the FSH level and aids in regulating the number of cells entering spermatogenesis. The Sertoli cells also produce a substance similar to LH-releasing factor that may function as an intercellular messenger between Sertoli cells and Leydig cells regulating cyclic Leydig cell activity that has been observed in rats.

Histochemical and morphological studies have indicated that the Sertoli cells undergo cyclic changes in their metabolic activity that are related to specific stages in the cycle of the seminiferous epithelium. These changes appear to be analogous to changes occurring in the granulosa cells during follicular growth and maturation in the ovary.

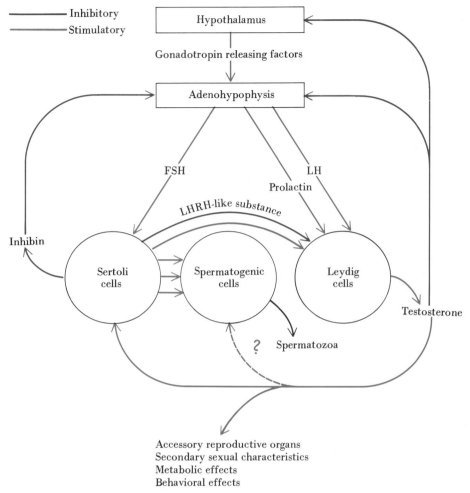

Inhibitory
Stimulatory

Hypothalamus

Gonadotropin releasing factors

Adenohypophysis

FSH

LH

Prolactin

LHRH-like substance

Inhibin

Sertoli cells

Spermatogenic cells

Leydig cells

Testosterone

?   Spermatozoa

Accessory reproductive organs
Secondary sexual characteristics
Metabolic effects
Behavioral effects

Figure 21.19. Diagram depicting the hormonal regulation of male reproductive function. **Red arrows** indicate inhibitory feedback; **blue arrows**, stimulatory. See text for explanation. (Modified from M. Dym, 1977.)

Factors Affecting Spermatogenesis

The spermatogenic cells are very sensitive to noxious agents. Degenerative changes, such as premature sloughing of the cells or formation of multinucleated giant cells, are readily apparent following exposure to such agents. Factors that affect spermatogenesis include: (1) dietary deficiencies; (2) general or local infections; (3) elevated testicular temperature; (4) hormones; (5) toxic agents such as mutagens, drugs, antimetabolites, and pesticides (particularly the short-chain halogenated hydrocarbons); and (6) irradiation. It should be noted that proliferating cells are particularly sensitive to mutagenic agents and the absence of essential metabolites. Therefore, the nondividing Sertoli and Leydig cells and the reserve stem cells, which demonstrate low mitotic activity, are much less vulnerable than the actively dividing, differentiating spermatogenic cells to such agents or nutritional deficiencies.

Administered hormones, such as corticosteroids, antiandrogens, androgens, and estrogens, can interfere with the normal hormonal regulation of spermatogenesis. Through the negative feedback mechanism, LH release may be inhibited, resulting in the atrophy of the Leydig cells and inhibition of spermatogenesis.

In species with scrotal testes, the spermatogenic cells are vulnerable to elevated temperature. In the human, the temperature differential between the scrotum and the core body temperature is 2°C. If the testis fails to descend into the scrotum (the condition is referred to as **cryptorchidism**), spermatogenesis is inhibited. After puberty in cryptorchid individuals, the Leydig cells demonstrate normal androgenic function, and normal numbers of Sertoli cells are present, but relatively few spermatogonia and occasional early spermatocytes populate the seminiferous epithelium.

GENITAL DUCT SYSTEM

Tubuli Recti and Rete Testis

At the ends of the seminiferous tubules are short, straight tubules, the *tubuli recti,* which are continuous with the *rete testis.* There is an abrupt narrowing and change in the epithelial lining of the tubule at the junction between the seminiferous tubule and the tubulus rectus. The epithelium, described as simple, low columnar or cuboidal, is devoid of spermatogenic cells.

The *rete testis* is a network of interconnected channels within the highly vascular connective tissue of the mediastinum (Fig. 21.20). The simple epithelium that lines these channels varies in height, but is generally described as cuboidal. The epithelium cells, like those of the tubuli recti, are relatively simple in ultrastructure. Each cell bears a single cilium and a few short microvilli on its luminal surface. The position of the rete testis shows species variation. In humans, it occupies a posterior position within the testis, but in many mammalian species it has a central or axial position.

Ductuli Efferentes

At the superior end of the mediastinum the *rete testis* terminates in 12 to 20 ducts, the *ductuli efferentes* (efferent ducts) that penetrate the tunica albuginea and pass from the testis to the epididymis (see Fig. 21.2). As the ducts exit the testis, they become highly coiled, forming 6 to 10 conical masses, the *coni vasculosi,* with their bases forming part of the head of the epididymis. The coni vasculosi, which are about 10 mm in length, contain convoluted ducts about 15 to 20 cm in length. At the base of the cones the efferent ducts open into a single channel, the *ductus epididymidis.*

The ductuli efferentes are lined with a pseudostratified columnar epithelium (Fig. 21.21). The epithelium consists primarily of alternating groups of tall columnar cells and cuboidal cells (cell

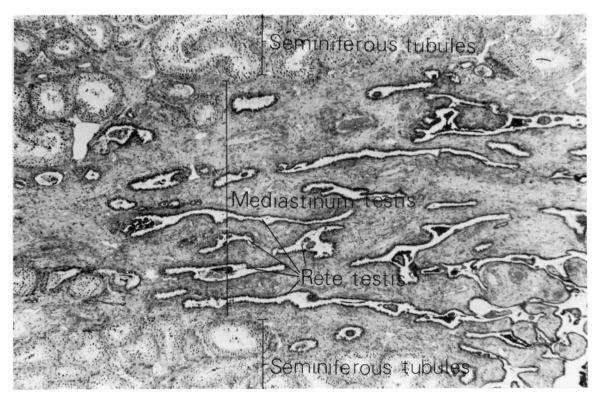

Figure 21.20. Photomicrograph of human testis. The section passes through the mediastinum of the testis. In this region the anastomosing channels of the rete testis are found. Seminiferous tubules can be seen in the region adjacent to the mediastinum. × 40.

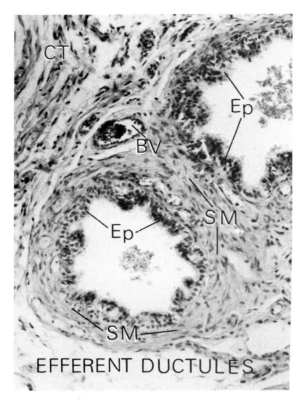

Figure 21.21. Photomicrograph of efferent ductules. The efferent ductules are lined with pseudostratified columnar epithelium (Ep). The luminal surface has an uneven or wavy appearance due to the presence of alternate groups of tall columnar and cuboidal cells. Cilia are present on some cells. The ductules surrounded by circularly arranged smooth muscle (SM) are embedded in the connective tissue (CT). × 160.

height varies from 15 μm to over 35 μm), but a few basal cells, intraepithelial lymphocytes, and macrophages are present. Ciliated and nonciliated cells are present. Generally, it is the tall columnar cells that are ciliated. The beat of the cilia, which is directed toward the epididymis, may aid in the transport of the spermatozoa and fluids in that direction. The nonciliated cells have microvilli on their luminal surface and appear to be actively involved in endocytosis. They have canalicular invaginations on their free surface and contain micropinocytotic vesicles, membrane-bound dense bodies, lysosomes, and other structures associated with endocytotic activity. Most of the fluids produced within the seminiferous tubules are absorbed by the epithelial cells of the ductuli efferentes and the epididymis.

The epithelium is surrounded by a thin layer of smooth muscle that becomes progressively thicker toward the epididymis. Activity of the muscular investment of this portion and the remainder of the genital duct system moves the nonmotile sperm along the duct.

Ductus Epididymidis

The ductuli efferentes join to form a single, highly convoluted *ductus epididymidis.* If this duct was straightened out, it would measure up to 6 m in length. The duct and surrounding smooth muscle, vascular connective tissue, and other supporting structures form a compact organ, the *epididymis,* measuring about 7.5 cm in length. By gross inspection, it is divided into three regions: a head *(caput);* a body *(corpus);* and tail *(cauda)* (see Fig. 21.2).

The epididymis plays an essential role in the development of the functional spermatozoa, providing both the essential environment and some of the molecular products required for their maturation. As the spermatozoa are released from the testis, they demonstrate limited motility (no directed movement) and are incapable of fertilizing ova. As they pass through the epididymis, they develop the capacity for forward motility and the ability to fertilize ova. These changes are accompanied by changes in the plasma membrane structure including the binding of surface glycoproteins of epididymal origin to the spermatozoa. These maturational events are androgen-dependent and require protein synthesis by the epididymis.

The ductus epididymidis is lined with a pseudostratified columnar epithelium consisting of two primary cell types, *principal cells* and *basal cells* (Figs. 21.22 and 21.23). Other minor cell types have been described, including *halo cells,* which have been identified as intraepithelial lymphocytes.

The *principal cells* are tall, columnar cells whose luminal surface is covered with long, slender, nonmotile microvilli called *stereocilia* (Fig. 21.23). The height of the principal cells is 60 to 80 μm in the initial segment and decreases to about half that in the tail region. The stereocilia show a similar decrease in size, having a maximum length of about 25 μm and a minimum of 5 to 10 μm. The principal cells demonstrate features typical of both secretory and absorptive cells. An absorptive function is indicated by the presence of numerous invaginations at the bases of the stereocilia, coated vesicles, multivesicular bodies, and lysosomes in the apical cytoplasm (Fig. 21.24). The uptake of dyes and electron-dense markers, such as horseradish peroxidase, have substantiated this view. A secretory function is indicated by the presence of numerous cisternae of rER around the basally located nucleus, scattered profiles of sER and rER

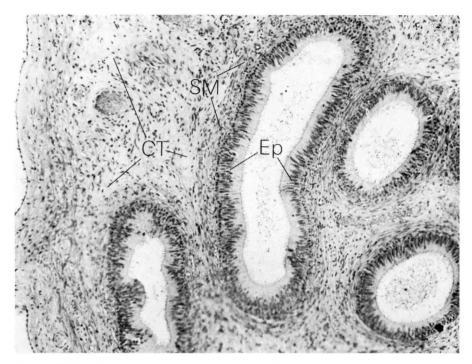

Figure 21.22. Photomicrograph of human epididymis. The section passes through the highly coiled ductus epididymidis in several places. The epithelium (Ep) which lines the epididymis is pseudostratified columnar. The duct, which is surrounded by smooth muscle (SM), is embedded in connective tissue (CT). × 80.

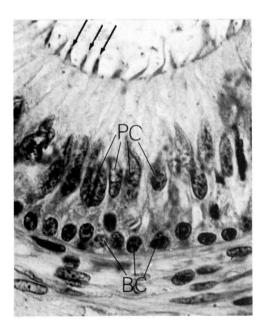

Figure 21.23. Photomicrograph of human epididymis. A portion of the tubular wall is shown. Two epithelial cell types can be identified, principal cells (PC) and basal cells (BC). Stereocilia **(arrows)** extend from the apical surface of the tall columnar principal cells. Nuclei of the basal cells are located adjacent to the basement membrane. × 640.

in the apical cytoplasm, and a remarkably large supranuclear Golgi complex. However, many of the specific functions of the cells remain to be elucidated.

The **basal cells** are located at the base of the epithelium. They are simple in structure, containing few cytoplasmic organelles and having a lightly stained cytoplasm.

The epithelium is surrounded by a thin lamina propria and an outer investment of smooth muscle. Through the head and body regions the muscle layer consists of smooth muscle cells oriented circumferentially around the duct. In the body region, a few bundles of longitudinally or obliquely oriented fibers form an incomplete outer layer. In the tail region, typical large smooth muscle cells increase in number distally along the duct. In the distal portion of the tail region, the muscle bundles are organized into three layers (inner longitudinal, middle circular, and outer longitudinal). Differences in the morphological organization of the muscle layers are correlated with differences in the muscular activity of the different regions. The head and body demonstrate spontaneous, rhythmic peristaltic contractions that serve to convey the sperm along the duct. Fewer such contractions are observed in the tail region, which is the principal site of sperm storage.

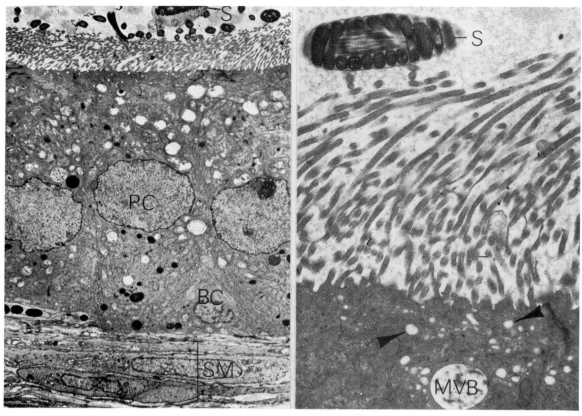

Figure 21.24(a). Electron micrograph of epididymal epithelium, showing principal cells (PC) extending to the lumen and a basal cell (BC) limited to the base of the epithelium. Smooth muscle (SM) is in the connective tissue below the epithelium. A portion of a sperm (S) is seen in the lumen. × 3,000. **(b)** Apical surface of the epithelial cell with its numerous microvilli. Again, a portion of a sperm (S) is evident in the lumen. The large, light circular object is a multivesicular body (MVB). The small, light circular profiles **(arrowheads)** are pinocytotic vesicles. × 13,000.

Sympathetic autonomic nerve fibers form an extensive network (the myenteric plexus) in the muscle layers around the duct in the distal region of the epididymis. The nerve plexus is even more extensive in the smooth muscle of the ductus deferens and seminal vesicles. Sympathetic (adrenergic) nervous stimulation of this musculature causes powerful contractions that expel the spermatozoa and seminal fluids at ejaculation.

Ductus Deferens (Vas Deferens)

The *ductus deferens* begins as a direct continuation of the ductus epididymidis and ends at the prostatic urethra (see Fig. 21.1). At its distal end it is joined by a duct from the seminal vesicle and then passes through the prostate gland to join the urethra. The dilated region of the ductus deferens just proximal to the site where it is joined by the duct of the seminal vesicle is called the *ampulla;* the narrowed region enclosed within the prostate is called the *ejaculatory duct.*

The wall of the duct is composed of an internal mucosa, an intermediate muscularis, and an external adventitia (Fig. 21.25). Longitudinal folds of the mucosa project into the lumen of the ductus deferens throughout most of its length. In the ampulla the mucosa is thrown into more slender and extensive, irregularly branching folds. The duct is lined by a pseudostratified columnar epithelium with stereocilia. The lamina propria underlying the epithelium contains numerous elastic fibers. The surrounding muscularis is about 1.0 to 1.5 mm in thickness and consists of three smooth muscle layers (inner longitudinal, middle circular, and outer longitudinal). Fibers of the three layers intermingle to some extent. The inner layer is thin and poorly defined in the distal region of the duct. An extensive network of autonomic nerve fibers is associated with the smooth muscle layer.

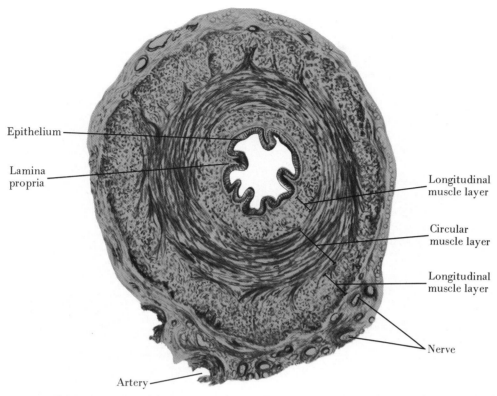

Epithelium

Lamina
propria

Longitudinal
muscle layer

Circular
muscle layer

Longitudinal
muscle layer

Nerve

Artery

Figure 21.25. Drawing of a cross-section through a human vas deferens. The thick muscularis is organized in three distinct smooth muscle layers—an inner longitudinal, middle circular, and outer longitudinal. Numerous elastic fibers are present in the lamina propria underlying the epithelium. × 30. (After Schaffer. In Bloom W, Fawcett, DW (eds): *A Textbook of Histology,* 10th ed. Philadelphia, WB Saunders, 1975.)

In the proximal region of the ejaculatory duct the epithelium is simple or pseudostratified columnar; in the distal region it often appears as transitional epithelium. The epithelial cells appear to have secretory activity and contain large numbers of yellow pigment granules. The mucosa of the ejaculatory duct is thrown into slender folds that extend into the lumen but are less elaborate than those of the ampulla. The lamina propria contains abundant elastic fibers. There is no muscularis in the wall of the ejaculatory duct. This portion of the ductus deferens is surrounded by the fibromuscular tissue of the prostate gland.

ACCESSORY SEX GLANDS

Seminal Vesicle

The *seminal vesicles* are elongated, contorted, sac-like structures that measure about 5 cm in length and lie between the posterior surface of the bladder and the rectum (see Fig. 21.1). Each gland consists of a single tube (about 3 to 4 mm in diameter and 10 to 15 cm in length) that is folded

upon itself. The lower portion of the gland becomes a narrow straight duct which joins the ductus deferens to form the ejaculatory duct. Since it develops as a diverticulum of the ductus deferens, it resembles it in structure.

The wall of the seminal vesicle is composed of three layers: a mucosa; an intermediate muscularis, which is thinner than that of the ductus deferens and is arranged in two smooth muscle layers, an inner circular layer and an outer longitudinal layer; and an external adventitia that is rich in elastic fibers (Fig. 21.26). Intricate folding of the mucosa forms numerous, irregularly shaped chambers or crypts that open into the large central cavity of the gland.

The pseudostratified epithelium of the mucosa is composed of small, rounded basal cells located between low columnar or cuboidal surface cells. The surface cells have distinct borders and contain large secretion granules and yellow lipochrome pigment that first appears at puberty and increases with age. The lamina propria is rich in elastic fibers and contains some smooth muscle cells in the mucosal folds.

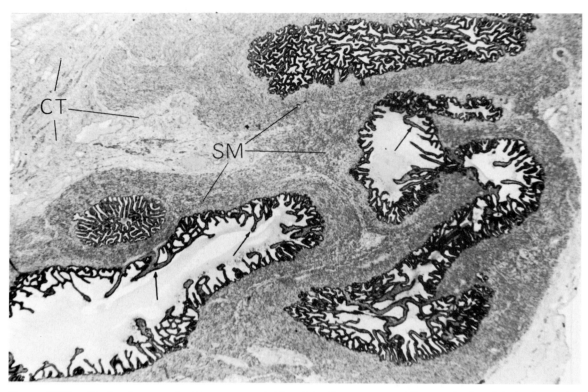

Figure 21.26. Photomicrograph of human seminal vesicle. The mucosa of the seminal vesicle is characterized by extensive folding **(arrows)**. The mucosa rests on a thick smooth muscle (SM) investment that is organized in two layers—an inner circular layer and an outer longitudinal layer. × 16.

The gland's secretory product is a yellowish, slightly alkaline, viscid substance that is rich in fructose. Measurement of the fructose content in the semen can provide an index of the secretory activity of the gland. The gland is androgen dependent. Reductions in the size of the gland and the height of its epithelium after castration can be reversed by injection of testosterone.

Prostate Gland

The *prostate,* the largest of the accessory reproductive glands, surrounds the initial portion of the urethra, the prostatic urethra (see Fig. 21.1). It is composed of fibromuscular and glandular tissue and is surrounded by a vascular capsule. It is described as being the size of a "horse chestnut" and weights about 20 g.

The glandular component of the organ consists of 30 to 50 tubuloalveolar glands. The ducts from the individual glands converge to form 16 to 32 terminal ducts that open directly into the prostatic urethra. Three groups of glands—mucosal, submucosal, and main prostatic—are arranged somewhat concentrically around the urethra (Fig. 21.27).

The structure of the glands, particularly the caliber of the lumen, is highly variable (Fig. 21.28). The glandular epithelium is most commonly identified as simple or pseudostratified columnar, but areas of low cuboidal or squamous epithelium may be seen. Typical basal cells are present. Transitional epithelium similar to that of the prostatic urethra is seen near the termination of the ducts. The epithelial cells contain secretion granules and lipid droplets. Histochemical studies demonstrate an abundance of acid phosphatase.

The stroma of the prostate contains numerous smooth muscle fibers and abundant fibroelastic tissue. Septa of this fibromuscular tissue extend from the capsule into the interior of the organ between the tubular alveolar glands. Numerous blood and lymphatic vessels and nerves are scattered in the interstitial connective tissue.

Spherical bodies called *prostatic concretions* normally occur in some of the alveoli (see Fig. 21.28). They vary greatly in size and may become calcified and exceed 1 mm in diameter. In sections, they appear as concentric lamellated bodies. They are believed to represent condensation of the secretory product.

The prostate gland secretes a slightly acid (pH

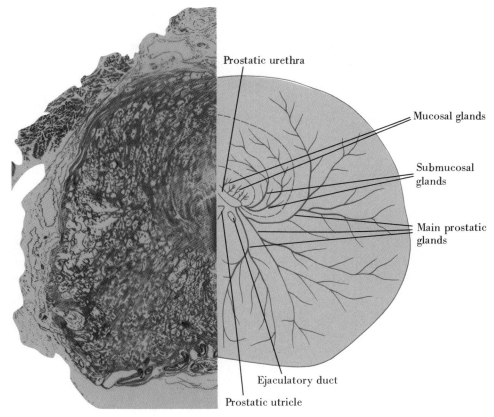

Prostatic urethra

Mucosal glands

Submucosal glands

Main prostatic glands

Ejaculatory duct

Prostatic utricle

Figure 21.27. Human prostate gland. The drawing on the left illustrates the basic morphology of the gland (see Fig. 21.28). The schematic diagram on the right illustrates the distribution of the glandular components within the prostate. The regions of the prostate containing mucosal, submucosal, and main prostate glands are indicated by **dashed lines**. (Modified from M. Dym, 1977.)

6.5), colorless fluid that is rich in citric acid and acid phosphatase. It also contains proteolytic enzymes including a fibrinolysin that functions in the liquefaction of the semen. The level of acid phosphatase and citric acid in the semen provides an index of prostatic function. Some of the acid phosphatase produced is released into the bloodstream. In patients with prostatic carcinoma the serum level of acid phosphatase may be useful in judging whether metastasis has occurred.

Bulbourethral Gland

The **bulbourethral glands,** or **Cowper's glands,** are paired structures about 1 cm in diameter. The excretory duct of each gland, which is about 3 cm in length, passes through the inferior fascia of the urogenital diaphragm and opens into the bulb of the urethra (see Fig. 21.1). Each gland is a compound tubuloalveolar gland made up of several lobules held together by fibrous connective tissue containing elastic fibers and smooth and skeletal

muscle fibers (Fig. 21.29). These fibrous components also contribute to the capsule. The ducts and glands are irregular in size and may have cyst-like enlargements.

The cells of the glandular epithelium vary in size and shape from columnar to low cuboidal depending on their functional state. They often appear flattened in large, distended alveoli. The cells have a spherical, basally located nucleus and contain various amounts of mucoid droplets and acidophilic spindle-shaped bodies in the apical cytoplasm. The collecting ducts within the gland are lined with simple columnar epithelium. The excretory ducts are lined with pseudostratified epithelium that resembles the epithelial lining of the urethra and may contain patches of secretory cells.

During erotic stimulation the bulbourethral glands secrete a clear, viscous, mucus-like substance that probably acts as a lubricant for the urethra. The substance is rich in sialoproteins and amino sugars.

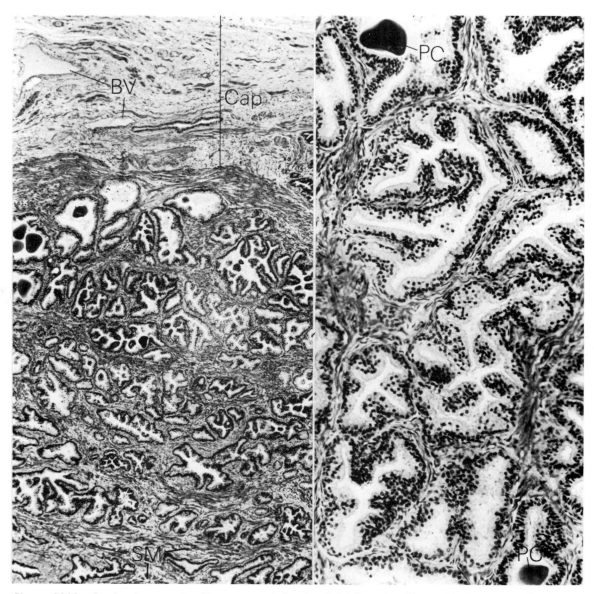

Figure 21.28. Photomicrograph of human prostate gland. **(a)** The gland has a thick capsule (Cap) that contains numerous large blood vessels (BV). Fibromuscular stroma composed of smooth muscle fibers (SM) and dense connective tissue surrounds the glandular component of the prostate. × 40. **(b)** Prostatic concretions (PC) are commonly seen in the lumen of tubuloalveolar glands. × 145.

PENIS

The **penis** consists primarily of a pair of dorsally placed **corpora cavernosa** and single, ventrally placed **corpus spongiosum** (Figs. 21.1 and 21.30). The corpus spongiosum, also known as the **corpus cavernosum urethrae,** surrounds the urethra and has an expanded distal portion, the **glans penis.** These three structures, composed of erectile tissue, are surrounded by loose connective tissue rich in elastic fibers and skin.

The erectile structures consist of numerous cavernous spaces created by a network of fine trabeculae. The spaces are lined with endothelium and are largest in the central region. The trabeculae contain fibroelastic tissue and smooth muscle. The penis becomes erect when these spaces are distended with blood; in the flaccid state the spaces contain a reduced amount of blood.

The corpora cavernosa are enclosed with a dense, fibroelastic connective tissue, the **tunica albuginea.** A fibrous septum of the tunica al-

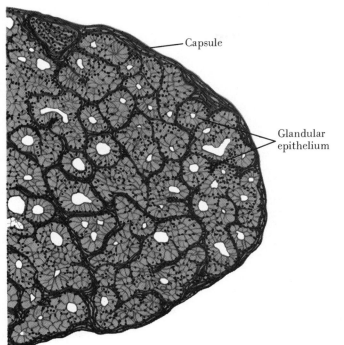

Figure 21.29. Drawing of a portion of a lobule of a bulbourethral gland. The variation in the height of the epithelial cells of this compound tubular alveolar gland reflects differences in their functional state. × 120. (After Stieve.)

Capsule

Glandular epithelium

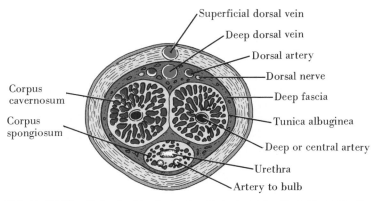

Superficial dorsal vein

Deep dorsal vein

Dorsal artery

Dorsal nerve

Corpus cavernosum

Deep fascia

Corpus spongiosum

Tunica albuginea

Deep or central artery

Urethra

Artery to bulb

Figure 21.30. Schematic diagram of a cross-section through the penis.

PROSTATE DISORDERS

The prostate is of major clinical interest because of the high incidence of *benign prostatic hyperplasia (BPH)* and carcinoma of the prostate. BPH is extremely rare in men under 40 years of age, but is common in men over 50. In men who live to be 80 years old, 80 percent will have BPH and approximately 10 percent will require surgery. Basically, BPH interferes with the flow of urine through the urethra leading to a number of secondary effects. Carcinoma of the prostate is the third leading type of cancer in the male. It accounts for 17 percent of all male cancers and is the second most common cause of death from carcinoma. About 5 percent of white males and 6 percent of nonwhite males will develop cancer of the prostate. It appears that BPH most commonly involves the periurethral mucosal glands. Carcinoma of the prostate most commonly originates in the periphery or both peripherally and centrally (that is, in the main prostatic or submucosal glands).

SEMEN

In addition to the spermatozoa, the semen contains contributions from the accessory sex glands. Ejaculation is initiated by sympathetic nerve stimulation of the smooth muscle bundles associated with the genital ducts and accessory sex glands. Contraction of these muscles forces the secretory products from the glands and propels the sperm and fluids along the duct system. At ejaculation the different components of the semen usually follow one another in a definite sequence. During arousal, mucus-like fluids are released from the bulbourethral gland and act as a lubricant. As ejaculation begins, the scant secretions of the bulbourethral gland are followed by the acid phosphatase and citric acid secretion of the prostate gland. These secretions are followed by the spermatozoa. The seminal vesicles then add the final component, a substance rich in fructose. These components are mixed during ejaculation.

The volume of the ejaculate in humans varies from 2 to 6 ml. About 95 percent of the volume is contributed by the accessory glands. The average sperm density is about 100 million/ml (the normal range is 20 to 250 million/ml). This tremendous number of spermatozoa is in dramatic contrast to the single egg contributed by the female. Only a few hundred sperm reach the ampulla region of the oviduct, where fertilization normally occurs. A single spermatozoon completes the process.

buginea separates the two corpora cavernosa in the proximal part of the penis. Distally, the septum is incomplete and the cavernous sinuses of both sides communicate. A much thinner investment of fibroelastic tissue, containing a layer of smooth muscle on its inner aspect, surrounds the corpus spongiosum. The cavernous spaces of the corpus spongiosum are uniform in size except in the glans where large anastomosing veins with thick muscle investments are present. The differences in the fibroelastic investments have functional significance in that the corpus spongiosum and glands do not attain the state of ridigity as that observed in the corpora cavernosa. This prevents the urethra from being occluded in full erection.

Blood may enter the cavernous spaces from capillaries in the trabeculae or arteries that empty directly into the spaces. The latter, called *helicine arteries,* are important in erection. During sexual stimulation, decreased muscle tone in the wall of the helicine arteries results in an increased blood flow through them, causing the cavernous sinuses to fill with blood and the penis to become rigid. The peripherally located veins become compressed against the internal aspect of the tunica albuginea, further contributing to maintenance of the erect state. (Some investigators believe that the restriction of venous return plays little role in erection, the important factor being the increase in blood flow into the cavernous spaces.) Sympathetic stimulation of the smooth muscle of the arteries at the end of ejaculation decreases blood flow and results in detumescence and return to the flaccid state.

The skin of the penis is thin and loosely attached to the underlying loose connective tissue, except at the *glans* where it is very thin and tightly attached. The subcutaneous tissue is free of adipose tissue, but contains a layer of smooth muscle that is continuous with the dartos tunic of the scrotum. The glans is covered by a fold of skin, the *prepuce,* which resembles a mucous membrane on its internal aspect. Sebaceous glands are present in the skin adjacent to the prepuce.

The penis is innervated by spinal, parasympathetic, and sympathetic nerves. Numerous sensory nerve endings are distributed throughout the tissue of the penis. Sympathetic and parasympathetic visceral motor fibers innervate the smooth muscle of the trabeculae and blood vessels. Both the sensory and the visceral motor fibers play essential roles in the sexual response, including the establishment and maintenance of the erection of the penis and the initiation of orgasm and ejaculation.

ATLAS PLATES

106–111

PLATE 106. Testis I

A section of the testis showing the seminiferous tubules and the tunica albuginea (**TA**), the capsule of the organ, is shown in **Figure 1.** Extending from the very thick capsule are connective tissue septa (**S**) that divide the organ into compartments. Each compartment contains several seminiferous tubules and represents a lobule (**L**). Blood vessels are present within the inner portion of the capsule, the part referred to as the tunica vasculosa, and in the connective tissue septa.

The seminiferous tubules are convoluted; thus, the profiles they present in a section are variable in appearance. Not infrequently, the wall of a tubule will be tangentially sectioned, thus, obscuring the lumen and revealing what appears to be a solid mass of cells (**X**).

Examination at higher magnification, as in **Figure 2,** reveals a population of interstitial cells that occur in small clusters and lie in the space between adjoining tubules. They consist mostly of Leydig cells (**LC**), the chief source of testosterone in the male. They are readily identified by virtue of their location and by their small round nucleus and eosinophilic cytoplasm. Macrophages are also found in close association with the Leydig cells, but in lesser number. However, they are difficult to identify in H&E sections.

Surrounding the epithelium of each seminiferous tubule, is a layer of closely apposed squamous cells that form a sheath-like investment around the tubule epithelium. [In man, several layers of cells invest the tubule epithelium.] The cells of this peritubular investment exhibit myoid features and account for the slow peristaltic activity of the tubules. Peripheral to the myoid layer is a broad lymphatic channel that occupies an extensive space between the tubules. However, in paraffin sections, the lymphatic channels are usually collapsed and, thus, unrecognizable. The cellular elements that surround the tubule epithelium are generally referred to as a lamina propria or as a boundary tissue. As a lamina propria, it is atypical. It is not a loose connective tissue. Indeed, under normal circumstances, lymphocytes and other cell types related to the immune system are conspicuously absent.

Examination of the tubule epithelium (**Fig. 2**) reveals two kinds of cells; a proliferating population of spermatogenic cells and a nonproliferating population, the Sertoli cells. The Sertoli cells are considerably fewer in number and can be recognized by their elongate, pale-staining nuclei (**Sn**) and by conspicuous nucleolus. The Sertoli cell cytoplasm extends from the periphery of the tubule to the lumen.

KEY

BV, blood vessels
L, lobule
LC, Leydig cells
LP, lamina propria
S, connective tissue septa
X, tangential section of tubule with lumen obscured

arrows, spermatid nuclei displaying early shape change
Sc, spermatocytes
Sg, spermatogonia
Sn, Sertoli nuclei
Sp, spermatids
TA, tunica albuginea

Fig. 1 (monkey), × 65

Fig. 2 (monkey), × 400

The spermatogenic cells consist of successive generations arranged in concentric layers. Thus the spermatogonia (**Sg, Fig. 2**) are found at the periphery. The spermatocytes (**Sc**), most of which have large round nuclei with a distinctive chromatin pattern (due to their chromatin material being reorganized), come to lie above the spermatogonia. The spermatid population (**Sp**) is comprised of one or two generations and occupies the site closest to the lumen. The tubules in **Figure 2** have been identified according to their stage of development. The tubule at the upper right can be identified as stage VI. At this stage, the mature population of spermatids (identified by their dark-blue heads and eosinophilic thread-like flagella protruding into the lumen) are in the process of being released (spermiogenesis). The younger generation of spermatids is comprised of round cells and exhibit round nuclei. Moving clockwise, the tubule indicated as stage VII is slightly more advanced. The mature spermatids are now gone. Progressing to stage VIII, the tubule at the bottom of the micrograph reveals that the spermatid population is undergoing a change in nuclear shape. Note the tapered nuclei (**arrows**). Further maturation of the spermatids is reflected in the tubule at the top of the micrograph, stage XI. Finally, the tubule marked as stage II, on the left, reveals slightly greater maturation of the luminal spermatids, and with the start of the new cycle (stage I) a newly formed spermatid population is now present. By examining the spermatid population and assessing the number of generations present, i.e., one or two, and the degree of maturation, it is possible with the aid of a chart to approximate the stage of a tubule.

PLATE 106

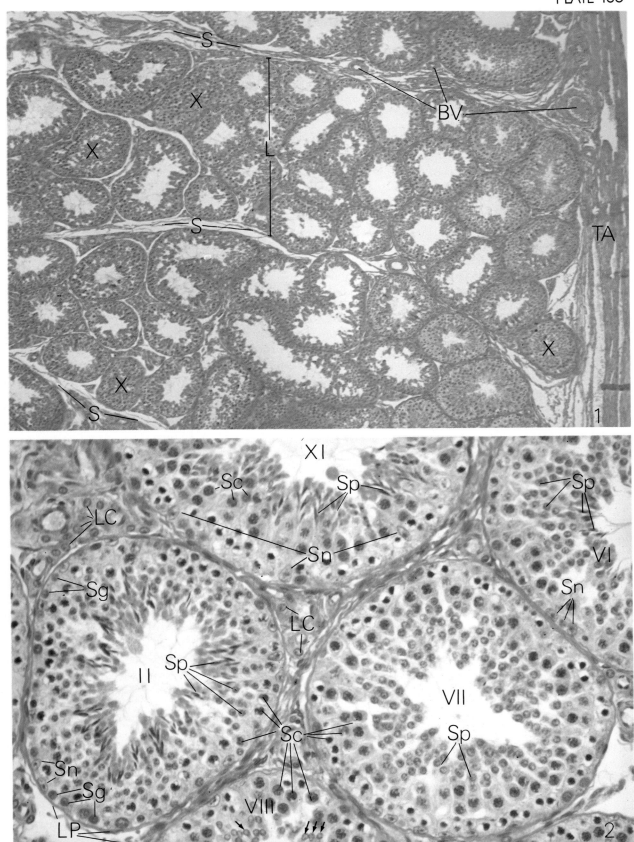

PLATE 107. Testis II

The prepubertal testis. The variety of germ cell types representative of spermatogenesis in the mature seminiferous tubules are not present in the testis before puberty or in the postpubertal undescended testis. Instead, the "tubules" are represented by cords of cells in which a lumen is lacking **(Fig. 1).** The seminiferous cords display the same tortuosity as in the adult; the tunica albuginea **(TA)** of the testis, though thinner, is of the same relative thickness.

The seminiferous cords are of considerably smaller diameter than the tubules of the adult and are comprised of two cell types, the gonocyte and a cell that resembles the Sertoli cell of the adult. The latter cell type predominates and comprises the bulk of the cord. The cells are columnar and their nuclei are close to the basement membrane. The gonocytes are the precursors of the definitive germ cells, or spermatogonia. They are round cells that have a centrally placed, spherical nucleus. The cytoplasm takes little stain and usually appears as a light ring around the nucleus. This gives the gonocyte **(G)** a distinctive appearance in histological sections **(Fig. 1, inset).** Generally, the gonocytes are found at the periphery of the cord, but many are also found more centrally placed. The gonocytes give rise to spermatogonia that begin to proliferate between the ages of 10 and 13 years. The seminiferous epithelium then becomes populated with cells at various stages of spermatogenesis, as is seen in the adult.

The epithelial cords are surrounded by one or two layers of cells with long processes and flat nuclei. They resemble fibroblasts at the ultrastructural level and give rise to the myoid peritubular cells of the adult.

The interstitial cells of Leydig are conspicuous in the newborn, a reflection of the residual effects of maternal hormones. However, the Leydig cells regress and do not become conspicuous again until puberty. In this preparation, the Leydig cells **(LC)** can be seen between the cords **(Fig. 1, inset).** They are ovoid or polygonal in the shape and are closely grouped so that adjacent cells are in contact with each other. Overall they have the same appearance as the Leydig cells of the adult.

Straight tubules and rete testes. In the posterior of the testis, the connective tissue of the tunica albuginea extends more deeply into the organ. This inward extension of connective tissue is called

KEY

AC, adipose cells
BV, blood vessels
G, gonocytes
LC, leydig cells
MT, mediastinum testis

RT, rete testis
ST, seminiferous tubules
TA, tunica albuginea
TR, tubulus rectus

Fig. 1, human, newborn × 180 inset, × 360
Fig. 2, monkey, × 65

Fig. 3, monkey, × 400.

the mediastinum testis. It contains a network of anastomosing channels called the rete testis **(Fig. 2).** Only a small portion of the mediastinum testes **(MT)** is evident in the figure. However, the area includes a few seminiferous tubules **(ST)** in the upper portion of the micrograph, and fortuitously it also includes the site where one of the seminiferous tubules terminates and joins the rete testis **(RT).** This can be recognized in the area delineated by the rectangle which is shown at higher magnification in **Figure 3.** As noted earlier, the seminiferous tubules are arranged in the form of a loop, with each end joining the rete testis. The seminiferous tubules open into the rete testis by way of a straight tubule, or tubulus rectus. The tubuli recti are very short and are lined by Sertoli-like cells; no germ cell component is present. The tubulus rectus **(TR)** in **Figure 3** appears to end on one side before it ends on the other. This is simply a reflection of the angle of section. However, when the straight tubule ends, the epithelial lining suddenly becomes cuboidal. This represents the rete testis, which constitutes an anastomosing system of channels that lead to the efferent ductules. The epithelial lining cells of the rete are sometimes more squamous than cuboidal or occasionally may be low columnar in appearance. Typically they possess a single cilium; however, this is difficult to see in routine H&E preparations.

The connective tissue of the mediastinum is very dense but exhibits no other special features, nor is smooth muscle present. Adipose cells **(AC)** and blood vessels **(BV),** particularly veins of varying size, are present within the connective tissue.

PLATE 107

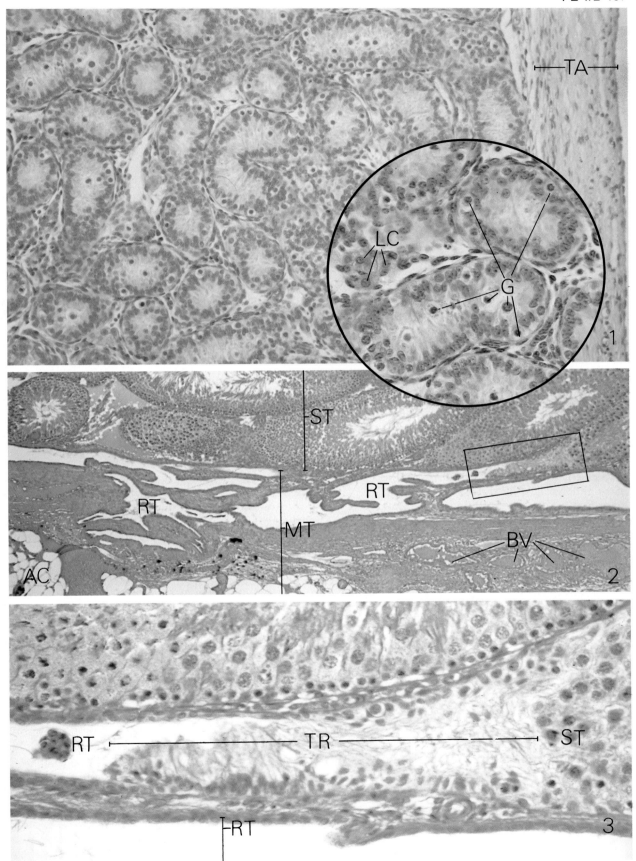

PLATE 108. Ductuli Efferents and Epididymis

Ductuli efferentes. About 12 to 20 efferent ductules leave the testis and serve as channels from the rete testis to the ductus epididymis. Each of the efferent ductules undergoes numerous spiral windings and convolutions to form a group of conical structures; together they constitute the initial part of the head of the epididymis. When examined in a tissue section, the ductules exhibit a variety of irregular profiles due to their twisting and turning. This is evident in **Figure 1,** on the right side of the micrograph.

The epithelium that lines the efferent ductules is distinctive in that groups of tall columnar cells aternate with groups of cuboidal cells, giving the lumenal surface an uneven contoured appearance. Thus, small cup-like depressions are created where the epithelium contains groups of cuboidal or low columnar cells. Typically, these shorter cells exhibit a brushborder-like apical surface due to the microvilli that they possess **(arrowhead, inset).** The basal surface of the ductule, in contrast, has a smooth contour **(Fig. 2** and **inset).** Some of the cells—generally the tall columnar cells—possess cilia **(C).** Whereas the ciliated cells aid in moving the contents of the tubule toward the epididymis, the cells with the microvilli are largely responsible for absorbing fluid from the lumen. In addition to the columnar and cuboidal cells, basal cells are also present, thus, the epithelium is designated pseudostratified columnar. The basal cells possess little cytoplasm and presumably serve as a reserve cell.

The efferent ductules possess a thin layer of circularly arranged smooth muscle cells **(SM, inset).** The muscle is close to the basal surface of the epithelial cells, being separated from it by only a small amount of connective tissue. Because of this close association, the smooth muscle may be overlooked or misidentified as connective tissue. Smooth muscle facilitates movement of luminal contents of the ductule to the ductus epididymidis.

Epididymis. The epididymis, by virtue of its shape, is divided into a head, body, and tail. The initial part of the head contains the ductus epididymidis, a single convoluted duct, into which the efferent ductules open. The duct at first is highly convoluted, but becomes less tortuous in the body and tail. A section through the head of the epididymis, as in **Figure 1,** cuts the ductus epididymidis in numerous places, and as in the efferent ductules, different-shaped profiles are observed.

The epithelium contains two distinguishable cell types: tall columnar cells and basal cells similar to those of the efferent ductules. The epithelium is thus also pseudostratified columnar. The columnar cells are tallest in the head of the epididymis and reduce in height as the tail is reached. The free surface of the cell possesses stereocilia **(SC, Fig. 2).** These are extremely long, branching microvilli. They evidently adhere to each other during the preparation of the tissue to form the fine tapering structures that are characteristically seen with the light microscope. The nuclei of the columnar cells are elongated and located a moderate distance from the base of the cell. They are readily distinguished from the spherical nuclei of the basal cells that lie close to the basement membrane. Other conspicuous features of the columnar cells include a very large supranuclear Golgi apparatus (not seen at the magnification offered here), pigment accumulations **(P),** and—demonstrable with appropriate techniques—numerous lysosomes.

Because of the unusual height of the columnar cells and, again, the tortuosity of the duct, an uneven lumen appears in some sites, indeed even "islands" of epithelium can be encountered in the lumen **(arrows, Fig. 1).** Such profiles are accounted for by sharp turns in the duct where the epithelial wall on one side of the duct is partially cut. For example, a cut in the plane of the **double-headed arrow** indicated in **Figure 2** would create such an isolated epithelial island.

A thin layer of smooth muscle circumscribes the duct and appears similar to that associated with the efferent ductules. However, in the terminal portion of the epididymis the smooth muscle acquires a greater thickness and longitudinal fibers are also present. Beyond the smooth muscle coat there is a small amount of connective tissue that binds the loops of the duct together and carries the blood vessels and nerves.

KEY

AT, adipose tissue
BV, blood vessel
C, cilia
CT, connective tissue
arrows, "islands" of epithelium in the lumen

arrowhead, inset, brush border
P, pigment
SC, stereocilia
SM, smooth muscle

Fig. 1, monkey, ×60

Fig. 2, monkey, ×180; inset, ×360.

PLATE 108

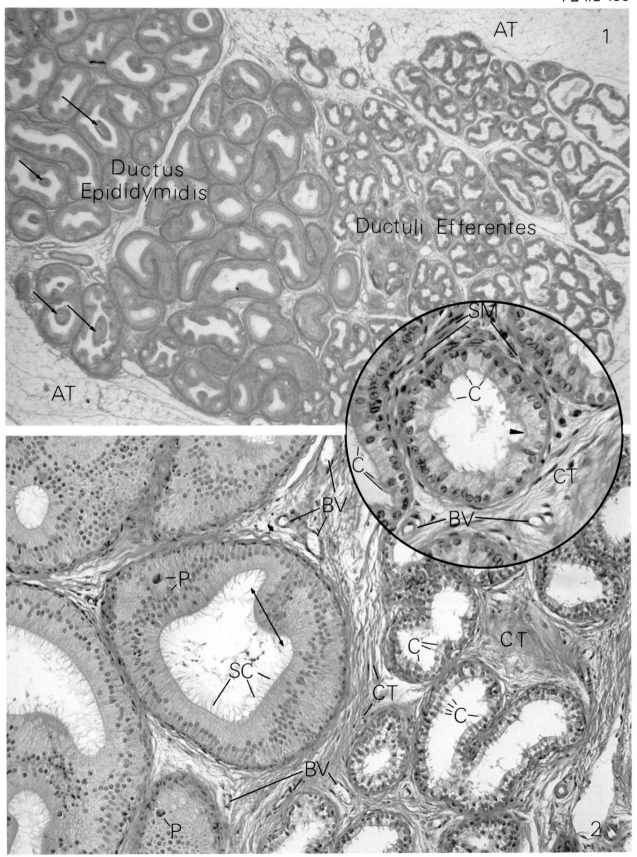

AT

1

Ductus
Epididymidis

Ductuli Efferentes

AT

SM

C

C

CT

BV

BV

P

SC

CT

C

CT

BV

P

C

2

PLATE 109. Spermatic Cord and Ductus Deferens

The ductus (vas) deferens continues from the duct of the epididymis as a thick-walled muscular tube that leaves the scrotum and passes through the inguinal canal as a component of the spermatic cord. At the deep inguinal ring, it continues into the pelvis and behind the urinary bladder it joins with the seminal vesicle to form the ejaculatory duct. The ejaculatory duct then pierces the prostate gland and opens into the urethra.

A cross-section through the ductus deferens and some of the vessels and nerves that accompany the duct in the spermatic cord is shown in **Figure 1.** The wall of the ductus deferens is extremely thick, owing mostly to the presence of a large amount of smooth muscle. The muscle contracts when the tissue is removed, causing the mucosa to form longitudinal folds. For this reason, in histological sections, the lumen usually appears irregular in cross-section.

The epithelial lining of the ductus deferens consists of pseudostratified columnar epithelium that may contain stereocilia **(arrowheads, Fig. 2).** It resembles the epithelium of the epididymis, but the cells are not as tall. The elongated nuclei of the columnar cells are readily distinguished from the spherical nuclei of the basal cells **(arrows).** The epithelium rests on a loose connective tissue **(CT),** which extends to the smooth muscle, and no submucosa is described.

The smooth muscle of the ductus deferens **(Fig. 1)** is arranged as a thick outer longitudinal layer **[SM(L)],** a thick middle circular layer **[SM(C)],** and a thinner inner longitudinal layer **[SM(L)].** Between the epithelium and the inner longitudinal smooth muscle layer there is a moderately thick cellular layer of loose connective tissue, the lamina propria **(LP).** The connective tissue immediately surrounding the ductus deferens con-

tains nerves and some of the smaller blood vessels that supply the duct. In fact, some of these vessels can be seen penetrating the outer longitudinal smooth muscle layer in **Figure 1 (asterisks).**

A unique feature of the spermatic cord is the presence of a plexus of atypical veins—the pampiniform plexus—which arise from the spermatic veins. These vessels receive the blood from the testis. (The pampiniform plexus also receives tributaries from the epididymis.) The plexus is an anastomosing vascular network that comprises the bulk of the spermatic cord. Portions of several of these veins **(BV)** are evident in the upper right of **Figure 1** along with a number of nerves **(N).** The unusual feature of the veins is their thick wall, which at a glance appears to be an artery rather than a vein. Careful examination of these vessels (see **inset**) shows that the bulk of the vessel wall is comprised of two layers of smooth muscle, an outer circular layer **SM(C)** and an inner longitudinal layer **SM(L).**

KEY

BV, blood vessels
CT, connective tissue
L, lumen of ductus deferens
LP, lamina propria
Lu, lumen of blood vessel
N, nerve
SM(C), circular layer of smooth muscle
SM(L), longitudinal layer of smooth muscle
arrows, Fig. 2, basal cell nucleus
arrowheads, stereocilia
asterisks, Fig. 1, small arteries supplying ductus deferens

Fig. 1, human, × 80
Fig. 2, human, × 320; inset, × 250.

PLATE 109

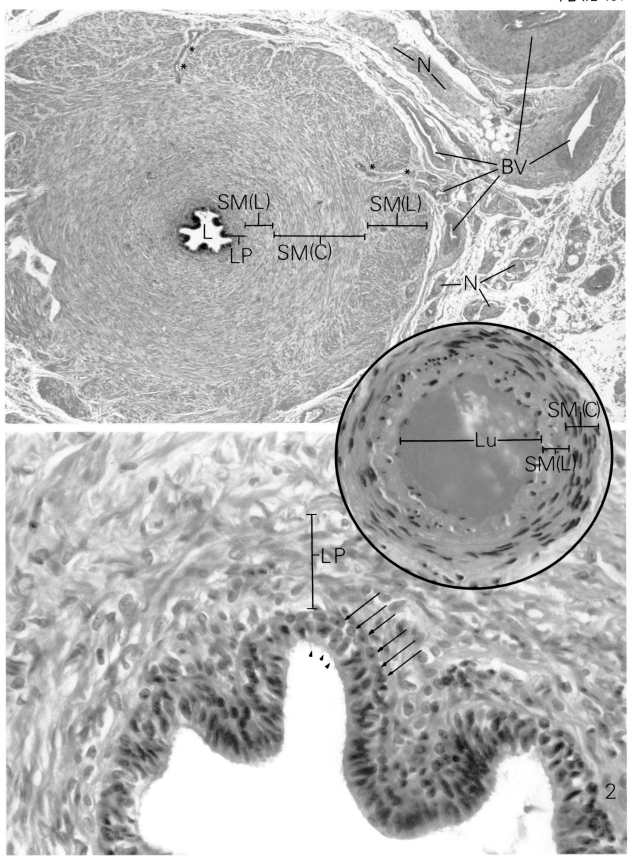

PLATE 110. Prostate Gland

The prostate gland surrounds the first part of the urethra. It consists of about 30 to 50 tubuloalveolar glands that are contained in a fibroelastic stroma. The stroma is characterized by the presence of numerous small bundles of smooth muscle so that it can also be described as a fibromuscular stroma. Surrounding the gland is a fibroelastic capsule that also contains small bundles of smooth muscle. Ducts from the gland empty into the urethra.

A section of the prostate gland is shown in **Figure 1.** The capsule **(Cap)** is in the upper part of the figure; the glandular components are in the lower part. The tubuloalveoli of the prostate gland vary greatly in form as evidenced in the illustration. They may appear as tubes, as alveoli, as alveoli with branches, or as tubes with branches. They may appear distended or they may be collapsed. Frequently, in older individuals, precipitates (prostatic concretions, **PC**) are present in the lumens. These stain with eosin and may have a concentric lamellar appearance. With time, they may become impregnated with calcium salts.

The area enclosed within the **large rectangle (Fig. 1)** is shown at higher magnification in **Figure 2** and shows some characteristic features of the tube-alveoli. In many places the epithelium bulges into the lumen; sometimes, the top of an epithelial fold is cut to give the impression of an island of cells in a lumen **(arrows).** Large numbers of closely packed nuclei are seen when a fold is cut obliquely or crosswise **(arrowheads).** This is one of the characteristic features of the prostate gland epithelium.

Figure 3 shows the epithelial cells at higher magnification. The epithelium consists mainly of columnar cells, although basal cells are also present. For this reason, the epithelium is classified as pseudostratified columnar. The columnar cells are described as containing secretion granules and lipid droplets, but these are not always evident.

Many cells possess apical cytoplasmic protrusions **(arrows)** that seemingly break off into the lumen.

The various tube-alveoli are surrounded by a fibroelastic stroma containing smooth muscle (fibromuscular stroma). The smooth muscle is not organized in a way that suggests that it belongs to any single tube or alveolus, as in the epididymis, but rather appears to be randomly dispersed in the stroma. In **Figure 1,** the staining of the muscle differs from the staining of the connective tissue. The muscle appears as the elongated dark fibers or as dark oval bodies **(SM),** in either case surrounded by a more extensive continuous phase of the lighter staining connective tissue. Some bundles of smooth muscle are also to be seen in the capsule. The **upper rectangle** in **Figure 1** is examined at higher magnification in **Figure 4.** This shows the smooth muscle cut in longitudinal [**SM(L)**] and cross-section [**SM(X)**], and also reveals the presence of a nerve bundle **(N).** The nerve stains very much like the connective tissue, but can be recognized by virtue of its organization and the presence of a perineurial sheath. These features would be more evident at higher magnifications.

PLATE 110

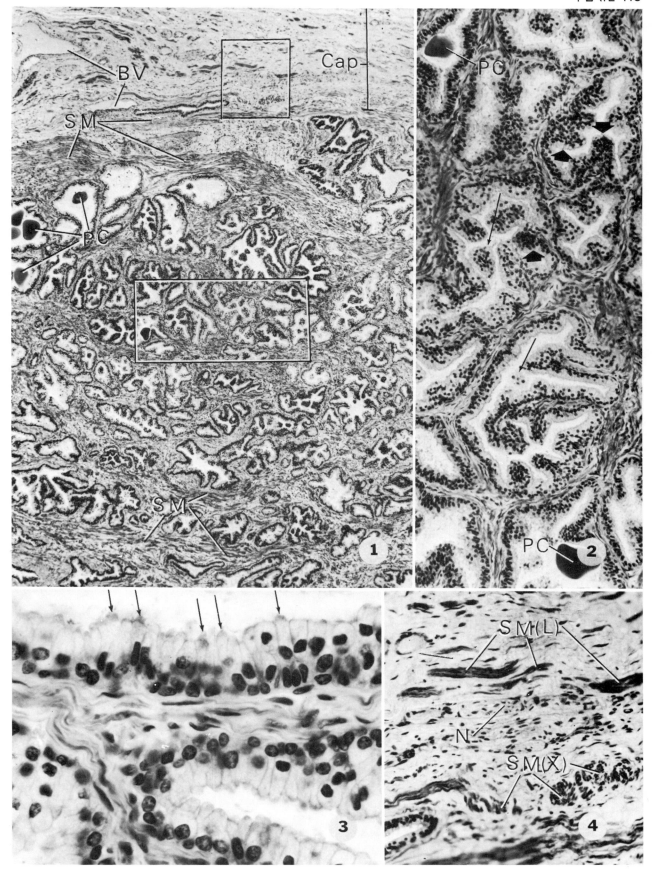

PLATE 111. *Seminal Vesicle*

The mucosa rests on a thick layer of smooth muscle **(SM).** The smooth muscle consists of an indefinite inner circular layer and an outer longitudinal layer, but these are difficult to distinguish. Beyond the smooth muscle is the connective tissue of the adventitia.

The seminal vesicles are paired elongated sacs. Each vesicle consists of a single tube folded and coiled upon itself with occasional diverticula in its wall. The upper extremity ends as a cul-de-sac; the lower extremity is constricted into a narrow straight duct that joins and empties into its corresponding ductus deferens.

Figure 1 shows a cross-section of a seminal vesicle. Due to the coiled nature of the vesicle, two almost distinct lumens, lying side by side, appear to be present. They are, however, connected so that, in effect, all of the internal spaces are continuous and what is seen here is actually a two-dimensional configuration reflecting a coiling of the tube.

The mucosa of the seminal vesicles is characterized by being extensively folded or ridged. The ridges vary in size and typically branch and interconnect with one another. The larger ridges may form recesses that contain smaller ridges, and when these are cut obliquely, they appear as mucosal arches which enclose the smaller folds **(arrows).** When the plane of section is normal to the surface, the mucosal ridges appear as "villi." In some areas, particularly the peripheral region of the lumen, the interconnecting folds of the mucosa appear as alveoli. However, it should be realized that each of these chambers is simply a pocket-like structure that is open and continuous with the lumen.

KEY

CT, connective tissue
Ep, epithelium
LP, lamina propria
SM, smooth muscle

arrows, mucosal arches
arrowhead, oblique
    section of epithelium

Fig. 1, human, × 30   **Fig. 2,** human, × 220

Figure 2, a higher magnification of the mucosal folds, reveals the epithelium **(Ep)** and the underlying loose connective tissue **(CT)** or lamina propria. The epithelium is described as pseudostratified. It is comprised of low columnar or cuboidal cells and small, round basal cells. The latter are randomly interspersed between the larger principal cells, but they are relatively sparse in number. For this reason, the epithelium may not be readily recognized as pseudostratified. In some areas, as in **Figure 2,** the epithelium appears thick **(arrowhead)** and based on the disposition of the nuclei would seem to be multilayered. This is due to a tangential section of the epithelium and is not a true stratification. The lamina propria of the mucosa is comprised of a very cellular connective tissue containing some smooth muscle cells and is rich in elastic fibers.

PLATE 111

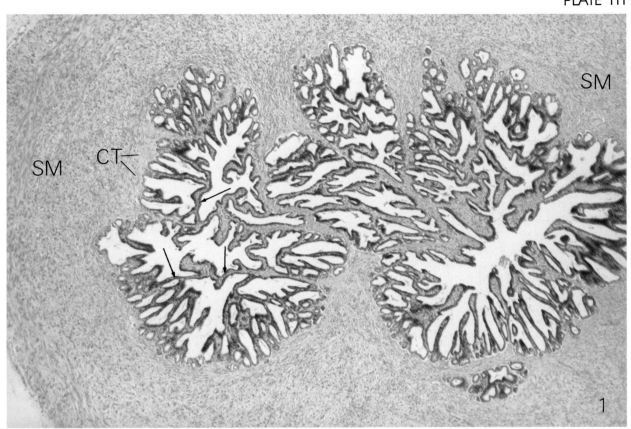

1

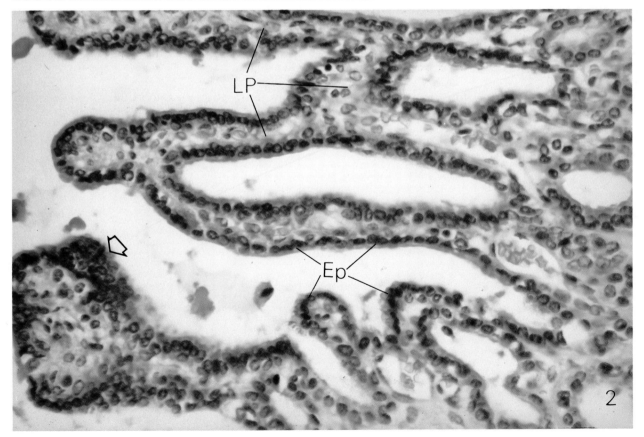

2

Female Reproductive System

22

The female reproductive system consists of a group of internal organs located in the pelvis and the external genitalia. The internal organs are the ovaries, oviducts, uterus, and vagina (Fig. 22.1). The external genitalia include the mons pubis, labia majora, labia minora, clitoris, vestibule of the vagina, and openings of the urethra and vagina. The mammary glands will be included in this chapter because their development and functional state is directly related to the hormonal activity of the female reproductive system.

The ovaries, oviducts, and uterus of the sexually mature female undergo marked structural and functional changes related to the menstrual cycle and pregnancy. Hormonal and neural mechanisms regulate these cyclic changes, as well as the development of the female reproductive system. The onset of the reproductive phase of life, which is marked by the initiation of the menstrual cycles and is referred to as the *menarche,* occurs in females between the ages of 9 and 14 years (average 13.5). Menarche marks the end of puberty and the beginning of the reproductive life span, which lasts about 30 to 40 years. During this phase of life, the *menstrual cycle* averages about 28 to 30 days in length. Between the ages of 45 and 55 years, the menstrual cycles become increasingly infrequent and then cease. This change in reproductive function is referred to as *menopause,* climacteric, or the "change of life." The reproductive organs cease function and atrophy at the termination of the menstrual phase.

OVARY

The ovaries have two interrelated functions: the production of gametes (*gametogenesis*) and the production of steroids (*steroidogenesis*). In the fe-male, the production of gametes is called *oogenesis.* Developing gametes are called *oocytes;* mature gametes are called *ova.* The steroid hormones secreted by the ovaries function in the regulation of the maturation of the oocytes and the development and maintenance of the secondary sex organs and the mammary glands.

The ovaries are paired, almond-shaped structures, measuring about 3 cm in length, 1.5 cm in width, and 1 cm in thickness. In postmenopausal women, the ovaries are about one-fourth the size observed during the reproductive period. The *hilus* of the ovary is attached to the posterior surface of the broad ligament by a peritoneal fold, the *mesovarium* (see Fig. 22.1). Ovarian vessels and nerves pass via a peritoneal fold, the *suspensory ligament* of the ovary, to the mesovarium and then to the hilus of the ovary. The medial pole of the ovary is attached to the uterus by the *ovarian ligament.*

The central portion of the ovary, the *medullary region,* or *medulla,* contains loose connective tissue, a mass of relatively large contorted blood vessels, lymphatic vessels, and nerves (Fig. 22.2). The peripheral portion of the ovary, the *cortical region,* or *cortex,* surrounds the medulla and contains the *ovarian follicles,* embedded in a compact, richly cellular connective tissue. Scattered smooth muscle fibers are present in the stroma around the follicles. The boundary between the medulla and cortex is indistinct. At the hilus, the cortex is interrupted and the mesovarium is continuous with the medulla. Small, irregular ducts, the *rete ovarii,* which are remnants of fetal structures, may be found in this region.

The surface of the ovary is covered by a single layer of cuboidal or squamous cells. This layer, known as the *germinal epithelium,* is continuous with the mesothelium that covers the mesovarium.

649

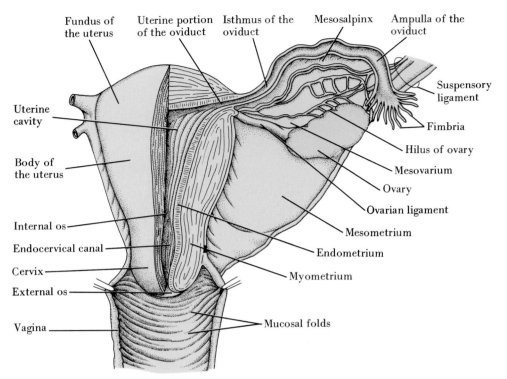

Figure 22.1. Schematic drawing of the components of the female reproductive system. (*Gray's Anatomy,* 1973.)

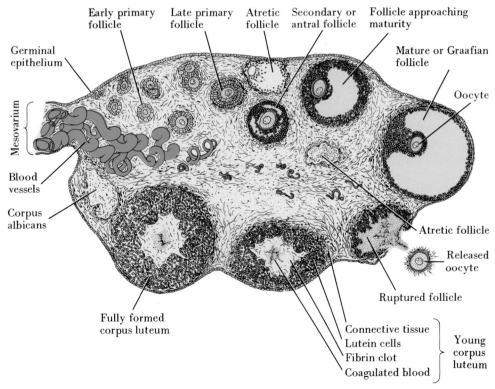

Figure 22.2. Schematic drawing of a section through the ovary. Highly coiled blood vessels are present in the hilum and medullary regions. (After C. E. Corliss.)

The germ *germinal epithelium* is a carryover from earlier days when it was incorrectly thought to be the site of germ cell formation. It is now known that the primordial germ cells are of extragonadal origin and that they migrate into the gonad where they differentiate into oogonia. A dense connective tissue layer, the *tunica albuginea,* lies between the germinal epithelium and the underlying cortex.

Ovarian Follicle

Ovarian follicles, each containing an oocyte, are embedded in the stroma of the ovarian cortex. The size of the follicle is indicative of the developmental state of the oocyte. Early stages of oogenesis occur during early fetal life with mitotic divisions of the oogonia (see section on oogenesis). The oocytes present at birth remain arrested in their development at the first meiotic division. As young girls pass through puberty, the ovaries begin a phase of reproductive activity characterized by the cyclic growth and maturation of small groups of follicles. The first ovulation generally does not take place for a year or more following menarche. A cyclic pattern of follicular maturation and ovulation then continues through a period of 30 to 40 years in parallel with the menstrual cycle. Normally, only one oocyte reaches full maturity and is released from the ovary during each menstrual cycle. Obviously, the maturation and release of more than one egg at ovulation may lead to multiple births. In her reproductive life-span, a woman produces only about 400 mature ova. Most of the estimated 400,000 oocytes present at birth fail to complete maturation and are gradually lost through *atresia.* The few oocytes that remain at menopause degenerate within a few years.

Three basic types of ovarian follicles can be identified: (1) primordial, (2) growing, and (3) mature, or Graafian (Fig. 22.3). The growing follicles can be further categorized as primary and secondary (or antral) follicles. Some histologists identify additional stages in follicular development. In the cycling ovary, follicles at all stages of development are found. The primordial follicles predominate.

Primordial follicle. The primordial follicles are found in the stroma of the cortex just beneath the tunica albuginea. A single layer of flattened or squamous *follicular cells* resting on a basement membrane surrounds the oocyte (Fig. 22.4). At this stage, the plasma membranes of the oocyte and the surrounding follicular cells are closely apposed to one another and are relatively smooth. The oocyte in the follicle measures about 30 μm in diameter and has a large, eccentric nucleus containing finely dispersed chromatin and one or more large nucle-

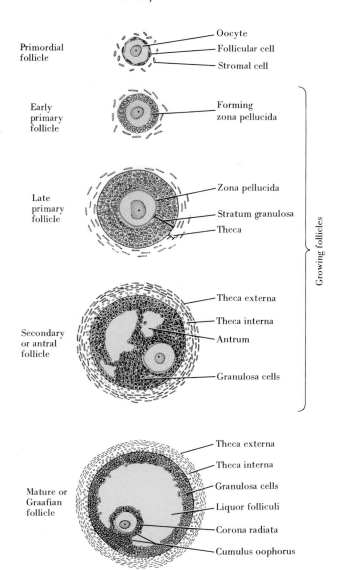

Figure 22.3. Schematic drawing of the stages in the development of ovarian follicles, beginning with the primordial follicle and ending with the mature, or Graafian, follicle. The secondary and mature follicle are drawn at reduced size, thus, the smaller appearing oocytes. The oocyte in a primordial follicle is arrested in the first meiotic prophase. As the follicle continues through its development, the oocyte progresses through the first meiotic division, which is completed just before the release of the oocyte from the mature follicle. The oocyte at this stage is referred to as a secondary oocyte (see text section on oogenesis and maturation of the ovum and fertilization). (Based on Junqueira LC, Carneiro J: *Basic Histology,* 3rd ed. Los Altos, CA, Lange, 1980.)

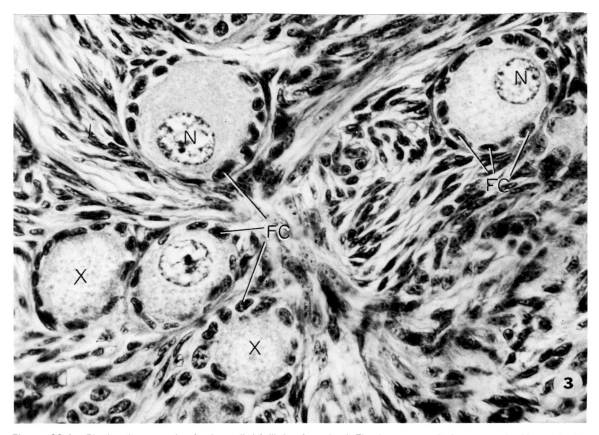

Figure 22.4. Photomicrograph of primordial follicles (monkey). The large oocyte is surrounded by a single layer of flattened follicle cells (FC). Usually, the large nucleus of the oocyte is in an eccentric position. Two oocytes are indicated (X) in which the nucleus is not included in the plane of section. × 640.

oli. A well-developed Golgi apparatus surrounded by numerous mitochondria is located near the nucleus. At the ultrastructural level the cytoplasm is seen to contain, in addition to other typical organelles, annulate lamellae[1] and numerous small vesicles that appear to be associated with the Golgi apparatus, but are also seen scattered through the cytoplasm. Pores in the nuclear envelope are numerous.

Growing follicle. As the primordial follicle makes the transition into the growing (active or maturing) follicle, changes occur in the follicular cells, oocyte, and adjacent stroma. Initially, the oocyte enlarges and the surrounding flattened follicular cells proliferate and become cuboidal in shape. At this stage, that is, with the follicular cells becoming cuboidal, the follicle is identified as a *primary follicle*. As the oocyte grows, a homogeneous, deeply staining, acidophilic, refractile layer called the *zona pellucida* appears between the oocyte and the adjacent follicular cells (Fig. 22.5). The zona pellucida is first apparent with the light microscope when the oocyte, surrounded by a single layer of cuboidal or columnar follicle cells, has grown to a diameter of 50 to 80 μm. The growing oocyte is responsible for the production of this gel-like, periodic acid-Schiff (PAS)-positive layer that is rich in glycosaminoglycans and proteoglycans.

Through rapid mitotic proliferation, the single layer of follicular cells gives rise to a stratified epithelium surrounding the oocyte and resting on a basement membrane. The follicular cells are then identified as *granulosa cells.* As the granulosa cells proliferate, the stromal cells immediately surrounding the follicle form a sheath of cells, the *theca folliculi,* just external to the basement membrane (Fig. 22.6). The theca folliculi further differentiates into two layers: the *theca interna,* an inner, highly vascularized layer of secretory cells, and the *theca externa,* an outer layer of connective tissue

_____

[1] Annulate lamellae occur in a limited number of cell types. They appear at the electron microscope level as a stack of nuclear envelope profiles. Each layer of the stack has the appearance of a segment of nuclear envelope including pore structures morphologically identical to nuclear pores.

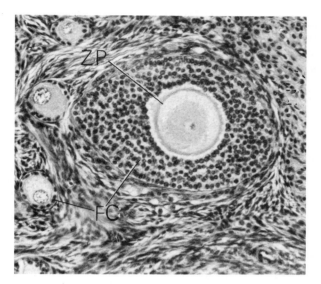

Figure 22.5. Photomicrograph of late primary follicle (monkey). In the late primary follicle, multiple layers of follicle cells (FC) surround the primary oocyte. At this stage, a homogeneous-appearing layer called the zona pellucida (ZP) is present between the oocyte and follicle cells. In the much smaller, adjacent primordial follicles, a single layer of flattened follicle cells can be seen. × 160.

cells. Boundaries between the thecal layers and between the theca externa and surrounding stroma are not distinct. However, the basement membrane between the granulosa layer and the theca interna establishes a distinct boundary separating these layers. It also separates the rich capillary bed of the theca interna from the granulosa layer, which is avascular during the period of follicular growth. When fully differentiated, the cells of the theca interna are cuboidal and possess ultrastructural features characteristic of steroid-producing cells.

The distribution of oocyte organelles changes as the oocyte matures. Multiple Golgi complexes, derived from the single juxtanuclear Golgi complex of the primordial oocyte, are scattered in the cytoplasm. There is an increase in the number of free ribosomes, small vesicles, and multivesicular bodies and in the amount of granular endoplasmic reticulum. Occasional lipid droplets and masses of lipochrome pigment can be seen. The oocytes of many species, including those of mammals, contain specialized secretory vesicles located just beneath the plasma membrane in the outer region, or ***cor-***

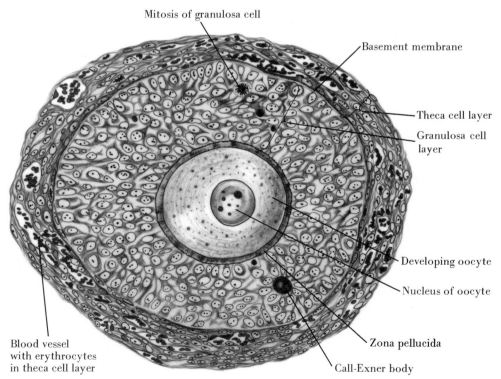

Figure 22.6. Drawing of growing follicle. A basement membrane separates the granulosa cell layer from the theca cell layer. The zona pellucida immediately surrounds the developing oocyte. × 375. (After Maximow AA: In Bloom W, Fawcett DW: *A Textbook of Histology,* 10th ed. Philadelphia, WB Saunders, 1975.)

tex, of the oocyte cytoplasm. These **cortical granules** release their contents by exocytosis when the egg is activated by the sperm (this is discussed in the section on oogenesis and fertilization). The contents of the granules interact with the plasma membrane and the coverings around the egg, the egg coat, so as to prevent other sperm from fusing with and entering the egg. Numerous irregular microvilli from the oocyte project into the space between the oocyte and the surrounding granulosa cells as the zona pellucida is deposited (Fig. 22.7). Slender processes from the granulosa cells develop at the same time and project toward the oocyte, intermingling with oocyte microvilli and, occasionally, invaginating into the oocyte plasma membrane. The processes may contact the plasma membrane, but do not establish cytoplasmic continuity between the cells. However, during follicular growth, extensive gap junctions, serving as channels for intercellular communication, develop between adjacent granulosa cells.

The primary follicle initially moves deeper into the cortical stroma as it increases in size, primarily through the proliferation of the granulosa cells. When the stratum granulosa reaches a thickness of 6 to 12 cell layers, fluid-filled cavities appear among the granulosa cells (Fig. 22.3). As the hyaluronic acid-rich fluid, called **liquor folliculi,** continues to accumulate among the granulosa cells, the cavities begin to coalesce, eventually forming a single crescent-shaped cavity, called the

antrum. The follicle is now identified as a **secondary** or **antral follicle.** The eccentrically positioned oocyte, which has attained a diameter of about 125 μm, undergoes no further growth. The follicle, which was 0.2 mm in diameter when the follicular fluid first appeared, continues to grow and will reach a size of 10 mm or more in diameter.

As the secondary follicle increases in size, the antrum, lined by several layers of granulosa cells, enlarges (Fig. 22.8). The stratum granulosa has a relatively uniform thickness except for the region associated with the oocyte. Here, the granulosa cells form a thickened mound, the **cumulus oophorus,** that projects into the antrum and surrounds the oocyte. Those cells of the cumulus oophorus that immediately surround the oocyte and remain with it at ovulation (see below) are also referred to as the **corona radiata.** Extracellular, densely staining material, called **Call-Exner bodies,** may be seen between the granulosa cells. With the PAS reaction, these bodies stain positively. Their role and nature is unknown.

Mature or Graafian follicle. A mature follicle has a diameter of 10 mm or more, extends through the full thickness of the ovarian cortex, and bulges from the surface of the ovary. As a follicle nears its maximum size, there is a decrease in the mitotic activity of the granulosa cells. The stratum granulosa appears to become thinner as the antrum increases in size. As the space between the granulosa cells continues to enlarge, the oocyte

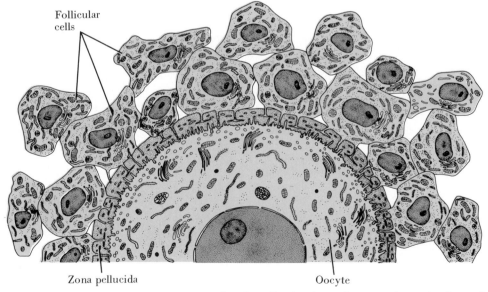

Follicular cells

Zona pellucida

Oocyte

Figure 22.7. Schematic drawing depicting the ultrastructure of an oocyte and adjacent follicular cells. Numerous microvilli from the oocyte and slender processes from the follicular cells extend into the zona pellucida which surrounds the oocyte. (Based on Junqueira LC, Carneiro J: In *Basic Histology*, 3rd ed. Los Altos, Lange, 1980.)

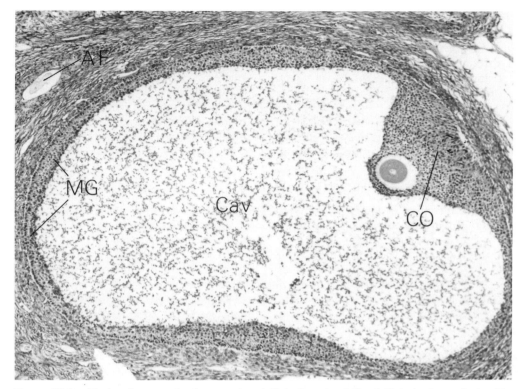

Figure 22.8. Photomicrograph of secondary follicle (monkey). The follicle is characterized by the presence of a large fluid-filled antrum, or follicular cavity (Cav). The oocyte is located at one end in a mound of granulosa cells called the cumulus oophorus (CO). The remaining follicle cells that surround the lumen are called the membrana granulosa (MG), or granulosa cells. An atretic follicle (AF, **upper left**), can be seen near the secondary follicle. × 65.

and cumulus cells are gradually loosened from the rest of the granulosa cells in preparation for ovulation. The cumulus cells immediately surrounding the oocyte form a single layer of cells, the *corona radiata,* just external to the zona pellucida. These cells and loosely arranged cumulus cells remain associated with the oocyte at the time of ovulation.

During this period of maturation of the follicle, the thecae folliculi become more prominent. Lipid droplets appear in the cytoplasm of the theca interna cells, and the cells demonstrate ultrastructural features associated with steroid-producing cells. The granulosa cells and thecal cells produce the ovarian hormones essential in normal reproductive function. In the human, luteinizing hormone (LH) stimulates the cells of the theca interna to secrete testosterone, which serves as the precursor for estrogens. The testosterone diffuses into the follicular stroma and reaches the granulosa cells. In response to follicle-stimulating hormone (FSH), the granulosa cells catalyze the conversion of testosterone to estrogen, which, in turn, stimulates the granulosa cells to proliferate and thereby increase the size of the follicle. As estrogen secre-

tion continues and blood estrogen levels increase, a surge in the release of LH is induced in the adenohypophysis. In response to the LH surge, the granulosa cells are down-regulated (or are desensitized) and no longer produce estrogens in response to LH. The granulosa and thecal cells then undergo luteinization and produce progesterone (this is discussed in section on the corpus luteum).

Ovulation

Ovulation is the process by which an oocyte is released from the ovarian follicle. It is inappropriate to refer to the oocyte at this stage as the ovum because it has not yet completed meiosis. Ovulation occurs through the rupture of the follicle at full maturity. Normally, only one follicle completes maturation and ruptures to release its oocyte at the middle of the menstrual cycle, on the 14th day of a 28-day cycle. Rarely, oocytes are released from other follicles that have reached full maturity during the same cycle, leading to the possibility of multiple births. Drugs, such as clomiphene citrate or human menopausal gonadotropins, given to stimulate ovarian activity greatly increase the possibility of multiple births by causing the simultaneous maturation of several follicles.

As ovulation approaches, follicular fluid appears to accumulate more rapidly in the antrum, causing the stratum granulosum, thecal layers, and overlying tunica albuginea to thin as the follicle bulges from the ovarian surface. The oocyte and the cumulus cells immediately surrounding it are freed from the follicular wall and float free in the antral fluid. Just before ovulation, blood flow stops in a small area of the ovarian surface overlying the bulging follicle. This area of the germinal epithelium, known as the **macula pellucida,** or **stigma,** becomes elevated and then ruptures. Within about 1 or 2 minutes, the oocyte, surrounded by the corona radiata and cells of the cumulus oophorus, is expelled from the ruptured follicle (Fig. 22.9). The oocyte then passes into the ostium of the oviduct. At the time of ovulation, the fimbriae of the oviduct become closely apposed to the surface of the ovary, directing the oocyte into the oviduct and not allowing it to pass into the peritoneal cavity.

Oogenesis, Maturation of the Ovum, and Fertilization

Primordial germ cells, which are first recognized among the endodermal cells of the yolk sac,

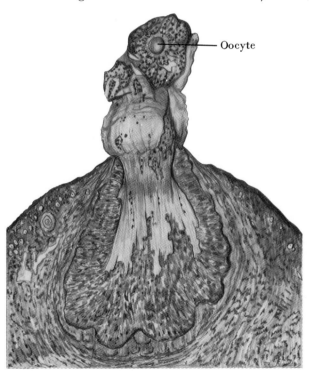

— Oocyte

Figure 22.9. Drawing of ovulation as observed in the rabbit. The oocyte, surrounded by the cumulus oophorus, is in the process of being expelled from the ruptured ovarian follicle. (L. Weiss and R. O. Greep, 1977.)

migrate to the genital ridges in the 6th week of embryonic development. During early fetal life, these primordial germ cells develop into oogonia and rapidly proliferate by mitotic division. Between 3 and 5 million oogonia enlarge to form primary oocytes. Primordial follicles are formed as the ovarian stromal cells form a flattened layer of follicular cells around each oocyte. Most of the primordial follicles are lost through atresia. Only about 400,000 follicles are present at birth. The primary oocytes within the primordial follicles begin the first meiotic division before birth, but the process is arrested at the diplotene stage (see section on meiosis in Chapter 21). At puberty, groups of follicles begin their cyclic development and resume the meiotic divisions. The completion of the first meiotic prophase does not occur until just before ovulation in the mature follicle. Therefore, some primary oocytes remain arrested in the first meiotic prophase for 45 years or more. It has been suggested that this long period of meiotic arrest may contribute to errors in the meiotic division such as nondisjunction, which results in chromosomal anomalies, such as trisomy of the 21st chromosome (Down's syndrome).

As the first meiotic division (reduction division) is completed in the mature follicle (Fig. 22.10), each daughter cell of the **primary oocyte** receives an equal share of the chromatin, but one daughter cell receives the majority of the cytoplasm and becomes the **secondary oocyte.** The other daughter cell receives a minimal amount of the cytoplasm and becomes the **first polar body.** As the secondary oocyte surrounded by the cells of the corona radiata leaves the follicle at ovulation, the second meiotic division (equatorial division) is in progress. This division is arrested at the second metaphase and is not completed unless the secondary oocyte is penetrated by a spermatozoon. If fertilization occurs, the secondary oocyte completes the second meiotic division and forms a mature **ovum** with the maternal pronucleus containing a set of 23 chromosomes. The other cell produced at this division is a **second polar body.** In the human, the first polar body does not divide; therefore, the fertilized egg can be recognized by the appearance of the second polar body. The polar bodies, which are not capable of further development, undergo degeneration. The nucleus of the sperm head that had entered the secondary oocyte forms a pronucleus containing 23 paternal chromosomes. After the fusion of the two pronuclei, the resulting **zygote** with its diploid ($2n$) complement of 46 chromosomes undergoes a mitotic division or first cleavage. This two-cell stage marks the beginning of the embryo.

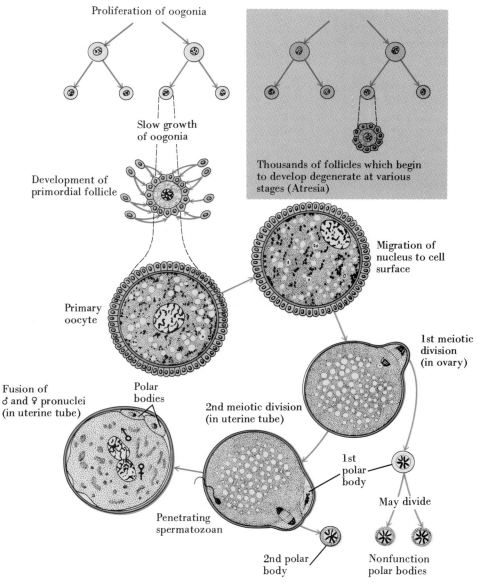

Proliferation of oogonia

Slow growth
of oogonia

Development of
primordial follicle

Thousands of follicles which begin
to develop degenerate at various
stages (Atresia)

Migration of
nucleus to cell
surface

Primary
oocyte

1st meiotic
division
(in ovary)

Fusion of
♂ and ♀ pronuclei
(in uterine tube)

Polar
bodies

2nd meiotic division
(in uterine tube)

1st
polar
body

May divide

Penetrating
spermatozoan

2nd polar
body

Nonfunction
polar bodies

Figure 22.10. Schematic diagrams illustrating changes that occur during the growth, maturation, and the fertilization of the oocyte. In the initial development of the primordial follicle shown above, stromal cells migrate to the oogonia and form a layer surrounding it, thus, forming the oocyte. Note that the primary oocyte remain arrested in prophase I of meiosis until just before ovulation. The first meiotic, or reductional, division is completed just before ovulation. The second meiotic, or equatorial, division is not completed unless the secondary oocyte is penetrated by a spermatozoon. (After C. E. Corliss.)

In order to fertilize an egg, a spermatozoon must pass through the corona radiata and zona pellucida and then penetrate the plasma membrane of the egg. Only a few hundred of the millions of spermatozoa present in an ejaculate reach the site of fertilization in the oviduct. Enzymes released from the acrosomes of the spermatozoa that do reach the site act to disperse the cells of the cumulus oophorus and the corona radiata and en-able the spermatozoa to penetrate the zona pellucida. Several spermatozoa may penetrate the zona pellucida, but normal development demands that only one spermatozoon penetrate the oocyte and complete fertilization, which culminates in the fusion of the egg and sperm pronuclei. As the fertilizing spermatozoon penetrates the plasma membrane of the egg, it is activated and the cortical granules move to the surface and release their contents by exocytosis (fusing with the plasma membrane). The contents of the granules interact with the plasma membrane and the coverings around the egg so as to prevent other sperm from fusing with and entering the egg.

After ovulation, the secondary oocyte remains viable for a period of approximately 24 hours. If fertilization fails to occur during this period, the secondary oocyte degenerates as it passes through the oviduct.

Corpus Luteum

Before ovulation, the basement membrane and thecal cells begin to fold into the layer of granulosa cells of the maturing follicle. At ovulation, the follicular wall, composed of the remaining granulosa and thecal cells, is thrown into deeper folds as the follicle collapses and is transformed into the *corpus luteum* (yellow body), or *luteal gland* (Fig. 22.11). Bleeding from the capillaries in the theca interna into the follicular lumen leads to the formation of a central clot. Some connective tissue from the stroma invades the former follicular cavity and then remains in the central region of the corpus luteum. The cells of the granulosa and theca interna layers then undergo dramatic morphological changes. These luteal cells increase in size and become filled with lipid droplets. A lipid-soluble pigment, lipochrome, in the cytoplasm of the cells gives them a yellow appearance in fresh,

unstained preparations. At the ultrastructural level, the cells demonstrate features associated with steroid-secreting cells—abundant smooth endoplasmic reticulum (sER) and mitochondria with tubular cristae (Fig. 22.12). Two types of luteal cells are usually identified: very large (about 30 μm in diameter), centrally located *granulosa lutein cells,* derived from the granulosa cells, and somewhat smaller (about 15 μm), more deeply staining, peripherally located *theca lutein cells,* derived from the cells of the theca interna layer. Some investigators argue that there is only one type of luteal cell and that the two types actually represent transitions in the differentiation of the luteal cell.

As the corpus luteum begins its formation, blood vessels and lymphatics from the theca interna rapidly grow into the granulosa layer. A rich vascular network is established within the corpus luteum. This highly vascularized structure located in the cortex of the ovary secretes progesterone and estrogens. These hormones stimulate the growth and secretory activity of the lining of the uterus, the *endometrium,* to prepare it for the implantation of the developing zygote, in the event that fertilization has occurred. If fertilization and implantation do occur, the corpus luteum increases in size to form the *corpus luteum of pregnancy.* The cyclic development of ovarian follicles is then blocked by the progesterone produced by the corpus luteum. *Human chorionic gonadotropin (HCG),* secreted by the trophoblasts of the chorion,

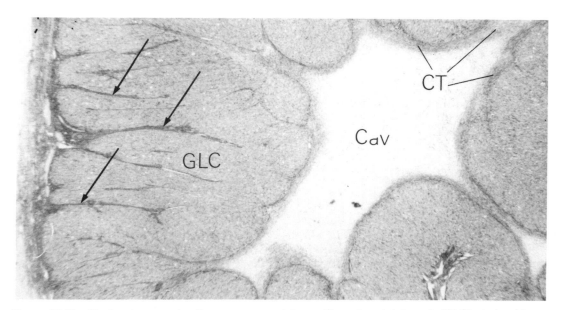

Figure 22.11. Photomicrograph of human corpus luteum. Granulosa lutein cells (GLC), derived from follicle cells, form a thick, folded layer around the former follicular cavity (Cav). Connective tissue (CT), which has invaded the follicular cavity and infoldings of theca interna **(arrows)**, can be seen in the corpus luteum. × 16.

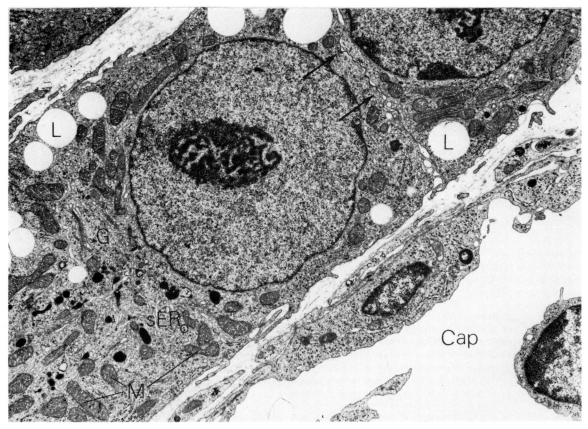

Figure 22.12. Theca lutein cells from a corpus luteum of a rhesus monkey at an early implantation stage (day 10.5 of gestation). Membrane-bound dense bodies are clustered near the Golgi region (G): most of the cytoplasm is packed with tubules of smooth endoplasmic reticulum (sER), lipid droplets (L), and mitochondria (M). Note the closely apposed cell membranes of adjoining cells (**arrows**) and the capillary (Cap) in the lower right. × 10,000. (Courtesy of Dr. C. Booher, 1984.)

stimulates the corpus luteum and prevents its degeneration. The corpus luteum reaches a size of 2 to 3 cm, is maintained for about 6 months, and then gradually declines over the remaining period of pregnancy. It remains active in the production of progesterone and estrogens throughout pregnancy, even though other tissues become the primary source of these hormones.

If fertilization and implantation do not occur, the corpus luteum remains active only for 14 days; in this case it is called the *corpus luteum of menstruation.* In the absence of chorionic gonadotropin, the rate of secretion of progesterone and estrogens declines and the corpus luteum begins to degenerate about 10 to 12 days after ovulation.

The corpus luteum degenerates and undergoes a slow involution after pregnancy or menstruation. The cells become loaded with lipid, decrease in size, and undergo autolysis. A white scar, the *corpus albicans,* is formed as intercellular hyaline material accumulates among the degenerating cells of the former corpus luteum (Fig. 22.13). The cor-

pus albicans sinks deeper into the ovarian cortex as it slowly disappears over a period of several months.

Follicular Atresia

As was previously stated, few of the ovarian follicles that begin their differentiation in the ovary are destined to complete their maturation. Most of the follicles degenerate and disappear through a process called *follicular atresia.* Large numbers of follicles undergo atresia during fetal development, early postnatal life, and puberty. After puberty, groups of follicles begin to mature each menstrual cycle, but only one follicle completes is maturation.

A follicle in any stage of its maturation may undergo atresia. The process becomes more complex as the follicle progresses further toward maturation. In the atresia of primordial and small growing follicles, the oocyte becomes smaller and

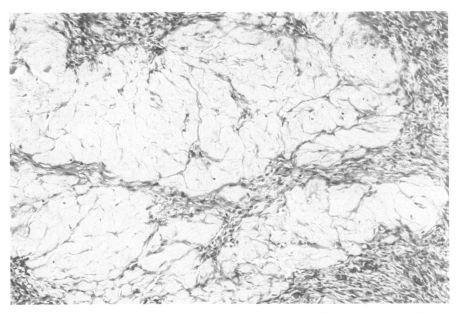

Figure 22.13. Photomicrograph of corpus albicans of human ovary. Large amounts of intercellular hyaline material can be seen among the degenerating cells of the former corpus luteum. The corpus albicans is surrounded by ovarian stroma. × 125.

degenerates, and then similar changes occur in the follicular cells. As the cells are resorbed and disappear, the surrounding stromal cells migrate into the space previously occupied by the follicle, leaving no trace of its existence. In the atresia of large growing follicles, the degeneration of the oocyte appears to occur secondarily to degenerative changes in the follicular wall, which includes the following sequential events: (1) invasion of the granulosa layer by strands of vascularized connective tissue, (2) sloughing of the granulosa cells into the antrum of the follicle, (3) hypertrophy of the theca interna cells, (4) collapse of the follicle as the degeneration continues, and (5) invasion of connective tissue into the cavity of the follicle. The oocyte undergoes typical changes associated with degeneration and autolysis and then disappears. The zona pellucida, which is resistant to the autolytic changes occurring in the cells associated with it, becomes folded and collapses as it is slowly broken down within the cavity of the follicle. Macrophages in the connective tissue are involved in the phagocytosis of the zona pellucida and remnants of the degenerating cells. The basement membrane, separating the follicular cells from the theca interna, may separate from the follicular cells and increase in thickness, forming a wavy hyaline layer called the *glassy membrane.* This structure is characteristic of follicles in late stages of atresia.

Enlargement of the cells of the theca interna occurs in some atretic follicles. These cells, which are similar to theca lutein cells, become organized into radially arranged strands, separated by connective tissue. A rich capillary network develops in the connective tissue. These atretic follicles, which resemble an old corpus luteum, are called *corpora lutea atretica.* As these follicles continue to degenerate, a scar with hyaline streaks develops in the center of the cell mass, giving it the appearance of a small corpus albicans. The follicle eventually disappears as the ovarian stroma invades the degenerating follicle. The strands of luteal cells do not degenerate immediately, but become broken up and scattered in the stroma. These cords of cells contribute to the *interstitial gland* of the ovary, producing steroid hormones.

Interstitial Gland

The ovaries of a number of mammals contain cells, scattered in the cortical stroma, which resemble theca lutein cells. These interstitial cells are collectively identified as the *interstitial gland.* The interstitial cells are believed to arise from the theca interna cells of atretic follicles. The development of the interstitial gland is most extensive in animal species that have large litters.

In the human ovary, there are relatively few interstitial cells. They occur in the largest numbers in the first year of life and during the early phases of puberty, corresponding to times of increased follicular atresia. At menarche there is involution of the interstitial cells and, therefore, few are present during the reproductive life-span and menopause. It has been suggested that, in the human, the interstitial cells are an important source of the estrogens that influence the growth and development of the secondary sex organs during the early phases of puberty. In other species, the interstitial cells have been shown to produce progesterone.

In the human, cells called *ovarian hilar cells* are found in the hilum of the ovary in association with vascular spaces and nonmyelinated nerve fibers. These cells, which structurally appear to be related to the interstitial cells of the testis contain Reineke crystalloids. The hilar cells appear to respond to hormonal change as evidenced by the fact that they are most easily identified during pregnancy or at the onset of menopause. It has been suggested that the hilar cells secrete androgens, since hyperplasia or tumors associated with these cells usually lead to masculinization.

Blood Supply, Lymphatic Drainage, and Innervation

The ovarian arteries, which pass to the ovaries through the suspensory ligaments, provide the principal arterial supply to the ovaries and oviducts. These arteries anastomose with the uterine arteries, which arise from the internal iliac arteries. Relatively large vessels arising from this region of anastomosis pass through the mesovarian ligament and enter the hilus of the ovary. These arteries are called helicine arteries because they branch and become highly coiled as they pass into the medulla (see Fig. 22.2). Veins accompany the arteries and form a plexus, named the *pampiniform plexus,* as they emerge from the hilus. The ovarian vein is formed from the plexus.

In the cortical region of the ovary, networks of lymphatic vessels in the thecal layers surround the large developing and atretic follicles and corpora lutea. The lymphatic vessels follow the course of the ovarian arteries as they ascend to lateral aortic lumbar lymph nodes.

Sensory and autonomic nerve fibers that supply the ovary are conveyed by the ovarian plexus and the uterine nerves. Although it is clear that the ovary receives both sympathetic and parasympathetic fibers, little is known of the actual distribution. Groups of parasympathetic ganglion cells are scattered in the medulla. Nerve fibers follow the arteries, supplying the smooth muscle in the walls of these vessels, as they pass into medulla and cortex of the ovary. Nerve fibers associated with the follicles apparently do not penetrate the basement membrane. Sensory nerve endings are scattered in the stroma. The sensory fibers, which reach the ovary via the ovarian plexus, have their cell bodies located in the dorsal root ganglia of the 10th or the 11th thoracic spinal nerves. Therefore, ovarian pain is referred over the distribution of these spinal nerves. At ovulation, many women experience low abdominal discomfort ("mittelschmerz"). This pain, typically described as dull aching, is felt in one of the lower abdominal quadrants and lasts from a few minutes to hours.

Hormonal Regulation of the Ovarian Cycle

During each menstrual cycle, the ovary undergoes cyclic changes, passing through a *follicular phase* and a *luteal phase,* which are separated by ovulation (Fig. 22.14). At the beginning of the follicular phase, a small number (10 to 20) of primary follicles begin to develop under the influence of FSH and LH, gonadotropic hormones released by the adenohypophysis. During the first 8 to 10 days of the cycle, FSH is the principal hormone influencing the growth of the follicles. It stimulates the granulosa and thecal cells, which begin to secrete steroid hormones, principally estrogens, into the follicular lumen. Late in the follicular phase, before ovulation, progesterone levels begin to rise under the influence of LH. Estrogens continue to accumulate in the follicular lumen, finally reaching a level that makes the follicle independent of FSH for its continued growth and development. The quantity of estrogens in circulating blood inhibits further production of FSH by the adenohypophysis. Follicles that have not reached a state of FSH-independent development undergo degeneration. As a result of this hormonally controlled development, only one of the maturing follicles normally reaches full maturation and is released from the ovary. Ovulation is induced by a sharp increase in the level of LH, which occurs concomitantly with a smaller increase in the FSH level.

The luteal phase begins immediately after ovulation, as the granulosa and thecal cells of the ruptured follicle undergo rapid morphological transformation as the corpus luteum is formed. Estrogens and large amounts of progesterone are secreted by the corpus luteum. Under the influence of both hormones, but primarily progesterone, the endometrium begins its secretory phase, which is essential for the preparation of the uterus for implantation in the event that the egg is fertilized. LH appears to be responsible for the development and maintenance of the corpus luteum during the menstrual cycle. If fertilization does not occur, the

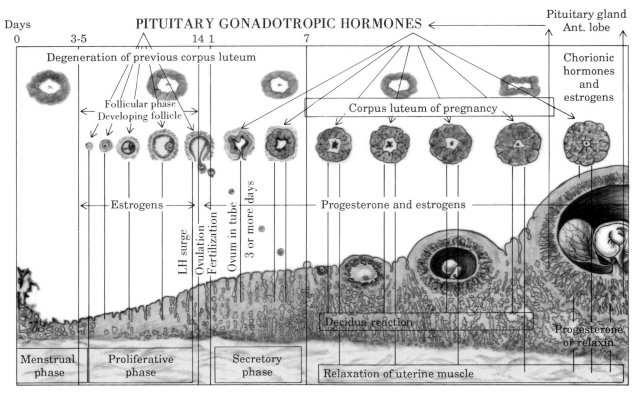

Figure 22.14. Schematic diagram illustrating the morphological changes in the endometrium and ovary during the menstrual cycle. The hormonal activities controlling these changes are indicated. For the purpose of this diagram, fertilization of the ovum is illustrated. Therefore, the decidua reaction is shown after the secretory phase of the endometrium. If fertilization had not occurred, the menstrual cycle would have followed the secretory phase and the cycle would have repeated itself. (Modified from Eastman NJ: *Williams' Obstetrics,* 11th ed. New York, Appleton, 1956.)

corpus luteum degenerates within a few days as the hormonal levels drop. If fertilization does occur, the corpus luteum is maintained and continues to secrete progesterone and estrogens. HCG, which is initially produced by the conceptus and later by the placenta, stimulates the corpus luteum and is responsible for its maintenance during pregnancy.

OVIDUCT

Paired tubes, the *oviducts,* supported by the mesosalpinx, a portion of the broad ligament, extend bilaterally from the uterus to the ovaries (see Fig. 22.1). The oviduct, which is also commonly referred to as the *uterine* or *fallopian tube,* transmits the ova from the ovary to the uterus and provides the necessary environment for fertilization and the initial development of the conceptus to the morula stage. One end of the tube is adjacent to the ovary and opens into the peritoneal cavity; the other end communicates with the uterine cavity.

The tube, which is approximately 10 to 12 cm long, can be divided into four segments by gross inspection: the infundibulum, ampulla, isthmus, and uterine segment. The *infundibulum* is the funnel-shaped segment of the tube adjacent to the ovary that opens into the ampulla. Fringed extensions, *fimbriae,* extend from the infundibulum toward the ovary. The *ampulla* is the longest segment of the tube, constituting about two-thirds the total length, and is the site of fertilization. The *isthmus* is the narrow, medial segment of the oviduct adjacent to the uterus. The *uterine* or *intramural* segment (*pars interstitialis),* measuring about 1 cm in length, is embedded in the uterine wall.

The oviduct wall resembles the wall of other hollow viscera, consisting of an internal mucosal layer, an intermediate muscular layer, and an external serosal layer. The serosa, or peritoneum, consists of a mesothelium and a thin layer of connective tissue. Throughout most of its length, the muscularis is organized into an inner, well-developed circular layer and an external, thinner longitudinal layer. The boundary between these layers is often indistinct. The muscularis is thickest in the isthmus, due to the thickness of the circular layer. An additional thin layer of longitudinal fibers is present in the uterine segment.

The mucosa of the oviduct consists of a simple columnar epithelium, composed of two kinds of cells, and a thin lamina propria (Fig. 22.15). Relatively thin longitudinal folds of the mucosa project into the lumen of the oviduct throughout its length. The folds, which are most numerous and complex in the ampulla (Fig. 22.16), become smaller in the isthmus and are reduced to small bulges in the uterine segment. The two cell types present in the epithelium are believed to be different functional states of a single cell type. *Ciliated cells* are most numerous in the infundibulum and ampulla. The wave of the cilia is directed toward the uterus. The *nonciliated, peg cells* are secretory cells that may provide nutritive material for the ovum. In some species, secretory cells provide substances that coat the egg. The epithelial cells undergo cyclic hypertrophy during the follicular phase and atrophy during the luteal phase in response to changes in the hormonal levels, particularly estrogens. At about the time of ovulation, the epithelium reaches a height of about 30 μm and then reduces to about one-half of that height just before the onset of menstruation.

The oviduct demonstrates active movements just before ovulation as the fimbriae become closely apposed to the ovary and localize over the region of the ovarian surface where rupture will occur. As the egg is released, the ciliated cells in the infundibulum sweep it toward the opening of the oviduct and, thus, prevent it from passing into the

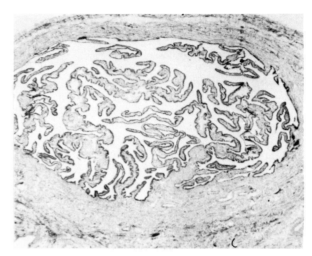

Figure 22.16. Photomicrograph of human uterine tube. The cross-section is through the ampulla region of the uterine tube. The mucosa is thrown into extensive folds that project into the lumen of the tube. The muscularis, composed of a thick inner layer of circular fibers and an outer layer of longitudinal fibers, can be seen. × 16.

peritoneal cavity. The egg is rapidly transported along the oviduct by peristaltic contractions. The mechanism by which spermatozoa and the egg are transported from opposite ends of the oviduct is not fully understood. Evidence suggests that both ciliary movements and peristaltic muscular activity are involved in the movements of the egg and spermatozoa. The movement of the spermatozoa is much too rapid to be accounted for by their intrinsic motility. Fertilization usually occurs in the ampulla near its junction with the isthmus. The egg remains in the oviduct for about 3 days before passing into the uterus.

UTERUS

The uterus is the part of the female reproductive system that receives the rapidly developing morula from the oviduct. All subsequent embryonic and fetal development occurs within the uterus, which undergoes dramatic increases in size and development. The human uterus is a hollow, pear-shaped organ, located in the pelvis between the bladder and rectum. In a woman who has never borne children (nulliparous), it weighs 30 to 40 g and measures 7.5 cm in length, 5 cm in width at its superior aspect, and 2.5 cm in thickness. Its lumen, which is also flattened, is continuous with the oviducts and the vagina.

Anatomically, the uterus is divided into two regions, the *body* and the *cervix,* by a constriction on its surface which corresponds to a narrowing of its cavity (see Fig. 22.1). The large upper portion is

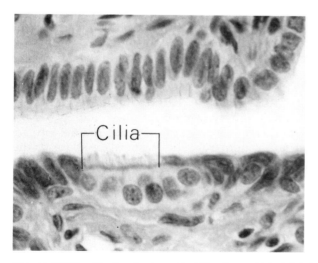

Figure 22.15. Photomicrograph of human uterine tube. The lumen of the tube is lined by simple columnar epithelium composed of ciliated and nonciliated cells. × 640.

the *body;* the upper, rounded part of the body is the *fundus.* The narrower lower portion is the *cervix.* The lumen of the cervix, the *endocervical canal,* has a constricted opening, or *os,* at each end. The *internal os* communicates with the cavity of the body, the *external os* with the vagina.

The uterine wall is composed of (1) an external layer, the serosa, or *perimetrium;* (2) a middle layer, the muscularis, or *myometrium;* and (3) an internal layer, the mucosa, or *endometrium.* The peritoneal or serous layer, consisting of a mesothelium and a thin layer of areolar tissue, covers only the upper part of the uterus. The surface of the uterus not covered by peritoneum is covered by connective tissue, or adventitia.

Myometrium

The myometrium is the thickest layer of the uterine wall, measuring about 10 to 15 mm in thickness. It is composed of three indistinctly defined layers of smooth muscle. The central muscle layer, containing numerous large blood vessels and lymphatics and called the *stratum vasculare,* is the thickest and has smooth muscle bundles oriented in a circular or spiral pattern. The smooth muscle bundles in the inner and outer layers are predominantly oriented in parallel to the long axis of the uterus.

In the nonpregnant uterus, the smooth muscle cells are about 50 μm in length. During pregnancy, the uterus undergoes enormous enlargement. The growth is due primarily to the hypertrophy of existing smooth muscle cells, which may reach more than 500 μm in length, and secondarily to the development of new fibers through the division of existing cells and the differentiation of undifferentiated cells. There is also an increase in the amount of connective tissue. The uterine wall becomes progressively thinner, stretching due to the growth of the fetus as pregnancy proceeds. After parturition, the uterus returns to near its original size. Some muscle fibers degenerate, but most return to their original size. The collage produced during pregnancy is enzymatically degraded. The uterine cavity remains larger and the muscular wall is thicker than before pregnancy.

Compared to the body of the uterus, the cervix has much greater amounts of connective tissue and less smooth muscle. Elastic fibers are abundant in the cervix, but are found in appreciable quantities only in the outer layer of the myometrium of the body of the uterus.

Endometrium

Throughout the reproductive life-span, the endometrium undergoes cyclic changes in its structure that prepare it for the implantation of the fertilized ovum and subsequent events necessary to support further embryonic and fetal development. During the cycle, which is controlled by ovarian hormones, the endometrium undergoes changes in its secretory activity and structure, which are correlated with the cyclic growth and maturation of ovarian follicles (see Fig. 22.14). The end of each cycle is characterized by the partial destruction and sloughing of the endometrium. Bleeding from vessels within the mucosa accompanies these changes. The discharge of the tissue and blood from the vagina, which usually continues for a period of 3 to 5 days, is referred to as *menstruation* or *menstrual flow.* The *menstrual cycle* is defined as beginning on the day when menstrual flow appears.

Two layers, or zones, which differ in structure and function, have been identified within the endometrium (Fig. 22.17). The thicker part of the endometrium, which is sloughed off at menstruation, is the *stratum functionale* or *functional layer.* The part retained at menstruation is the *stratum basale* or *basal layer.* This layer serves as the source for the regeneration of the stratum functionalis.

During the phases of the menstrual cycle, the endometrium varies from 1 to 6 mm in thickness. It is lined with a simple columnar epithelium with a mixture of secretory and ciliated cells. The surface epithelium invaginates into the underlying lamina propria, the *endometrial stroma,* forming *uterine glands.* These simple tubular glands, containing fewer ciliated cells, occasionally branch in the deeper aspect of the endometrium. The surface and glandular epithelium rests on a basal lamina. The endometrial stroma, which resembles mesenchyme, is highly cellular and contains abundant intercellular ground substance. No submucosa separates the endometrium from the myometrium.

The endometrium contains a unique system of blood vessels, which undergo development each menstrual cycle to prepare them to support development of the conceptus if implantation occurs. The uterine artery gives off six to ten arcuate arteries that penetrate the stratum vasculare of the myometrium and anastomose with one another. Branches from these arteries, the *radial arteries,* pass into the basal layer of the endometrium where they give off small arteries, the *straight arteries,* which supply this region of the endometrium. As the main branch of the radial arteries continues upward, it becomes highly coiled and is referred to as the *spiral artery.* The spiral arteries give off numerous arterioles that often anastomose with one another as they supply a rich capillary bed. The capillary bed includes thin-walled dilated units

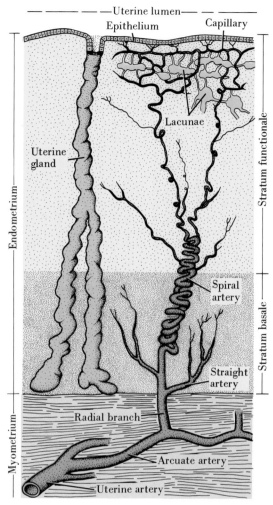

Figure 22.17. Schematic diagram illustrating the blood supply to the two layers—stratum basale and stratum functionale—of the endometrium. (Based on Weiss L, Greep RO: *Histology,* 4th ed. New York, McGraw-Hill, 1977.)

Figure 22.18. Photomicrograph of human cervix. The plane of section passes through the long axis of the cervix. The vaginal canal (VC) is present at the **top** of the photomicrograph; the cervical canal (CC) is on the **right**. The portion of the cervix that projects into the vagina, called the portio vaginalis, is covered with stratified squamous epithelium (see Fig. 22.19). The portion of the cervical mucosa (Muc) that faces the cervical canal is covered with columnar epithelium. An abrupt change in the surface epithelium occurs at the ostium of the uterus (see Fig. 22.20a). Cervical glands, which extend from the surface of the cervical canal into the underlying connective tissue, commonly develop into cysts (Cy) owing to obstruction in their ducts. × 10.

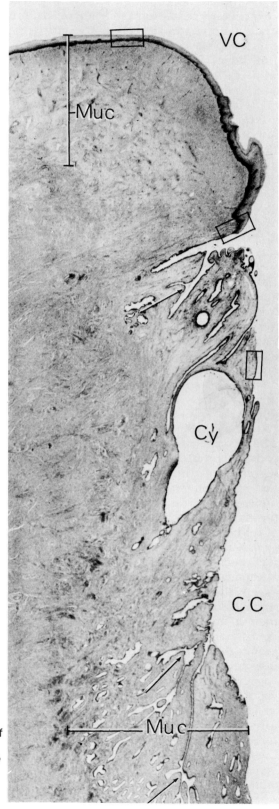

called *lacunae.* Lacunae may also occur in the venous system that drains the endometrium. The straight arteries and the proximal part of the spiral arteries do not change during the menstrual cycle. The distal portion of the spiral arteries, under the influence of estrogens and progesterone, undergoes cyclic regeneration with each menstrual cycle.

The cervical mucosa, which measures about 2 to 3 mm in thickness, differs dramatically from the rest of the uterine endometrium in that it contains large, branched glands and lacks spiral arteries (Fig. 22.18). It undergoes little morphological change during the menstrual cycle and is not sloughed during the period of menstrual flow. Blockage of the openings of the mucosal glands results in the retention of their secretions and the formation of dilated cysts within the cervical mucosa, called *Nabothian cysts.*

During each menstrual cycle, the cervical glands undergo important functional changes that are related to the transport of spermatozoa within the female reproductive tract. The amount and properties of the mucus secreted by the gland cells vary during the menstrual cycle under the influence of the ovarian hormones. At midcycle, there is a ten-fold increase in the amount of mucus produced. This mucus is less viscous and appears to provide a more favorable environment for sperm migration. The cervical mucus at other times in the cycle restricts the passage of sperm into the uterus. Thus, hormonal mechanisms ensure that ovulation and changes in the cervical mucus are coordinated, thereby increasing the possibility that fertilization will occur since freshly ejaculated spermatozoa and the egg will arrive simultaneously at the site of fertilization in the oviduct.

The portion of the cervix that projects into the vagina, the *portio vaginalis,* is covered with a stratified squamous epithelium (Fig. 22.19). There is an abrupt transition just outside the external os between the squamous epithelium of the portio vaginalis and the mucus-secreting columnar epithelium of the cervical canal (Fig. 22.20a,b). Alterations in this transition zone may occur, more commonly after childbearing, leading to the formation of patches of columnar epithelium on the portio vaginalis. These patches, called *erosions,* are susceptible to inflammatory reaction. It is believed that untreated chronic inflammation associated with the erosions may be a predisposing or contributing factor to cancer of the cervix.

The epithelial cells of the cervix are constantly being released, or exfoliated, into the vagina. Stained preparations of the cervical cells (Pap smears) can be used in the diagnosis of cancer of the cervix.

Cyclic Changes in the Endometrium

The endometrium passes through a sequence of morphological and functional changes each menstrual cycle. For descriptive purposes, these are identified as three successive phases, the *proliferative, secretory,* and *menstrual* phases (see Fig. 22.14). It should be remembered that the phases are part of a continuous process, and that there is no abrupt change from one to the next. The proliferative phase occurs concurrently with follicular maturation and is influenced by the estrogens being produced. The secretory phase coincides with functional activity of corpus luteum and is primarily influenced by the progesterone being produced. The menstrual phase commences as hormone production by the ovary declines with the degeneration of the corpus luteum.

Proliferative Phase. At the end of the menstrual phase, the endometrium consists of a thin band of connective tissue, about 1 mm thick, containing the basal portion of the uterine glands and the lower portion of the spiral arteries (Fig. 22.21). This layer is the stratum basale; the layer that was sloughed off is the stratum functionale. Under the influence of estrogens, the stromal and epithelial cells in the stratum basale begin to proliferate by

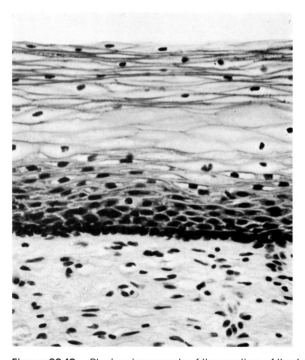

Figure 22.19. Photomicrograph of the portion of the human cervix that faces the vaginal canal. (The **upper rectangle** in Fig. 22.18 indicates the area shown in this figure.) This surface of the cervix is covered with stratified squamous epithelium. × 300.

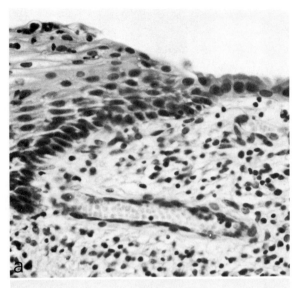

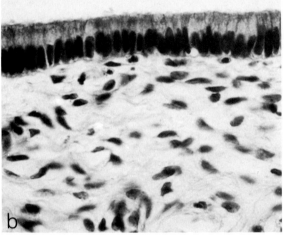

Figure 22.20(a). Photomicrograph of the surface epithelium of the cervix at the ostrium of the cervix. The **middle rectangle** in Figure 22.18 indicates the area shown in this figure. The abrupt transition from stratified squamous epithelium to columnar epithelium can be seen. × 300. **(b)** The columnar epithelium shown here came from the **lower rectangle** in Figure 22.18.

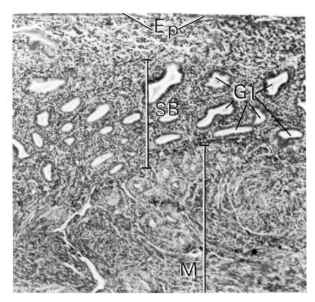

Figure 22.21. Photomicrograph of human uterus. The endometrium is comprised of a simple columnar epithelium and an extremely cellular connective tissue. A portion of the endometrium, the stratum functionale, undergoes dramatic change and is eventually sloughed during each menstrual cycle. The tissue shown is at an early phase following sloughing. The resurfacing of the epithelium (Ep) is almost complete. The underlying stratum basale (SB), which does not slough, contains glands (Gl) that give rise to new epithelium. Large numbers of blood vessels can be seen in the myometrium (M), the muscle layer underlying the endometrium. × 40.

numerous mitotic divisions, and the following changes can be seen: (1) the epithelial cells in the basal portion of glands rapidly proliferate, reconstituting the glands and migrating to cover the denuded endometrial surface, (2) the stromal cells proliferate and ground substance accumulates, and (3) the spiral arteries lengthen as the endometrium is replenished, but these arteries are only slightly coiled and do not extend into the upper third of the endometrium.

The proliferative phase continues for 1 day after ovulation, which occurs at about day 14 of a 28-day cycle. At the end of this phase, the endometrium has reached a thickness of about 3 mm. The glands have narrow lumens and are relatively straight, having a slightly wavy appearance (Fig. 22.22). Accumulations of glycogen are present in the basal portion of the epithelial cells.

Secretory Phase. Under the influence of progesterone, dramatic changes occur in the stratum functionale beginning a day or two after ovulation. The endometrium becomes edematous and may eventually reach a thickness of 5 to 6 mm. The glands enlarge and become corkscrew-shaped, and their lumens become sacculated as they fill with secretory products from the epithelial cells (Fig. 22.23). The mucoid fluid being produced by these cells is rich in nutrients, particularly glycogen, required to support development if implantation occurs. Mitoses are rare because the growth seen at this stage results from hypertrophy of the epithelial cells and an increase in vascularity and edema of the endometrium. The spiral arteries lengthen and become more coiled during this phase. They extend nearly to the surface of the endometrium.

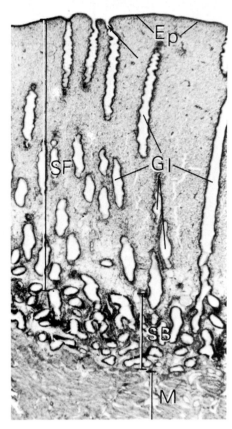

Figure 22.22. Photomicrograph of monkey uterus. The endometrium is at the proliferative phase of the cycle. During this phase the stratum functionale (SF) greatly thickens. Long, slightly wavy glands (Gl) extend from the stratum basale (SB) to the surface epithelium (Ep). The junction between a gland and the surface epithelium is indicated by an **arrow**. × 16.

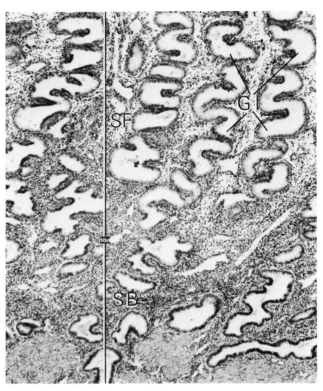

Figure 22.23. Photomicrograph of human uterus. The endometrium is at the secretory phase of the cycle. Glands (Gl) within the stratum functionale (SF) assume a corkscrew shape as the endometrium further increases in thickness. The stratum basale (SB) demonstrates less dramatic changes in its morphology. × 65.

The sequential influence of estrogens and progesterone on the stromal cells makes them capable of undergoing transformation into *decidual cells.* The stimulus for the transformation is the implantation of the blastocyst. Large pale cells rich in glycogen result from this transformation. Although the precise function of these cells is not known, it is clear that they provide a favorable environment for the nourishment of the conceptus and that they create a specialized layer, which facilitates the separation of the placenta from the uterine wall at the termination of pregnancy.

Menstrual Phase. The corpus luteum remains active in hormone production for only about 10 days if fertilization does not occur. As the hormone levels rapidly decline, changes occur in the blood supply to the stratum functionale. Initially, periodic contractions of the walls of the spiral ar-

teries, lasting for several hours, cause the stratum functionale to become ischemic, the glands to stop secreting, and the endometrium to shrink in height as the stromal cells become more densely packed. After about 2 days, extended periods of contraction, with only brief periods of blood flow, cause disruption of the surface epithelium and rupture of the blood vessels. It is important to note that when the spiral arteries close off, blood flows into the stratum basale, but not into the stratum functionale. Blood, uterine fluid, and sloughing stromal and epithelial cells from the stratum functionale, thus, appear in the vaginal discharge. As patches of tissue separate from the endometrium, the torn ends of veins, arteries, and glands are exposed. The desquamation continues until only the stratum basale remains. Clotting of blood if inhibited during this period of menstrual flow. Arterial blood flow is restricted except for the brief periods of relaxation of the walls of the spiral arteries. The period of menstrual flow normally lasts about 5 days. Blood continually seeps from the open ends of the veins. The average blood loss in the menstrual phase is 35 to 50 ml. Blood flow through the straight arteries maintains the stratum basale.

As we have said, this is a cyclic process. Figure 22.14 shows a single cycle of the endometrium, and then demonstrates a gravid state as it is established at the end of a secretory phase. In the absence of fertilization, a cessation of bleeding would accompany the growth and maturation of new ovarian follicles. The epithelial cells rapidly proliferate and migrate out to restore the surface epithelium as the proliferative phase of the next cycle begins.

In the absence of ovulation (such a cycle is referred to as an *anovulatory cycle*), a corpus luteum does not form and progesterone is not produced. In the absence of progesterone, the endometrium does not enter the secretory phase and continues in the proliferative phase until menstruation. In cases of infertility, biopsies of the endometrium can be used to diagnose such anovulatory cycles, as well as other diseases of the ovary and disorders of the endometrium.

Gravid Cycle. If fertilization and subsequent implantation occur, decline of the endometrium is delayed until after parturition. As the blastocyst becomes embedded in the uterine mucosa in the early part of the second week, cells in the *chorion* begin to secrete HCG. HCG maintains the corpus luteum and stimulates it to continue the production of progesterone and estrogens. Thus, the decline of the endometrium is prevented and the endometrium undergoes further development during the first few weeks of pregnancy.

Implantation

The fertilized human ovum undergoes a series of changes as it passes through the oviduct and into the uterus in preparation for becoming embedded in the uterine mucosa. The zygote undergoes cleavage, a series of mitotic divisions without cell growth, resulting in a rapid increase in the number of cells. The resulting cell mass is known as a *morula,* the individual cells as *blastomeres.* On about the 3rd day after fertilization, the morula, which has reached a 12- to 16-cell stage and is still surrounded by the zona pellucida, enters the uterine cavity. The centrally located morula cells, the *inner cell mass,* will give rise to the tissues of the embryo proper; the surrounding layer of cells, the *outer cell mass,* will form the trophoblast and then the *placenta* (Fig. 22.24). As the morula enters the uterine cavity, fluid passes through the zona pellucida into the morula forming a fluid-filled cavity, the *blastocyst cavity.* This event marks the beginning of the *blastocyst.* As the blastocyst remains free in the uterine lumen for 1 or 2 days undergoing further mitotic divisions, the zona pellucida disappears. The outer cell mass is now called the *trophoblast,* and the inner cell mass is referred to as the *embryoblast.*

In the human, it is believed that the attachment of the blastocyst to the endometrial epithelium occurs at about 5½ to 6 days after fertilization. As contact is made by the trophoblastic cells over the embryoblast pole, the trophoblasts rapidly proliferate and begin to invade the endometrium.

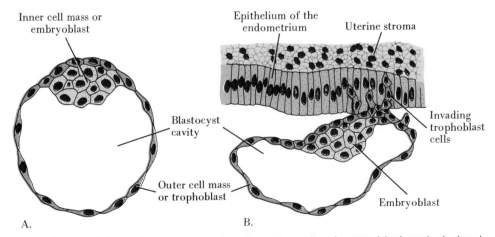

Inner cell mass or embryoblast

Epithelium of the endometrium

Uterine stroma

Blastocyst cavity

Invading trophoblast cells

Outer cell mass or trophoblast

Embryoblast

A.

B.

Figure 22.24. Schematic diagrams of sections through a human blastocyst at about 4½ days of development **(A)** and through a monkey blastocyst at about 9 days of development **(B)**. The human blastocyst was recovered from the uterine lumen. At 9 days, the trophoblastic cells of the monkey blastocyst have begun to invade the epithelial cells of the endometrium. In the human, the blastocyst begins to invade the endometrium at about the 5th or 6th day of development. (After Langman, 1975.)

The invading trophoblast differentiates into the **syncytiotrophoblast** and the **cytotrophoblast.** The cytotrophoblast is a mitotically active inner cell layer producing cells that fuse with the syncytiotrophoblast, the outer erosive layer. The syncytiotrophoblast is not mitotically active and consists of a multinucleate cytoplasmic mass; it actively invades the epithelium and underlying stroma of the endometrium. Through the activity of the trophoblast, the blastocyst is entirely embedded within the endothelium by about the 11th day of development.

As the trophoblastic layers develop during this period, small spaces, called **lacunae,** appear in the syncytiotrophoblast (Fig. 22.25). Maternal blood, liberated from vessels eroded by the invading syncytiotrophoblast, fill the lacunae and provide the initial nourishment for the embryo. The differential pressure between the arterial and venous channels that communicate with the lacunae establishes directional flow from the arteries into the veins, thereby establishing a primitive uteroplacental circulation. Numerous pinocytotic vessels present in the syncytiotrophoblast are indicative of the transfer of nutrients from the maternal vessels to the embryo.

Ultrastructural studies of the syncytiotrophoblast have demonstrated the presence of well-developed Golgi complexes, abundant smooth and rough endoplasmic reticulum, numerous mitochondria, and relatively large amounts of lipid. Such findings are consistent with the suggested role of the syncytiotrophoblast in producing progesterone, estrogens, chorionic gonadotropin, and lactogen.

During pregnancy, the portion of the endometrium that undergoes morphological changes is called the **decidua** or **decidua graviditatis.** The decidua includes all but the deepest layer of the endometrium. Stromal cells differentiate into large, rounded **decidual cells.** The uterine glands enlarge and become more coiled during the early part of pregnancy and then become thin and flattened as the growing fetus fills the uterine lumen. Three different regions of the decidua are identified by their relationship to site of implantation (Fig. 22.26). The **decidua basalis** is the portion of the endometrium that underlies the implantation site. The **decidua capsularis** is a thin portion of endometrium that lies between the implantation site and the uterine lumen. The **decidua vera** includes the remaining endometrium of the uterus and cervix. By the end of the 3rd month the fetus grows to the point that the overlying decidua capsularis fuses with the decidua vera, thereby obliterating the uterine cavity.

By the 13th day of development, an extra-embryonic space, the **chorionic cavity,** has been established (see Fig. 22.25). The cell layers that form the outer boundary of this cavity are collectively referred to as the **chorion.** The inner-most membranes enveloping the embryo are called the **amnion** (Fig. 22.26).

Placenta

Structure and Development. The placenta consists of a fetal portion, formed by the **chorion,** and a maternal portion, formed by the **decidua basalis.** The two parts are involved in physiological

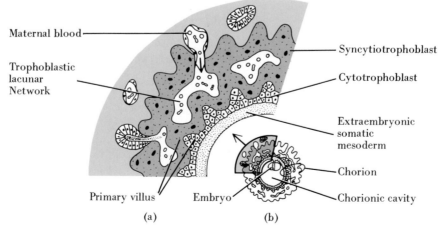

Figure 22.25. Schematic diagrams of sections through a human conceptus at 14 days of development. The relationship of the embryo to the chorionic sac is illustrated in **(b)**. A more detailed diagram of a section through the wall of the chorionic sac is shown in **(a)**. (After Moore, 1977.)

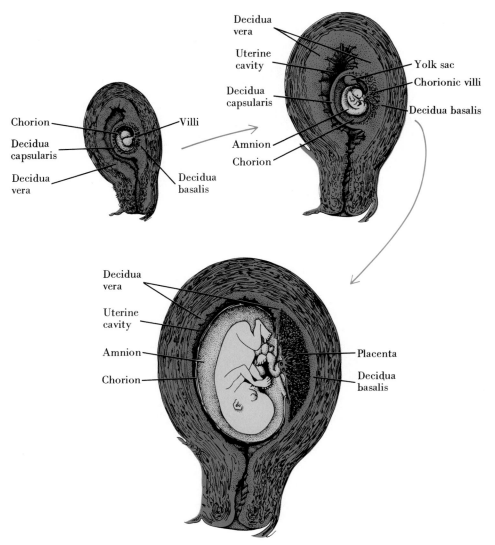

Figure 22.26. Schematic drawing of stages of human pregnancy depicting the development of the placenta. Note that there is a gradual obliteration of the uterine lumen and disappearance of the decidua capsularis as the definitive discoid placenta is established. (After J. Williams, 1927.)

exchange of substances between the maternal and fetal circulation.

Beginning about the 13th day, the cytotrophoblast proliferates rapidly, sending cords or masses of cells, called ***primary chorionic villi,*** into the syncytiotrophoblast (see Fig. 22.25). Shortly after forming, these villi begin to branch as chorionic mesoderm invades at their bases, forming a central core of loose connective tissue in which embryonic blood vessels will gradually form. These ***secondary villi,*** composed of a core of mesenchyme surrounded by an inner layer of cytotrophoblast and an outer layer of syncytiotrophoblast, cover the entire surface of the chorionic sac (Fig. 22.27). The

villi become ***tertiary villi*** after blood vessels have developed in the cores.

As the tertiary villi are forming, cytotrophoblastic cells in the villi continue to grow out through the syncytiotrophoblast. As they meet the maternal endometrium, they grow laterally and meet similar processes growing from neighboring villi. Thus, a thin layer of cytotrophoblastic cells, called the ***trophoblastic shell,*** is formed around the syncytiotrophoblast. The trophoblastic shell is interrupted only at sites where maternal vessels communicate with the intervillous spaces. Future growth of the placenta is accomplished by interstitial growth of the trophoblastic shell.

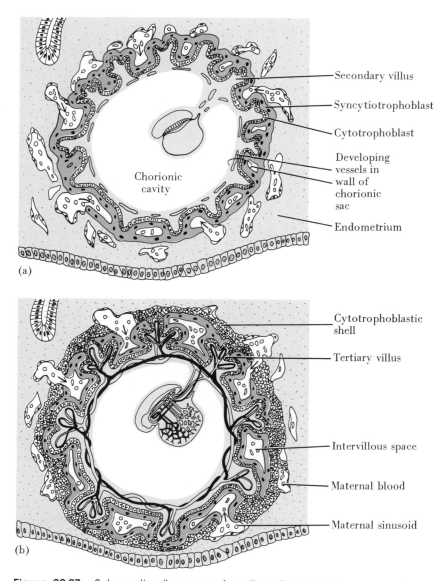

Secondary villus

Syncytiotrophoblast

Cytotrophoblast

Developing vessels in wall of chorionic sac

Endometrium

Chorionic cavity

(a)

Cytotrophoblastic shell

Tertiary villus

Intervillous space

Maternal blood

Maternal sinusoid

(b)

Figure 22.27. Schematic diagrams of sections through a human embryo, chorionic sac, and placenta at 16 **(a)** and 21 **(b)** days of development. The diagrams illustrate the separation of the fetal and maternal blood vessels by the placental membrane composed of the endothelium of the capillaries, mesenchyme, cytotrophoblast, and syncytiotrophoblast. (After Moore, 1977.)

Two types of cells are recognized in the stroma of the villi, the fibroblast and the **_Hofbauer cell_** (Fig. 22.28). The role of the Hofbauer cells, which are more common in early placenta, is not known, but morphologically they have characteristics of macrophages. The vacuoles in these cells contain lipids, mucopolysaccharides, and mucoproteins.

Early in development, the blood vessels of the villi become connected with vessels from the embryo. Blood begins to circulate through the primitive cardiovascular system and the villi at about 21

days. The intervillous spaces provide the site of exchange of nutrients, metabolic products and intermediates, and wastes between the maternal and fetal circulatory systems.

Through the first 8 weeks, villi cover the entire chorionic surface, but as the growth continues, villi on the decidua capsularis begin to degenerate, producing a smooth, relatively avascular surface called the **_chorion laeve._** The villi adjacent to the decidua basalis rapidly increase in size and number and become highly branched. This region of the chorion, which is the fetal component of the pla-

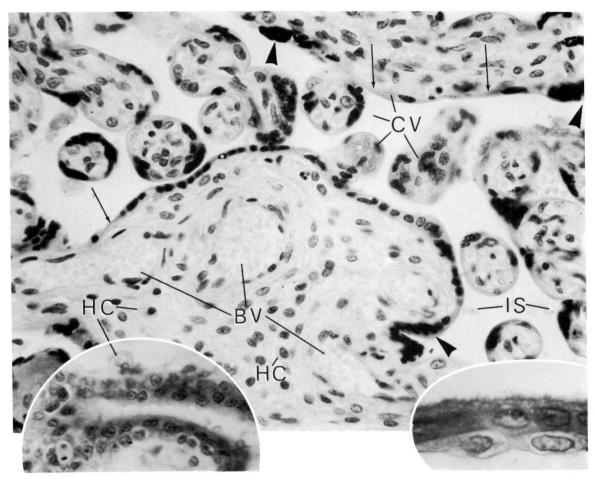

Figure 22.28. Photomicrograph of human placenta. The section is through the substance of a term placenta. Chorionic villi (CV) of various sizes and surrounding intervillous spaces (IS) can be seen. The connective tissue core of the villi contains branches and tributaries of the umbilical arteries and veins (BV). Only capillaries are present in the smallest villi. The villi are covered by two cell layers **(insets)**. The outer layer is the syncytiotrophoblast; immediately under this is the layer composed of the cytotrophoblasts. Phagocytic cells, called Hofbauer cells (HC), can be seen within the villi. **Arrowheads** indicate clusters of syncytial trophoblast nuclei; **arrows** indicate attenuated syncytial cytoplasm. × 280 **(inset,** × 300).

centa, is called the *chorion frondosum* or *villous chorion.* The layer of the placenta from which the villi project is called the *chorionic plate.* The decidua basalis forms a compact layer, known as the *basal plate,* which is the maternal component of the placenta. Vessels within this part of the endometrium supply blood to the intervillous spaces. Except for relatively rare rupturing of capillary walls, which is more common at delivery, there is separation of the fetal and maternal blood. The separation of the fetal and maternal blood, referred to as the *placental barrier,* is maintained primarily by the layers of fetal tissue. Starting at the 4th month, these layers become very thin to facilitate the exchange of products across the placental barrier. The thinning of the wall of the villus is due, in part, to the degeneration of the inner cytotrophoblast layer.

The final shape of the placenta is determined by the arrangement of the villi that persist in the decidua basalis. The placenta is usually circular in shape and covers approximately 25 to 30 percent of the luminal surface of the uterus. During the period of rapid growth of the chorion frondosum, at about the 4th to 5th month, the fetal part of the placenta is divided into 10 to 38 areas, called *cotyledons.* Wedge-shaped areas of decidual tissue form the boundaries of the cotyledons as groups of villi grow into the decidua basalis.

The placenta, which measures about 15 to 20 cm in diameter and 2 to 3 cm in thickness and weighs 500 to 600 g at full term, is released from the uterus approximately 30 minutes after the birth of the child. The entire fetal portion of the placenta and the intervening projections of decidual tissue are released. Gross inspection of the maternal side of the placenta reveals 10 to 38 bulging areas, the **cotyledons.** The **basal plate** and the cytotrophoblastic shell can be identified. Most of the decidua basalis is sloughed from the basal layer of endometrium during the period of uterine bleeding that follows childbirth.

Placental circulation and function. Blood flow through the placenta is intimately related to its primary functions, the production of metabolites and hormones and the exchange of gases and metabolic products between the maternal and fetal circulatory systems.

Fetal blood enters the placenta through a pair of **umbilical arteries** (Fig. 22.29). As they pass into the placenta, these arteries branch into several radially disposed vessels, which give numerous branches in the chorionic plate. Branches from these vessels pass into the villi, forming extensive capillary networks in close association with the intervillous spaces. Exchange of gases and metabolic products occurs across the thin fetal layers that separate the two bloodstreams at this level. Fetal blood returns through a system of veins that parallel the arteries, except that they converge upon a single **umbilical vein.**

Maternal blood is supplied to the placenta through 80 to 100 spiral endometrial arteries that penetrate the basal plate. These are derived from the arcuate branches of the uterine arteries. Blood from the spiral arteries flows into the intervillous spaces. In the mature placenta, these spaces contain about 15 ml of maternal blood that is exchanged three or four times per minute. The spiral arteries enter at the base of the intervillous spaces. The blood pressure in the spiral arteries is much higher than that in the intervillous spaces.

FETAL CIRCULATION

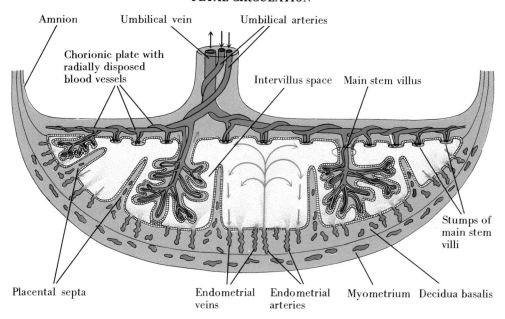

MATERNAL CIRCULATION

Figure 22.29. Schematic diagram of mature human placenta. The placenta is divided into subdivisions, called cotyledons, by placental septa that are formed by invaginations of the decidua basalis. Maternal blood enters the placenta through numerous endometrial spiral arteries that penetrate the basal plate. As the blood enters the intervillus space, it is directed deep into the space (**arrows**). It then passes over the surface of the villi where exchange of gases and metabolic products occurs. The maternal blood finally leaves the intervillus space through endometrial veins. The fetal blood enters the placenta through umbilical arteries which divide into several radially disposed arteries within the chorionic plate. Branches from these vessels pass into the main stem villi and there form extensive capillary networks. The veins within the villi then carry the blood back through a system of veins that parallels the fetal arteries. As was noted above, exchange of gases and metabolic products occurs as the maternal blood flows over the surface of the villi in close approximation to the fetal placental capillary beds within the villi. (After Moore, 1977.)

As blood is injected into these spaces at each pulse, it is directed deep into the spaces. As the pressure decreases, the blood flows back over the surfaces of the villi and eventually enters endometrial veins located in the base of the spaces. Exchange of gases and metabolic products occurs as the blood passes over the villi. Normally, water, carbon dioxide, metabolic waste products, and hormones are transferred from the fetal blood to the maternal blood, and water, oxygen, metabolites, electrolytes, vitamins, hormones, and some antibodies pass in the opposite direction. The placental barrier does not exclude many potentially dangerous agents, such as viruses, drugs, hormones, and metals. Therefore, a woman must be extremely careful to avoid exposure to or ingestion of such agents to reduce the risk of injury to the embryo or fetus.

During the early phases of pregnancy, the forming placenta plays an essential role in providing nourishment to the developing embryo. Before the establishment of blood flow through the placenta, the growth of the embryo is supported, in part, by metabolic products that are synthesized by or transported through the trophoblast. The syncytiotrophoblast synthesizes glycogen, cholesterol, fatty acids, as well as other nutrients utilized by the embryo.

Placental hormones. The placenta also functions as an endocrine organ. The human placenta is known to produce two steroid hormones and four peptide hormones. Immunocytochemical studies indicate that the syncytiotrophoblast is the site of synthesis of these hormones. The steroid hormones, progesterone and estrogen, have essential roles in the maintenance of pregnancy. As pregnancy proceeds, the placenta takes over the major role in the secretion of these steroids from the corpus luteum. The placenta produces enough progesterone by the end of the 4th month to maintain pregnancy if the corpus luteum is removed or fails to function. In the production of placental estrogen, the fetal adrenal cortex plays an essential role providing the precursors needed for estrogen synthesis. Because the placenta lacks the enzymes needed for the production of the estrogen precursors, a cooperative *fetoplacental (endocrine) unit* is established. (Clinically, the monitoring of estrogen production during pregnancy can be used as an index for fetal development.) The peptide hormones produced by the placenta are human chorionic gonadotropin (HCG), human chorionic somatomammotropin (HCS), human chorionic thyrotropin (HCT), and relaxin. HCS, also known as human placental lactogen (HPL), is closely related to human growth hormone. HCS promotes general growth, as well as development of the maternal breast. Although the full role of HCG in pregnancy has not been defined, it is known to function in the maintenance of the corpus luteum during the early period of pregnancy. Relaxin is a hormone of pregnancy that is involved in the softening of the cervix and the pelvic ligaments in preparation for parturition.

VAGINA

The vagina is the fibromuscular sheath extending from the cervix to the vestibule, which is the area between the labia minora. In the virgin, the opening into the vagina is surrounded by the hymen, folds of mucous membrane extending into the vaginal lumen. The extent and shape of this structure if highly variable. The vaginal wall consists of an inner mucosal layer, an intermediate muscular layer, and an outer adventitia (Fig. 22.30).

The vaginal mucosa has numerous transverse folds, or rugae (see Fig. 22.1). The mucosa is lined with stratified squamous epithelium, which is about 150 to 200 μm thick (Fig. 22.31). Connective tissue papillae from the underlying lamina propria project into the epithelial layer. In humans and other primates, keratohyaline granules may be present in the epithelial cells, but under normal conditions keratinization does not occur. Therefore, nuclei can be seen in epithelial cells throughout the thickness of the epithelium.

The mucosa contains no glands. The vaginal

The examination of vaginal smears is a valuable diagnostic tool in evaluating the estrogenic stimulation of the vaginal mucosa. The synthesis and release of glycogen into the uterine lumen appears to be related directly to changes in the pH of the vaginal fluid. The pH of the vaginal fluid, which is normally low, becomes more acid near midcycle as lactic acid-forming bacteria in the vagina metabolize the glycogen. An alkaline environment is favorable for the growth of infectious agents such as staphylococci, *Trichomonas vaginalis,* and *Candida albicans.* Estrogen therapy is often effective in the treatment of such infections, particularly in postmenopausal women and children, because it stimulates growth of epithelium and synthesis of glycogen. The metabolism of the glycogen results in the lowering of the pH and the creation of an environment that retards the growth of the infectious agents.

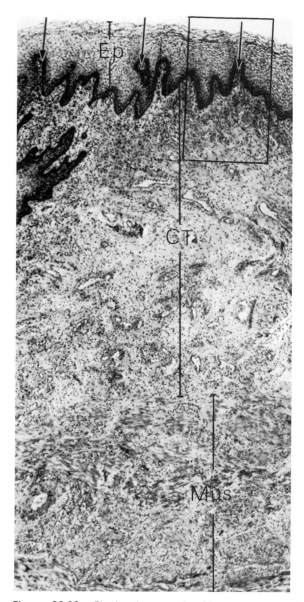

Figure 22.30. Photomicrograph of human vagina. The vaginal wall consists of three layers: a mucous membrane, a muscular layer (Mus), and an outer adventitia. The mucous membrane is composed of a stratified squamous epithelium (Ep) and an underlying connective tissue layer (CT). Connective tissue papillae project into the undersurface of the epithelium **(arrows)**. × 40.

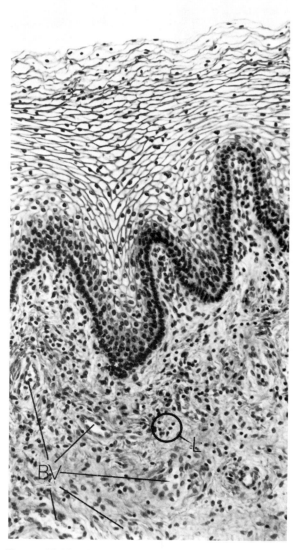

Figure 22.31. Photomicrograph of human vaginal mucosa. The **rectangle** in Figure 22.30 indicates the area shown in this figure. Projection of connective tissue papillae into the epithelium gives the connective tissue–epithelial junction a very uneven appearance. Numerous blood vessels (BV) and leukocytes (L) are present in the connective tissue. The number of leukocytes varies with the ovarian cycle. The greatest number is found around the time of menstruation. × 180.

surface is lubricated by mucus from the cervix. The epithelium undergoes cyclic changes during the menstrual cycle. Under the influence of estrogens, during the follicular phase, the epithelial cells synthesize and accumulate glycogen as they migrate toward the surface. Cells are continuously desquamated, but near or during the menstrual phase the superficial layer of the vaginal epithelium may be shed.

The lamina propria exhibits two distinct regions. The outer region is a moderately dense connective tissue. The deeper region, adjacent to the muscular layer, is less dense and may be considered a submucosa. A large number of thin-walled veins, which simulate erectile tissue during sexual excitement, are present in the deeper region. Abundant elastic fibers are present immediately below the epithelium, and some of the fibers extend into the muscular layer. Numerous lymphocytes and leukocytes (particularly neutrophils) are found in the lamina propria and many are seen migrating into the epithelium. Solitary lymphatic nodules may also be present. The number of lymphocytes and leukocytes in the mucosa and vaginal lumen dramatically increases around the time of menstrual flow.

The vaginal muscularis is organized in two, sometimes indistinct, intermingling smooth muscle layers, an outer longitudinal layer and an inner circular layer. The outer layer, which is continuous with the corresponding layer in the uterus, is much thicker than the inner layer. Striated muscle fibers of the bulbospongiosus muscle are present at the vaginal opening.

The vaginal adventitia is organized into an inner dense connective tissue layer, adjacent to the muscularis, and an outer loose connective tissue layer that blends with the adventitia of the surrounding structures. The inner layer contains numerous elastic fibers that contribute to the elasticity and strength of the vaginal wall. The outer layer contains numerous blood and lymphatic vessels and nerves.

The vaginal mucosa has few general sensory nerve endings. The sensory nerve endings that are more plentiful in the lower third of the vagina are probably associated primarily with pain and stretch sensations.

EXTERNAL GENITALIA

In the female, the external genitalia are referred to as the **vulva.** Its parts are the **mons pubis, labia minora** and **majora, clitoris, vestibule** of the vagina and its glands, and openings of the urethra and vagina. The surface of all these structures is covered with stratified squamous epithelium.

The **mons pubis,** the rounded prominence

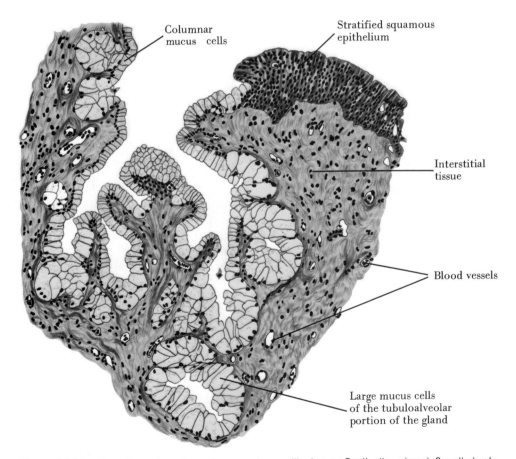

Figure 22.32. Drawing of section of a greater vestibular, or Bartholin, gland. Small ducts lined with columnar mucus cells extend from the tubuloalveolar terminal portions of the glands. Patches of stratified columnar epithelium are present in the larger ducts. × 185. (After Maximow AA: In Bloom W, Fawcett DW: *A Textbook of Histology,* 10th ed. Philadelphia, WB Saunders, 1975.)

over the pubic symphysis, is formed by subcutaneous adipose tissue. Extending from the mons pubis are two large longitudinal folds of skin, the **labia majora,** which form the lateral boundaries of the urogenital cleft. The labia majora are homologous to the scrotum and contain a thin layer of smooth muscle, resembling the dartos muscle of the scrotum, and a large amount of subcutaneous adipose tissue. The outer surface, like the mons pubis, is covered with pubic hair. The inner surface is smooth and devoid of hair. Numerous sebaceous and sweat glands are present on both surfaces.

The **labia minora** are paired, hairless folds of skin that border the vestibule. Abundant pigment is present in the cells of the deeper epithelial layers. The core of connective tissue within each fold is devoid of fat, but does contain numerous blood vessels and fine elastic fibers. Numerous large sebaceous glands are present in the stroma.

The **clitoris** is an erectile structure that is homologous to the penis. The body of the clitoris is composed of two small erectile bodies, the **corpora cavernosa;** the **glans clitoris** is a small, rounded tubercle of erectile tissue. The skin over the glans is very thin and contains numerous sensory nerve endings.

The **vestibule** is lined with stratified squamous epithelium. Numerous small mucous glands, the **small vestibular glands** (also called **glandulae vestibulares minores,** lesser vestibular glands, or **Skene's glands**), are present primarily near the clitoris and around the urethral opening. The large, paired **greater vestibular glands** (also called **glandulae vestibulares majores** or **Bartholin's glands**) are homologous to the male bulbourethral glands. These glands, which are about 1 cm in diameter, are located in the lateral wall of the vestibule posterior to the bulb of the vestibule. The greater vestibular glands are tubuloalveolar glands that secrete a lubricating mucus (Fig. 22.32). The ducts of these glands open into the vestibule near the vaginal opening at the base of the hymen.

Numerous sensory nerve endings are present in the external genitalia. **Meissner's corpuscles** are particularly abundant in the skin over the clitoris. **Pacinian corpuscles** are distributed in the deeper layers of the connective tissue and are found in the labia majora and in association with the erectile tissue. The sensory signals from these nerve endings play an important role in the physiological response during sexual arousal.

MAMMARY GLANDS

Mammary glands, or breasts, are a distinguishing feature of mammals. They have evolved as milk-producing organs to provide nourishment for the offspring. During embryological development, there is growth and development of the breast in both sexes. Paired glands develop along paired lines, the **milk lines,** between the limb buds of the upper and lower extremities. In the human, normally only one group of cells develops into a breast on each side. An extra breast (polymastia) or nipple (polythelia) may occur as an inheritable condition in about 1 percent of the female population. These relatively rare conditions may also occur in the male. When present, the supernumerary breast or nipple usually forms along the milk lines; about one-third of the affected individuals have multiple extra breasts or nipples. In the male, there is normally little additional development in postnatal life and the glands remain rudimentary. In the female, the mammary glands undergo further development under hormonal influence. They are also influenced by changes in the ovarian hormone levels during each menstrual cycle. The actual secretion and production of milk is induced by prolactin from the pituitary and somatomammotropin from the placenta. With the change in the hormonal environment at menopause, the glandular component of the breast regresses, or involutes, and is replaced by fat and connective tissue.

Inactive Mammary Gland

The adult mammary gland is composed of 15 to 20 irregular lobes of branched tubuloalveolar glands (Fig. 22.33). The lobes, separated by fibrous bands of connective tissue, radiate from the **mammary papilla** or **nipple,** and are further subdivided into numerous lobules. Some of the fibrous bands, called **suspensory** or **Cooper's ligaments,** connect with the dermis. Abundant adipose tissue is present in the dense connective tissue of the interlobular spaces. The intralobular connective tissue is much less dense and contains little fat.

The tubuloalveolar glands, derived from modified sweat glands in the epidermis, lie in the subcutaneous tissue. Each gland ends in a **lactiferous duct** (2 to 4 mm in diameter), which opens through a constricted orifice (0.4 to 0.7 mm in diameter) onto the nipple. Beneath the **areola** (the pigmented area surrounding the nipple), each duct has a dilated portion, the **lactiferous sinus.** Near their openings the lactiferous ducts are lined with stratified squamous epithelium. The epithelial lining of the duct shows a gradual transition to two layers of cuboidal cells in the lactiferous sinus and then becomes a single layer of columnar or cuboidal cells through the remainder of the duct system.

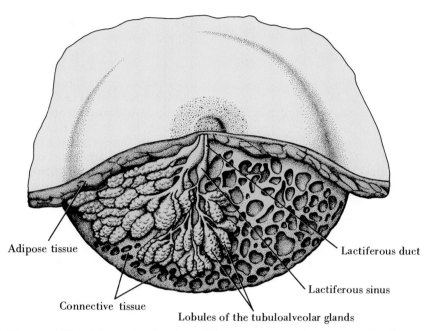

Adipose tissue

Lactiferous duct

Lactiferous sinus

Connective tissue

Lobules of the tubuloalveolar glands

Figure 22.33. Schematic drawing of the human breast as seen during lactation. The breast is composed of branched tubuloalveolar glands. (*Gray's Anatomy,* 36th ed.)

Myoepithelial cells of ectodermal origin lie within the epithelium between the surface epithelial cells and the basal lamina. These cells, arranged in a basket-like network, are present in the secretory portion of the gland, but are more apparent in the larger ducts.

The morphology of the secretory portion of the mammary gland varies greatly with age, pregnancy, and lactation. In the inactive gland, the glandular component is sparse and consists chiefly of duct elements (Fig. 22.34). Most investigators believe that the secretory units in the inactive breast are not organized as alveoli and consist only of ducts. During the menstrual cycle, the inactive breast undergoes slight cyclic changes. Early in the cycle, the ducts appear as cords with little or no lumen. Under estrogen stimulation, at about the time of ovulation, secretory cells increase in height, lumens appear in the ducts as small amounts of secretions accumulate, and fluids accumulate in the connective tissue.

Nipple and Areola

The epidermis of the nipple and areola is highly pigmented and somewhat wrinkled and has long dermal papillae invading into its deep surface (Fig. 22.35). It is covered by keratinized stratified squamous epithelium. At puberty, this skin becomes pigmented and the nipple becomes more prominent. During pregnancy, the areola becomes larger and the degree of pigmentation increases. Deep to the areola and nipple, bundles of smooth muscle fibers are arranged radially and circumferentially in the dense connective tissue and longitudinally along the lactiferous ducts. These muscle fibers allow the nipple to become erect in response to various stimuli.

The areola contains sebaceous glands, sweat glands, and modified mammary glands (glands of Montgomery). These glands, which are described as having a structure intermediate between sweat glands and true mammary glands, produce small elevations on the surface of the areola. Numerous sensory nerve endings are present in the tip of the nipple. The areola contains few sensory nerve endings.

Active Mammary Glands— Pregnancy and Lactation

The mammary glands undergo dramatic proliferation and development during pregnancy in preparation for lactation. These changes in the glandular tissue are accompanied by decreases in the amount of connective and adipose tissue. Plasma cells, lymphocytes, and eosinophils infiltrate the fibrous component of the connective tissue as the breast develops. The development of the glandular tissue is not uniform and variation in the degree of development is seen even within a single lobule. The cells vary in shape from flattened to

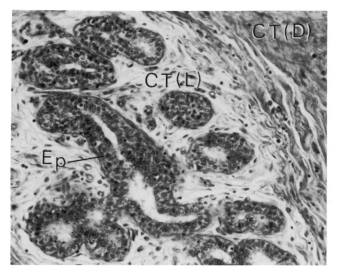

Figure 22.34. Photomicrograph of inactive or resting human mammary gland. The epithelial (Ep) or glandular elements are embedded in loose connective tissue [CT(L)]. The epithelial cells within the lobule are primarily duct elements. The lobule is surrounded by dense connective tissue [CT(D)]. × 160.

low columnar. As the cells proliferate by mitotic division, the ducts branch and alveoli begin to develop. In the later stages of pregnancy, alveolar development becomes more prominent (Fig. 22.36). The actual proliferation of the glandular cells declines and subsequent enlargement of the breast occurs through hypertrophy of the secre-

tory cells and accumulation of secretory product in the alveolar ducts.

The secreting cells contain abundant granular endoplasmic reticulum, a moderate number of large mitochondria, a supranuclear Golgi complex, and a number of dense lysosomes (Fig. 22.37). Depending on the secretory state, large lipid droplets and secretory granules may be present in the apical cytoplasm. The secretory cells produce two distinct products that are released by different mechanisms. The protein component of the milk is synthesized in the granular endoplasmic reticulum, packaged in membrane-limited secretory granules for transport in the Golgi apparatus, and released from the cell by fusion of the granule's limiting membrane with the plasma membrane. This type of secretion is referred to as **merocrine secretion.** The fatty or lipid component of the milk arises as lipid droplets free in the cytoplasm. The lipid coalesces to form large droplets that pass to the apical region of the cell and project into the lumen of the acinus. The droplets are invested with an envelope of the plasma membrane as they are released. A thin layer of cytoplasm is trapped between the plasma membrane and lipid droplet and is released with the lipid, but it should be emphasized that the cytoplasmic loss in this process is minimal. This type of secretion is classically known as **apocrine secretion.**

The milk released in the first few days after childbirth is known as **colostrum.** It has a low lipid content, but is believed to contain considerable

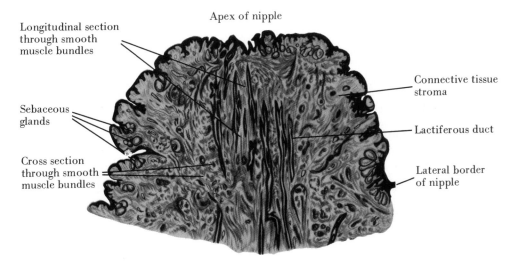

Figure 22.35. Drawing of a perpendicular section through the nipple of a female breast. Keratinized stratified squamous epithelium covers the somewhat wrinkled surface of the nipple and areola. Bundles of smooth fibers are embedded in the dense connective tissue that surrounds the lactiferous ducts located deep to the areola and nipple. × 6. (After Schaffer, in Bloom W, Fawcett DW: *A Textbook of Histology,* 10th ed. Philadelphia, WB Saunders, 1975.)

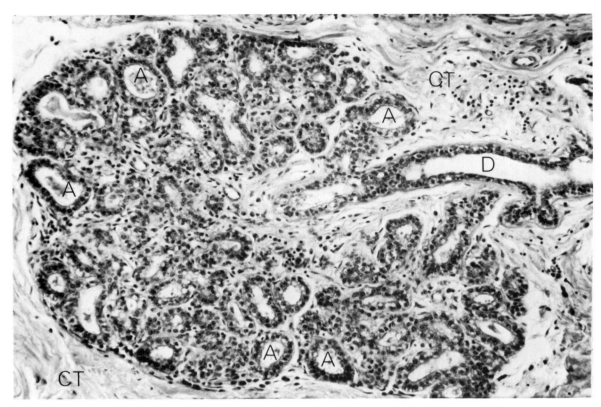

Figure 22.36. Photomicrograph of proliferative human mammary gland. During the early proliferative period the development of the alveolar elements of the gland becomes conspicuous (compare Fig. 22.35). Distinct alveoli (A) are present. Within a lobule all these alveoli are joined to a duct. Loose, highly cellular connective tissue (CT) surrounds the alveoli. Dense connective tissue septa separate the individual lobules. × 160.

amounts of antibodies that may provide the newborn with some degree of passive immunity. The colostrum is believed to be produced, in part, by the lymphocytes and plasma cells infiltrated into the stroma of the breast during its proliferation and development. As these wandering cells decrease in number, the production of colostrum stops and lipid-rich milk is produced.

Hormonal Regulation of the Mammary Gland

The initial growth and development of the mammary gland at puberty occurs under the influence of estrogens and progesterone being produced by the maturing ovary. Subsequent to this initial development, slight changes in the morphology of the glandular tissue occur during each ovarian cycle. During pregnancy, the corpus luteum and placenta continuously produce estrogens and progesterone. This hormonal stimulation causes proliferation and development of the mammary gland. It is now believed that the growth of the

mammary glands is also dependent upon the presence of prolactin, produced by the adenohypophysis; somatomammotropin (lactogenic hormone), produced by the placenta; and adrenal corticoids.

At parturition, the level of circulating estrogens and progesterone falls abruptly with the degeneration of the corpus luteum and loss of the placenta. The secretion of milk is then brought about by the increased production of prolactin and secretion of adrenal cortical steroids. The high level of prolactin secretion is dependent upon a neurohormonal reflex. The act of suckling initiates impulses from receptors in the nipple to the hypothalamus. The impulses inhibit the release of prolactin-inhibiting factor and prolactin is released from the adenohypophysis. The impulses also cause the release of oxytocin in the neurohypophysis. The oxytocin stimulates the myoepithelial cells of the mammary glands, causing them to contract and eject the milk from the glands. In the absence of suckling, secretion of milk ceases and the mammary glands begin to regress. The glandular tissue then returns to an inactive condition.

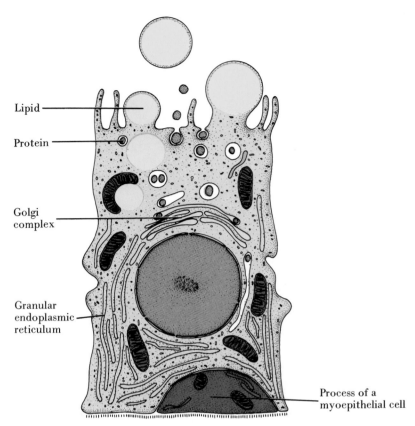

Lipid

Protein

Golgi
complex

Granular
endoplasmic
reticulum

Process of a
myoepithelial cell

Figure 22.37. Schematic diagram of a secretory epithelial cell from a lactating mammary gland. The large milk lipid droplets (shown in yellow) and a thin layer of adjacent cytoplasm are enclosed with an envelope of plasma membrane as the droplets are released (apocrine secretion). The protein component of the milk (shown in blue), which is synthesized in the granular endoplasmic reticulum and packaged in the Golgi complex, is released from the cell by fusion of the granule's limiting membrane with the plasma membrane (merocrine secretion). (Redrawn after Bloom W, Fawcett DW: *A Textbook of Histology,* 10th ed., Philadelphia, WB Saunders, 1975.)

The mammary gland atrophies, or involutes, after menopause. In the absence of ovarian hormone stimulation, the secretory cells of the alveoli degenerate and disappear, but some ducts may remain. The connective tissue also demonstrates degenerative changes, marked by a decrease in the number of stromal cells and collagen fibers.

Blood Supply, Lymphatic Drainage, and Innervation

The arteries that supply the breast are derived from thoracic branches of the axillary artery, the internal thoracic (or mammary) artery, and intercostal arteries. Branches of the vessels pass primarily along the path of the alveolar ducts as they reach capillary beds surrounding the alveoli. Veins basically follow the path of the arteries as they return to the axillary and internal thoracic veins.

Lymphatic capillaries are located in the connective tissue surrounding the alveoli. Lymphatic vessels may drain into axillary, subclavicular, or parasternal lymph nodes.

The nerves that supply the breast are anterior and lateral cutaneous branches from the fourth, fifth, and sixth intercostal nerves. The nerves convey afferent and sympathetic fibers to the breast. The secretory function is primarily under hormonal control, but afferent impulses associated with suckling are involved in the reflex secretion of prolactin and oxytocin.

ATLAS PLATES

112–124

PLATE 112. Ovary I

The ovaries are small ovoid solid structures whose dimensions are roughly 3.0 × 1.5 × 1 cm. They possess a hilus on one edge for the transit of neurovascular structures. On this same edge they are attached to a mesovarium that joins them to the broad ligament. The ovaries produce oocytes and female sex hormones.

The outer part of the ovary contains numerous primordial follicles that are already present at the time of birth and that remain quiescent until sexual maturation. At this time, under the influence of pituitary hormones, the ovaries undergo cyclical changes designated the ovarian cycles. During each ovarian cycle, the ovaries produce an oocyte (usually only one) that is ready for fertilization, and also the hormones estrogen and progesterone, which bring about uterine cycles, and, in the human, menstruation. Thus, the ovarian cycles are directly correlated with the uterine and other cyclical changes that accompany the menstrual cycle.

The cortex of an ovary from a sexually mature individual is shown in **Figure 1.** On the surface there is a single layer of epithelial cells designated the germinal epithelium **(Gep).** This epithelium is continuous with the serosa (peritoneum) of the mesovarium. Contrary to the implication inherent in its name, the epithelium does not give rise to the germ cells. The germinal epithelium covers a dense fibrous connective tissue layer, the tunica albuginea **(TA),** and under the tunica albuginea are the primordial follicles **(PF).** At the beginning of the ovarian cycle, under the influence of a pituitary hormone (follicle-stimulating hormone FSH), some of the primordial follicles begin to undergo changes that lead to the development of a mature (Graafian) follicle. These changes include a proliferation of cells and total enlargement of the follicle. Although several primordial follicles begin this series of developmental changes, usually only one reaches maturity and yields an oocyte. The discharge of the oocyte and its adherent cells is called ovulation. The other follicles that began to proliferate at the same time degenerate—a process referred to as atresia. Thus, it is not unusual to see follicles at various stages of development or atresia in the ovary. In **Figure 1,** along with the large number of primordial follicles, there are four growing follicles **(SF),** an atretic follicle **(AF),** and part of a large follicle on the right. The region of the large follicle shown in the figure includes the theca interna **(TI),** granulosa cells **(GC),** and part of the antrum **(A).**

Figure 2 shows several primordial follicles at higher magnification. Each follicle consists of an

KEY

A, antrum
AF, atretic follicle
F, follicle cells, primordial
FC, follicle cells
GC, granulosa cells
GEp, germinal epithelium
N, nucleus of oocyte

arrowhead, follicle cells in face view
PF, primordial follicles
SF, growing follicles
TA, tunica albuginea
TI, theca interna
X, oocyte in which nucleus was missed
ZP, zona pellucida

Fig. 1, × 120

Figs. 2–4, × 450; all monkey.

oocyte surrounded by a single layer of squamous follicular cells **(F).** The nucleus **(N)** of the oocyte is typically large, but the oocyte itself is so large that often the nucleus is not included in the plane of section, as in the oocyte marked **X.** The group of epithelioid cells marked by the **open arrowhead** are follicular cells of a primordial follicle that has been sectioned in a plane that just grazes the follicular surface. In this case, the follicular cells are seen in face view.

When a primordial follicle begins the changes leading to the formation of a mature follicle, the layer of squamous follicular cells becomes cuboidal; in addition, the cells proliferate and become multilayered. A follicle undergoing these early changes is called a primary follicle. Thus, a primary follicle may be unilaminar **(Fig. 3),** but it is surrounded by cuboidal cells, and this distinguishes it from the more numerous unilaminar primordial follicles that are surrounded by more flattened cells. The primary follicle in **Figure 4** shows a multilayered mass of follicular cells **(FC)** surrounding the oocyte. Moreover, the innermost layer of follicular cells is now columnar and adjacent to a thick eosinophilic layer of extracellular homogeneous material called the zona pellucida **(ZP).** At the same time, the oocyte has also enlarged slightly. It should be realized that the entire structure surrounded by the zona pellucida is the oocyte.

Surrounding the follicles are elongate cells of the highly cellular connective tissue, referred to as stromal cells. The stromal cells surrounding a secondary follicle become disposed into two layers designated the theca interna **(TI)** and the theca externa. As seen in **Figure 1,** stromal cells become epitheloid in the cell-rich theca interna.

PLATE 112

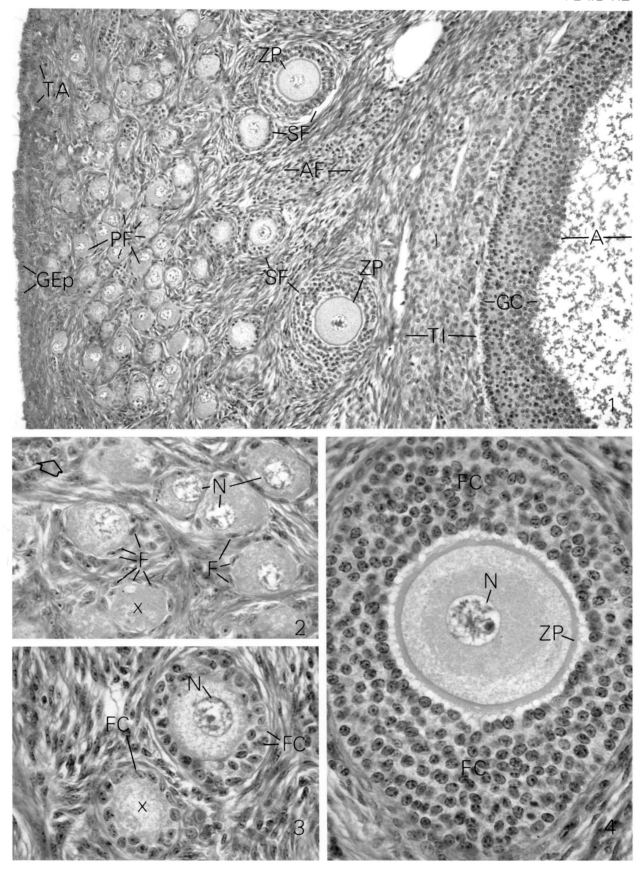

PLATE 113. Ovary II

Two follicles growing under the influence of FSH are shown in **Figure 1.** The more advanced follicle is a secondary follicle. The oocyte in this follicle is surrounded by several layers of follicular cells **(FC)**, which, at this stage, are identified as granulosa cells. At a slightly earlier time, small lakes of fluid formed between the follicular cells and these have now fused into a well-defined larger cavity called the follicular antrum **(FA)** that is evident in the figure. The antrum is also filled with fluid and stains with the PAS reaction, although only lightly. The substance that stains with the PAS reaction has been retained as an eosinophilic precipitate in the antrums of the secondary follicles shown in **Figs. 1 and 2.** Immediately above the obvious secondary follicle is a slightly smaller follicle. Because no antral spaces are evident between the follicular cells, it is appropriate to classify it as a primary follicle. In both follicles, but particularly in the larger follicle with the antrum, the surrounding stromal cells have become altered to form distinctive layers designated as the theca interna **(TI)** and the theca externa **(TE)**. The theca interna is a more cellular layer and the cells are epithelioid. With the electron microscope, they display the characteristics of endocrine cells, in particular, steroid-secreting cells. In contrast, the theca externa is a connective tissue layer. Its cells are more or less spindle-shaped.

A later stage in the growth of the secondary follicle is shown in **Figure 2.** The antrum **(FA)** is larger and the oocyte is off to one side surrounded by a mound of follicular cells called the cumulus oophorus. The remaining follicular cells that surround the antral cavity are referred to as the membrana granulosa **(MG)** or simply as granulosa cells.

Atresia of follicles is a regular event in the ovary. Follicles of various stages can be seen undergoing atresia. In all cases, the follicular cells show pyknosis of their nucleus and dissolution of the cytoplasm, and the follicle is invaded by macrophages and other connective tissue cells. The oocyte degenerates, leaving behind the prominent zona pellucida. This may be folded inwardly or collapsed but it usually retains its thickness and staining characteristics. Thus, when included in the plane of section, a partially disrupted zona pellucida serves as a reliable diagnostic feature of an atretic follicle. Atretic follicles **(AF)** are shown in **Figure 3** and at higher magnification in **Figure 4.**

KEY

AF, atretic follicle
FA, antrum of follicle
FC, follicle cells
MG, Fig. 2, membrana granulosa
MG, Fig. 4, persisting theca interna cells
TE, theca externa

TI, theca interna
ZP, zona pellucida
open arrowhead, persisting theca interna cells
arrows, glassy membrane

Fig. 1, × 120
Fig. 2, × 120
Fig. 3, ×65

Fig. 4, × 120
Fig. 5, × 120; all monkey

The two smaller atretic follicles **(Fig. 3)** can be identified by virtue of the retained zona pellucida **(ZP, Fig. 4).** The two larger, more advanced follicles do not display the remains of a zona pellucida, but they do display other features of follicular atresia.

In the atresia of a more advanced follicle, the follicular cells tend to degenerate more rapidly than the cells of the theca interna and the basement membrane separating the two becomes thickened to form a hyalinized membrane—the glassy membrane **(Fig. 4).** This glassy membrane **(arrows)** separates an outer layer of remaining theca interna cells **(TI)** from the degenerating inner follicular cells. Moreover, the remaining theca internal cells may show cytological integrity and experimental data indicate that these intact theca cells remain temporarily functional in steroid secretion. (In some ovaries, including the human ovary, clusters of epithelioid cells are observed in the ovarian cortex. These are referred to collectively as interstitial glands. They are thought to be remnants of theca cells of large degenerating follicles, as in **Fig. 4.**)

Additional atretic follicles **(AF)** are shown in **Figure 5.** Again, some show remnants of a zona pellucida **(ZP)** and two show a glassy membrane **(arrows).** Note that even though the atresia in these follicles is well advanced, some of the cells external to one of the glassy membranes still retain their epithelioid character **(open arrowhead).** These are persisting theca interna cells.

686

PLATE 113

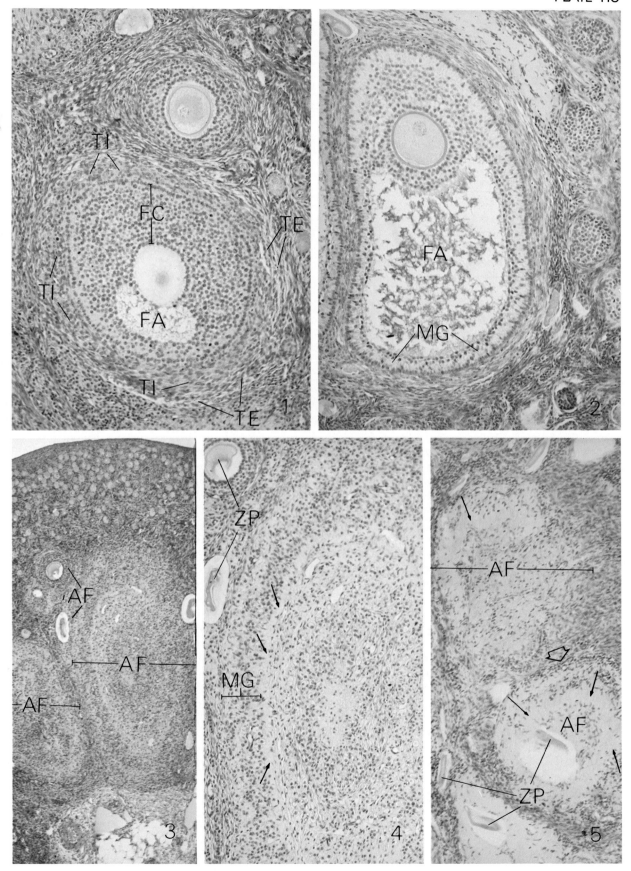

PLATE 114. Corpus Luteum

After the oocyte and surrounding cumulus cells are discharged from the mature ovarian follicle (ovulation), the remaining follicle cells (membrana granulosa) and the adjacent theca interna undergo changes that result in the formation of a new functional unit, the corpus luteum. **Figure 1** depicts these tissues shortly after ovulation. The **arrowhead** points toward the surface of the ovary where the ovulation occurred. The cavity (**FC**) of the former follicle has been invaded by connective tissue. In addition, the membrana granulosa becomes plicated at the same time that the granulosa cells become transformed into cells of the corpus luteum now called granulosa lutein cells. This plication of the membrana granulosa begins just before ovulation and it continues as the corpus luteum develops. As the corpus luteum becomes more plicated, the former follicular cavity becomes reduced in size. At the same time, blood vessels (**BV**) from the theca of the follicle invade the former cavity and the transforming membrana granulosa cells (**TC**). Cells of the theca interna follow the blood vessels into the outermost depressions of the plicated structure. These theca interna cells become transformed into cells of the corpus luteum called theca lutein cells.

A portion of a fully formed corpus luteum is shown in **Figure 2**. The main mass of endocrine cells are the granulosa lutein cells (**GLC**). These form a folded cell mass that surrounds the remains of the former follicular cavity (**FC**). External to the corpus luteum is the connective tissue of the ovary (**CT**). It should be kept in mind that the theca interna was derived from the connective tissue stroma of the ovary. The location of theca lutein cells reflects this origin and these cells (**TLC**) can be found in the deep outer recesses of the glandular mass, adjacent to the surrounding connective tissue.

A segment of the plicated corpus luteum is shown in **Figure 3** at higher magnification. As already noted, the main cell mass is comprised of granulosa lutein cells (**GLC**). On one side of this cell mass is the connective tissue (**CT**) within the former follicular cavity; on the other side are the

KEY

BV, blood vessels
CT, connective tissue
FC, former follicular cavity
GLC, granulosa lutein cells

TC, cells transforming into the corpus luteum
TLC, theca lutein cells

Fig. 1, × 20
Fig. 2, × 20

Fig. 3, × 65
Fig. 4, × 240; all human

theca lutein cells. As evident in **Figure 4,** the granulosa lutein cells (**GLC**) contain a large spherical nucleus (**GLC, Fig. 4**) and a large amount of cytoplasm. The cytoplasm contains pigment, therefore the name corpus luteum. However, the pigment is not evident in routine H&E paraffin sections. Theca lutein cells also contain a spherical nucleus (**TLC**), but the cells are smaller; thus, when identifying the two cell types, aside from location, it should be noted that the nuclei of adjacent theca lutein cells generally appear to be closer than nuclei of adjacent granulosa lutein cells. The connective tissue (**CT**) and small blood vessels that invaded the granulosa lutein cells can be identified as the flattened and elongated components between the granulosa lutein cells.

The changes whereby the ruptured ovarian follicle is transformed into a corpus luteum occur under the influence of a pituitary hormone. In turn, the corpus luteum itself secretes a hormone—progesterone—which has a profound effect on the estrogen-primed uterus. If pregnancy occurs, the corpus luteum remains functional; if pregnancy does not occur, the corpus luteum regresses after having reached a point of peak development, roughly 2 weeks after ovulation. The regressing cellular components of the corpus luteum are replaced by fibrous connective tissue, and the structure is then called a corpus albicans.

PLATE 114

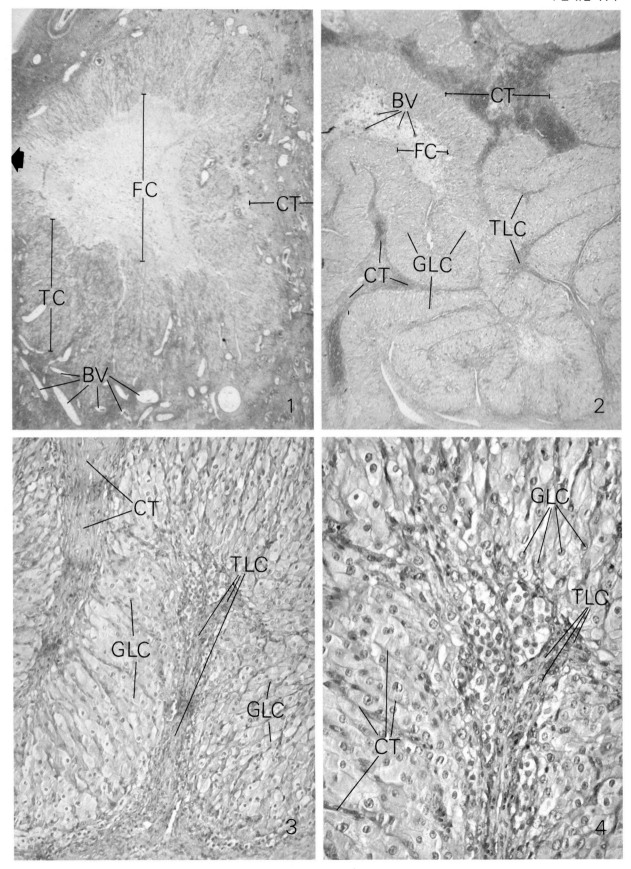

PLATE 115. Oviduct-Uterine Tube

The oviducts (uterine tubes) are joined to the uterus and extend to the ovaries where they present an open flared end for entry of the ovum. Fertilization of the ovum usually occurs in the oviduct and, for the first several days, the developing embryonic cells are contained in the tube as they travel to the uterus. The oviduct undergoes cyclical changes along with those of the uterus, but they are not nearly as pronounced. The tubal changes primarily involve the epithelial cells. They increase in height during the middle of the cycle, just about the time the ovum will be passing through the tube, but they become reduced during the premenstrual period. Some of the epithelial cells are ciliated; the number of ciliated cells increases during the follicular phase of the ovarian cycle.

The uterine tube varies in size and degree of mucosal folding along its length. The mucosal folds are more numerous near the open end and less numerous near the uterus. Near the uterus the tube is narrow and referred to as the isthmus. Then, for about two-thirds of its length it is an expanded form and is referred to as the ampulla. Near the opening the tube flares outward and is called the infundibulum. It has fringed folded edges that are called fimbria.

A cross-section through the ampulla of the tube is shown in **Figure 1.** Many mucosal fold project into the lumen and the complicated nature of the folds is evident by the variety of profiles that are seen. In addition to the mucosa, the remainder of the wall consists of a muscularis **(Mus)** and connective tissue.

The area enclosed by the rectangle in **Figure 1** is shown at higher magnification in **Figure 2.** The specimen shows a longitudinal section through a lymphatic vessel **(Lym).** In other planes of section, the lymphatic vessels are difficult to identify. The fortuitously sectioned lymphatic vessel is seen in the core of the mucosal fold, along with a highly cellular connective tissue **(CT)** and the blood ves-

sels **(BV)** within the connective tissue. The epithelium lining the mucosa is shown in the **inset.** The ciliated cells are readily identified by the presence of well-formed cilia **(C).** Nonciliated cells, also called peg cells **(PG),** are also readily identified by the absence of cilia; moreover, they have elongate nuclei and sometimes appear to be squeezed between the ciliated cells.

The ciliated cells depend on the ovaries for their viability. Experimental studies show that removal of ovaries in mature animals leads to atrophy of the epithelium and loss of ciliated cells.

The connective tissue **(CT)** contains cells whose nuclei are arranged in a typically random manner. They vary in shape, being elongated, oval, or round. Their cytoplasm cannot be distinguished from the intercellular material **(inset).** The character of the connective tissue is essentially the same from the epithelium to the muscularis and, for this reason, no submucosa is described.

The muscularis **(Mus)** consists of smooth muscle that forms a relatively thick layer of circular fibers and a thinner outer layer of longitudinal fibers **(Fig. 1).** The layers are not clearly delineated and no sharp boundary separates the two.

KEY	
BV, blood vessels	L, lumen
C, cilia	Muc, mucosa
CT, connective tissue	Mus, muscularis
Ep, epithelium	PC, peg cells

Fig. 1, × 40	Fig. 2, × 160; inset, × 320; all human

PLATE 115

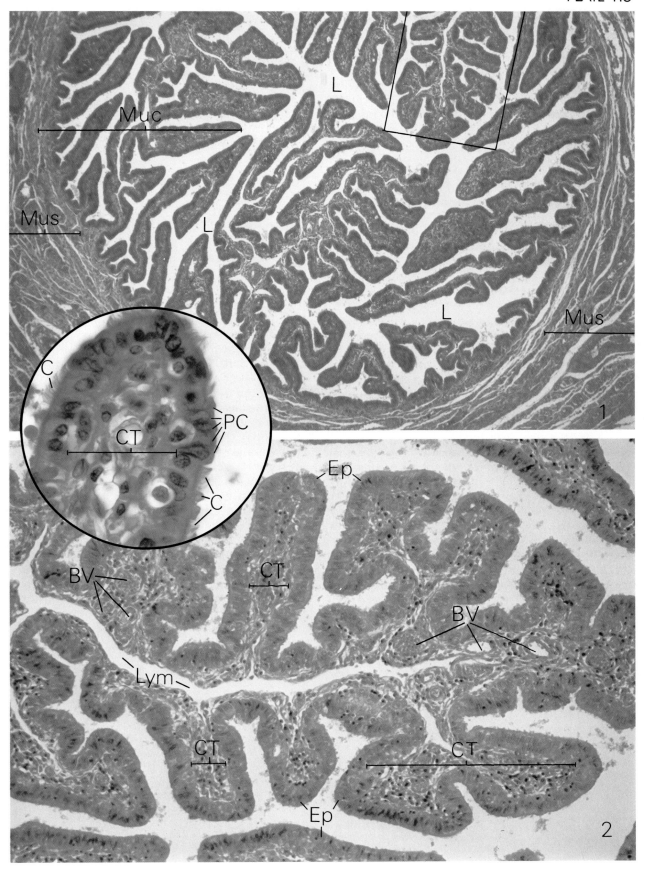

L

Muc

Mus

L

L

Mus

C

PC

CT

C

1

Ep

CT

BV

BV

Lym

CT

CT

Ep

2

PLATE 116. Uterus I

The uterus is a hollow, pear-shaped organ with a thick muscular wall and, in the nonpregnant state, a narrow cavity. The uterine wall is comprised of a mucosa, referred to as the endometrium; a muscularis, referred to as the myometrium; and externally a serosal cover, the visceral peritoneum. The serosa presents no special features. The myometrium consists of smooth muscle and connective tissue and contains the larger blood vessels. A small portion of the thickness of the myometrium (**M**) is shown at low power in **Figure 1.** A higher power of the interlacing bundles of smooth muscle cells is illustrated in Figure 4 of Atlas section, Plate 27.

The uterus undergoes cyclical changes that are largely manifested by the changes that occur in the endometrium. If implantation of an ovum does not occur after preparation for this event, the state of readiness is not maintained and much of the endometrium degenerates and is sloughed off, constituting the menstrual flow. The part of the endometrium that is lost is referred to as the stratum functionale. The part that is retained is called the stratum basale. The stratum basale is the deepest part of the endometrium and adjoins the myometrium.

After the stratum functionale is sloughed off, resurfacing of the raw tissue occurs. The epithelial resurfacing comes from the glands that remain in the stratum basale. The gland epithelium simply proliferates and grows over the surface. **Figure 1** shows the endometrium as it appears when resurfacing is complete. The area inscribed in the **upper small circle** is shown at higher magnification in the **inset** of **Figure 1** (on the **right**). Note the simple columnar epithelium (**SEP**) that covers the endometrial surface and its similarity to the glandular epithelium (**GI**). The endometrium is relatively

thin at this stage and over half of it consists of the stratum basale (**SB**). The area inscribed by the **lower circle,** located in the region of the stratum basale, is shown at higher magnification in **Figure 2** (on the **left**). The glandular epithelium (**GI**) of the deep portion of the glands is similar to that of the endometrial surface. Below the endometrium is the myometrium (**M**), in which a number of large blood vessels (**BV**) are present.

Under the influence of estrogen, the various components of the endometrium proliferate (proliferative stage) so that the total thickness of the endometrium is increased (**Fig. 2**). The glands (**GI**) become rather long and follow a fairly straight course within the stratum functionale (**SF**) to reach the surface. The stratum basale (**SB**) remains essentially unaffected by the estrogen and appears much the same as in **Figure 1**. The stratum functionale (**SF**), on the other hand, increases in thickness and comes to constitute about four-fifths of the endometrial thickness as shown in **Figure 2.**

PLATE 116

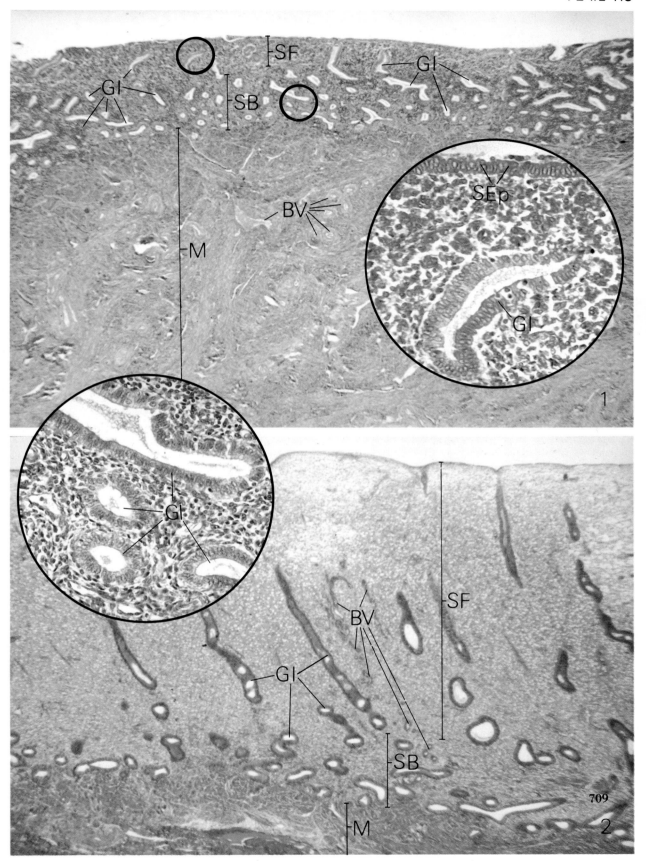

PLATE 117. Uterus II

After estrogen brings about the uterine events designated as the proliferative stage, another hormone, progesterone, influences additional uterine changes that constitute the secretory stage of the uterine cycle. This hormone brings the endometrium to a state of readiness for implantation, and as a consequence of its actions, the thickness of the endometrium increases further. There are conspicuous changes in the glands; these changes are primarily in the stratum functionale.

A view of the endometrium in the secretory stage is shown in **Figure 1.** This shows the stratum functionale **(SF),** the stratum basale **(SB),** and in the **lower left** of the photomicrograph, a small amount of the myometrium **(M).** The uterine glands have been cut in a plane that is close to their long axes, and one gland **(arrow)** is seen opening at the uterine surface. Except for a few glands near the center of the diagram that resemble those of the proliferative stage, most of the glands **(Gl)** in this figure, including those that are labeled, show numerous shallow sacculations that give the profile of the glandular epithelium a serrated appearance. This is one of the distinctive features of the secretory stage. It is seen most advantageously in areas where the plane of section is close to the long axis of the gland, as in **Figure 1.** In contrast to the characteristic sinuous course of the glands in the stratum functionale, glands of the stratum basale more closely resemble the appearance they displayed in the proliferative stage. They are not oriented in any noticeable relationship to the uterine surface and many of their long profiles are even parallel to the plane of the surface.

The slightly higher magnification of the stratum functionale **(Fig. 2)** shows essentially the same characteristics of the glands **(Gl)** described above; it also shows other modifications that occur during the secretory stage. One of these is that the endometrium becomes edematous. The increase in endometrial thickness due to edema is reflected by the presence of empty spaces between cells and other formed elements. Thus, many areas of **Figure 2,** especially the area within and near the circle, show histological signs of edema.

In addition, the glandular epithelial cells be-

gin to secrete a mucoid fluid that is rich in glycogen. This product is secreted into the lumen of the glands and these become dilated. Typically, the glands of the secretory endometrium are more dilated than those of the proliferative endometrium, and this point can be readily discriminated by comparing **Figures 1 and 2** of this plate with **Figure 2** of the preceding plate. The **small circle** in **Figure 2** inscribes two glands that are shown at higher magnification in the **circular inset.** Each one of these glands contains some substance within the lumen. The mucoid character of the substance within one of the glands can be surmised by its blue staining. While not evident in H&E paraffin sections, the epithelial cells also contain glycogen during the secretory stage and, as already mentioned, this becomes part of the secretion. The **arrowheads** indicate stromal cells; some of these cells undergo enlargement late in the secretory stage. These modified stromal cells, called decidual cells, play a role in implantation.

As mentioned previously, if fertilization of the ovum and implantation of the embryonic cells do not occur, the stratum functionale is sloughed off, but the stratum basale remains behind. Associated with this partial loss of endometrium are vascular changes that occur in the stratum functionale but not in the stratum basale. The specialized nonreacting arterial branches that supply the stratum basale are called straight arteries.

KEY

Gl, glands
M, myometrium
SB, stratum basale

SF, stratum functionale
arrowheads, stromal cells

Fig. 1, human, × 25

Fig. 2, × 30; inset, × 120; all human.

PLATE 117

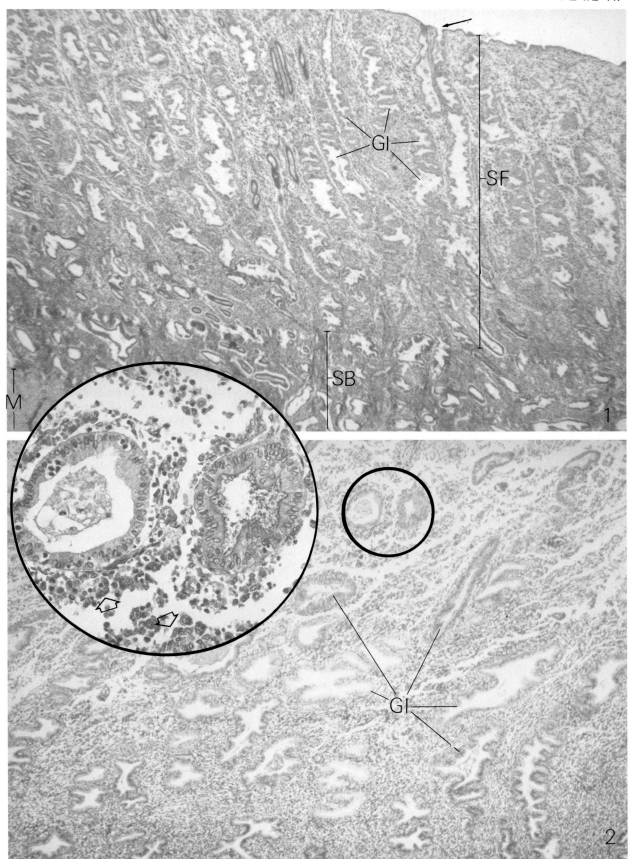

PLATE 118. Cervix

The cervix is the narrow or constricted portion of the uterus, part of which projects into the vagina. A cavity referred to as the cervical canal traverses the cervix and provides a channel connecting the vagina and the uterine cavity. In its general features, the structure of the cervix resembles the remainder of the uterus in that it consists of a mucosa (endometrium) and a myometrium. There are, however, some differences in the mucosa.

The portion of the cervix that projects into the vagina, the portio vaginalis, is represented by the upper two-thirds of **Figure 1**. The lower third of the micrograph reveals the supravaginal portion of the cervix (portio supravaginalis). **Figure 2** shows the supravaginal cervix at a slightly higher level as compared with **Figure 1**. The plane of section in both figures passes through the long axis of the cervical canal. The cervical canal (**CC**) is narrowed and cone-shaped at its two ends. The upper end, the **internal os,** communicates with the uterine cavity and the lower end, the **external os (OS),** communicates with the vagina. (For purposes of orientation it should be realized that only one side of the longitudinal section of the cervix is shown in **Figures 1 and 2** and that the actual specimen, as seen in a section, would present a similar image on the other side of the cervical canal.)

The mucosa (**Muc**) of the cervix differs according to the cavity it faces. The **two small circles** in **Figure 1** delineate representative areas of the mucosa that are shown at higher magnification in **Figures 3 and 4**. The portio vaginalis is surfaced by stratified squamous epithelium (**Fig. 3**). The epithelial-connective tissue junction presents a relatively even contour in contrast to the irregular profile seen in the vagina. In other respects, the epithelium has the same general features as the vaginal epithelium. Another similarity is that the epithelial surface of the portio vaginalis undergoes cyclical changes similar to those of the vagina in response to ovarian hormones. The mucosa of the portio vaginalis, like that of the vagina, is devoid of glands.

The mucosa of the supravaginal portion of the cervix, the portion that includes the cervical canal, is surfaced by columnar epithelium. An abrupt change from stratified squamous epithelium to columnar epithelium occurs at the opening of the

---

KEY

BV, blood vessels
CC, cervical canal
CEp, columnar epithelium
Gl, cervical glands
Muc, mucosa

Os, ostium of the uterus
SSEp, stratified squamous epithelium
asterisk, Figure 5, tangential cut of the epithelial surface

Figs. 1 and 2, human, × 15
Figs. 3 and 4, human, × 240

Fig. 5, human, × 500

---

cervical canal. The **lower circle** in **Figure 1** marks this site. The encircled area is shown at higher magnification in **Figure 4**. Note the abrupt change in the epithelium at the point indicated by the **diamond-shaped marker,** as well as the large number of lymphocytes present in this region (compare with **Fig. 3**).

Figure 2 emphasizes the nature of the cervical glands (**Gl**). The glands differ from those of the uterus in that they extensively branch. They secrete a mucous substance into the cervical canal that serves to lubricate the vagina. The circle in **Figure 2** identifies portions of a gland that is shown at high magnification in **Figure 5**. Note the tall epithelial cells and the lightly staining supranuclear cytoplasm, a reflection of the mucin dissolved out of the cell during tissue preparations. The crowding and change in shape of the nuclei (**asterisk**) seen at the bottom of one of the glands in **Figure 5** is due to a tangential cut through the wall of the gland as it passed out of the plane of section. (It is not uncommon for cervical glands to develop into cysts owing to obstruction in the duct. Such cysts are referred to as Nabothian cysts.)

The endometrium of the cervix does not undergo the cyclical loss of tissue that is characteristic of the body and fundus of the uterus. However, the amount and character of its mucous secretion varies at different times of the uterine cycle. The myometrium forms the major thickness of the cervix. It consists of interweaving bundles of smooth muscle cells situated in a more extensive, continuous network of fibrous connective tissue.

PLATE 118

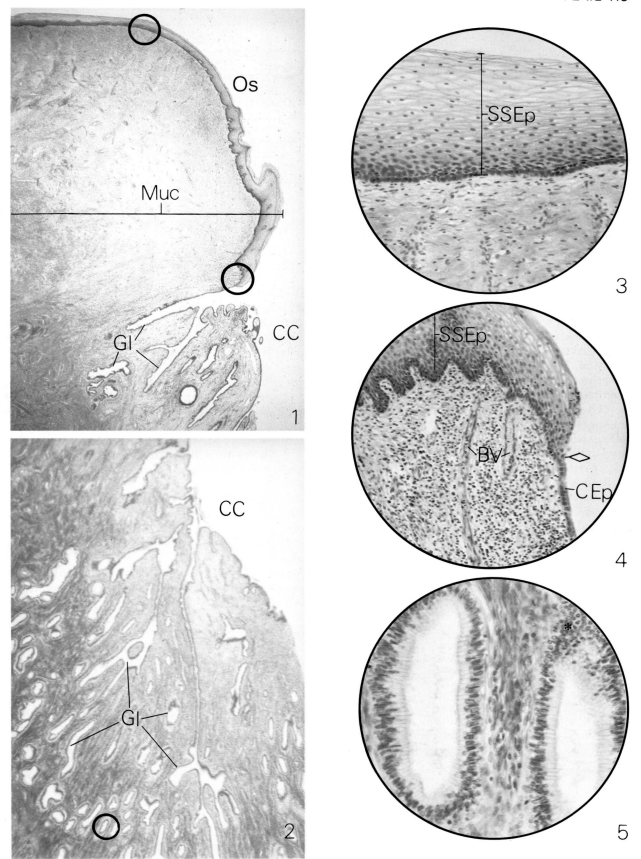

PLATE 119. Placenta I

The placenta is a discoid-shaped organ that serves for the exchange of materials between the fetal and maternal circulations during pregnancy. It develops primarily from embryonic tissue; however, it also has a component derived from the uterus, namely, the stratum basale.

One side of the placenta is embedded in the uterine wall; the other side faces the amniotic cavity that contains the fetus. After birth, the placenta separates from the wall of the uterus and is discharged along with the contiguous membranes of the amniotic cavity.

A section extending from the amniotic surface into the substance of the placenta is shown in **Figure 1.** This includes the amnion **(A),** the chorionic plate **(CP),** and the chorionic villi **(CV).** The amnion consists of a layer of simple cuboidal epithelium and an underlying layer of connective tissue. The connective tissue of the amnion is continuous with the connective tissue of the chorionic plate as a result of their fusion at an earlier time. The plane of fusion, however, is not evident in H&E sections; the separation **(asterisks)** in parts of **Figure 1** in the vicinity of the fusion is an artifact.

The chorionic plate is a thick connective tissue mass that contains the ramifications of the umbilical arteries and vein. These vessels **(BVp)** do not have the distinct organizational features characteristic of arteries and veins; rather, they resemble the vessels of the umbilical cord. While their identification as blood vessels is relatively simple, it is difficult to distinguish which vessels are branches of an umbilical artery and which are tributaries of the vein.[1]

---

[1] The umbilical cord contains two arteries that carry blood to the placenta and a vein that returns blood to the fetus. The umbilical arteries have thick muscular walls. These are arranged as two layers, an inner longitudinal and an outer circular. Elastic membranes are poorly developed in these vessels and, indeed, may be absent. The umbilical vein is similar to the arteries, also having a thick muscular wall arranged as inner longitudinal and outer circular layers. Near its connection to the fetus, the umbilical cord may contain remnants of the allantois and yolk sac.

KEY

A, amnion
BVp, blood vessel in chorionic plate
BVv, blood vessel in chorionic villi
CP, chorionic plate

CV, chorionic villi
DC, decidual cells
SC, stratum basale
asterisk, see text

Fig. 1, human, × 16

Fig. 2, human, × 70 (inset, × 370)

The main substance of the placenta consists of chorionic villi of different sizes (see Plate 120). These emerge from the chorionic plate as large stem villi that branch into increasingly smaller villi. Branches of the umbilical arteries and vein **(BVv)** enter the stem villi and ramify through the branching villous network. Some villi extend from the chorionic plate to the material side of the placenta and make contact with the maternal tissue; these are called ***anchoring villi.*** Other villi, the *free villi,* simply arborize within the substance of the placenta without anchoring onto the maternal side.

The maternal side of the placenta is shown in Figure 2. The ***stratum basale*** **(SB)** is on the right side of the illustration. This is the part of the uterus to which the chorionic villi anchor. Along with the usual connective tissue elements, the stratum basale contains specialized cells called ***decidual cells*** **(DC).** The same cells are shown at higher magnification in the **inset.** Decidual cells are usually found in clusters and they have an epithelial appearance. Because of these features they are easily identified.

Septa from the stratum basale extend into the portion of the placenta that contains the chorionic villi. The septa do not contain the branches of the umbilical vessels and, on this basis, they can frequently be distinguished from stem villi or their branches.

PLATE 119

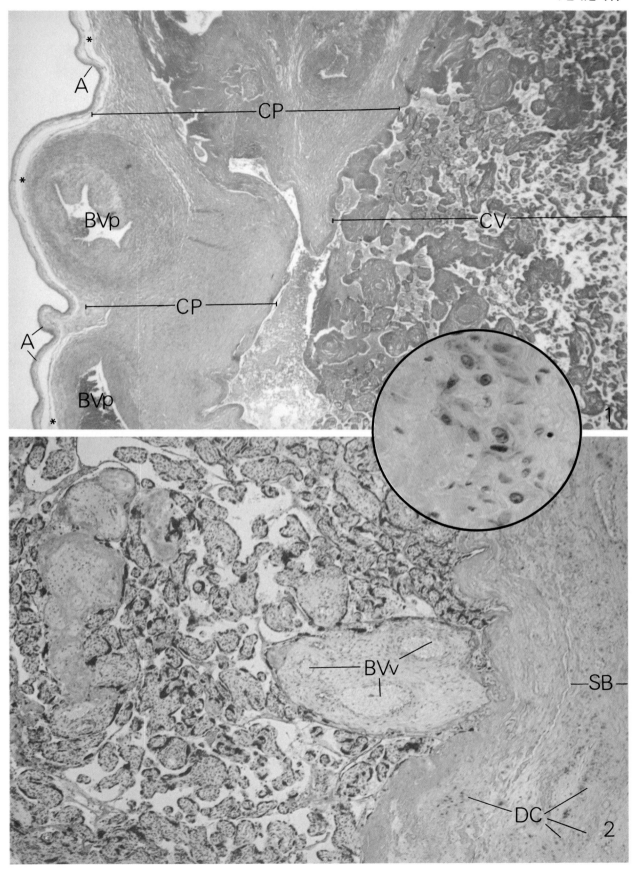

PLATE 120. Placenta II

Chorionic villi consist of a connective tissue core and a two-layered cellular covering. The outermost cellular layer is the syncytiotrophoblast; immediately under this is another layer of cells referred to as cytotrophoblasts. The latter are numerous in the early placenta; however, relatively few are present in the placenta of late pregnancy.

The syncytiotrophoblast covers not only the surface of the chorionic villi, but also extends from the anchoring villi onto the surface of the stratum basalis and onto the placental septa. As a consequence, the entire compartment in which maternal blood is contained is walled by syncytiotrophoblast.

A section through the substance of a full term placenta is shown in the figure. This shows chorionic villi **(CV)** of different size, and the surrounding intervillous space **(IS).** The connective tissue of the villi contains branches and tributaries of the umbilical arteries and vein **(BV).** The smallest villi contain only capillaries; larger villi contain correspondingly larger blood vessels. The intervillous space contains maternal blood. Maternal blood was drained from the specimen before its preparation and, therefore, few maternal blood cells are seen in the section.

The nuclei of the syncytiotrophoblast may be more or less evenly distributed, giving this layer an appearance in H&E sections similar to that of cuboidal epithelium. There are, however, sites where the nuclei are gathered in clusters **(arrowheads),** as well as regions of syncytium relatively free of nuclei **(arrows).** These stretches of syncytium may be so attenuated as to give the impression that the villous surface is devoid of a covering. It is thought that the nuclear clusters and the vicinal cytoplasm may separate from the villus and enter the maternal blood pool.

The syncytiotrophoblast contains microvilli

KEY	
BV, blood vessels	**arrows,** attenuated
CV, chorionic villi	syncytial cytoplasm
Cy, cytotrophoblasts	**asterisk,** tangentially
HC, Hofbauer cells	sectioned villus
IS, intervillous space	
arrowheads, clusters of	
syncytial trophoblast	
nuclei	

Fig., human, × 280

that project into the intervillous space. These may appear as a striated border in paraffin sections; however, they are not always adequately preserved and many not be evident.

In earlier placentas, the cytotrophoblasts **(Cy)** form an almost complete layer of cells immediately deep to the syncytiotrophoblast. Cytotrophoblasts are the source of syncytial trophoblasts. Cell division occurs in the cytotrophoblast layer and the newly formed cells become incorporated into the syncytial layer. In this full-term placenta, only occasional cytotrophoblasts **(Cy)** can be discerned.

Most of the cells within the core of the villus are typical connective tissue fibrocytes and fibroblasts. The nuclei of these cells stain well with hematoxylin; but the cytoplasm cannot be distinguished from the delicate intercellular fibrous material. Other cells have a recognizable amount of cytoplasm surrounding the nucleus. These are considered to be phagocytic and are named Hofbauer cells. The Hofbauer cells **(HC)** shown in the figure do not contain any distinctive cytoplasmic inclusions.

PLATE 120

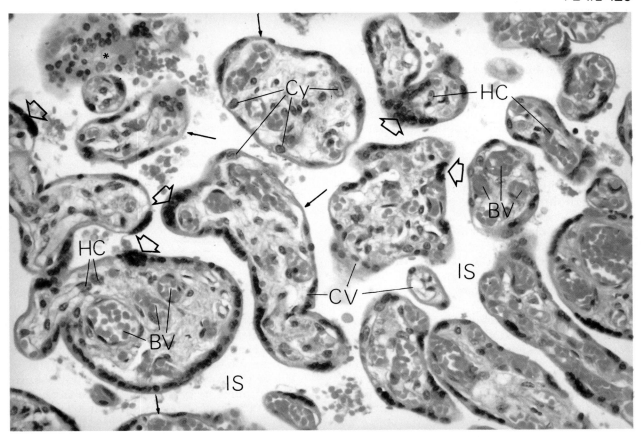

PLATE 121. Vagina

The vagina is a fibromuscular tube that forms the opening of the female reproductive tract to the exterior. The wall of the vagina (**Fig. 1**) consists of three layers: a mucous membrane, a muscular layer, and an outer adventitia. The mucous membrane, in turn, consists of stratified squamous epithelium (**Ep**) and an underlying connective tissue (**CT**). The boundary between the two is readily identified, owing to the more intense staining of the deep portion of the epithelium. Connective tissue papillae project into the undersurface of the epithelium, giving the epithelial-connective tissue junction an uneven appearance. The papillae (**arrows**) may be cut obliquely or in cross-section, and appear as connective tissue islands within the epithelium.

The muscular layer (**Mus**) of the vaginal wall is made up of smooth muscle. The smooth muscle is arranged in two ill-defined layers, the outer one being somewhat longitudinal. The area marked by the **circle** in the upper left of **Figure 1** is shown at higher magnification in the **inset** to illustrate the smooth muscle cells. They are organized as small interlacing bundles surrounded by connective tissue. At the lower end of the vagina, the opening is surrounded by the erectile tissue of the bulb of the vestibule. A relatively thin layer of striated muscle fibers, the bulbospongiosus muscle, lies just external to the bulb of the vestibule.

The **rectangle** in **Figure 1** marks an area of vaginal epithelium and connective tissue that is examined at higher magnification in **Figure 2**. The epithelium is characteristically thick. Although keratohyaline granules may be present in the superficial cells, keratinization (in the human) does not occur. In this connection, nuclei can be observed throughout the entire thickness of the vaginal epithelium.

One of the features of vaginal epithelium that aids in its identification is that, except for the deepest layers, the cells have an empty appearance. This is due, in part, to the fact that the cells accumulate glycogen as they migrate toward the surface, and in the preparation of routine H&E sections, the glycogen is lost.

Vaginal epithelium is influenced by ovarian hormones and undergoes cyclical changes that correspond to the ovarian cycle. In rodents, these changes are manifest by marked alterations in the cells. In the human, however, the epithelial changes are less pronounced, but nevertheless evident. For example, the amount of glycogen increases under the influence of estrogen; moreover, the desquamation, which the epithelium continuously undergoes, increases under the influence of progesterone.

The connective tissue immediately under the vaginal epithelium contains large numbers of cells, most of which are lymphocytes (**L**). The lymphocytes are characterized by their deep-staining, round nuclei. The number of lymphocytes varies during the ovarian cycle.

Lymphocytes invade the epithelium around the time of menstruation and they appear along with the epithelial cells in vaginal smears. The connective tissue includes large amounts of elastic material in addition to collagen fibers; however, this is not evident in H&E sections. The connective tissue also characteristically contains a large number of blood vessels (**BV**).

Histological study of the vagina should take into account the following points: (1) the epithelium does not keratinize and, except for the deepest layers, the cells appear to be empty in routine H&E sections; (2) the mucous membrane contains neither glands nor a muscularis mucosae; and (3) the muscle is chiefly smooth and not well ordered. (In contrast, the muscle of the oral cavity, pharynx, and upper part of the esophagus is striated; in its more distal portion, where the esophagus contains smooth muscle, it can be easily distinguished from the vagina by the presence of a muscularis mucosae.)

KEY

BV, blood vessels
CT, connective tissue
EP, epithelium
L, lymphocytes

Mus, muscular layer
arrows, connective tissue papillae

Fig. 1, human, × 40 (inset, × 250)

Fig. 2, human, × 180

PLATE 121

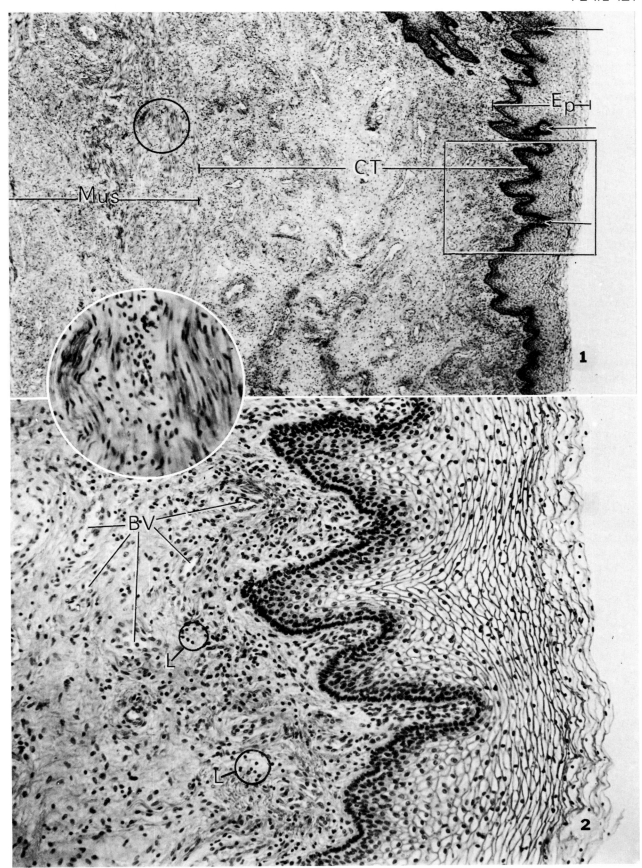

Ep

CT

Mus

1

BV

L

L

2

PLATE 122. Mammary Glands

The mammary glands are branched tubuloalveolar glands that develop from the epidermis and come to lie in the subcutaneous tissue (superficial fascia). They begin to develop at puberty in the female, but do not reach a full functional state until after pregnancy. The glands also develop in the male at puberty; however, the development is limited and the glands usually remain in a stabilized state.

Figure 1 is a section through an inactive gland. The parenchyma is sparse and consists mainly of duct elements. Several ducts (**D**) are shown in the center of the field. A small lumen can be seen in each. The ducts are surrounded by a loose connective tissue [**CT(L), Fig. 2**]. and together the ducts and surrounding connective tissue constitute a lobule. Two lobules (**L**) are bracketed in **Figure 1.** Beyond the lobule, the connective tissue is more dense [**CT(D)**]. The two connective tissues can be distinguished at the low magnification of **Figure 1.**

Additional details are evident at higher magnification in **Figure 2.** In distinguishing between the loose and dense connective tissue, it should be recalled that both extracellular and cellular features show differences (**Fig. 2** and **inset**). Note the thicker collagenous fibers in the dense connective tissue in contrast to the much thinner fibers of the loose connective tissue. The loose connective tissue, contains far more cells per unit area and a greater variety of cell types. **Figure 2** shows a cluster of lymphocytes (**L**), and at still higher magnification (**inset**) one can identify plasma cells (**P**) and individual lymphocytes (**L**). Both plasma cells and lymphocytes are cells with a rounded shape, but plasma cells are larger and show more cytoplasm. In addition, regions of plasma cell cytoplasm display basophilia. Elongate nuclei in spindle-shaped cells belong to fibroblasts. In contrast, while the cell types in the dense connective tissue may also be

diversified, a simple examination of equal areas of loose and dense connective tissue will show relatively fewer cells by far in the dense connective tissue. Characteristically, the dense connective tissue contains numerous aggregates of adipocytes (**A**).

The epithelial cells within the resting lobule are regarded as being chiefly duct elements. It is usually found that alveoli are not present; however, their precursors are represented as cellular thickenings of the duct wall. The epithelium of the resting lobule is cuboidal and, in addition, myoepithelial cells are present. Re-examination of the **inset** shows a thickening of the epithelium in one location, presumably the precursor of an alveolus, and myoepithelial cells (**M**) at the base of the epithelium. As elsewhere, the myoepithelial cells are on the epithelial side of the basement membrane. During pregnancy, the glands begin to proliferate. This can be thought of as a dual process in which ducts proliferate and alveoli spring from the ducts.

KEY

A, adipocytes
CT(D), dense connective tissue
CT(L), loose connective tissue
D, ducts

L, Fig. 1, lobules
L, Fig. 2 and inset, lymphocytes
M, myoepithelial cells
P, plasma cells

Fig. 1, × 80

Fig. 2, × 200; inset, × 400; all human

PLATE 122

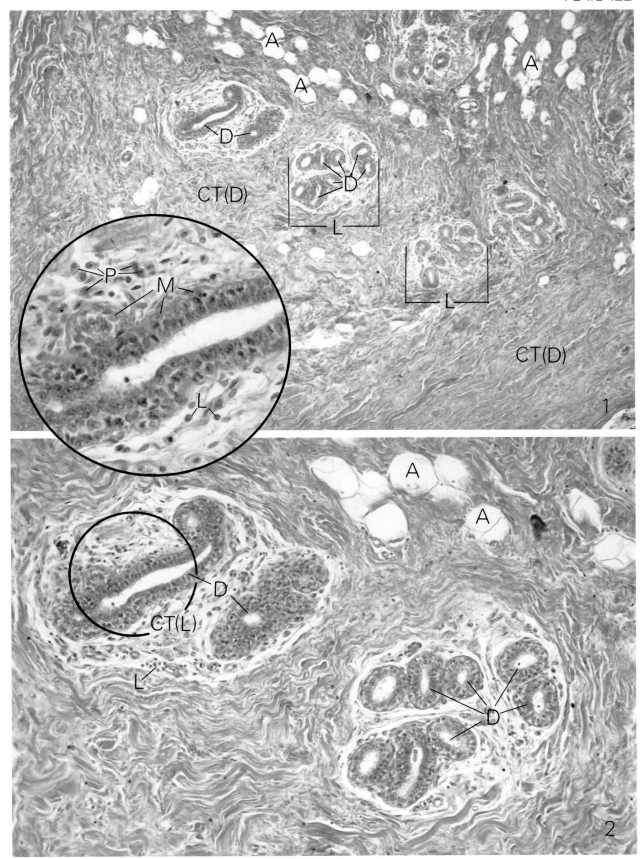

PLATE 123. Mammary Gland, Proliferative

Whereas the development of the duct elements in the mammary gland is well marked during the early proliferative period, the development of the alveolar elements becomes conspicuous at a later time. **Figure 1** shows several lobules **(L)** at a later stage of proliferation than is shown in the preceding plate. Distinct alveoli **(A)** can now be recognized. These are all joined to a duct **(D),** although the connections are usually not seen in a two-dimensional section. Lobules are separated by dense connective tissue septa **(S),** and some ducts can be recognized as being in an interlobular location. Although alveolar development is well under way **(Fig. 1),** some regions of the gland are still in a relatively early stage of proliferation. For example, the **inset (Fig. 1)** shows where epithelial sprouting is occurring along the length of a duct **(arrowheads).**

A higher magnification of one of the proliferating lobules is in **Figure 2.** Numerous alveoli **(A)** are evident. The alveoli consist of a single layer of cuboidal epithelium as well as myoepithelial cells. A small amount of precipitate is located in the lumen of some of the alveoli. This represents the early secretory activity of the cells.

The duct **(D)** through which the alveoli will discharge their product is shown on the left, almost

like a stalk. It can be recognized because of its location and its elongated profile. Some of the flattened nuclei that are at the epithelial-connective tissue junction of the duct belong to myoepithelial cells.

The connective tissue **(CT)** surrounding the alveoli is loose and contains delicate collagenous fibers and large numbers of round cells **(arrows).** The identity of these cells is difficult to establish at this magnification, though most are probably lymphocytes.

KEY	
A, alveoli	arrowheads, epithelial
CT, connective tissue	sprouts
D, duct	arrows, round
L, lobule	connective tissue cells
S, septa	
Fig. 1, human, × 65 (inset, × 160)	Fig. 2, human, × 160

PLATE 123

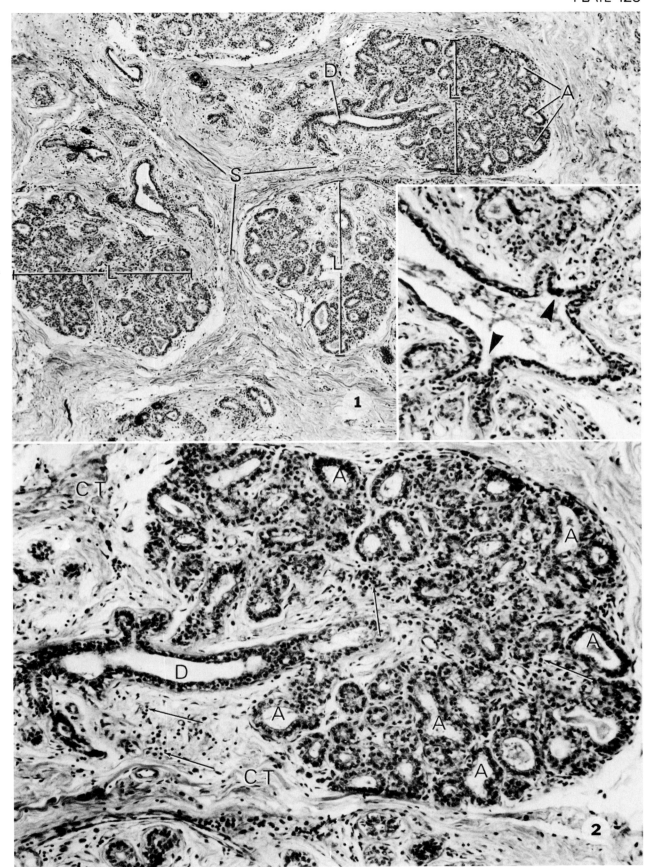

PLATE 124. Mammary Gland, Lactating

The lactating mammary gland is characterized by the presence of large numbers of alveoli (**Fig. 1**). Many of these appear as oval or spherical profiles and, in this respect, on cursory examination, the gland is easy to confuse with the thyroid gland. However, all of the alveoli in the mammary gland are joined to a duct and often the place where several alveoli open into a central channel can be seen. These connections represent branchings of a terminal duct system. The presence of connected alveoli (**asterisks**) enable one to identify the lactating mammary gland and distinguish it from thyroid tissue even if the duct elements are not conspicuous. Sections of mammary blands usually include duct elements, but the small ducts are difficult to identify because they resemble the alveoli.

A large duct (**D**), easily recognized by its size, is in the upper left of the figure. A number of connective tissue septa (**S**) separate the alveoli of neighboring lobules. Large blood vessels (**BV**) are within the connective tissue septa.

Figure 2 shows several alveoli at higher magnification. The alveoli of lactating mammary glands are made up of cuboidal epithelium and myoepithelial cells. Frequently, some precipitated product can be seen within the lumen of the alveolus. Only a small amount of connective tissue separates the neighboring alveoli. Capillaries (**Cap**) can be seen in this connective tissue.

Figure 3 is a special preparation showing some of the lipid that is present in the mammary secretion. The lipid appears as the black spheres of various size within the alveolar lumen as well as within most of the cells. In its production, the lipid first appears as small droplets within the cells. These droplets become larger and ultimately they are discharged into the alveolar lumen.

The lymphatic vessels of the mammary glands, which are important clinically, are not usually evident in histological sections.

KEY

BV, blood vessels
Cap, capillaries
D, duct

S, septa
asterisks, branchings of
  terminal duct system

Fig. 1, human, × 160

Figs. 2 and 3, human, × 640

PLATE 124

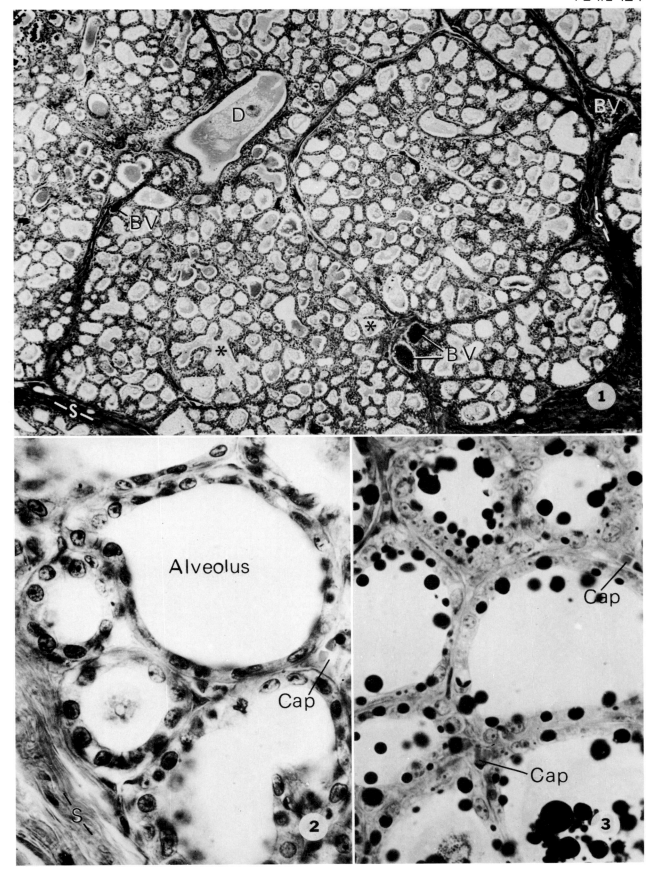

The paired eyes are complex, highly developed organs that provide us with sense of sight. Functionally, the eyes are often compared to a simple camera with a lens to capture and focus the light and film to record the image. In the eye, the *lens* concentrates and focuses light on the *retina.* Photoreceptors in the retina detect the intensity and color of the light striking them and encode the various parameters for transmission to the brain. Form and motion reflect the pattern and duration of the stimulation of the photoreceptors as the image is interpreted by the brain. Since vertebrates have evolved a pair of eyes, two different images are sent to the brain. In the evolution of many vertebrates including primates, the visual fields of the eyes have come to overlap and complex neural mechanisms have developed to coordinate the movements of the eyes and to perform the interpretation of the slightly different images. Binocular vision enables us to perceive depth and distance as in a three-dimensional image.

The study of the eye may be divided into the analysis of the eye itself, its adjacent structures, and the more distant structures that are functionally related to the eye. The eye is an easily accessible organ whose structure is the focal point of the field of ophthalmology. The ophthalmologist routinely assesses the details of the structure of the eye that can be revealed by the slit-lamp and the ophthalmoscope. A basic understanding of the structure of the eye is essential to the medical student who will routinely evaluate the eye as part of the physical examination.

GENERAL STRUCTURE OF THE EYE

The eye measures nearly 2.5 cm in diameter and lies suspended by six extrinsic ocular muscles in the (periorbital) fat that largely fills the *orbit,* a four-sided, pyramid-shaped space bordered by bones of the skull. The slightest pull of the extrinsic muscles that insert into the eye will rotate it about its own center. The eye is separated by only a few millimeters from the converging bony walls of the orbit that provide protection on all but its anterior surface, where the convex corneal window lies.

Layers of the Eye

The eye consists essentially of three separate concentric layers (Fig. 23.1): (1) an outer or fibrous layer, the *corneoscleral coat,* that consists of the *sclera* and the *cornea;* (2) the middle layer or vascular coat, the *uvea,* that consists of the *choroid, ciliary body,* and *iris;* and (3) the innermost layer, the *retina,* that consists of an outer pigment epithelium and an inner neural retina. Anteriorly, these layers are modified to admit and regulate the passage of light. The neural retina communicates with the central nervous system through the *optic nerve.* The internal cavity of the eye is filled with a transparent jelly, the *vitreous body,* that, along with the coverings of the eye, serves to maintain shape and turgor pressure.

Corneosclera. This layer, consisting of the transparent *cornea* over its anterior one-sixth and the white opaque *sclera* (Gr. *scleros,* hard) over its posterior five-sixths (Fig. 23.1a), is composed of dense fibrous connective tissue. The sclera, constituting the "white" of the eye (rather bluish in children and yellowing in old age), is protective in function and provides attachment for the extrinsic muscle of the eye. The surface of the eye has an anterior prominence or convexity in the window-like corneal region. The corneosclera encloses the

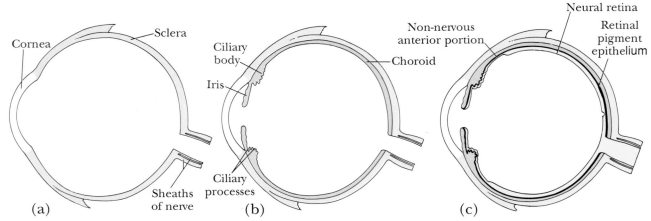

Figure 23.1. Schematic diagram of the layers of the eye. The layers are organized in three separate concentric layers: an outer supporting layer, the *corneoscleral coat* (a), a middle vascular coat, the *uvea* (b), and an inner photosensitive layer, the *retina* (c). (Modified from Cormack DH: In *Ham's Histology*, 9th ed. Philadelphia, JB Lippincott, 1987.)

inner two layers except posteriorly where it is penetrated by the optic nerve.

Uvea. This layer consists principally of the *choroid,* a nutrient vascular bed supporting the retina (Fig. 23.1b). The choroid has an intense dark brown color due to the presence of a large amount of the pigment melanin, which absorbs scattered or reflected light and minimizes glare within the eye. The choroid, containing many venous plexuses and layers of capillaries, is firmly attached to the retina; however, it can be stripped easily from the sclera. The anterior rim of the uveal layer continues forward where it forms the *ciliary body* and *iris.* The ciliary body is a ring-like thickening of the anterior end of the uvea that extends inward at the corneoscleral junction. Within the ciliary body is the ciliary (intraocular) muscle that is responsible for lens accommodation. The smooth muscle of the ciliary muscle pulls on the periphery of the lens to change its shape in order to bring light rays from different distances to focus on the retina. The iris, a thin continuation of the uveal layer from the ciliary body, is a contractile diaphragm that extends over the anterior surface of the lens. The iris also contains smooth muscle and melanin-containing pigment cells scattered among the connective tissue. The central circular aperture of the iris is the pupil, that appears black because one looks through the lens toward the heavily pigmented back of the eye. The size of the pupil varies to control the amount of light that passes through the lens to reach the retina.

Retina. The *retina* is a thin, delicate layer consisting of two discrete subdivisions or layers (Fig. 23.1c): (1) the innermost layer of the retina, known as the *neural retina,* contains light sensitive

receptors and complex neuronal networks that encode the visual information and send the information to the brain via impulses conveyed through the optic nerve and (2) the outer layer of the retina, known as the *retinal pigment epithelium,* consists of a simple cuboidal pigment epithelium that is associated with the neural layer. Externally, the retina is associated with the choroid; internally, it is associated with the vitreous body. The neural retina largely consists of *photoreceptor cells,* called retinal *rods* and *cones,* together with interneurons.

Chambers of the Eye

The basic components of the eye include a wall composed of three concentric layers that are described above and a biconvex transparent lens held in place by a circular system of fibers, the *zonule of Zinn.* These structures define the boundaries of the three compartments contained within the eye (Fig. 23.2): (1) the *anterior compartment* occupying the space between the cornea and the iris and lens; (2) the *posterior compartment* bordered by the iris, ciliary processes, zonular attachments, and the lens; and (3) the *vitreous space* lying behind the lens and bordered posterolaterally by the retina. The *vitreous body,* a transparent jelly-like substance containing hyaluronic acid, widely dispersed collagen fibrils, and other proteins, fills the vitreous space.

Refractile Media

As light rays pass through the components of the eye to reach the photoreceptors of the retina, they are refracted in order to bring them to focus. Four transparent components of the eye, that alter

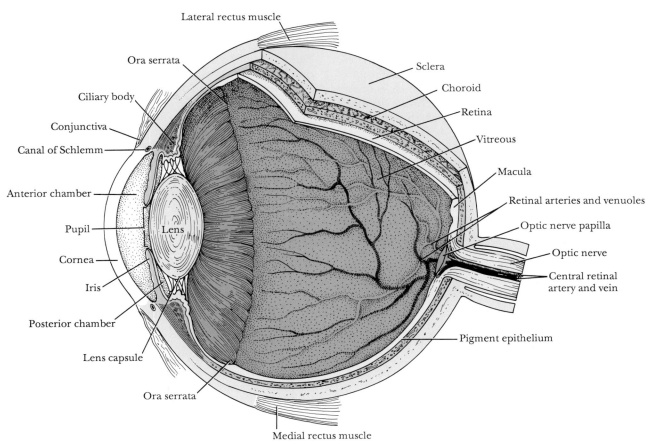

Lateral rectus muscle

Ora serrata

Ciliary body

Conjunctiva

Canal of Schlemm

Anterior chamber

Pupil

Lens

Cornea

Iris

Posterior chamber

Lens capsule

Ora serrata

Medial rectus muscle

Sclera

Choroid

Retina

Vitreous

Macula

Retinal arteries and venuoles

Optic nerve papilla

Optic nerve

Central retinal artery and vein

Pigment epithelium

Figure 23.2. Schematic diagram illustrating the internal structures of the human eye. (Modified from an original drawing by Paul Peck in: *The Anatomy of the Eye*, Lederle Laboratories).

the path of the light rays, are often described as the ***refractile (or dioptric) media*** of the eye. These components are: (1) the ***cornea,*** the anterior window of the eye; (2) the ***aqueous humor,*** a watery fluid located in the anterior chamber immediately behind the cornea and in the posterior chamber; (3) the ***lens,*** a transparent crystalline structure suspended from the inner surface of the ciliary body; and (4) the ***vitreous body (or humor).***

The cornea is the chief refractive element of the eye. It has a refractive index of 1.376; air, an index of 1.0. The lens is second in importance to the cornea in the refraction of light rays. The unique importance of the lens is that, due to its elasticity, it can undergo a slight shape change in response to the pull of the ciliary muscles. The shape change is important in accommodation for proper focusing on near objects. The aqueous humor and the vitreous humor have only minor roles in the refraction of light rays. An important role of the aqueous humor is to provide necessary nutrients to two avascular structures, the lens and inner region of the cornea. Aqueous humor contains a

relatively high concentration of bicarbonate, sodium, and chloride ions and free amino acids and ascorbic acid. The vitreous body, while serving primarily as a supporting structure for the lens and iris, permits light to pass freely from the lens to the photoreceptors of the retina.

Blood Supply of the Eye

Two essentially independent arterial systems, arising from the ophthalmic artery, supply blood to the eye. One system, which can be visualized with an ophthalmoscope, supplies the optic nerve and inner surface of the retina. The second system supplies the outer coverings of the eye and the vascular layer. The outer portions of the retina, including the photoreceptor cells and the outer pigment layer, receive blood from the choriocapillary layer of the vascular layer.

Development of the Eye

The tissues of the eye are derived from three sources: neuroectoderm, surface ectoderm, and mesoderm. The developing eyes are first evident as shallow grooves, the *optic sulci* or *grooves,* in the neural folds at the cranial end of the human embryo at about 22 days. As the neural tube closes, the paired grooves form outpocketing called *optic vesicles* (Fig. 23.3A). As each optic vesicle grows laterally, the connection to the forebrain becomes constricted into an optic stalk and the overlying surface ectoderm thickens and forms a lens placode. As development continues, there is concomitant invagination of both the optic vesicles and the lens placodes. The invagination of the optic vesicle results in the formation of the double layer *optic cup* (Fig. 23.3B). The inner layer becomes the neural retina; the outer layer becomes the retinal pigment epithelium. Invagination of the central re-

gion of each lens placode results in the formation of the *lens vesicles.* By the 5th week of development, the lens vesicle loses its contact with the surface ectoderm and comes to lie in the mouth of the optic cup. Grooves, in which blood vessels derived from mesenchyme form, develop along the inferior surface of each optic cup and stalk. The grooves, known as the *choroid fissures,* enable the hyaloid artery to reach the inner chamber of the eye to supply the inner chamber of the optic cup, the lens vesicle, and mesenchyme within the optic cup. The hyaloid vein returns blood from these structures. The distal portions of the hyaloid vessels degenerate, but the proximal portions remain as the *central artery* and *vein of the retina.* By the end of the 7th week, the edges of the choroid fissue

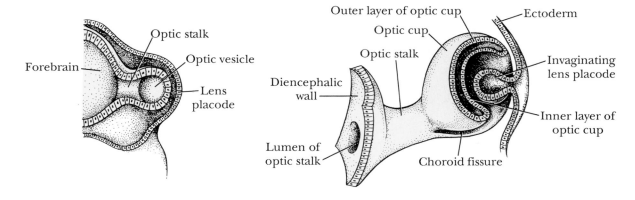

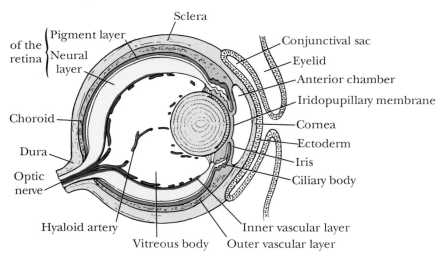

Figure 23.3. Schematic drawings illustrating the development of the eye. In **A,** for forebrain and developing optic vesicles are shown as they are seen in a 4-mm embryo. In **B,** the bilayered optic cup and invaginating lens vesicle are shown as they would be seen in a 7.5-mm embryo. The optic stalk connects the developing eye to the brain. In **C,** the eye is shown as it would ap-

pear in a 15-week fetus. All the layers of the eye are established and the hyaloid artery can be seen traversing the vitreous body from the optic disc to the posterior surface of the lens. (Modified from Sadler, *Langman's Medical Embryology,* 5th ed. Baltimore, Williams & Wilkins, 1985.)

TABLE 23.1. Embryonic Origins of the Individual Structures of the Eye

SOURCE	DERIVATIVE
Surface ectoderm	Lens; epithelium of the cornea, conjunctiva, and lacrimal gland and its drainage system
Neural ectoderm	Vitreous body (derived partly from neural ectoderm of the optic cup and partly from mesenchyme); epithelium of the retina, iris, and ciliary body; muscle of pupillary sphincter and dilator; optic nerve
Mesoderm	Sclera; stroma of the cornea, conjunctiva, ciliary body, iris, and choroid; extraocular muscles, eyelids (except epithelium and conjunctiva), hyaloid system (most of which degenerates before birth), coverings of the optic nerve; connective tissue and blood vessels of the eye, bony orbit, and vitreous

fuse and form a round opening, the future pupil, enclosing the lens vesicle.

The outer layer of the optic cup forms a single layer of pigmented cells. Pigmentation begins at about the end of the 5th week. The inner layer undergoes complicated differentiation into the outer nine layers of the retina. The photoreceptor (rod and cone) cells, as well as the bipolar, amacrine, and ganglion cells and nerve fibers are present by the 7th month. The macular depression begins to develop during the 8th month and is not complete until about 6 months after birth.

During the 3rd month, growth of the optic cup results in extension of its rim, the future iris, lying in front of the lens as a double row epithelium. The mesoderm located external to this region becomes the stroma of the iris. Both epithelial layers of the iris become pigmented, in contrast to the ciliary body where only the outer layer is pigmented. In fair-skinned individuals, pigment is usually not present at birth, so that the iris is light blue in color. The dilator and sphincter pupillary muscles develop during the 6th month as derivatives of the neuroectoderm of the outer layer of the optic cup.

Components of the middle (uveal) and external (corneoscleral) layers of the eye are derivatives of the surrounding mesoderm. The cornea consists of: (1) an outer layer derived from surface ectoderm; (2) the stroma, or substantia propria, derived from mesoderm and continuous with the sclera; and (3) an inner epithelial layer formed by vacuolization of the mesoderm bordering the anterior chamber of the eye. The embryonic origins of individual eye structures are summarized in Table 23.1.

EXTERNAL LAYERS—CORNEOSCLERA

Cornea

The cornea forms the transparent anterior pole of the eye (see Figs. 23.1 and 23.2, and Atlas section, Plate 125). Its radius of curvature is slightly less than the eye as a whole causing it to protrude anteriorly. It is only 0.5 mm thick at its center and about 1 mm thick peripherally.

Three cell layers, that are quite distinct both in appearance and origin, are recognized in the cornea. These layers are separated from one another by two important lamellae that appear structureless when viewed with the light microscope. Thus, collectively, the five layers of the cornea that are seen in a transverse section are: the corneal epithelium, Bowman's membrane, the stroma, Descemet's membrane, and the endothelium (see Atlas section, Plate 128).

Corneal Epithelium. The corneal epithelium is nonkeratinized stratified squamous and consists of five or six layers of cells. It measures about 50 μm in average thickness and is continuous with the conjunctival epithelium that overlies the adjacent sclera. The corneal cells adhere to neighboring cells via desmosomes that are present in short interdigitating processes. The cornea has remarkable regenerative capacity with a turnover time of approximately 7 days. As is typical of other stratified epithelium, such as that in the skin or conjunctiva, the cells proliferate from a columnar basal layer and become flat as they approach the surface. The basal layer consists of low columnar cells with oval nuclei; the intermediate layer (two or three cells in thickness), of polyhedral "wing cells" with horizontally flattened nuclei; and the surface layer (one or two cells thick), of very flat nonkeratinized cells that have retained their nuclei. As the cells migrate to the surface, the cytoplasmic organelles gradually disappear, indicating a progressive decline in metabolic activity.

The numerous free nerve endings present in the cornea provide it with extreme sensitivity to touch. Stimulation of these nerves elicits blinking of the eyelids and the flow of tears. Microvilli present on the surface epithelial cells help retain the tear film over the entire corneal surface. Drying of the corneal surface may cause it to ulcerate. Minor injuries of the corneal surface heal rapidly by the migration of cells to fill the defect.

Bowman's Membrane. The corneal epithelium rests on a rather homogeneous, faintly fibrillar lamina, approximately 8 μm in thickness, called *Bowman's membrane* or *layer*. With transmission electron microscopy, randomly oriented collagen fibrils with a diameter of about 18 nm have been identified. Bowman's membrane does not extend into the sclera; it ends abruptly at the limbus. Bowman's membrane offers resistance to infection and other injury; however, it does not regenerate. Therefore, if it is damaged, an opaque scar will result and vision will be impaired.

Substantia Propria. The *substantia propria* or *stroma,* constituting 90% of the corneal thickness, is composed of about 60 thin lamellae of parallel bundles of collagen fibrils and associated fibroblasts. In each successive layer, the direction of the collagen fibrils changes. The fibrils, measuring approximately 23 nm in diameter, cross at various angles in the successive layers, forming a crystalline-like lattice in a ground substance that contains sulfated glycosaminoglycans (chiefly, keratan sulfate with some chondroitin sulfate) covalently bound to protein known as *corneal proteoglycans.*

In contrast to the sclera, the cornea lacks any vessels or pigments. Scattered between the lamellae are slender flattened fibroblasts and a number of lymphocytes that migrate from vessels located at the corneal limbus. During an inflammatory response involving the cornea, enormous numbers of neutrophilic leukocytes and lymphocytes migrate between the lamellae of the stroma.

Descement's Membrane. *Descemet's membrane* (the posterior elastic membrane) is a 5- to 10-μm thick, homogeneous acellular layer that separates the substantia propria from the endothelium. It is produced by the corneal endothelial cells. In common with Bowman's membrane, Descemet's membrane serves as a barrier for the spread of infections but (unlike Bowman's membrane), it readily regenerates after injury. Descemet's membrane extends peripherally beneath the sclera as a meshwork known as the *pectinate ligament*. Strands from the pectinate ligament insert into the ciliary muscle and the sclera.

Corneal Endothelium. The *corneal endothelium* is a single layer of flattened granular polygonal shaped cells with centrally located nuclei. This layer is continuous with the endothelium that covers the anterior surface of the iris. The cells are joined on their inner aspect to neighboring cells by a zona occludens. The endothelial cells function both in the transport of water from the cornea and in the diffusion of nutrients from the aqueous humor to the avascular cornea. In order for the cornea to remain transparent, water (as tissue fluid) must be constantly removed from the stroma. Evidence clearly suggests that the endothelial cells are responsible for this transport process. Injury to this layer may result in corneal edema, local clouding of the cornea, or if severe enough, corneal opacity.

Sclera

The *sclera* consists of dense connective tissue made of flat collagen bundles that pass in various directions in parallel to the surface, fine networks of elastic fibers interspersed between the collagen bundles, a moderate amount of ground substance, and relatively few flat, elongated fibroblasts. It is pierced by four vortex veins (just posterior to the equator between the rectus muscles), the anterior ciliary nerves and vessels just behind the corneoscleral junction, the long and short ciliary nerves and vessels, and posteriorly at the lamina cribrosa by the optic nerve (Fig. 23.2). The sclera is 1 mm thick posteriorly, 0.3 to 0.4 mm thick at the equator, and 0.7 mm thick at the corneoscleral margin or "limbus." The opacity of the sclera is primarily due to its higher water content as compared to the cornea.

Three rather ill-defined layers of fibers have been defined in the sclera. The *episclera* is the external layer of loose fibrous tissue containing fine capillaries and located adjacent to the periorbital fat. Fine strands from the episclera connect it with the investing fascia of the eye or *sclera proper* (also called *Tenon's capsule*), which is composed of a dense network of collagen fibers. *Tenon's (or the episcleral) space* is located between episclera and Tenon's capsule. This space and the surrounding periorbital fat allow the eye to rotate freely within the orbit. The tendons of the extraocular muscles, whose fibers differ from those of the sclera in being parallel and not interlacing, attach to Tenon's capsule. The orientation of the collagen fibers in the sclera is determined by the intraocular pressure and the pull of the muscles. A third layer, the *lamina fusca,* is identified on the inner aspect of the sclera adjacent to the choroid. Here the fiber bundles are smaller and an increasing number of pigment cells and elastic fibers are present.

The *corneoscleral junction* or *limbus cornea* is a 1-mm wide transitional zone between cornea and sclera. At this point, Bowman's membrane ends abruptly and the overlying epithelium thickens from the five cell layers of the cornea to the 10 to 12 cell layers of the conjunctiva. There is also a transition at this point as the corneal lamellae becomes less regular, as they merge with the circular and oblique bundles of collagen fibers of the sclera. There is also an abrupt transition form the avascular cornea to the well-vascularized sclera.

It is the limbus region that contains the apparatus for the outflow of aqueous humor. In the stromal layer, endothelium-lined channels, called the trabecular meshwork (or **spaces of Fontana**), merge to form the **canal of Schlemm,** a canal that encircles the eye (Fig. 23.4). The aqueous humor is produced by the ciliary processes that border the lens in the posterior chamber of the eye. The fluid passes from the posterior chamber into the anterior chamber through the valve-like potential opening between the iris and lens. The fluid then passes through the openings in the trabecular meshwork in the limbus region as it continues on its course to enter the canal of Schlemm. Collecting trunks in the sclera, called **aqueous veins** because they convey aqueous humor instead of blood, transports the aqueous humor to veins located in the sclera.

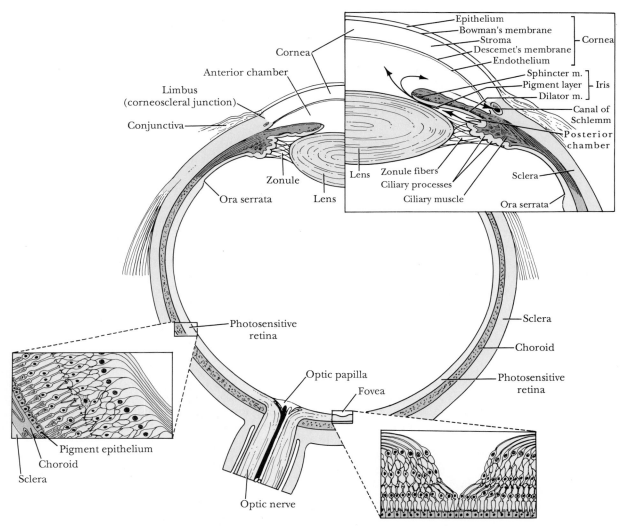

Figure 23.4. Schematic diagram of the structure of the eye. The upper enlargement depicts the anterior and posterior chambers in more detail and illustrates the direction of the flow of aqueous humor. The lower enlargements illustrate the organization of the cells of the retina in the retina proper (on the **left**) and the fovea (on the **right**). (Modified from Ham AW, Cormack DH: In *Ham's Histology,* 8th ed. Philadelphia, JB Lippincott, 1979.)

Glaucoma is a clinical condition resulting from the impedance of the normal drainage of aqueous humor within the eye. Nourishment of the internal tissues of the eye, particularly the retina, is dependent upon the diffusion of oxygen and nutrients from the intraocular vessels. In order to have normal flow of blood through these vessels (including the capillaries and veins), the hydrostatic pressure within the vessels must exceed the intraocular pressure. If the drainage of the aqueous humor is impeded, the intraocular pressure becomes elevated because the coverings of the eye do not allow the wall to expand. This increased pressure interferes with normal retinal nourishment and function. Visual deficits associated with glaucoma include blurring of vision, impaired dark adaptation, and halos around lights (symptoms that indicate loss of normal retinal function). If the condition is not treated, the retina will be permanently damaged and blindness will occur. Treatments are directed at decreasing the rate of production of aqueous humor or at eliminating the cause of the obstruction of normal drainage.

VASCULAR LAYER OR UVEA

The intermediate coat of the eye is a vascular layer, called the uvea or uveal tract (Fig. 23.1). It consists of the *iris, ciliary body,* and *choroid.* The latter two structures are adherent to the sclera. In contrast, the iris is separated from the overlying cornea by the anterior compartment of the eye. As was explained, the posterior chamber is a very shallow space bordered by the iris, ciliary processes, zonular attachments, and the lens.

Iris

The iris is the anterior continuation of the uveal layer that forms a contractile diaphragm over the anterior surface of the lens (see Atlas section, Plate 127). The iris arises from the anterior border of the ciliary body, that is attached to the sclera about 2 mm posterior to the corneoscleral junction. The pupil is the central aperture of this thin disc. The iris lies against the lens and is pushed slightly forward as it constantly changes in size in response to light intensity. The size of the pupil is controlled by the contraction of the pupillary sphincter or dilator muscles (comparable to the varible aperture of a camera) so that only the appropriate amount of light enters the eye. The sphincter pupillae is a circular band of smooth muscle located at the pupillary margin. It is supplied by parasympathetic fibers associated with the oculomotor nerve (cranial nerve III). Contraction of the sphincter pupillae, in response to bright light, causes the pupil to diminish in size. (Failure of the pupil to respond when light is shined into the eye—"pupil fixed and dilated"—is a sign of the lack of nerve or brain function). The dilator pupillae consists of less well-defined thin sheets of smooth muscle that lie near the posterior border of the iris and are radially oriented. Contraction of these muscles, which are innervated by sympathetic nerve fibers arising from the superior cervical ganglion, cause the pupil to increase in size as the pupillary margin is drawn laterally.

When viewing the iris at the gross anatomical level, one is struck by its vibrant coloration in most individuals. Distinct markings are also evident on its anterior surface, including a line concentric with and about 1.5 mm from the pupillary margin. This line separates the pupillary zone from the wider ciliary zone. (As can be seen in Fig. 23.2, the thickness of the iris diminishes at its ciliary and pupillary margins). Irregularly arranged contraction furrows are also evident and are particularly prominent when the pupil is dilated. When the posterior surface of the iris is viewed from behind (Fig. 23.2), it appears as a smooth dark brown layer with fine radial lines.

Microscopically, five layers of cells can be seen in the iris. The first layer consists of a discontinuous layer of fibroblasts and melanocytes covering the anterior surface. The surface of this layer is rough and irregular and is marked with ridges and grooves. The second layer is a thin layer of stroma that is devoid of blood vessels, the *anterior stromal sheet* or *lamella.* The third layer, constituting the main mass of the iris, is a layer rich in blood vessels that are embedded in loose connective tissue. The fourth layer consists of a discontinuous layer of smooth muscle, called the *posterior membrane.* The fifth layer, or posterior surface of the iris, is a layer of epithelial pigment that is a direct continuation from the two layers of the retinal epithelium (Fig. 23.1). The inner layer (located adjacent to the lens) is continuous with the nonpigmented layer of the retina. However, it becomes a heavily pigmented region in the iris (see Atlas section, Plate 128). The outer layer (or anterior layer as it is oriented relative to the iris) is continuous with the pigmented layer of the retina and is also a pigmented layer of the iris.

Two muscles, the sphincter pupillae and dilator pupillae, form the posterior membrane, that is located between the pigment epithelium and the vascular stroma of the iris. These muscles are derived embryologically from the anterior layer of the optic cup. The distinct innervation and orientation of the muscles is described above. The cells of the dilator pupillae, located immediately adjacent to the anterior layer of the pigment epithelium, are derived from this layer and are called (*pigmented*) *myoepithelial cells.*

The function of the pigment-containing cells in the eye is to eliminate stray light rays. In the iris, they are responsible for its color (that is, eye color). The number of melanocytes in the stroma is responsible for variation in eye color. If there are relatively few melanocytes in the stroma, eye color is derived from light reflected from the pigment present in the cells of the posterior surface of the iris giving it a blue appearance. As the amount of pigment present in the stroma increases, the color changes from blue to shades of greenish-blue, gray, and finally brown.

Ciliary Body

The *ciliary body* is located between the iris and choroid (see Atlas section, Plate 127). It extends for about 6 mm from the root of the iris, posterolaterally, to the *ora serrata* (Fig. 23.2). As seen from behind, the lateral edge of the ora serrata bears 17 to 34 grooves or crenulations, which mark the anterior limit of both the retina and choroid. The anterior third of the ciliary body has about 75 radial ridges or ciliary processes. The fibers of the zonule arise from the grooves between the ciliary processes.

The layers of the ciliary body are similar to those of the iris, consisting of a stroma and an epithelium. The stroma has an outer layer of smooth muscle, the *ciliary muscle,* which makes up the bulk of the ciliary body, and an inner vascular region, which extends into the ciliary processes. The epithelial layer covering the internal surface of the ciliary body is a direct continuation from the two layers of the retinal epithelium (Fig. 23.1).

Ciliary Muscle. The ciliary body consists of smooth muscle organized in three groups of fibers: (1) bundles of muscle fibers (*tensor portion*) that are oriented longitudinally or meridionally and border the scleral surface, these fibers (also known as Brucke's fibers) function chiefly in stretching the choroid; (2) bundles of muscle fibers (*radial portion*) that radiate in a fan-like fashion from their attachment on the scleral spur to insert into the circular portion of the ciliary muscle; (3) bundles of muscle fibers (*circular portion*) that are located most internally, occupying the inner and anterior

part of the ciliary body, and are oriented in a circular pattern forming a sphincter. The pull of the circular and radial fibers combine to reduce the tension on the zonule so that the lens becomes more spherical in shape. Forces generated by the longitudinal fibers on the scleral spur may also open the angle of Schlemm and facilitate drainage of the aqueous humor.

Ciliary Processes. The ciliary processes are thickenings of the inner vascular region of the stroma that are continuous with the vascular layers of the choroid. Scattered chromatophores and elastic fibers are present in the ciliary processes that measure about 2 mm in length, 1 mm in width, and 0.5 mm in height.

A double lamina, the continuation of Bruch's membrane of the choroid is present between the stroma and the epithelium. The inner layer of the lamina bears elevations that pass between the basal epithelial cells and apparently serve as an attachment site for the suspensory ligament so that the two epithelial layers are not pulled apart when stress is applied.

Ciliary Epithelium. The epithelium covering the inner surface of the ciliary body is composed of two layers of single cells that are continuous with the two pigmented layers of the iris. However, in the ciliary body, only the outer layer that is continuous with the retinal pigment epithelium is pigmented. The cells in the two layers are associated such that their apical portions are adjacent to each other and their basal regions that rest on a basal lamina are directed away from each other. Discontinuous intercellular spaces, called *ciliary channels,* separate the two layers. The basal lamina of the outer, pigmented layer is continuous with the basal lamina of the retinal pigment epithelium; that of the inner, nonpigmented layer is continuous with the limiting membrane of the retina and borders the posterior chamber of the eye. The fibers of the zonule that attach to and suspend the lens have their origin in the basal lamina of the inner cell layer.

Embryologically, the two epithelial layers are derived from the inner and outer layers of the optic cup. In the ciliary body, the two apposed cell layers are firmly fixed together; in contrast to the retina where the cells of pigment epithelium and sensory retina are not adherent to each other. In general, the nonpigmented cells of the inner layer are columnar in shape. However, they are cubical over the ciliary processes and are more flattened in shape near the ora serrata. The pigmented cells contain large numbers of melanin granules that essentially fill the cytoplasm leaving little space for other organelles. They have an apically located nu-

The choroid layer in the eyes of elasmobranch fishes and many mammals contains an intermediate layer of fibers or flattened cells, with highly refractile crystals, called tapetum. This additional layer is responsible for the brightly luminous color that is reflected from the eyes of horses, dogs, and cats or the silvery glistening that emanates from the eyes of a shark.

cleus, a small Golgi apparatus, and a moderate number of mitochondria and bundles of filaments. The epithelial cells in both the pigmented and nonpigmented layers are joined at their apical, lateral border to neighboring cells by desmosomes and elaborate tight junction. The nonpigmented cells have a centrally located nucleus, a well-developed Golgi apparatus, numerous profiles of rough and smooth endoplasmic reticulum, and extensive interdigitating processes on their basal lateral surface. These features of the nonpigmented cells are characteristic of epithelia engaged in the transport of water and ions. The cells of this layer are responsible for the production of the *aqueous humor,* a fluid similar in ionic composition to plasma but containing less than 0.1 percent protein (compared to 7 percent protein in plasma). The aqueous humor passes from the ciliary body toward the lens, then between the iris and lens before it reaches the anterior chamber of the eye (Fig. 23.4). In the anterior chamber of the eye, the aqueous humor passes laterally to the angle formed between the cornea and iris where it penetrates the tissues of the limbus as it enters the labyrinthine spaces and finally reaches the canal of Schlemm that communicates with the vessels of the sclera.

Choroid

The *choroid* is a dark brown vascular sheet, only 0.25 mm thick posteriorly and 0.1 mm thick anteriorly, that separates the sclera from the retina (Fig. 23.1). At the margin of the optic nerve, the choroid is attached firmly to the sclera. A potential space, the *perichoroidal space* (between the sclera and retina), is traversed by thin lamella or strands that run obliquely and loosely connect the sclera to the choroid. These lamellae form a layer called the *suprachoroid lamina.* The lamellae consist of large flat melanocytes scattered between connective tissue elements including collagen and elastic fibers, fibroblasts, macrophages, lymphocytes, plasma cells, and mast cells. The lamellae of the suprachoroid pass inward to surround the vessels in the remainder of the choroid layer. Free smooth muscle cells, not associated with blood vessels, have been identified in this tissue. Lymphatic channels, called *epichoroid lymph spaces,* and the long and short posterior ciliary vessels and nerves on their

way to the front of the eye are also present in the suprachoroid lamina.

Vascular Layers. Most of the choroid consists of vessels that decrease in size as the retina is approached. The largest vessels continue forward beyond the ora serrata into the ciliary body. These vessels can be seen with an ophthalmoscope. The large vessels are mostly veins that course about in whorls before passing obliquely through the sclera as vortex veins. The inner layer of vessels, arranged in a single plane, is called the *choriocapillary layer.* This layer is essential in providing nutrients to the cells of the retina. The capillaries are lined with fenestrated endothelium and have lumens that are large and irregular in shape. The choriocapillary layer is thicker and the capillary network is denser in the region of the fovea. This layer ends at the ora serrata.

Bruch's Membrane. Between the choriocapillary layer and the pigment epithelium of the retina is a thin refractile layer, called the *lamina vitrea* or *Bruch's membrane.* In the light microscope, it appears as an amorphous layer, 1 to 4 μm in thickness. With the electron microscope, five different layers have been identified in Bruch's membrane: (1) the basal lamina of the endothelial cells of the choriocapillary layer; (2) a layer of collagen fibers approximately 0.5 μm thick; (3) a layer of elastic fibers approximately 2 μm thick; (4) a second layer of collagen fibers (thus, forming a sandwich around the intervening elastic tissue layer); and (5) the basal lamina of the retinal epithelial cells.

RETINA

The retina, derived from the inner and outer layers of the optic cup, is the most internal of the three layers of the eye (Fig. 23.1C). The outer layer of the retina, which rests upon and is firmly attached to the choriocapillary layer of the choroid, consists of a pigmented epithelial layer, the *retinal pigment epithelium.* The inner layer containing the photoreceptors is the *neural retina* or *retina proper.* A potential space exists between the two layers of the retina. The two layers may be separated mechanically from each other in the preparation of histological specimens. Separation of the layers, "retinal detachment," may also occur in the living state as a result of eye disease or trauma to the eye.

Two regions or portions of the retina, that differ in function, are recognized: (1) a nonphotosensitive region, located anterior to the ora serrata, that lines the inner aspect of the ciliary body and the posterior surface of the retina (this portion of the retina has been described in the sections on the iris and ciliary body) and (2) the photosensitive region that lines the whole inner surface of the eye posterior to the ora serrata, except where it is pierced by the optic nerve (this is the location of the *optic papilla* or *disc*). Because the optic papilla is devoid of photoreceptors, it is a blind spot in the visual field (see Atlas section, Plate 126). In contrast, the *fovea centralis,* located about 2.5 mm lateral to the optic disc, is the area of greatest visual acuity. The visual axis of the eye passes through the fovea, a shallow round depression surrounded by a yellow pigmented zone called the *macula lutea.* In relative terms, this region of the retina contains the greatest concentration and most precisely ordered arrangement of the visual elements. Peripheral to this region the visual elements are less ordered and are fewer in number.

Layers of the Retina

The proliferation and differentiation of cells during development results in the establishment of ten layers within the retina consisting of cells and cellular processes (Fig. 23.5 and Atlas section, Plate 126). The cells of the neural retina can be divided

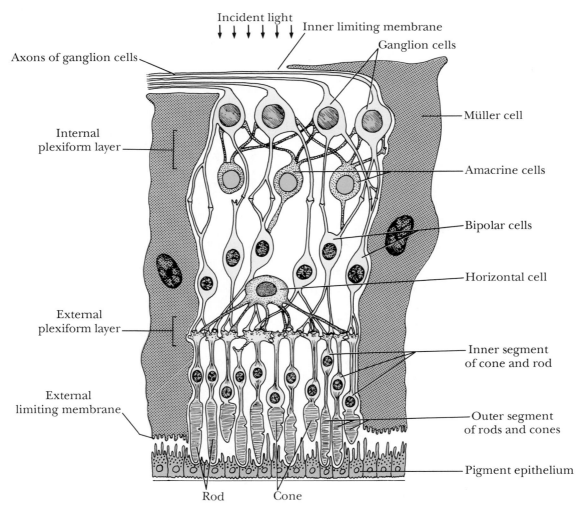

Figure 23.5. Schematic drawing of the layers of the retina. The interrelationship of the neurons is indicated. Light would enter the retina and pass through the internal layers of the retina before reaching the photoreceptors of the rods and cones that are closely associated with the pigment epithelium. (Modified from Boycott and Dowling; *Proc R Soc Lond [Biol]* 1966; 166:80).

into four groups: (1) photoreceptors—the retinal rod and cones; (2) direct conducting neurons—bipolar and ganglion cells; (3) association and other neurons—horizonal, centrifugal, and amacrine; and (4) supporting cells—Müller's cells and neuroglial cells. The specific arrangement and association of the nuclei and processes of these cells results in the retina being organized in well-defined layers that are seen with the light microscope. The layers are, from outside inward:

1. *Pigment epithelium*—outer layer of the retina that is not part of the neural retina but is associated with it
2. *Layer of rods and cones*—containing outer and inner segments of photoreceptors
3. *External (or outer) limiting membrane*—apical boundary of Müller's cells
4. *Outer nuclear layer*—containing cell bodies (nuclei) of retinal rods and cones
5. *Outer plexiform layer*—containing processes of retinal rods and cones and processes of horizonal, amacrine, and bipolar cells
6. *Inner nuclear layer*—containing cell bodies (nuclei) of horizonal, amacrine, bipolar, and Müller's cells
7. *Inner plexiform layer*—containing processes of horizonal, amacrine, and bipolar cells and processes of ganglion cells
8. *Ganglion cell layer*—containing cell bodies (nuclei) of ganglion cells
9. *Layer of optic nerve fibers*—containing processes of ganglion cells
10. *Internal (or inner) limiting membrane*—composed of the basal lamina of Müller's cells.

1. Pigment Epithelium. The *pigment epithelium,* derived from the outer wall of the optic cup, is a single layer of hexagon-shaped cells, about 14 μm wide and 10 to 14 μm tall. The cells rest on Bruch's membrane, which is considered to be part of the choroid layer even though the basal lamina adjacent to the pigment cells is produced by them. Adjacent pigment epithelial cells are connected by a junctional complex consisting of gap junctions and elaborate zonulae occludentes and adherentes. The junctional complex is the site of the "blood-retinal barrier." The pigment cells have cylindrical sheaths on their apical surface that are associated with but do not directly contact the tip of the photoreceptor processes of the adjacent rod and cone cells. Complex cytoplasmic processes, typical of cells involved in active transport, project for a short distance between the photoreceptors of the rods and cones. Numerous elongated melanin granules, unlike those found elsewhere in the eye and aggregated on the side of the cell nearest the rods and cones, are the most prominent feature of the cells. The nucleus is located near the basal plasma membrane, that is, adjacent to Bruch's membrane and has many convoluted infoldings. A supranuclear Golgi apparatus and a rather extensive network of smooth endoplasmic reticulum that surrounds the melanin granules and residual bodies are present in the cytoplasm. The pigment cells are tallest in the fovea and adjacent region, thus, accounting for the darker color of this region. The cells also contain material, phagocytized from the processes of the photoreceptors, in the form of lamellar debris contained in residual bodies, or phagosomes.

The retinal pigment epithelium serves several important functions including: (1) absorption of light passing through the neural retina preventing reflection and the resultant glare; (2) isolation of the retinal cells from blood borne substances, as it serves as a component of the *blood-retina barrier* via tight junctions between the lateral borders of adjacent cells within the retinal pigment epithelium; (3) restoration of photosensitivity to visual pigments that were dissociated in response to light; and (4) phagocytosis and disposal of membranous discs from the retinal photoreceptor cells.

2. Layer of Rods and Cones. The *rods and cones* are the outer segments of photoreceptor cells, whose nuclei form the outer nuclear layer of the retina (Fig. 23.6). It is important to recognize that the light that reaches the photoreceptors must pass through all of the other more internal layers of the neural retina. The rods and cones are arranged in a palisade manner so that, with the light microscope, they appear as vertical striations. In the human eye, there are approximately 125 million rods measuring about 2 μm in thickness and 50 μm length (ranging from about 60 μm at the fovea to 40 μm peripherally) and 7 million cones that vary in length from 85 μm at fovea to 25 μm at the periphery of the retina. Functionally, the rods are extremely sensitive to light and are the receptors used during periods of low light intensity (for example, at dusk or during the night). The visual image provided is one composed of gray tones ("a black and white picture"). In contrast, the cones exist in three forms that cannot be distinguished morphologically. They are less sensitive to low light and have maximal sensitivity to the red, green, or blue region of the visual spectrum. They provide a visual image composed of color and one that is believed to permit better visual acuity. [The specificity of the cones provides a functional basis

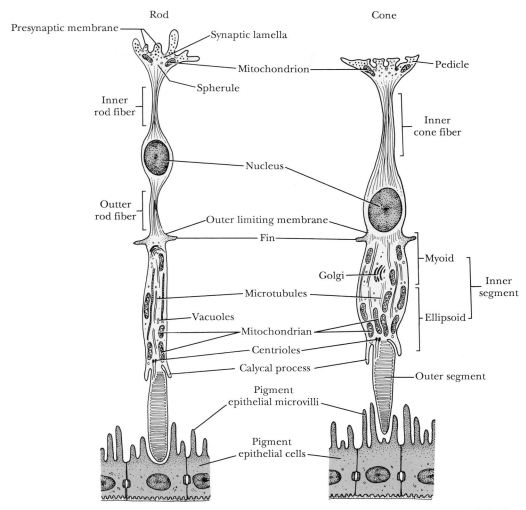

Figure 23.6. Schematic diagram of the ultrastructure of rod and cone cells. The outer segments of the rods and cones as closely associated with the adjacent pigment epithelium. (Modified from Cormack DH: *Ham's Histology*, 9th ed. Philadelphia, JB Lippincott, 1987.)

to explain color blindness that is believed to result from the lack of red-, green-, or (much less commonly) blue-sensitive cones].

Each rod and cone photoreceptor consists of three parts: an outer segment, a connecting stalk, and an inner segment. (1) The outer segment is roughly cylindrical or conical in shape (hence, the descriptive name rod or cone). This portion of the photoreceptor is intimately related to villi projecting from the adjacent pigment epithelial cells. (2) The connecting stalk contains a cilium composed of nine peripheral microtubule doublets extending from a basal body. The connecting stalk is seen as the constricted region of the cell that joins the inner to the outer segment. It should also be noted that, in this same region, a thin, tapering process

called the ***calycal process*** extends from the distal end of the inner segment to surround the upper portion of the outer segment (Fig. 23.6). (3) The inner segment is divided into an outer ***ellipsoid*** and an inner ***myoid*** portion and contains a typical complement of organelles associated with a cell actively synthesizing proteins. A prominent Golgi apparatus, rough endoplasmic reticulum, and free polysomes are concentrated in the myoid region. Mitochondria are most numerous in the ellipsoid region. Microtubules are distributed throughout the inner segment. In the outer segments of rods, cross-striated fibrous rootlets may extend from the basal body among the mitochondria. (In teleostean fishes and amphibians, the inner cone segment is contractile and shortens in response to bright light, thus, reflecting the use of the descriptive term myoid for this cell region). In terms of function, the outer segment is the site of photosensitivity and the inner segment contains the metabolic machinery providing the energy to support the activity of the photoreceptors.

The outer segment is often considered to be a highly modified cilium because it is joined to the inner segment by a short **connecting stalk** containing a cilium. In electron micrographs, each outer segment is recognized to contain between 600 and 1000 horizontal discs that are regularly spaced along the length of this region of the cell (Fig. 23.7). In rods, these discs are membrane-bound structures measuring about 2 μm in diameter and are enclosed within the plasma membrane of the

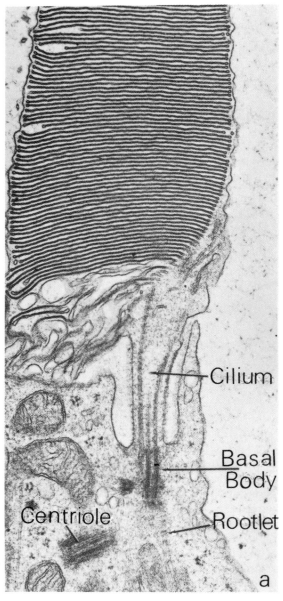

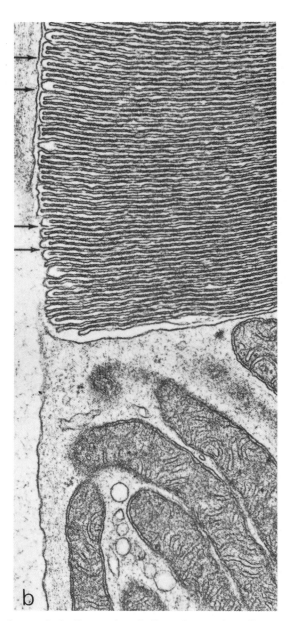

Figure 23.7. Transmission electron micrographs of portions of the inner and outer segments of a rod cell (a) and a cone cell (b). The outer segments contain the horizontally flattened discs. The interior of the discs of the cones have continuity with the extracellular space (arrows). In the rod cell, the plane of section passes through the connecting stalk and cilium. A centriole, cilium, basal body, and ciliary rootlet are identified. (Courtesy of T. Kuwabara.)

outer segment (Fig. 23.7a). The parallel membranes of the discs are about 6 nm in thickness and are continuous at their ends. The central enclosed space is about 8 nm across. In both rods and cones, the plasma membrane in the region of the outer segment near the cilium has undergone repetitive transverse infolding to form the membranous discs. Autoradiographic studies have demonstrated that rods form new discs by infolding of the plasma membrane through out their life-span. Discs are formed in cones in a similar manner but they are not replaced on a regular basis. Rod discs lose their continuity with the plasma membrane from which they were derived soon after they are formed and then pass like a stack of plates down the length of the cylindrical portion of the outer segment until they are eventually phagocytosed by the pigment epithelial cells. Thus, each rod disc is a membrane-enclosed compartment within the cytoplasm. In contrast, the discs of cones are not replaced on a regular basis and demonstrate continuity with the plasma membrane (Fig. 23.7b). *Thus, the interior of the discs of cones is continuous with the extracellular space.*

The basic difference in the structure of the rod and cone discs, that is, continuity with the plasma membrane, is correlated with the slightly different means by which the visual pigments are renewed in rods and cones. Newly synthesized rhodopsin is incorporated into the membrane of the rod disc as the disk is being formed. It then takes several days for the disc to reach the tip of the outer segment. In contrast, although labeled visual proteins are constantly being produced in retinal cones just as they are in the retinal rods, these proteins are incorporated into cone discs located anywhere in the outer segment. Thus, newly synthesized photopsin as well as other membrane proteins are incorporated at multiple sites in the cone membrane.

In the rod cells, the flattened discs contain the pigment called *visual purple* or *rhodopsin.* This substance initiates the visual stimulus as it is bleached by light. Rhodopsin is present in globular form on the outer surface of the lipid bilayer (that is, on the cytoplasmic side) of the membranous discs. In the cone cells, the only visual pigment that has been isolated from the membranous discs at this time is the photopigment called *iodopsin.* Yet, it is known that, functionally, the cones are specialized to respond maximally to one of the three colors (red, green, or blue). The visual pigments, rhodopsin and iodopsin, are molecules that have a membrane-bound subunit called *opsins* and second component called a *chromophore.* The opsin of rods is *scotopsin;* the opsins of cones are *photop-*

sins. The chromophore of the rods is a vitamin A-derived carotenoid called *retinal.*[1]

In simplistic terms, vision is a process by which the light striking the retina is converted into electrical impulses that are conveyed by an elaborate network of nerves to the brain where a visual image is produced. The conversion of the incident light into nerve impulses is called transduction and involves primary and secondary steps. The primary step is a photochemical reaction that occurs in the outer segment of the rod and cone receptors as absorbed light energy causes conformational changes in the chromophores. The second step consists of changes in the concentration of internal transmitters within the cytoplasm of the inner segment of the photoreceptors. These changes influence the ionic permeability of the plasma membrane and cause the photoreceptor to become hyperpolarized, thus, initiating the impulses that are conveyed to the brain.

The photochemical process has been most fully defined in the rods. Here, absorbed light energy causes conformational changes in the retinal (changing it to retinol) and resulting in its detachment from the scotopsin; the reaction is called "bleaching." This causes the cell to become hyperpolarized as calcium diffuses from the receptor and it reduces its permeability to sodium. The visual pigment is then reassembled and calcium is transported back into the cell. The energy for this process is provided by the mitochondria located in the inner segment. The Müller's cells and the pigment epithelial cells also participate in the interconversion of retinal-retinol and the reactions necessary for the resynthesis of rhodopsin.

During the normal functioning of the photoreceptors, the membranous discs of the outer segment are shed and phagocytized by the pigment epithelial cells (Fig. 23.8). It is estimated that each of these cells is capable of phagocytosing and disposing of about 7500 shed discs per day. The discs are constantly turning over and the production of new discs must be equal to the rate of disc shedding. Discs are shed from both rods and cones. In rods, there is a burst of disc shedding each morning, when, after a period sleep, light first enters the eye. The time of disc shedding in cones is more variable in the animal models that have been used to study this phenomenon. The shedding of discs in cones also enables the receptors to eliminate superfluous membrane. Although not fully understood, the shedding process in cones must alter the

---

[1] An adequate intake of vitamin A is essential for normal vision. A prolonged dietary deficiency of vitamin A leads to the inability to see in dim light ("night blindness").

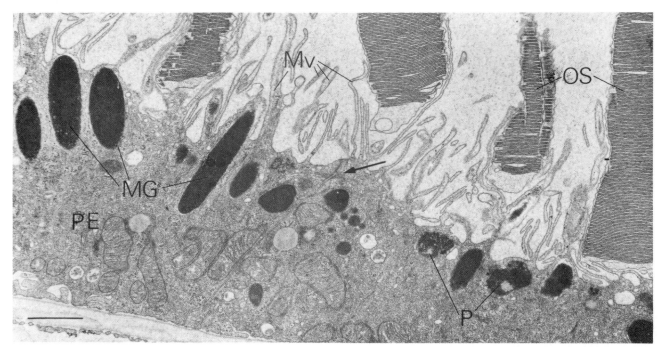

Figure 23.8. Transmission electron micrograph of the outer segments of rods and cones in association with the pigment epithelium. The pigment epithelium cells (PE) contain numerous elongated melanin granules (mel) that are aggregated against the side of the cell where microvilli (Mv) extend from the surface toward the outer segments (OS) of rod and cone cells. The pigment epithelial cells contain numerous mitochondria and phagosomes (P). The **arrow** indicates the location of the junctional complex between adjacent pigment epithelial cells. (Courtesy of T. Kuwabara.)

size of the discs so that the conical form is maintained as discs are released from the apical end of the process.

3. External (or Outer) Limiting Membrane. The outer limiting membrane is not a true membrane. It is a row of zonulae adherentes between the apical end of the Müller's cells, which are directed toward the pigmented epithelial cells, and the adjacent surface of the retinal rods and cones. Since the Müller's cells end at the base of the inner segments of the receptors, they mark the location of this layer. Thus, in a sense, the supporting processes of Müller's cells on which the rods and cones rest is pierced by the inner and outer segments of the photoreceptors.

4. Outer Nuclear Layer. The outer nuclear layer contains the nuclei of the retinal rods and cones. The region of the cytoplasm of the rods containing the nucleus is separated from the inner segment by a tapering process of the cytoplasm; in cones, the nuclei are located close to the outer segments and similar tapering is not seen. The cone nuclei stain lightly and are larger and more oval than rod nuclei. Rod nuclei are surrounded by only a thin rim of cytoplasm in contrast to a relatively thick investment around the cone nuclei.

5. Outer Plexiform Layer. The outer plexiform layer is formed by the processes of retinal rods and cones and the processes of horizonal, amacrine, and bipolar cells. The processes allow the photoreceptor cells to be coupled electrically to these specialized interneurons via synapses. A thin process extends from the region of the nucleus of each rod or cone to an inner expanded portion with several lateral processes. The expanded portion is called a *spherule* in a rod or a *pedicle* in a cone. Many photoreceptors converge onto one bipolar cell and also interconnect with one another. Cones located in the fovea synapse with a single bipolar cell. The fovea is also unique in that the compactness of the inner neural layers of the retina cause the photoreceptors to be oriented obliquely. Horizonal cell dendritic processes synapse with photoreceptors throughout the retina and further contribute to the elaborate neuronal connections in this layer.

6. Inner Nuclear Layer. This layer consists essentially of the nuclei of the horizontal, amacrine, and bipolar cells. The nuclei of Müller's cells are also found at this level as these cells form the scaffolding for the whole retina. The Müller's cell processes invest the other cells of the retina so completely that they essentially fill all of the extracellular space. The basal and apical ends of the Müller's cells form the internal and external limiting membranes, respectively; and the microvilli extending from their apical border lie between the photoreceptors of the rods and cones. Capillaries from the retinal vessels extend to this layer. The more external layers are avascular; the rods and cones receiving their blood supply from the choriocapillaris.

The three types of conducting cells—*bipolar, horizonal,* and *amacrine*—found in this layer have distinct orientation (Fig. 23.5). The processes of *bipolar cells* extend to both the inner and outer plexiform layers. Through these connections, the bipolar cells establish synaptic connections with multiple cells in each layer, except in the fovea where the number of interconnected cells is reduced to provide greater visual acuity. The processes of *horizonal cells* extend to the external plexiform layer where they intermingle with processes of bipolar cells. The cells have synaptic connections with rod spherules, cone pedicles, and bipolar cells. This electrical coupling of cells is thought to affect the functional threshold between rods and cones and bipolar cells. The processes of *amacrine cells* branch extensively to provide sites of synaptic connections with axonal endings of bipolar cells and dendrites of ganglion cells.

In the peripheral regions of the retina, the axons of bipolar cells pass to the inner plexiform layer where they synapse with several ganglion cells; in the fovea, they may synapse with a single ganglion cell reflecting the greater visual acuity in this region. Amacrine cell processes pass inward contributing to a complex interconnection of cells as they synapse in the inner plexiform layer with bipolar, ganglion, as well as other amacrine cells (Fig. 23.5).

7. Inner Plexiform Layer. This layer consists of the complex intermingling of the processes of the amacrine, bipolar, and ganglion cells. The processes have a course that parallels the inner limiting membrane, thus, giving the appearance of horizontal striations to this layer.

8. Ganglion Cell Layer. This layer is composed of large multipolar nerve cells, up to 30 μm in diameter. They have lightly staining round nuclei with prominent nucleoli and have Nissl bodies in their cytoplasm. An axonal process emerges from the rounded cell body containing the nucleus, passes into the nerve fiber layer, and then into the optic nerve. The dendrites extend from the opposite end of the cell to ramify in the inner plexiform layer. In the peripheral regions of the retina, a single ganglion cell may synapse with a

hundred bipolar cells. In marked contrast, in the macular region, surrounding the fovea, the bipolar cells are smaller (some authors refer to them as "midget" bipolar cells) and there tends to be a single connection between a midget bipolar cell and a ganglion cell. Over most of the retina, the ganglion cells are only a single layer of cells. However, at the macula, they are piled up to eight deep, but are absent over the fovea itself. Scattered among the ganglion cells are small neuroglial cells with densely staining nuclei.

9. Layer of Optic Nerve Fibers. This layer contains the axonal processes of the ganglion cells. They occur in a flattened layer running parallel to the retinal surface, which increases in depth as the axons converge at the optic disc. The axons are thin, nonmyelinated processes measuring up to 5 μm in diameter.

10. Internal (or Inner) Limiting Membrane. This layer consists of the thin lamina separating the retina from the vitreous body. It is essentially the basal lamina of the Müller's cells.

Specialized Regions of the Retina

The *fovea* appears as a shallow depression, located at the posterior pole of the optical axis of the eye. Its central region, known as the *fovea centralis,* is about 200 μm in diameter. Most of the layers of the retina are markedly reduced or are absent in this region, except for the layer of the photoreceptors (Fig. 23.5). Here it is composed entirely of cones that are longer and are more slender and rod-like than they are elsewhere. The adjacent pigment epithelial cells and choriocapillaris are also thickened in this region.

The *macula lutea* is the area surrounding the fovea. It appears yellowish after death due to the presence of yellow pigment (xanthophyl). Retinal vessels are absent in this region. Here the retinal cells and their processes, especially the ganglion cells, are heaped up on the sides of the fovea, so that light may pass uninterrupted to this most sensitive area of the retina.

Vessels of the Retina

The *central retinal artery* and *vein,* the vessels that can be seen and assessed with an ophthalmoscope, pass through the center of the optic nerve to enter the bulb of the eye at the optic disc (see Fig. 23.2 and the section on the developing eye). The artery immediately branches into upper and lower branches, each of these divides again. Veins undergo a similar pattern of branching. The vessels initially lie between the vitreous body and inner limiting membrane. As the vessels pass laterally, they pass deeper within the inner retinal layers. Branches from these vessels form a capillary plexus that does not extend beyond the inner nuclear layer. The branches of the central retinal artery do not anastomose with each other and, therefore, are classified as anatomical end arteries. Evaluation of the retinal vessels and optic disc during the physical examination of a patient not only provides important information on the state of the eye, but also provides early clinical signs of a number of conditions including elevated intracranial pressure, hypertension, and diabetes.

CRYSTALLINE LENS

The lens is a transparent, avascular, biconvex structure. It is suspended between the edges of the ciliary body by the *zonule* or *suspensory ligament.* The pull of zonule fibers causes the lens to flatten. With age, the lens becomes less elastic, thus, limiting its usefulness in focusing light on the retina. Therefore, it is common for individuals in their 40s to discover that they are required to wear glasses for reading. Loss of transparency of the lens or its capsule is also a relatively common condition associated with aging. This condition is called *cataract.* The development of a cataract may be related to disease processes, metabolic or hereditary conditions, trauma, or exposure to a deleterious agent (such as ultraviolet radiation).

In understanding the histology of the lens, it is helpful to examine its development. The lens arises embryologically as an invagination of the epithelium overlying the optic cup. The cavity, the lens vesicle, is then obliterated by elongation of the layer of cells forming its posterior surface (Fig. 23.3). This results in the anterior surface of the lens being covered by a single layer of cuboidal cells, whereas the remainder of the lens is composed of elongated cells with their long axis oriented in an anterior to posterior plane. In the adult, three basic components of the lens are identified (see Atlas section, Plate 128, Fig. 3).

1. Lens Capsule. The lens capsule is a layer approximately 10 to 20 μm thick that represents a greatly thickened basal lamina produced by the anterior lens cells and the lens fibers. It is elastic and is composed primarily of type IV collagen. It is thickest at the equator where the fibers of the zonule attach to it. In transmission electron microscopy, the capsule exhibits a lamellar structure, suggesting that it develops by the laying down of consecutive layers of basal lamina.

2. Subscapular Epithelium. This consists of the cuboidal layer of cells present only on the anterior surface of the lens. These cells, connected by gap junctions, have few cytoplasmic organelles and stain lightly. The apical region of the cell is directed toward the internal aspect of the lens and the lens fibers with which they form junctional complexes. The lens increases in size during normal growth and then continues, at an ever decreasing rate, the production of new lens fibers throughout life. The new lens fibers develop from the subcapsular epithelial cells located near the equator. Cells in this region increase in height and then differentiate into lens fibers.

3. Lens Fiber. Lens fibers are structures derived from subcapsular epithelial cells. They have become highly elongated and appear as thin, flattened structures. During their differentiation, they lose their nuclei and other organelles as they become filled with a group of proteins called *crystallins.* They attain a length of 7 to 10 mm, a width of 8 to 10 μm, and a thickness of 2 μm.

VITREOUS

The posterior four-fifths of the eye is filled with *vitreous humor,* a transparent jelly-like substance. The vitreous humor is loosely attached to the surrounding structures including the limiting membrane of the retina. The main body of the vitreous is a homogeneous gel containing about 99 percent water, collagen, and glycosaminoglycans (principally hyaluronic acid). The hyaloid canal (or Cloquet's canal) runs through the center of the vitreous from the optic disc to the posterior lens capsule. In the fetus, the hyaloid artery was present in this space.

ACCESSORY STRUCTURES OF THE EYE

Conjunctiva

The conjunctiva is a thin, transparent mucous membrane that extends from the lateral surface of the cornea and covers the internal surface of the eyelids. It consists of a stratified columnar epithelium containing numerous goblet cells and rests upon a lamina propria composed of loose connective tissue.

Eyelids

The primary function of the eyelids (Fig. 23.9) is to protect the eye. The skin of the lids is loose and elastic to accomodate their movement. Within each eyelid is a flexible support, the *tarsal plate,* consisting of dense fibrous and elastic tissue. The undersurface of the tarsal plate is covered by conjunctiva.

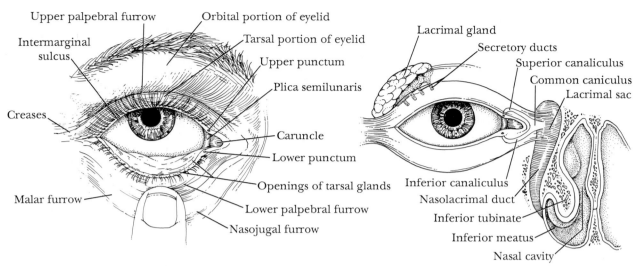

Figure 23.9. Schematic diagrams of the eye and its accessory structures. The drawing on the right shows a coronal section passing through the lacrimal bone and associated bones bordering the nasal cavity. The components of the lacrimal drainage system are shown.

The eyelid contains three types of glands. (1) The *meibomian glands* are long sebaceous glands embedded in the tarsal plates. They appear as vertical yellow streaks in the tissue deep to the conjunctiva and have no communication with the hair follicles. About 25 glands are present in the upper eyelid and 20 in the lower eyelid. The sebaceous secretion of the meibomian glands produces an oily layer on the surface of the tear film that delays the evaporation of the normal tear layer. (2) The *glands of Zeis* are small modified sebaceous glands that are connected with and empty their secretion into the follicles of the eyelashes. (3) The *glands of Moll* are sweat glands with unbranched sinuous tubules that begin as a simple spiral.

Lacrimal Gland and Associated Structures

Tears are produced by the *lacrimal gland* located beneath the conjunctiva on the upper lateral side of the eye and *accessory tear glands* (or *tarsal glands*) located on the inner surface of the upper and lower eyelids and opening of their free margins (Fig. 23.9). These glands develop within the conjunctiva as compound serous tubuloalveolar type glands. Their lumens are usually distended.

The secretory product is slightly alkaline and contains lysozyme, a bactericidal enzyme. The tears function to moisten and lubricate the adjacent surfaces of the eye and eyelids and to flush foreign substances from these surfaces. The lacrimal gland consists of several separate glandular lobes. They end on 6 to 12 excretory ducts that open along the internal lateral surface of the upper eyelid. The serous cells of the gland are column-shaped and contain lightly staining secretory granules. Myoepithelial cells surround the secretory unit of the glands and aid in the release of tears. After the fluid produced by the lacrimal and tarsal glands passes over the surface of the eye and conjunctiva, it drains into the *superior* and *inferior lacrimal canaliculi* through openings called *lacrimal puncta*. The puncta are about the 0.5 mm in diameter and are located on the medial inner surface of the upper and lower eyelids (Fig. 23.9). The canaliculi, lined with a thick stratified squamous epithelium, join to form a common canaliculus before opening into the *lacrimal sac*. The lacrimal sac and its continuation, the *nasolacrimal duct,* allow the tears to drain into the nasal cavity through an opening located in the inferior nasal meatus below the inferior turbinate. A pseudostratified ciliated epithelium lines the lacrimal sac and the nasolacrimal duct.

PLATE 125. Eye I

A section through the eyeball is shown in Plate 125. The micrograph illustrates most of the structural features of the eye at low magnification and provides orientation for the micrographs that follow.

The wall of the eyeball consists of three layers: the retina, the uvea, and an outer fibrous layer (corneoscleral coat). Innermost is the retina **(R),** which is comprised of several layers of cells. Among these are receptor cells (rods and cones), neurons (e.g., bipolar and ganglion cells), supporting cells, and a pigmented epithelium (see Atlas section, Plate 126). The receptor components of the retina are situated in the posterior three-fifths of the eyeball. At the anterior boundary of the receptor layer, the ora serrata **(OS),** the retina becomes reduced in thickness and nonreceptor components of the retina continue forward to cover the posterior or inner surface of the ciliary body **(CB)** and the iris **(I).** This anterior nonreceptor extension of the inner layer is highly pigmented and the pigment (melanin) is evident as the black inner border of these structures.

The uvea, the middle layer of the eyeball, consists of the choroid, the ciliary body, and the iris. The choroid is a vascular layer; it is relatively thin and difficult to distinguish in the accompanying figure, except by location. On this basis, it is identified **(Ch)** as being just external to the pigmented layer of the retina. The choroid is also highly pigmented; the choroidal pigment is evident as a discrete layer in several parts of the section.

Anterior to the ora serrata, the uvea is thickened; here, it is called the ciliary body **(CB).** This contains the ciliary muscle (see Atlas section, Plate 127), which brings about adjustments of the lens for the focusing of light. The ciliary body also contains processes to which the zonular fibers are at-

tached. These fibers function as suspensory ligaments of the lens. The iris **(I)** is the most anterior component of the uvea and contains a central opening, the pupil.

The outermost layer of the eyeball, the fibrous layer, consists of the sclera **(S)** and the cornea **(C).** Both of these contain collagenous fibers as their main structural element; however, the cornea is transparent and the sclera is opaque. The extrinsic muscles of the eye insert into the sclera and affect movements of the eyeball. These are not included in the preparation except for a small piece of a muscle insertion **(arrow)** in the upper left of the illustration. Posteriorly, the sclera is pierced by the emerging optic nerve **(ON).**

The lens **(L)** will be considered in Atlas section, Plate 128. Just posterior to the lens is the large cavity of the eye, the vitreal cavity, which is filled with a thick jelly-like material, the vitreous humor or body. Anterior to the lens are two additional chambers of the eye, the anterior **(AC)** and posterior chambers **(PC),** separated by the iris.

KEY

AC, anterior chamber
C, cornea
CB, ciliary body
Ch, choroid
I, iris
L, lens

ON, optic nerve
OS, ora serrata
PC, posterior chamber
R, retina
S, sclera

Fig., human, × 7

PLATE 125

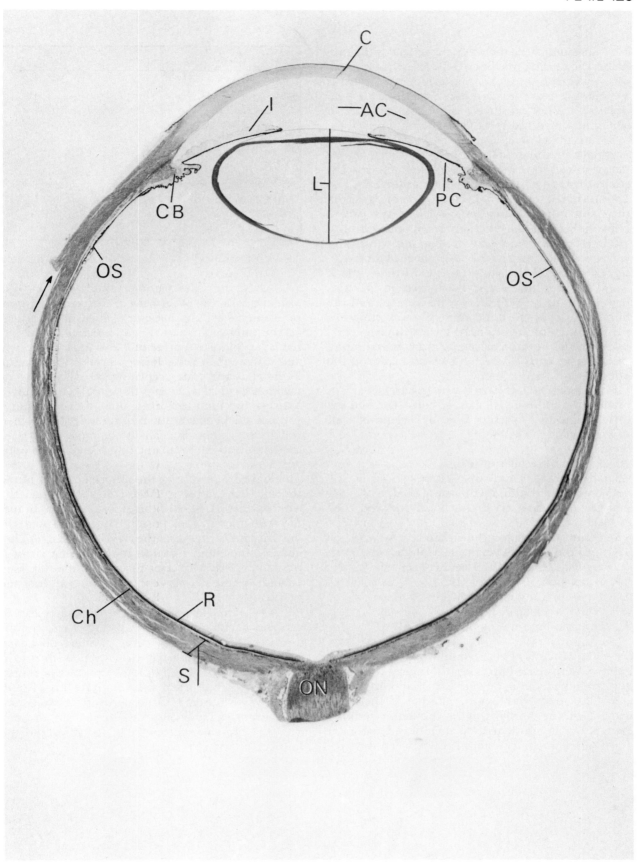

PLATE 126. Eye II

The site where the optic nerve leaves the eyeball is called the optic disc (**OD**). It is characteristically marked by a depression, evident in **Figure 1.** Receptor cells are not present at the optic disc and because it is not sensitive to light stimulation, it is sometimes referred to as the blind spot.

The fibers that give rise to the optic nerve originate in the retina, more specifically, in the ganglion cell layer (see below). They traverse the sclera through a number of openings (**arrows. Fig. 1**) to form the optic nerve. The region of the sclera that contains these openings is called the lamina cribrosa (**LC**). The optic nerve contains a central artery and vein (not seen in **Fig. 1**), which also traverse the lamina cribrosa. Branches of these vessels (**BV**) supply the inner portion of the retina.

The optic nerve and retina are, in effect, a projection of the central nervous system, and the fibrous cover of the optic nerve is an extension of the meninges of the brain. As a consequence, pressure within the cranial cavity, transmitted along this channel, can be detected by examination of the optic disc.

On the basis of structural features that are readily evident in histological sections, the retina is divided into ten layers as listed below and labeled in **Figure 2.**

1. Pigment epithelium (**PEp**)
2. Layer of rods and cones (**R&C**)
3. External limiting membrane (**ELM**)
4. Outer nuclear layer (nuclei of rod and cone cells, **ONL**)
5. Outer plexiform layer (**OPL**)
6. Inner nuclear layer (nuclei of bipolar, horizontal, amacrine, and Müllers cells, **INL**)
7. Inner plexiform layer (**IPL**)
8. Layer of ganglion cells (**GC**)
9. Nerve fiber layer (**NFL**)
10. Internal limiting membrane (**ILM**)

The Müller's cells are supporting cells comparable to neuroglia. Processes of Müller's cells ramify virtually through the entire thickness of the retina. The inner limiting membrane is the basal lamina of the Müller's cells; the outer limiting membrane is not actually a membrane, rather it represents junctional complexes between the pro-

---

KEY

BV, blood vessels
Ch, choroid
FC, fovea centralis
LC, lamina cribrosa
LV, lamina vitrea

OD, optic disc
arrows, openings in sclera (lamina cribrosa)

Fig. 1, human, × 65
Fig. 2, human, × 325

Fig. 3, human, × 440

---

cesses of Müller's cells and photoreceptor cells (rods and cones).

Aside from the pigment epithelium and the Müller's cells, the other cells of the retina are neural elements arranged sequentially in three layers: (1) the rods and cones; (2) an intermediate neuronal layer (bipolar, horizontal, and amacrine cells); and (3) ganglion cells. Nerve impulses originating in the rods and cones are transmitted to the intermediate layer and then to the ganglion cells. Synaptic connections occur in the inner and outer plexiform layers, resulting in some degree of neuronal integration. Finally, the ganglion cells send their axons to the brain as components of the optic nerve.

Figure 2 also shows the innermost layer of the choroid (**Ch**). This is a cell-free membrane, the lamina vitrea (**LV**), also called Bruch's membrane. Electron micrographs reveal that it corresponds to the basement membrane of the pigment epithelium. Immediately external to the lamina vitrea is the capillary layer of the choroid (lamina choriocapillaris). These vessels supply the outer part of the retina.

The posterior portion of the retina (see **Fig. 3**) contains a small depression called the fovea centralis (**FC**). This part of the retina contains only cone cells. The depression of the fovea is due to a spreading apart of the inner layers of the retina, leaving the cone elements relatively uncovered. The fovea centralis is associated with acute vision. As one moves from the fovea toward the ora serrata, the number of cone cells decreases and the number of rod cells increases.

PLATE 126

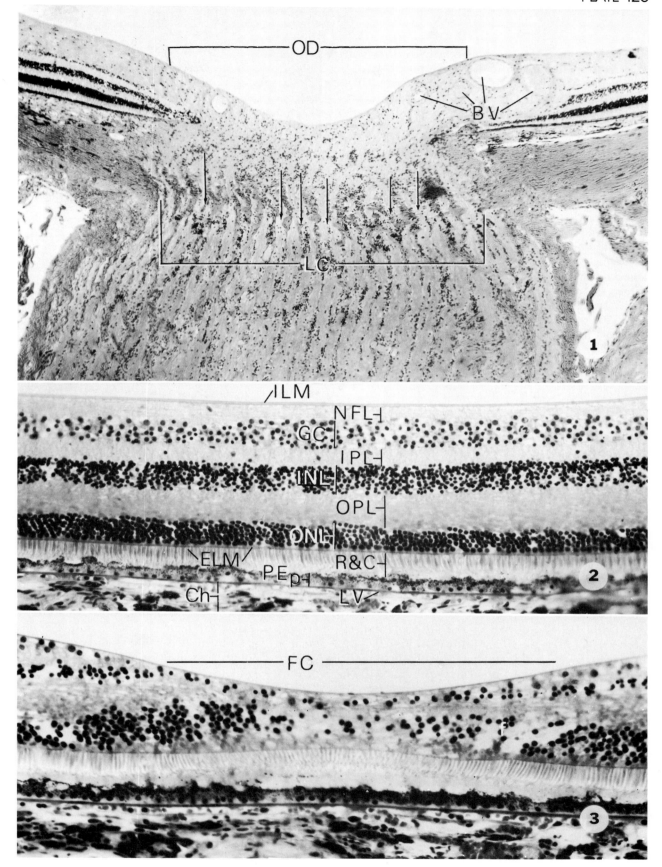

PLATE 127. Eye III

A portion of the anterior of the eye is shown in **Figure 1.** Included in the illustration are parts of the cornea **(C),** sclera **(S),** iris **(I),** ciliary body **(CB),** anterior chamber **(AC),** posterior chamber **(PC),** lens **(L),** and zonular fibers **(ZF).** The zonular fibers function as a suspensory ligament of the lens.

The cornea is considered in detail in Atlas section, Plate 128. However, the relationship of the cornea to the sclera is illustrated to advantage in **Figure 1.** The junction between the two **(arrows)** is marked by a change in staining, the substance of the cornea appearing lighter than that of the sclera. The corneal epithelium **(CEp)** is continuous with the epithelium **(CjEp)** that covers the sclera. (The junction between these is marked by the **small circle** in **Fig. 1** and shown at higher magnification in the **inset.)** However, the latter is separated from the dense fibrous component of the sclera by a loose vascular connective tissue. Together, this connective tissue and its covering epithelium constitute the conjunctiva **(Cj).** The epithelial-connective tissue junction of the conjunctiva is irregular; in contrast, the undersurface of the corneal epithelium presents an even profile.

Just lateral to the junction of the cornea and sclera is a canal, seen in cross-section, the canal of Schlemm **(CS, Fig. 2).** This canal takes a circular route about the perimeter of the cornea. It communicates with the anterior chamber through a loose trabecular meshwork of tissue called the spaces of Fontana. These spaces can only be seen adequately in ideal preparations and they are not evident in **Figures 1 or 2.** The canal of Schlemm also communicates with episcleral veins. By means of its communications, the canal of Schlemm provides a route for the fluid in the anterior and posterior chambers to reach the bloodstream. The canal may form more than one channel as it encircles the cornea.

Immediately internal to the anterior margin of the sclera **(S)** is the ciliary body **(CB, Fig. 2).** The inner surface of this forms radially arranged, ridge-shaped elevations, the ciliary processes **(CP),** to which the zonular fibers **(ZF)** are anchored. From the outside in, the components of the ciliary body are: the ciliary muscle **(CM),** the connective tissue (vascular) layer **(VL),** the lamina vitrea **(LV),**

KEY	
AC, anterior chamber	LV, lamina vitrea
C, cornea	nP, non-pigmented
CAV, circular artery and	layer of the ciliary
vein	epithelium
CB, ciliary body	P, pigmented layer of
CEp, corneal epithelium	the ciliary epithelium
CiEp, ciliary epithelium	PC, posterior chamber
Cj, conjunctiva	S, sclera
CjEp, conjunctival	VL, vascular layer (of
epithelium	ciliary body)
CM, ciliary muscle	ZF, zonular fibers
CP, ciliary processes	arrows, junction
CS, canal of Schlemm	between cornea and
I, iris	sclera
L, lens	
Fig. 1, human, × 30	**Fig. 2,** human, × 65
(inset, × 300)	(inset, × 570)

and the ciliary epithelium **(CiEp).** The ciliary epithelium consists of two layers **(inset),** the pigmented layer **(P)** and the nonpigmented layer **(nP).** The ciliary epithelium plays a role in the formation of the aqueous humor. The lamina vitrea is a continuation of the same layer of the choroid: It is the basement membrane of the pigmented ciliary epithelial cells.

The ciliary muscle is arranged in three patterns. The outer layer is immediately deep to the sclera. These are the meridionally arranged fibers of Brücke. The outermost of these continues more posteriorly into the choroid and is referred to as the tensor muscle of the choroid. The middle layer is the radial group. It radiates from the region of the sclerocorneal junction into the ciliary body. The innermost layer of muscle cells is circularly arranged. These are seen in cross-section. The circular artery and vein **(CAV)** for the iris, also cut in cross-section, are just anterior to the circular group of muscle cells.

The iris and lens are considered in the Atlas section, Plate 128. The **rectangles in Figure 1** mark those areas of the lens which are shown in Atlas section, Plate 128 **(Fig. 3** and its **inset).**

PLATE 127

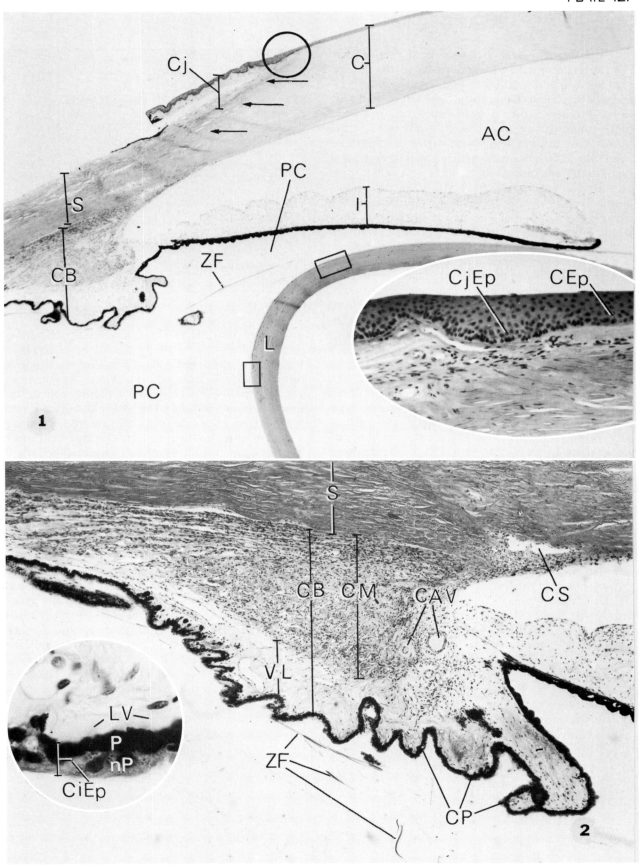

PLATE 128. Eye IV

The cornea is the transparent portion of the eye, anterior to the iris. It consists of five layers, three of which are cellular. The layers are: the epithelium; Bowman's membrane, which is acellular; the substantia propria (corneal stroma); Descemet's membrane, also acellular; and the endothelium. The full thickness of the cornea is illustrated in **Figure 1,** and the two surfaces, at higher magnification, in the **insets.**

The epithelium (**Ep**) is stratified squamous, about five or six cells in thickness. The basal cells exhibit a columnar or polyhedral shape, but they become progressively flattened as they migrate toward the surface. They do not keratinize and, accordingly, each cell contains a nucleus. The cells are joined by desmosomes that appear as "intercellular bridges" (**arrow**) in light micrographs (**inset**).

The undersurface of the corneal epithelium presents a smooth profile. It rests on a homogeneous-appearing substance called Bowman's membrane (**BwM**). The substantia propria (**SP**) forms most of the thickness of the cornea. It consists of regularly arranged sheets, or lamellae, of collagen fibers and fibroblasts. The collagen fibers within each lamella are parallel to each other, but at right angles to the fibers of adjacent lamellae. This orientation contributes to the transparency of the cornea. Indeed, opaqueness due to scarring of the cornea (e.g., after a wound), is accompanied by a failure to reestablish the normal orientation. The substantia propria is separated from the corneal endothelium by Descemet's membrane (**DM**). Like Bowman's membrane, this appears homogeneous with the light microscope. The endothelium (**En**) consists of a single layer of cuboidal cells whose lateral cell margins are sometimes evident. The cornea is devoid of blood vessels. During inflammation, white blood cells migrate into the cornea from the vessels in the sclera. Even in noninflammatory states, lymphocytes are seen in the cornea. The corneal epithelium is richly supplied with nerve endings; however, these are not evident in H&E sections.

The pupillary margin of the iris is shown at higher magnification in **Figure 2.** The major portion of the iris consists of connective tissue (**CT**) which contains pigment cells (**PC**) to a varying de-

gree (only in the albino are these absent). The posterior surface of the iris consists of two layers of pigmented epithelial cells (**PE**). The cells located immediately adjacent to the anterior of these two layers contain myofilaments and are called pigmented myoepithelial cells (**PMyE**) because they are derived from the cells of the anterior layer. These cells make up the radial, or dilator, muscle fibers of the iris. The myoid character of these cells is largely obscured by the pigment. In addition, the iris contains smooth muscle cells arranged circularly around the pupil. These are seen in cross-section in **Figure 2 [SM(C)].** These circularly arranged muscle cells make up the pupillary constrictor of the iris.

The lens consists entirely of epithelial cells (**Fig. 3**) surrounded by a homogeneous capsule (**LCap**) to which the zonular fibers (**ZF**) are joined. On the anterior surface of the lens, the cells have a cuboidal shape. However, all the lateral margin, the cells are extremely elongated (**inset**) and their cytoplasm extends toward the center of the lens. These elongated columns of epithelial cytoplasm are also referred to as lens fibers (**LF**). New cells are produced at the margin of the lens and displace the older cells toward the center. As the cell differentiate, the older cells (called lens fibers) lose their nucleus.

KEY

BwM, Bowman's membrane
CT, connective tissue
DM, Descemet's membrane
En, corneal endothelium
Ep, corneal epithelium
LCap, lens capsule
LF, lens "fibers"
PC, pigment cells

PE, pigmented epithelium
PMyE, pigmented myoepithelial cells
SM(C), circular smooth muscle
SP, substantia propria
ZF, zonular fibers
arrows, intercellular bridges

Fig. 1, human, × 135 (inset, × 600)
Fig. 2, human, × 250

Fig. 3, human, × 800 (inset, × 250)

PLATE 128

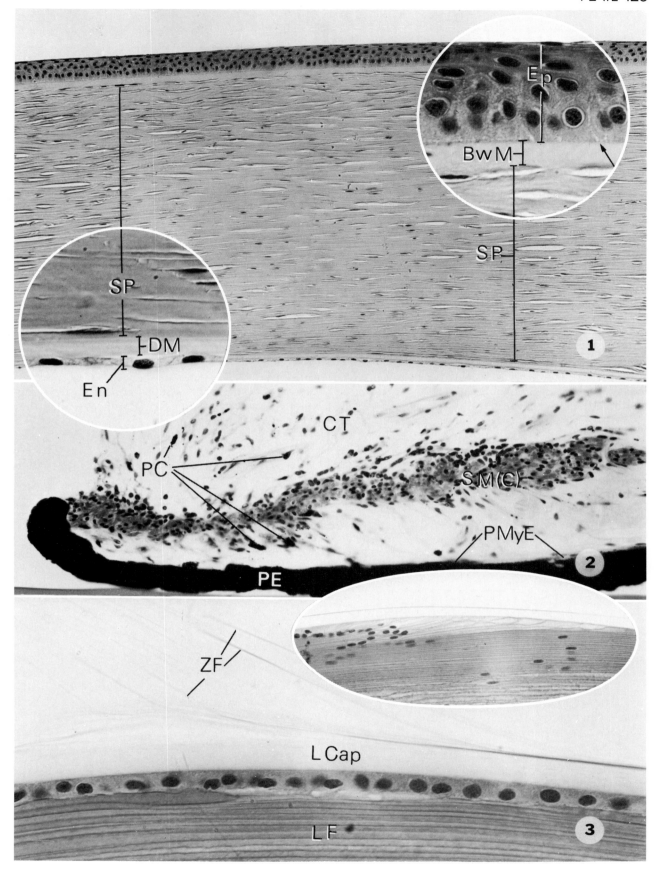

Ep

BwM

SP

SP

DM

En

1

CT

PC

SM(C)

PMyE

PE

2

ZF

L Cap

LF

3

The Ear

The ear is a compound organ that consists of the *auditory system,* which is involved in the detection of sound, and the *vestibular system,* which is involved with static and dynamic equilibrium. Each division of the ear (*external ear, middle ear,* and *inner ear*) is an integral component of the auditory system (Fig. 24.1). The external ear and middle ear collect and convey sound energy to the inner ear where auditory sensory receptors transform the energy into neural impulses. Sensory receptors of the vestibular system, which are responsive to gravity and to movements of the head, are located also in the inner ear and function independently of both the external ear and middle ear.

EXTERNAL EAR

The external ear is composed of an *auricle* and *external auditory meatus.* The *auricle* (or *pinna*) is shaped and formed by a single irregular plate of elastic cartilage. The skin overlying the cartilage is thin, containing fine hairs and sebaceous glands. Sweat glands are also present in the skin covering the posterior aspect of the auricle. In humans, the auricle is considered to be a vestigial structure, but for many other mammals, it is an essential component in sound localization and amplication.

The *external auditory meatus* (or canal) extends from the auricle to the tympanic membrane (eardrum) of the middle ear. The slightly S-shaped course of the external auditory canal is approximately 25 mm in length. Its outer one-third is formed by elastic cartilage that is continuous with the cartilage of the auricle. The inner two-thirds of the canal wall is formed by the temporal bone. The external auditory meatus is lined by skin that con-

tains numerous hairs and both sebaceous and ceruminous glands, which are greatest in number in the outer one-third of the canal. The ceruminous gland is a modified sweat gland with a coiled tubular apocrine architecture. Secretions of the ceruminous and sebaceous glands combine with desquamated cells to form *cerumen* (earwax). Cerumen protects the skin from desiccation (drying) and, along with the meatal hairs, helps to prevent foreign bodies from entering the ear. An excessive accumulation of cerumen can occlude the canal, resulting in a conductive hearing impairment.

MIDDLE EAR

The middle ear consists of the *tympanic cavity* (middle ear space) and its components, namely, the *tympanic membrane* (eardrum), three small bones (*ossicles*) and associated muscles, and the *auditory tube* (eustachian tube). Functionally, the middle ear converts air vibrations (sound waves) from within the external ear canal into mechanical vibrations that are conveyed to the inner ear.

Tympanic Cavity

The *tympanic cavity* is an irregular, air-filled space that lies within the temporal bone (Fig. 24.2). In most regions, the tympanic cavity is lined by simple squamous to low cuboidal epithelium. Near the opening of the auditory tube, the surface epithelial cells are ciliated and columnar. The lateral wall of the cavity is formed primarily by the tympanic membrane. The medial wall of the cavity is a common wall shared with the inner ear. Two important openings are present in this wall, the *ves-*

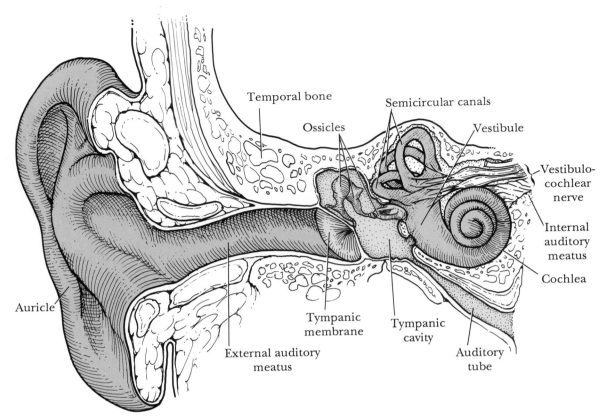

Figure 24.1. Schematic illustration of the three divisions of the ear: external ear (auricle and external auditory meatus), middle ear (tympanic cavity, ossicles, tympanic membrane, and auditory tube), and inner ear (vestibule, semicircular canals, and cochlea).

tibular (oval) window and the *cochlear (round) window*. The significance of these windows in the transmission of vibrations is described below.

Ossicles

Three small bones (*ossicles*), the *malleus (hammer)*, the *incus (anvil)*, and the *stapes (stirrup)* form a chain of levers that link the external ear to the inner ear (Fig. 24.3). The malleus is attached to the inner aspect of the tympanic membrane. The stapes is oriented at a right angle to the incus and is secured by a fibrous (annular) ligament into the oval window of the inner ear. The malleus and the incus are suspended from the roof of the cavity by suspensory ligaments. The three ossicles, composed of compact bone, are joined to one another by synovial joints. The ossicles are covered by epithelium that is continuous with the epithelium that lines the tympanic cavity.

Sound waves that impinge upon the tympanic membrane are transmitted to the malleus as mechanical vibrations. The mechanical vibrations are conveyed from the malleus to the incus and then to the stapes, which moves like a piston, leading to fluid displacement within the inner ear. Associated with the three ossicles are two small striated muscles, the Tensor tympani, attached to the malleus, and the Stapedius, attached to the stapes. These two muscles adjust the tension of the tympanic membrane in order to convey vibrations to the inner ear and dampen ossicular movement. During exposure to extremely loud noises they protect the delicate auditory receptors of the inner ear. The latter is principally a function of the Stapedius.

Tympanic Membrane

In *tympanic membrane* is a thin, somewhat rigid, semitransparent membrane that is ovoid in shape. The tension, created by the attachment of the malleus to the center of the tympanic membrane, causes the membrane to appear as an inwardly directed cone. The tympanic membrane consists of a central core of connective tissue covered by an inner and an outer epithelial layer. The

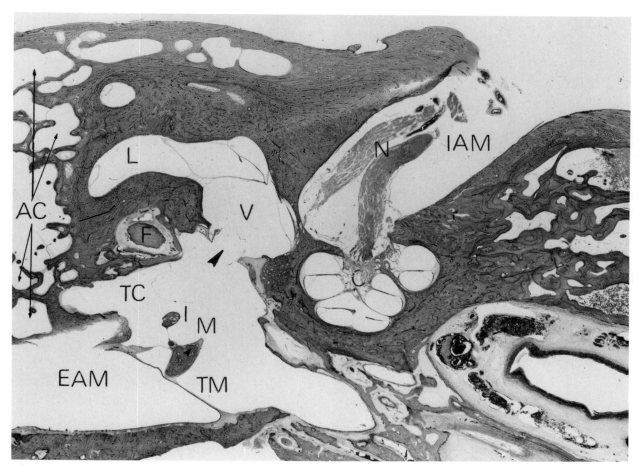

Figure 24.2. Horizontal section of a human temporal bone. The relationships of the three divisions of the ear within the temporal bone can be observed. The tympanic membrane (TM) separates the external auditory meatus (EAM) from the middle ear space (tympanic cavity, TC). Within the tympanic cavity cross-sections of the malleus (M) and incus (I) can be seen. The posterior wall of the tympanic cavity is associated with the mastoid air cells (AC). The lateral wall of the cavity is formed principally by the tympanic membrane. The opening into the inner ear (oval window, arrow) is seen in the medial wall of the cavity (the stapes has been removed). The facial (F) nerve can be observed near the oval window. The cochlea (C), the vestibule (V), and a portion of the lateral semicircular canal (L) of the inner ear are identified. The cochlear and vestibular divisions of the eighth cranial nerve (N) also can be observed within the internal auditory meatus (IAM). × 6.5.

core is composed of fibrocytes, layers of radiating fibrous filaments, and elastic fibers (Fig. 24.4). A simple low cuboidal epithelium, which is continuous with the lining of tympanic cavity, covers the inner surface of the tympanic membrane (Fig. 24.5); stratified squamous epithelium, which is devoid of hair and is continuous with the epithelium of the external auditory meatus, covers the external surface.

The tympanic membrane is divided into two parts. The lower four-fifths of the tympanic membrane (*pars tensa*) has a more organized core of connective tissue. One layer of collagen fibers courses radially and another layer of fibers courses circularly. The upper one-fifth of the membrane (*pars flaccida, Shrapnell's membrane*) lacks the fibrous middle layer and is more flexible than the pars tensa. Perforations of the tympanic membrane can produce a conductive hearing loss.

Auditory Tube

The *auditory tube* (eustachian tube) extends from the anterior wall of the tympanic cavity to the nasopharynx. The tube, which has a flattened vertical lumen, is approximately 3.5 cm in length. The

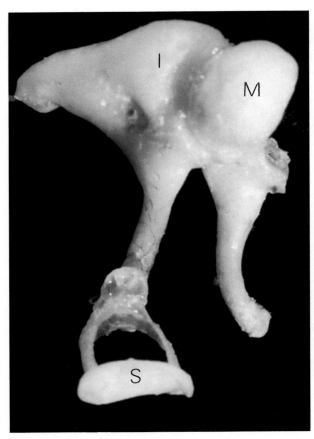

Figure 24.3. Photomicrograph of the three articulated human middle ear ossicles: malleus (M); incus (I); stapes (S). × 10.

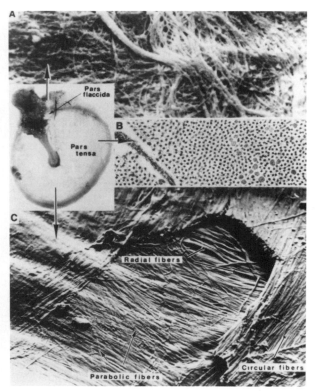

Figure 24.4. Electron micrographs of the tympanic membrane. **(A)** Scanning electron micrograph that demonstrates the irregular arrangement of collagen and elastic fibers in the upper one-fifth region of the membrane (pars flaccida). **(B)** Cross-section of fibers of the lower four-fifths of the tympanic membrane (pars tensa). The majority of fibers seen in this region are round collagen fibers. **(C)** Scanning electron micrograph of a partially dissected human tympanic membrane. Observe the arrangement of fibers in the pars tensa. (Courtesy of D. Lim, from Lim DJ: Scanning electron microscope morphology of the ear. In Paparella, Shumrick (eds): *Otolaryngology.* Chapt. 18. Philadelphia, WB Saunders, 1980.)

lateral one-third of the walls of the auditory tube is formed by bone. The medial two-thirds of its walls is formed by elastic cartilage, except at its opening into the nasopharynx where it becomes hyaline cartilage. These walls are normally apposed to one another. The auditory tube is lined by ciliated epithelium that varies from simple low columnar near the tympanic cavity to pseudostratified columnar near the nasopharynx and the epithelium rests on a lamina propria (Fig. 24.6). Toward the pharyngeal end of the auditory tube, tubuloalveolar (seromucous) glands, composed of goblet cells interposed among columnar epithelial cells, extend into the lamina propria.

The primary function of the auditory tube is to equalize the air pressure between the tympanic cavity and external environment. Equilibration of the air pressure occurs during swallowing and yawning when the walls of the tube are separated, allowing air to enter the tympanic cavity from the nasopharynx. Clinically, dysfunction of the auditory tube, particularly in children, is a causative

factor by which infections of the upper respiratory airway can invade the middle ear cavity and cause infection (otitis media).

A system of air cells (*mastoid air cells*), which vary in number and size, projects into the mastoid portion of the temporal bone from the tympanic cavity. The mastoid air cells replace marrow of the mastoid portion of the temporal bone. Each mastoid air cell is lined by mucous membrane that is continuous with the epithelium of the tympanic cavity and that rests on a thin periosteum. The epithelial cells lining the air cells are more squamous in shape than those lining the tympanic cavity. The continuity of the middle ear cavity with the mastoid air cells enables infections to spread from

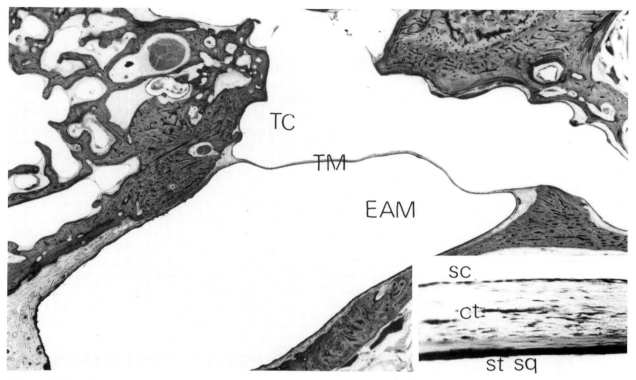

Figure 24.5. Cross-section through a human tympanic membrane. The tympanic membrane (TM), external auditory meatus (EAM), and tympanic cavity (TC) can be seen. × 9. Inset, higher magnification of the tympanic membrane. The outer epithelial layer of the membrane consists of stratified squamous epithelium (st sq) and the inner epithelial layer of the membrane consists of low simple cuboidal (sc) epithelium. A middle layer of connective tissue (ct) lies between the two epithelial layers. × 190.

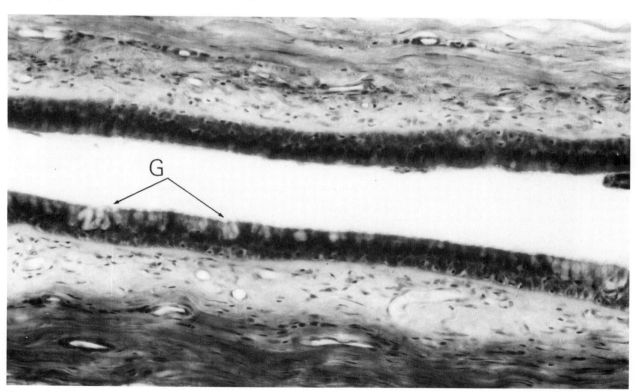

Figure 24.6. Photomicrograph of a human auditory tube near the nasopharynx. In this region, the auditory tube is lined by ciliated, pseudostratified columnar epithelium. Goblet cells (G) are seen interspersed among the epithelial cells. × 180.

743

the middle ear into these air cells (resulting in an inflammation called mastoiditis).

INNER EAR

The inner ear consists of a series of membranous sacs and ducts (***membranous labyrinth***) (labyrinth = maze) that are encased within a series of bony cavities and canals (***bony labyrinth***) located deep within the petrous portion of the temporal bone.

Bony Labyrinth

The ***bony labyrinth*** consists of the ***vestibule,*** the ***semicircular canals,*** and the ***cochlea*** (Fig. 24.7a). The walls of the bony labyrinth are composed of an outer periosteal layer, a middle endochondral layer, and an inner endosteal layer.

Vestibule. The central portion of the bony labyrinth is a bony cavity, called the ***vestibule.*** It has an elliptical recess and a spherical recess for two membranous sacs, the utricle and the saccule, respectively. The lateral wall of the vestibule has the vestibular (oval) window, in which the footplate of the stapes is inserted. The membranous endolymphatic duct lies in an opening of a small canal (vestibular aqueduct) in the medial wall of the vestibule.

Semicircular Canals. Three ***semicircular canals*** extend posteriorly from the vestibule. These semicircular canals, derive their names [***superior, lateral (horizontal),*** and ***posterior***] from their orientation to one another. Each canal forms about two-thirds of a circle and is located at approximately a right angle to the other two canals. The lateral or horizontal semicircular canals of both ears lie in the same plane of the head. The supe-

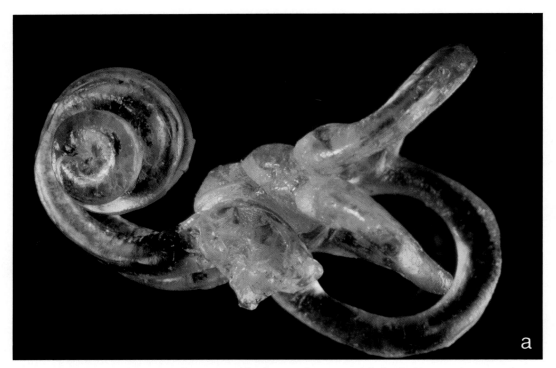

Figure 24.7. Photograph and diagrams of the human inner ear. **(a).** Cast of human inner ear bony labyrinth. The cochlear portion of the labyrinth is indicated by the green color, and the regions of the vestibular bony labyrinth are indicated by the orange color. (Courtesy of Dr. Merle Lawrence.) **(b).** Components of the bony labyrinth. Divisions of the bony inner ear labyrinth are the vestibule, cochlea, and three semicircular canals. The openings of the oval window and the round window can be observed. Lateral view of left bony labyrinth. **(c).** Diagram of the membranous inner ear labyrinth lying within the bony labyrinth. The cochlear duct can be seen spiraling within the bony cochlea. The saccule and utricle are positioned within the vestibule and the three semicircular ducts are lying within their respective canals. This is a medial view of the right membranous labyrinth, allowing the endolymphatic duct and sac to be observed from this perspective. **(d).** Diagram of the sensory regions of the inner ear for equilibrium and hearing. These regions are the macula of the utricle, macula of the saccule, cristae ampullaris of the three semicircular ducts and the organ of Corti of the cochlear duct. Medial view of right membranous labyrinth.

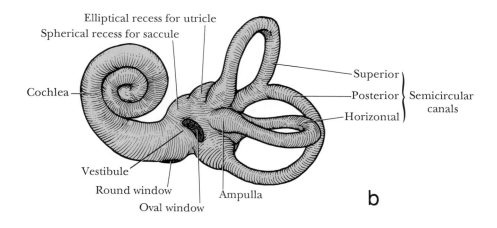

Elliptical recess for utricle
Spherical recess for saccule
Cochlea
Superior
Posterior
Horizontal
Semicircular canals
Vestibule
Round window
Ampulla
Oval window

b

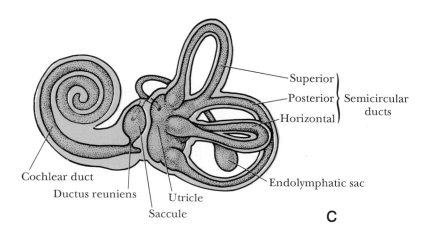

Superior
Posterior
Horizontal
Semicircular ducts
Cochlear duct
Ductus reuniens
Utricle
Saccule
Endolymphatic sac

c

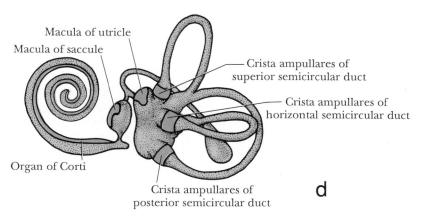

Macula of utricle
Macula of saccule
Crista ampullares of superior semicircular duct
Crista ampullares of horizontal semicircular duct
Organ of Corti
Crista ampullares of posterior semicircular duct

d

Figure 24.7 (b), (c), (d).

rior semicircular canal of one ear is in the parallel plane of the head with the posterior semicircular canal of the opposite ear. At one end of each semicircular canal is a dilation, the **ampulla.** The three semicircular canals open into the vestibule by five openings. One of the five openings, the **common**

crus, is shared by both the superior and posterior semicircular ducts.

Cochlea. The **cochlea** is a complex bony canal that coils like a snail shell approximately two and three-quarter turns around a central pillar of bone, the **modiolus.** Projecting from the modiolus is a partial shelf of bone, the *osseous spiral lamina,* which partially divides the cochlear canal. One opening of the canal, the *cochlear (round) window,* is covered by a thin membrane. An additional opening, the *cochlear canaliculus (aqueduct),* is located in the more basal turn of the cochlear canal. The cochlear canaliculus is patent during the early decades of life and allows communication between the subarachnoid space and the cochlear canal.

Membranous Labyrinth

The epithelial-lined sacs (*utricle, saccule,* and *endolymphatic sac*) and ducts (*semicircular ducts, endolymphatic duct,* and *cochlear duct*) of the *membranous labyrinth* form a closed system within the bony labyrinth (Fig. 24.7b). All of the components of the membranous labyrinth communicate with each other. Within this closed system of the membranous labyrinth is fluid that has a high concentration ratio of K^+ to Na^+ ions. This fluid, known as *endolymph,* is similar to intracellular fluids. External to the membranous labyrinth is the second fluid of the inner ear, *perilymph.* The ionic concentration of perilymph is the reverse of that for endolymph, having a high Na^+ to K^+ ratio similar to other extracellular body fluids. Maintenance of the ionic gradients between endolymph and perilymph is necessary for proper transduction of neural impulses from the sensory receptors of the inner ear.

Associated with the vestibular system are five regions of sensory receptors located in the utricle, the saccule, and the three semicircular ducts (Fig. 24.7c). An additional region of the sensory receptors is associated with the auditory system and is located in the duct of the cochlea. As will be described later, all six regions of sensory receptors share similar characteristics despite having different functions.

Utricle. Located on the medial wall of the vestibule is an irregular, oblong membranous sac called the *utricle.* Its nonsensory walls are composed of connective tissue lined internally by a simple squamous to cuboidal epithelial layer that rests on a typical basal lamina. The connective tissue layer contains fibrocytes, a small number of melanocytes, and blood vessels.

The sensory region of the utricle, the *macula* (macula = spot) is ovoid in shape and is oriented in a horizontal plane (Fig. 24.8). There are three principal cell types within the macula. One cell type is a tall, columnar supporting (sustentacular) cell that has short microvilli on its apical surface and contains numerous secretory granules. The other two cell types of the macula are sensory cells

that are classified as either *type I* or *type II* non-neuronal, mechanoreceptors. Type I cells are piriform in shape with a rounded base and a thin neck. The basal aspect of each type I cell is surrounded by an afferent nerve chalice and some efferent nerve fibers. Type II cells are cylindrical in shape and have afferent and efferent bouton nerve endings synapsing basally.

Each sensory cell has one *kinocilium* (a modified cilium, 9 + 2 pattern of microtubules) and 30 to 100 *stereocilia* (modified microvilli containing actin filaments) on its apical surface (Fig. 24.9). Collectively, the stereocilia have a pipe-organ arrangement, i.e., the taller stereocilia are proximate to the kinocilium while the more shorter stereocilia are located farther away from the kinocilium. Because of the presence of the stereocilia, these cells are referred to as sensory hair cells.

The stereocilia and kinocilia of the sensory hair cells of the utricle and saccule are embedded in a sheet-like gelatinous membrane, the *otolithic membrane,* which resides atop the sensory hair cells. The matrix of the membrane is produced by the supporting cells of the macula. On the surface of the otolithic membrane are otoconia (otoliths), minute crystalline bodies, which are composed of calcium carbonate and protein (Fig. 24.10). Each otoconium is 3 to 5 μm in length and has a rounded body with three-headed ends. As the otoconia respond to gravity, they interact with underlying cells in the macula of both the utricle and the saccule to detect positional changes during movements of the body.

On the utrical wall opposite that of the macula, there is a specialized region of epithelial cells, called *dark cells,* due to the electron density of their cytoplasm. Each dark cell contains numerous supranuclear vesicles and mitochondria. The apical surfaces of these cells have microvilli and pinocytotic invaginations. Because of the presence of ion-transporting enzymes and their morphological similarity to known ion-transporting cells in other organ systems (e.g., basolateral infoldings), the dark cells are thought to be involved in the elaboration and/or maintenance of endolymph. The semicircular ducts and the ductus utriculosaccularis connect the utricle with the endolymphatic sac.

Saccule. Located in the medial wall of the bony vestibule is a second membranous sac called the *saccule.* It is flattened and irregular in shape and is oriented perpendicular to the utricle. Histologically, the walls of the saccule are similar to the walls of the utricle. The sensory region, *macula of the saccule,* is positioned in a vertical plane, perpendicular to the macula of the utricle. The sac-

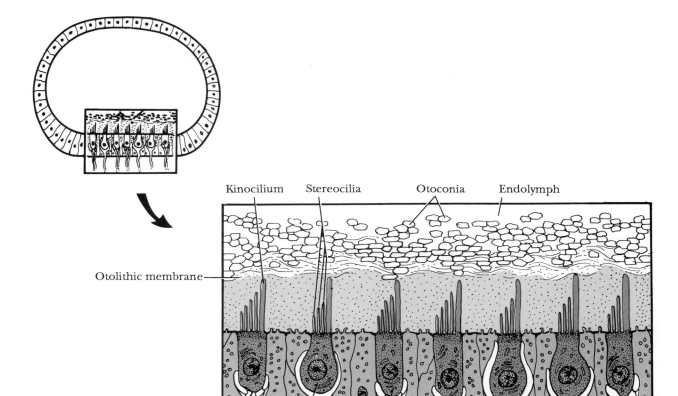

Figure 24.8. Diagram of a cross-section of the utricle. A more detailed cellular organization of the macula of the utricle can be observed in the insert. Supporting cells can be seen lying between the two principle types of sensory hair cells (type I and type II). The stereocilia and kinocilium of each sensory hair cell is embedded in the otolithic membrane on which otoconia are lying.

cule, like the utricle, is composed of supporting cells and sensory hair cells (type I and type II). The stereocilia of the hair cells of the macula of the saccule also are embedded in an otolithic membrane containing otoconia.

There are two openings of the saccule. One opening is a small duct that unites with the ductus utriculosaccularis of the utricle to form the endolymphatic duct. The other opening communicates with the duct of the cochlea through the ductus reuniens.

Semicircular Ducts. The *superior, lateral,* and *posterior semicircular ducts* are located within their respective bony semicircular canals. Each duct is approximately one-fourth of the size of its bony canal and is about 10 to 15 mm in length and 0.1 mm in diameter. The cellular organization of the walls of each semicircular duct is similar in composition to the nonsensory walls of the utricle and saccule. At the end of each duct is a dilated region, the *ampulla* (1 mm in diameter), which contains a sensory region, the *crista ampullaris* (crista = crest). The crista ampullaris lies perpendicular to the plane of the duct (Fig. 24.11) and contains supporting cells and sensory hair cells (type I and type II) like those in the maculae of the utricle and saccule. The sensory hair cells of the crista ampullaris are embedded in a gelatinous membrane, the *cupula.* Unlike the otolithic membrane, the cupula is tall and extends toward the wall opposite the crista ampullaris. There are no otoconia associated with the cupula.

Endolymphatic Sac. Extending from both the utricle and saccule is a membranous duct, the

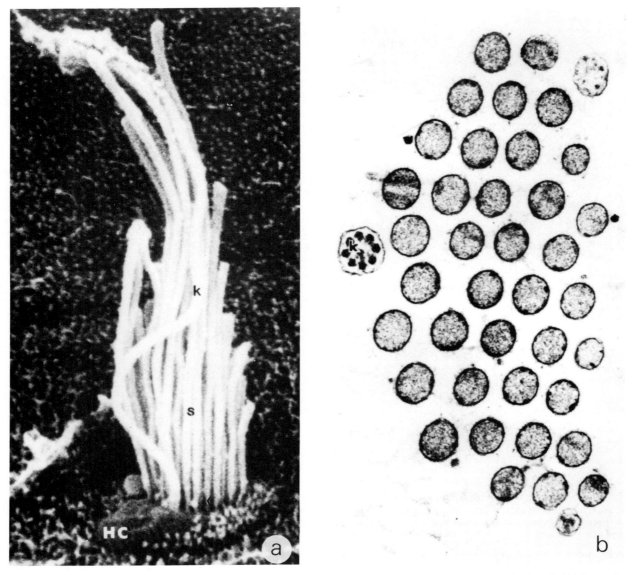

Figure 24.9. Electron micrographs of the kinocilium and stereorcilia of a vestibular sensory hair cell. **(A)** Scanning electron micrograph of apical surface of sensory hair cell (HC) from macula of the utricle. Note the relationship of the kinocilium (k) to the stereocilia (s). **(B)** Transmission electron micrograph of kinocilium and sterocilia of vestibular hair cell in cross-section. The kinocilium (k) has a greater diameter than the stereocilia. × 47,500. (Courtesy of Hunter-Duvar and Hinojosa, from Hunter-Duvar IM, Hinojosa R: Vestibule: Sensory epithelia. In Friedmann I, Ballantyne J (eds): *Ultrastructural Atlas of the Inner Ear.* Chapt. 9. London, Butterworths, 1984.)

endolymphatic duct, which opens into the endolymphatic sac (Fig. 24.7b). The endolymphatic duct is lined by squamous to cuboidal epithelial cells and lies in the bony vestibular aqueduct. The *endolymphatic sac* is located in a small bony depression on the posterior aspect of the temporal bone and between the dura mater of the posterior cranial fossa (Fig. 24.7b). The endolymphatic sac is divided into three portions: a proximal portion that lies within the temporal bone and is lined by tall epithelial cells, an intermediate portion that lies partially within the temporal bone and partially within the dura mater (the cell types found here are described below), and a distal portion that lies within the dura mater overlying the sigmoid venous dural sinus and is lined by cuboidal epithelial cells.

The intermediate portion of the endolymphatic sac consists of two principal cell types: light

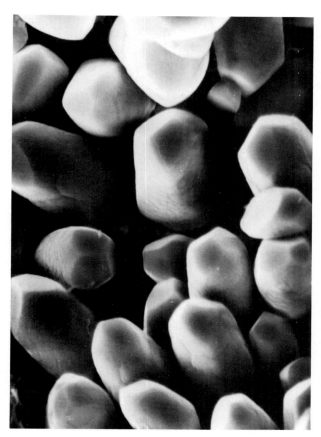

Figure 24.10. Scanning electron micrograph of human otoconia. Each otoconium has a long cylindrical body with a three-headed facet on each end of its body. × 5000.

FUNCTIONAL ASPECTS OF THE VESTIBULAR SYSTEM

The characteristic arrangement of the kinocilium and stereocilia on the apical surface of each sensory hair cell results in a distinct morphological pattern within each sensory region of the vestibular system (Fig. 24.12). All kinocilia of the macula of the utricle are oriented toward the midline, while those of the saccule are oriented away from the midline. In the cristae ampullares, the kinocilia face either away from the utricle in the superior and posterior semicircular ducts or toward the utricle in the horizontal semicircular ducts.

The morphological pattern within these vestibular sensory regions creates a functional polarization. Displacement of stereocilia toward the kinocilium results in *depolarization* (excitation) of the sensory hair cell, while bending of the stereocilia away from the kinocilium results in hyperpolarization (*inhibition*) of the hair cell (Fig. 24.13).

Stimulation of the hair cells in the maculae of the utricle and saccule is different from that in the cristae ampullaris of the semicircular ducts. The sensory hair cells of the utricle and the saccule are embedded in the otolithic membrane that is covered by otoconia. The weight of the otoconia on the maculae of the utricle and saccule effectively makes these structures behave like gravity receptors. They detect linear acceleration. Changes in position of the head result in changes in position of the otolithic membrane. In turn, these pressure changes stimulate the macular sensory hair cells, creating ionic movement in the apical regions of the sensory hair cells. This results in the discharge of neural impulses at the base of the hair cells. Maximum stimulation of the macula of the utricle occurs when the head is bent forward or backward. Maximum stimulation of the macula of the saccule occurs when the head is bent side to side.

Movement of endolymph fluid within each semicircular duct causes displacement of the cupula. Displacements may cause either depolarization or hyperpolarization of the sensory hair cells. Hair cells of the cristae ampullaris are responsive to angular acceleration. Semicircular ducts in the same plane, but on opposite sides of the head,

cells and dark cells. Each cell type is tall and cylindrical in shape. The light cells have a lightly staining cytoplasm containing numerous pinocytotic vesicles and vacuoles and have microvilli on their apical surfaces. The dark cells also possess apical microvilli but have densely staining cytoplasm containing pinocytotic vesicles. The intermediate portion of the endolymphatic sac is thought to be actively involved in absorption of the endolymph. Recent data suggest that this portion may also be the site of immunological defense, that is, the site of the immune response to antigens that gain access to the inner ear.

Movement of endolymph within the vestibular labyrinth can be induced by creating a temperature gradient. A simple clinical procedure, the bithermal caloric procedure, makes use of this effect for evaluating the functional integrity of the vestibular system. Briefly, this procedure involves irrigating the external ear canal of each ear, in turn, with warm water and cool water to induce convection currents within the endolymph. These currents displace the sensory structures and cause stimulation of the vestibular neuroepithelial regions. Thus, this caloric stimulation produces a vestibular-ocular reflex, producing measurable eye movements (nystagmus).

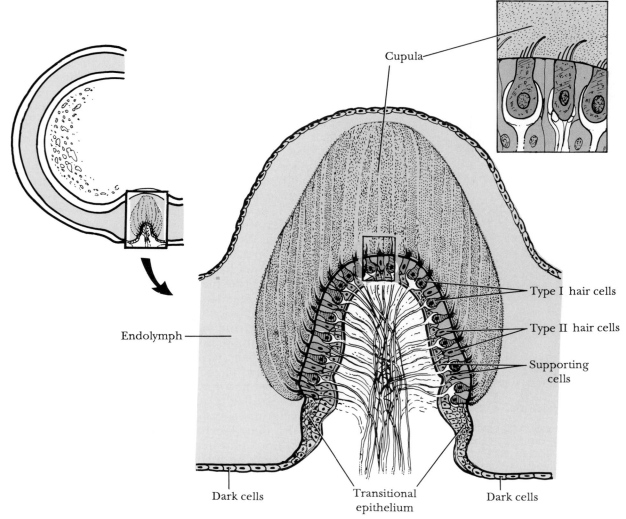

Figure 24.11.   Diagram of a typical semicircular duct within its canal. The cellular organization of the sensory region, crista ampullaris, of a semicircular duct can be observed in the insert. The crista is composed of both type I and type II sensory hair cells and supporting cells. The stereocilia and kinocilium of each hair is embedded in the cupula that projects toward the nonsensory wall of the ampulla.

work antagonistically. For example, a rotation of the head to the right causes stimulation of hair cells of the crista ampullaris of the right horizontal semicircular duct and inhibition of hair cells in the crista ampullaris of the left horizontal semicircular duct.

DUCT OF THE COCHLEA

The duct of the cochlea is composed of connective tissue that is lined internally by epithelial cells. The duct lies in the bony cochlear labyrinth between the osseous spiral lamina and the external

wall of the bony cochlea. It spirals around the modiolus two and three-quarters turns. The basal aspect of the duct communicates with the saccule by the ductus reuniens. Apically, the cochlear duct terminates as a blind sac, cupular cecum.

The cochlear duct along with the osseous spiral lamina divides the cochlea into two spaces, the *scala vestibuli* (scala = stairway) and the *scala tympani* (Fig. 24.14). The scala vestibuli and scala tympani are only continuous with one another at the blind end of the bony cochlea, the **helicotrema.** The scala vestibule and scala tympani are filled with perilymph. The *scala media,* the space within the cochlear duct, contains endolymph.

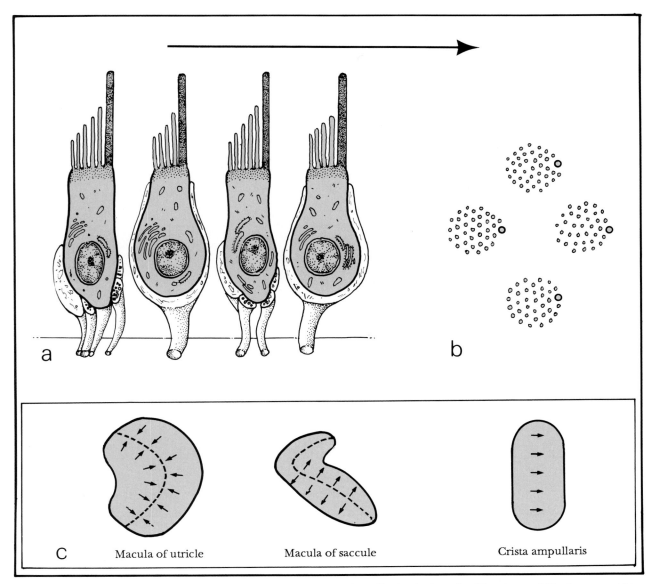

a

b

c   Macula of utricle   Macula of saccule   Crista ampullaris

Figure 24.12. Diagram of the morphological polarization of vestibular hair cells. (Courtesy of Lindenman, HH: Anatomy of the otolith organs. *Adv Oto Rhinol Laryngol* 20:405–433, 1973.)

The duct of the cochlea is triangular in appearance unlike the more oval appearance of other portions of the inner ear membranous labyrinth. One side of the triangular duct attaches to the tympanic lip of the osseous spiral lamina and extends laterally to the bony wall of the cochlea. This region of the duct is called the **basilar membrane.** The basilar membrane is composed of a connective tissue layer that contains collagen-like filaments embedded in homogenous ground substance. The side of the basilar membrane facing the scala tympani is lined by mesothelial cells. A distinct basement membrane separates the connective tissue

components of the basilar membrane from the overlying supporting and sensory cells that comprise the organ of Corti. The width and stiffness of the basilar membrane vary from the basal aspect of the cochlea to its apex. It is more narrow (80 μm) and has a greater degree of stiffness in the basal portion of the cochlea and is wider (500 μm) and more flexible apically. It is 100 times more compliant at the apex than at the base. These physical properties of the basilar membrane enable us to discrimant sounds of different frequencies as will be discussed below.

The second side of the triangular cochlear

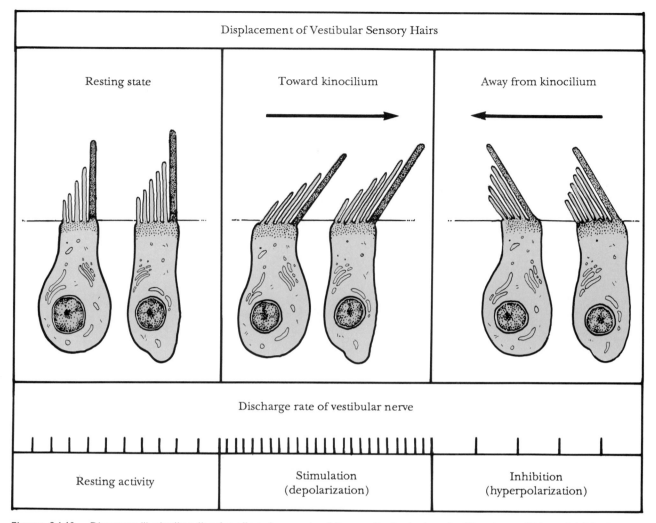

Figure 24.13. Diagram illustrating the functional aspects of the vestibular hair cells. (Courtesy of Wersall J. Modified from Wersall J. Gleisner L, Lundquist P-G: Ultrastructure of the vestibular end organs. In DeReuck AVS, Knight J (Eds): *Myotatic, Kinesthetic and Vestibular Mechanisms.* Boston, Little, Brown & Co., 1967.)

duct is attached to the external bony wall of the cochlea. This region is known as the *lateral cochlear wall.* It consists of the *spiral ligament* and several epithelial regions (the *stria vascularis,* the *spiral prominence,* and the *external sulcus cells*) that line the internal surface of the spiral ligament.

The third side of the triangular cochlear duct is the *vestibular (Reissner's) membrane.* It attaches obliquely from the vestibular lip of the spiral limbus to the spiral ligament above the stria vascularis.

The three regions of the cochlear duct—the organ of Corti, the lateral cochlear wall, and the vestibular membrane—have distinctive histological characteristics (Fig. 24.14). These regions are described in more detail in the following sections.

Organ of Corti

The *organ of Corti* is a collection of sensory and supporting epithelial cells that rests partially on the tympanic lip of the osseous spiral lamina and on the basilar membrane (Fig. 24.14). The cellular constituency of the organ of Corti is similar to sensory regions of the vestibular membranous labyrinth (that is, they are divided into sensory cells and supporting cells), however, the epithelial cells of the organ of Corti are arranged in a more complicated manner.

Sensory Cells. The sensory cells of the organ of Corti are classified as *inner hair cells* and *outer hair cells.* In the human ear, there are ap-

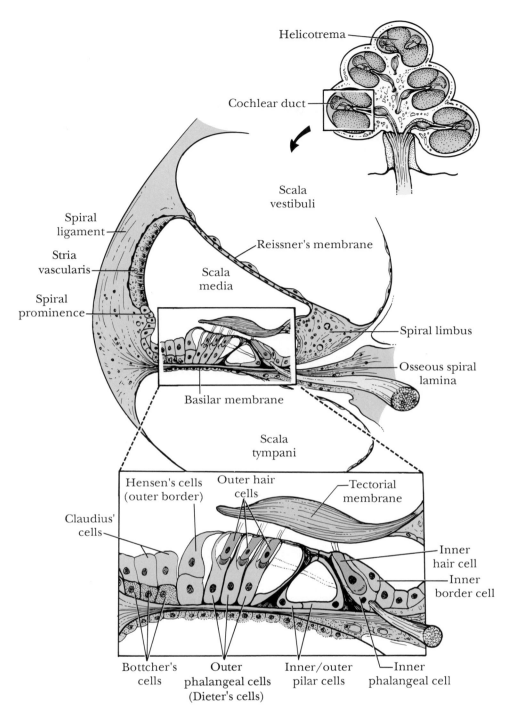

Figure 24.14. Schematic diagram of a midmodiolar section of the cochlea that illustrates the position of the cochlear duct within the two and three-quarter turns of the bony cochlea. M, modiolus, SM, scala media, ST, scala typmanic, SV, scala vestibuli, CD, cochlear duct. Observe that the scala vestibuli and scala tympani are continuous apically (helicotrema). Cross-section of basal cochlear duct. The cochlear duct and the osseous spiral lamina divide the cochlea into the scala vestibuli and the scala tympani, which contain perilymph. The scala media is the space within the cochlear duct that is filled with endolymph. Diagram of the sensory and supporting cells of the organ of Corti. The sensory cells are divided into an inner row of sensory hair cells and three rows of outer sensory hair cells. The supporting cells are: inner and outer pillar cells, inner and outer (Deiter's) phalangeal cells, border cells, Hensen's cells, Claudius' cells, and Boettcher's cells. (Modified from Goodhill V: *Ear; Diseases, Deafness, and Dizziness.*)

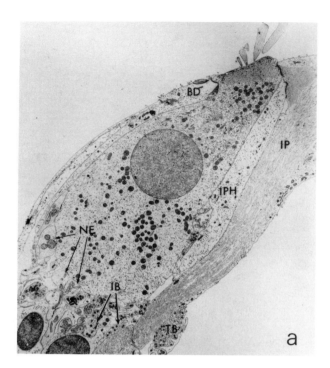 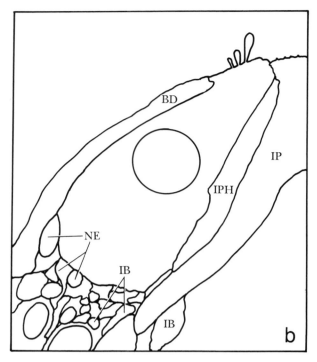

Figure 24.15. Electron micrograph and accompanying diagram of an inner sensory hair cell. Observe the rounded base and constricted neck of the inner hair cell. Nerve endings (NE) from afferent nerve fibers to inner hair cells (IB) are seen basally. Afferent nerve fibers to outer hair cells (IB) are seen in a tunnel lateral to inner pillar cell (IP). (IPH, inner phalangeal cell; BD, border cell; NE, nerve endings). × 6300. (Courtesy of Kimura RS: Sensory and accessory epithelia of the cochlea. In Friedmann I, Ballantyne J: *Ultrastructural Atlas of the Inner Ear.* Chapt. 5. London, Butterworths, 1984.)

proximately 3500 inner hair cells and 12,000 outer hair cells. The inner hair cells have a rounded base and a short neck, similar in appearance to type I hair cells of the vestibular labyrinth (Fig. 24.15). The inner hair cells lie in a single row along the length of the basilar membrane and are surrounded completely by supporting cells. The outer hair cells are cylindrical in shape (similar to type II hair cells) and lie in three to five rows along the basilar membrane (Fig. 24.16). Only the apical and basal surfaces of the outer hair cells are surrounded by supporting cells. The midexternal surfaces of the outer hair cells are bathed by fluid. This exposure of the outer hair cell membranes to surrounding fluid has been thought to make the outer hair cells more susceptible to injury by toxic agents than the inner hair cells to cell injury and death.

Each sensory hair cell has stereocilia on its apical surface. There are 100 to 300 stereocilia on the apical surface of each outer hair cell. The stereocilia are arranged in three to four rows and shaped in a 'v' or 'w' configuration (Fig. 24.17). Each inner hair cell has 50 to 70 stereocilia on its apical surface. The height of each stereocilia increases from the inner row of hair cells to the outer row of hair cells and from base to apex of the cochlear duct. The height of the stereocilia on an outer hair cell in the apex of the cochlea is three times that of one in the basal region. The cochlear sensory hair cells do not have kinocilia. These structures are lost during fetal development and are represented by vestigial basal bodies in differentiated cells.

The stereocilia of the outer row of hair cells are embedded in a gelatinous membrane, the ***tectorial membrane.*** This membrane arises from the vestibular lip of the spiral limbus, and is composed of fibrils embedded in dense amorphous ground substance. The tectorial membrane extends over the sensory hair cells to supporting cells, called ***Hensen's cells.*** Only the stereocilia of the outer hair cells are in contact with the membrane; the stereocilia of the inner hair cells are free. The structural relationships and support of the sensory cells influence their response. The outer hair cells are affected by vibration of the tectorial membrane and the basilar membrane. The inner hair cells are more passive mechanoreceptors, transducing the

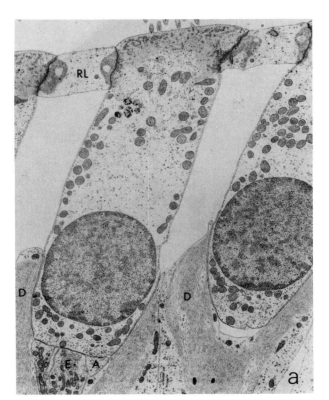
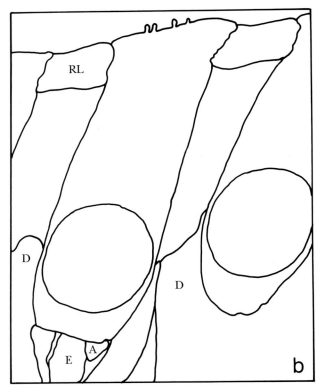

Figure 24.16.   Electron micrograph and accompanying diagram of outer sensory hair cells. Afferent (A) and efferent (E) nerve endings are seen basally. Deiter's (outer phalangeal, (D) cells are seen surrounding the outer hair cells basally. Their apical projections form the reticular lamina (RL). Observe that the midexternal surfaces of the outer hair cells are not surrounded by supporting cells. × 6300. (Courtesy of Kimura RS: Sensory and accessory epithelia of the cochlea. In Friedmann I, Ballantyne J: *Ultrastructural Atlas of the Inner Ear,* Chapt. 5. London, Butterworths, 1984.)

motion of their stereocilia into intracellular receptor potentials.

Supporting Cells.   The supporting cells of the organ of Corti are classified as *inner* and *outer pillar cells, inner* and *outer phalangeal (Deiter's) cells, border cells, Hensen's cells, Claudius' cells,* and *Boettcher's cells* (Fig. 24.14). The *inner* and *outer pillar cells* have broad basal and apical surfaces that form a broad plate. The inner pillar cell rests on the tympanic lip of the osseous spiral lamina and the outer pillar cell rests on the basilar membrane. Each cell contains well-organized microtubules for support. The inner and outer pillar cells form a triangular-shaped tunnel (tunnel of Corti) between them. The *inner* and *outer phalangeal cells* support more directly the inner and outer rows of sensory hair cells. Each phalangeal cell has a flat base resting on the basilar membrane, an elongated body, and an extended head that lies between the apical surfaces of the hair cells. Each cell contains numerous microtubules for internal support, and is positioned between a sensory hair cell and the basilar membrane. This configuration does not allow an individual sensory hair cell to

touch the basilar membrane. The inner phalangeal cells lie close to the inner hair cells and project their processes toward the apical surface. These processes form a plate around the inner hair cell. The outer phalangeal cells support the outer rows of hair cells. Each outer phalangeal cell sends an upward projection toward the apical surface and forms an apical plate, the reticular lamina, around an outer hair cell (Fig. 24.18). Tight junctions, located at the apical lateral borders between the cells of the reticular lamina and the sensory hair cells, seal the endolymphatic surface of the organ of Corti from the inferior extracellular spaces.

The remaining supporting cells associated with the organ of Corti are located either more medially or more laterally to the sensory hair cells and, therefore, are less involved in direct support of the sensory hair cells (Fig. 24.14). The columnar shaped inner *border cells* lie between the inner row of hair cells and the cells of the internal sulcus on the tympanic lip of the osseous spiral lamina. The tall columnar, *Hensen's cells,* which lie lateral to the outer phalangeal cells, constitute the outer border of the organ of Corti. These cells have a lightly

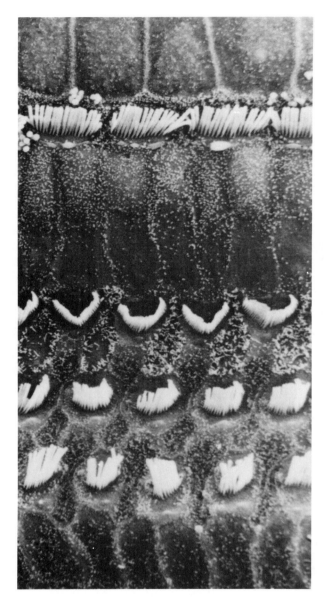

Figure 24.17. Scanning electron micrograph illustrating the configuration of stereocilia on the apical surfaces of the inner row and three outer rows of cochlear sensory hair cells. × 3250.

staining cytoplasm with few organelles and some apical microvilli. Lateral to the Hensen's cells are cuboidal cells known as the *cells of Claudius.* They have a lightly staining cytoplasm and lie adjacent to cells of the external sulcus. They are similar in cytoplasmic appearance to the cells of the inner sulcus. *Boettcher's cells* are found in clusters beneath the cells of Claudius. They have large oval nuclei and their cytoplasm is more densely staining than that of the adjacent cells. Boettcher's cells rest on the basement membrane of the basilar membrane

and their apical surfaces do not reach the endolymphatic fluids of the scala media. The function of the Boettcher cells is not known, but their structure suggests that they may function in secretion and absorption.

Lateral Cochlear Wall

The *spiral ligament* is not a true ligament because it is not composed of organized dense connective tissue. The spiral ligament consists of fibrocytes associated with a meshwork of intercellular fibrils and blood vessels. Portions of the spiral ligament form lateral boundaries of the perilymph-containing spaces of the scala vestibuli and scala tympani.

The *external sulcus cells* lie between the epithelial cells of the organ of Corti and the cells of the spiral ligament. They have an irregular shape and send cytoplasmic extensions into the stroma of the spiral ligament. Each cell has a rich ribosomal cytoplasm. The external sulcus cells are involved in fluid absorption and phagocytosis.

The *spiral prominence* is a region of the lateral cochlear wall that lies between the external sulcus cells and the stria vascularis. The spiral prominence is lined by cuboidal epithelial cells with densely staining cytoplasm and contains a complex capillary network. Cells of the spiral prominence are thought to be involved in homeostasis of the cochlear fluids.

The *stria vascularis,* characterized by the presence of numerous capillaries, is also a region of the lateral cochlear wall. This region lies between the cells of the spiral prominence and the cells forming Reissner's membrane (Figs. 24.14 and 24.19). Three cell types can be identified in the stria vascularis: epithelial (marginal) cells, intermediate cells, and basal cells. The marginal cells are hexagonal in appearance and have microvilli on their apical surfaces. They have a densely staining cytoplasm containing numerous mitochondria. The apical aspect of these cells is bathed by the endolymph; their basal aspect demonstrates basolateral infoldings that interdigitate with infoldings of the intermediate cells. The plasma membrane in the region of these basolateral infoldings of the marginal cells contains Na-K-ATPase and other enzymes that are involved in ion and fluid regulation. The intermediate cells assist the marginal cells. The basal cells seal the stria vascularis from the cells of the spiral ligament.

Vestibular (Reissner's) Membrane

The *vestibular (Reissner's) membrane* is a delicate structure composed of two cellular layers that

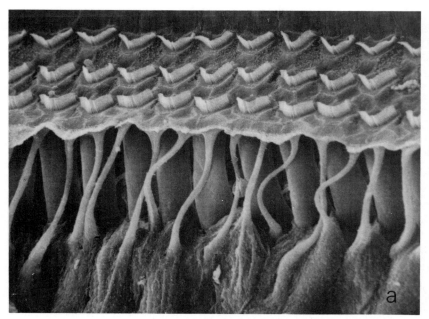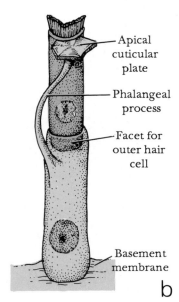

Figure 24.18. Scanning electron micrograph and accompanying diagram that illustrate the architecture of Deiter's cells. Each Deiter's cell cups the basal surface of an outer sensory hair cell and extends its phalangeal process apically to form an apical plate which supports the outer sensory hair cells. × 2400.

has a total thickness of only 2 to 3 μm (Figs. 24.14 and 24.20). The cellular layer that faces toward the scala vestibuli is composed of mesothelial cells, which are continuous with those lining the scala vestibuli. The layer of cells that faces the scala media is composed of squamous epithelial cells. These cells are hexagonal in appearance and have microvilli on their surface. The epithelial cells are held together by zonula occludens. A basal lamina separates the epithelial layer from the mesothelial layer of cells. The cells of Reissner's membrane form a structure that runs obliquely from the spiral ligament above the stria vascularis to the vestibular lip of the osseous spiral lamina. The vestibular membrane separates the perilymphatic space of the scala vestibuli from the endolymph space of the scala media.

The *spiral limbus* is an elevation of tissue that overlies the osseous spiral lamina (Fig. 20.14). It has two projections, a vestibular lip and a tympanic lip. The inner sulcus cells lie in a groove between the two tissue projections. The spiral limbus is composed of loose connective tissue and blood vessels. Vertically positioned collagen fibers within the limbus produce "auditory teeth" (of Huschke). The surface of the spiral limbus is lined by epithelial cells, the interdental cells, which secrete the matrix of the tectorial membrane. The phalangeal portions of the interdental cells cover the endolymphatic surface of the spiral limbus and serve as an anchor for the tectorial membrane. Cells of the spiral limbus have been hypothesized to be involved in fluid maintenance.

FUNCTIONAL ASPECTS OF THE AUDITORY SYSTEM

The auditory system has a large dynamic range for detecting sound energy that consists of waves of alternating compression and rarefaction of molecules in a transmitting medium (e.g., air, water, etc.). For sound energy to be perceived, it must be transformed efficiently into neural impulses that are transmitted to the auditory cortex. To accomplish this, two obstacles must be overcome. First, air-borne vibrations collected in the external ear must be conveyed into the dense fluid of the inner ear with the least loss of energy. This is a major obstacle because air and water have vastly differing resistance to the passage of sound energy (impedance). Normally, 99.9 percent of sound energy is reflected back at an air-fluid interface and only 0.1 percent of the sound energy is transmitted into the fluid medium. The middle ear components perform the role of reducing the reflection of sound energy at the air-fluid interface (impedance matching). This is accomplished by the middle ear matching the acoustic properties of air to the more dense fluid of the inner ear.

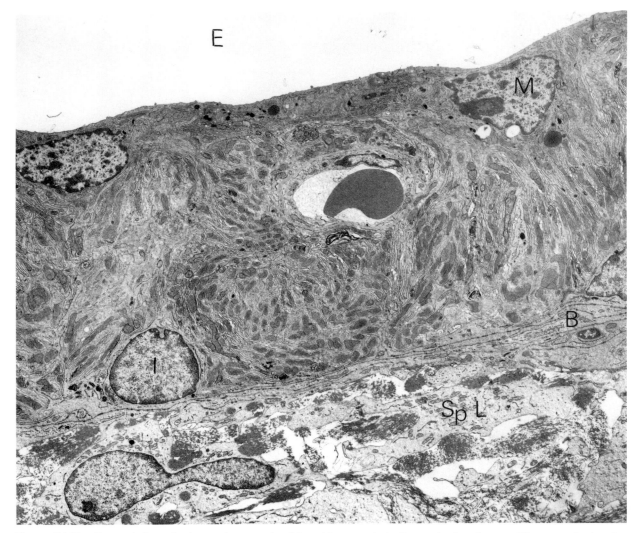

Figure 24.19. Transmission electron micrograph of the stria vascularis. The apical surfaces of the marginal cells (M) of the stria are bathed by endolymph (E). Intermediate cells (I) are positioned between the marginal cells and basal cells (B), which separates the other cells of the stria vascularis from the spiral ligament (SpL). × 4700.

The second obstacle for efficient transfer of sound energy from the external ear to the inner ear is that the vibrations must have access to the sensory receptors that are bathed in fluid, which is encased in bone and is, therefore, potentially incompressible. In order to overcome this obstacle, there has to be one opening of the inner ear for the vibrations to enter and another opening to act as a release valve. This release valve mechanism is accomplished by expansion (or pushing out) of the round window membrane as the base of the stapes rocks in and out against the oval window (Fig. 24.21). As this occurs, the fluid vibrations are transmitted across the cochlear duct to the organ of Corti. Sound vibration of a given frequency causes movement of the basilar membrane with an equal frequency. The lower the frequency of the sound wave, the farther from the oval window is the location of maximum displacement of the basilar membrane. Each site of maximum displacement is correlated with a specific frequency of the sound wave. Low frequencies of sound are detected toward the apex of the cochlea and high frequencies are detected in the basal portion of the cochlea. The perception of pitch is related to differences in the location of the site of maximum displacement along the basilar membrane in response to different frequencies of sound. Additionally, with greater displacements of the basilar membrane, greater numbers of sensory receptors and neurons are stimulated, leading to increase sound intensity.

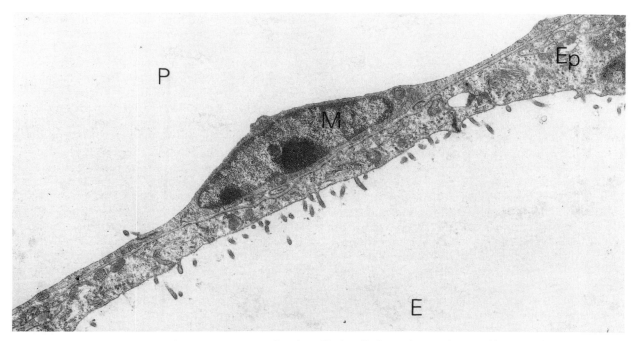

Figure 24.20. Transmission electron micrograph of vestibular (Reissners) membrane. Two cell types can be observed: (1) a mesothelial cell (M) that faces the scala vestibuli and is bathed by perilymph (P) and (2) an epithelial cell (Ep) that faces the scala media and is bathed by endolymph (E). × 8400.

Because the sensory hair cells lie on the basilar membrane and the stereocilia of the outer row of hair cells are embedded in the overlying tectorial membrane, fluid displacement in the inner ear causes a bending action of the hair cells resulting in mechanical deformation at the apical portions of the sensory hair cells. This deformation initiates electrochemical events within the hair cells that are transmitted to synaptic regions in basal regions of the cells. Release of neurotransmitters in the synapses leads to the production of action potentials and the discharge of neural impulses.

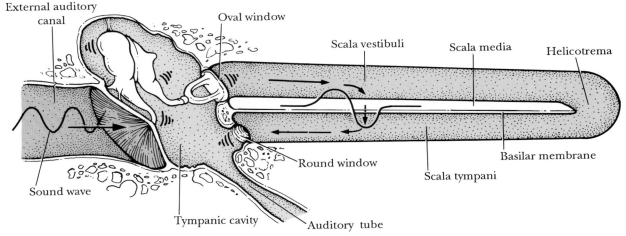

Figure 24.21. Schematic diagram that illustrates the dynamics of the three divisions of the ear. Sound waves are collected and transmitted from the external ear to the middle ear where they are converted into mechanical vibrations. The mechanical vibrations are then converted at the oval window into fluid vibrations within the inner ear. Fluid vibrations cause displacement of the basilar membrane on which rests the auditory sensory hair cells. Such displacement leads to stimulation of the hair cells and a discharge of neural impulses from them. (Modified from Karmody CS: *Textbook of Otolaryngology.* Philadelphia, Lea & Febiger, 1983.)

INNERVATION OF THE SENSORY REGIONS OF THE INNER EAR

The vestibulocochlear, eighth cranial, nerve innervates the sensory regions of the inner ear membranous labyrinth. The eighth cranial nerve is divided into a vestibular division, which innervates the sensory receptors associated with the vestibular system, and a cochlear division, which innervates the sensory receptors associated with the auditory system (Fig. 24.22).

The vestibular nerve is further subdivided into a superior division and an inferior division. The superior division innervates the macula of the utricle, part of the macula of the saccule, and the crista ampullaris of the superior and lateral semicircular ducts. The inferior division innervates the macula of the saccule and the crista ampullaris of the posterior semicircular duct.

Bipolar neurons of the vestibular division have their cell bodies (ganglion of the vestibular nerve, Scarpa's ganglion) located in the internal auditory meatus. Dendritic processes of the vestibular nerve fibers synapse at the base of the vestibular sensory hair cells, either as a chalice around a type I hair cell or as a bouton associated with a type II hair cell. The axons of the vestibular nerve fibers enter the brainstem and terminate in the vestibular nuclei. Some secondary neuronal fibers travel to the cerebellum, to the nuclei of the third, fourth, and sixth cranial nerves that innervated muscles of the eye. Other secondary fibers descend into the cervical segments of the spinal cord as the vestibulospinal tracts.

Nerve fibers of the cochlear nerve division enter the bony cochlea through the modiolus from the internal auditory meatus. Neurons of the cochlear nerve fibers also are bipolar and have their cell bodies located in the spiral ganglion within the modiolus. Dendritic processes of the afferent cochlear nerve fibers exit the modiolus through foraminae nervosa and enter the organ of Corti. The dendritic processes are divided into two branches. Fifteen to twenty dendritic processes of one branch will innervate only one inner-row sensory hair cell. Ninety-five percent of all afferent neurons will make up this branch. Dendritic processes of the other branch innervate the sensory hair cells of the outer rows. One dendritic nerve fiber of this branch will innervate ten outer-row hair cells. The axons of the cochlear nerve fibers enter the brainstem and terminate in the cochlear nuclei of the medulla. Nerve fibers from these nuclei pass to the geniculate of the thalamus and then to the auditory cortex of the temporal lobe.

Efferent fibers conveying impulses from the brain pass parallel to the ascending afferent nerve fibers of the vestibulocochlear nerve. Efferent nerve fibers from the brainstem pass through the vestibular nerve and synapse either on afferent endings of the inner hair cell (or type I hair cell) or on the basal aspect of an outer hair cell (or type II

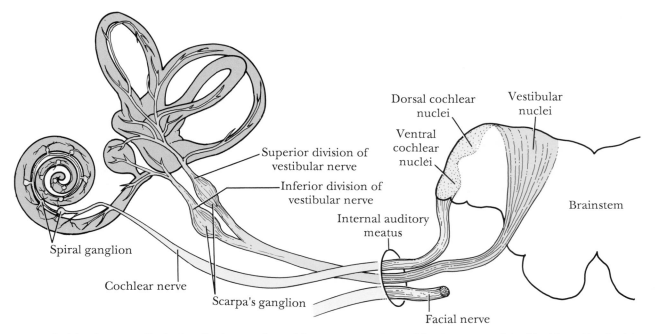

Figure 24.22. Diagram illustrating the innervation of the sensory regions of the inner ear. (Modified from Hawke M, Keene M, Alberti PW: In: *Clinical Otoscopy. A Text and Colour Atlas.* Edinburgh, Churchill Livingstone, 1984.)

hair cell). Efferent fibers are thought to affect control of auditory and vestibular input to the central nervous system, presumably enhancing some afferent signals while suppressing other signals.

BLOOD VESSELS OF THE MEMBRANOUS LABYRINTH

The blood supply to the external ear, middle ear, and the bony labyrinth of the inner ear is derived from vessels associated with the external carotid arteries. The arterial blood supply to tissues of the membranous labyrinth of the inner ear is derived intracranially from the labyrinthine artery, a common branch of the anterior inferior cerebellar or basilar artery. The labyrinthine artery is a terminal artery in that it has no anastomosis with other surrounding arteries. Importantly, interruption of blood flow in this artery can have severe consequences for the inner ear function. Experimental disruption of blood flow for only 15 seconds can cause the loss of electrical potentials and excitable nerve fibers of the inner ear. Irreversible loss of fibers and cells can result from the prolonged occlusion of the arterial supply.

The labyrinthine artery lies in the internal auditory canal where it divides into the common cochlear artery and the anterior vestibular artery (Fig. 24.23). The common cochlear artery divides into the main cochlear artery and the vestibulocochlear artery. The vestibulocochlear artery branches into the posterior vestibular artery and the cochlear branch. The main cochlear artery distributes to three-fourths of the cochlea whereas the cochlear branch supplies the basal one-fourth of the cochlea. The anterior vestibular artery supplies the macula of the utricle, a part of the macula of the saccule, and the crista ampullaris of the superior and lateral semicircular ducts. The posterior vestibular artery supplies the macula of the saccule and the crista ampullaris of the posterior semicircular duct.

Radiating arterioles arise from the main arterial divisions and distribute to various regions of the membranous labyrinth. In the cochlear tissues, arterioles are distributed to the spiral limbus, to the basilar membrane, and to the lateral cochlear wall. Importantly, there are no arterioles distributed to the tissues of the organ of Corti. Oxygen and nutrients to the sensory hair cells must be diffused from vessels in the surrounding tissues.

Venous drainage from the cochlea is by the posterior and anterior spiral modiolar veins (Fig. 24.24) that form the common modiolar vein. The common modiolar vein and the vestibulocochlear vein form the vein of the cochlear aqueduct. The latter empties into the inferior petrosal sinus. The anterior vestibular vein drains blood from the utricle and superior and lateral semicircular ducts, while the posterior vestibular vein drains the saccule and posterior semicircular duct. The anterior and posterior vestibular veins join the vein of the round window to form the vestibulocochlear vein. The semicircular canals and the endolymphatic duct and sac are drained by the vein of the vestibular aqueduct that drains into the sigmoid venous sinus.

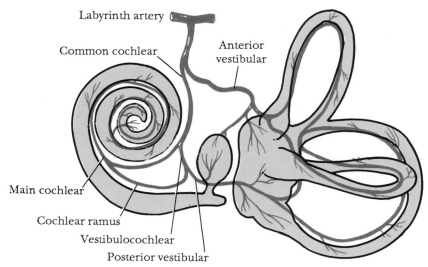

Labyrinth artery

Common cochlear

Anterior vestibular

Main cochlear

Cochlear ramus

Vestibulocochlear

Posterior vestibular

Figure 24.23. Diagram of the arterial supply of the membraneous labyrinth of the inner ear. (Modified from Schuknecht HF: *Pathology of the Ear.* Cambridge, MA, Harvard University Press, 1974.)

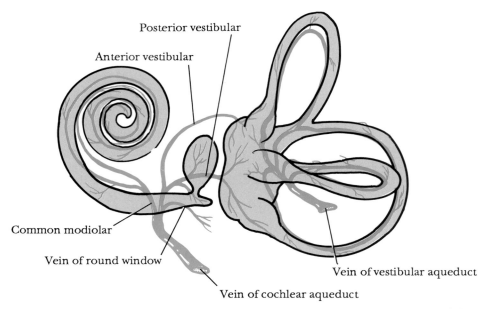

Figure 24.24. Diagram of the venous drainage of the membranous labyrinth of the inner ear. (Modified from Schuknecht HF: *Pathology of the Ear.* Cambridge, MA, Harvard University Press, 1974.)

HEARING LOSS—VESTIBULAR DYSFUNCTION

There are several types of disorders that can affect the auditory and vestibular system, resulting in deafness and/or dizziness (vertigo). Auditory disorders are classified as either conductive or sensorineural in nature. Conductive hearing loss results when sound waves are impeded mechanically from reaching the auditory sensory receptors within the inner ear. This type of hearing loss principally involves the external ear or structures of the middle ear. One example of a conductive hearing loss is the disease of otosclerosis, which is characterized by the growth of new spongy bone within the bony labyrinth near the oval window. This spongy bone growth can cause the fixation of the base of the stapes (ankylosis) in the oval window, thereby decreasing the efficiency of sound conduction to the inner ear.

Sensorineural hearing impairment may also occur after injury to the auditory sensory hair cells within the inner ear or to cochlear division of the eighth cranial nerve. Such hearing losses may be congenital or acquired. Causes of acquired sensorineural hearing loss include infections of the membranous labyrinth (e.g., meningitis, chronic otitis media), acoustic trauma (i.e., exposure to excessive noise for long periods of time), and administration of certain classes of antibiotics and diuretics).

A third example of sensorineural hearing loss is that which often occurs during the process of aging. A loss of the sensory hair cells and/or associated nerve fibers occurs beginning in the basal turn of the cochlea and progressing apically over time. The characteristic impairment is a high-frequency hearing loss. This type of hearing loss is termed Presbycusis.

The sense of rotation without equilibrium (dizziness, vertigo) is the major clinical sign of dysfunction of the vestibular system. Causes of vertigo range from the administration of specific drugs to a tumor (acoustic neuroma), which develops in or near the internal auditory meatus and exerts pressure on the vestibular division of the eighth cranial nerve or branches of the labyrinthine artery. Vertigo can be produced normally in individuals by excessive stimulation of the semicircular ducts. Similarly, excessive stimulation of the utricle can produce motion sickness (sea-sickness, car-sickness, or air-sickness) in some individuals.

Some diseases of the inner ear affect both hearing and equilibrium. For example, patients who are diagnosed as having Meniere's disease initially complain of episodes of dizziness, tinnitus (ringing), and later develop a low-frequency hearing loss. Although the etiological agent of Menieres' disease has not been determined, it is known that the membranous labyrinth becomes distended (endolymphatic hydrops). This distension is thought to be a result of malabsorption of endolymph within the endolymphatic sac.

ATLAS PLATES

129–130

PLATE 129. The Ear

The inner ear consists of a system of chambers and canals in the temporal bone, which contain a network of membranous channels. These are referred to, respectively, as the bony labyrinth and membranous labyrinth. In places, the membranous labyrinth forms the lining of the bony labyrinth; in other places, there is a separation of the two. Within the space lined by the membranous labyrinth is a water fluid, called endolymph. External to the membranous labyrinth, that is, between the membranous and bony labyrinths, is additional fluid, called perilymph.

The bony labyrinth is divided into three parts: the cochlea, semicircular canals, and the vestibule. The cochlea and semicircular canals each contain membranous counterparts of the same shape; however, the membranous components of the vestibule are more complex in their form, being comprised of ducts and two chambers, the utricle and saccule. The cochlea contains the receptors for hearing, the organ of Corti; the semicircular canals contain the receptors for movement; and the saccule and utricle contain receptors for position.

A section through the inner ear is shown in **Figure 1.** Bone surrounds the entire inner ear cavity. Because of its labyrinthine character, in sections, the inner ear appears as a number of separate chambers and ducts. These, however, are all interconnected (except that the perilymphatic and endolymphatic spaces remain separate). The largest chamber is the vestibule (**V).** The **left side** of this chamber (**black arrow)** leads into the cochlea (**C).** Just below the **black arrow** and to the right is the oval ligament (**OL)** surrounding the base of the stapes (**S).** Both structures have been cut obliquely and are not seen in their entirety. The facial nerve (**FN)** is in an osseous tunnel to the left of the oval ligament. The communication of the vestibule with one of the semicircular canals is marked by the **white arrow.** At the upper right are cross-sections through components of the duct system (**DS)** of the membranous labyrinth.

The cochlea is a spiral structure having the general shape of a cone. The specimen illustrated in **Figure 1** makes three and one-half turns (in man, there are two and three-quarters turns). The section goes through the central axis of the cochlea. This consists of a bony stem called the mo-

KEY

C, cochlea
CN, cochlear nerve
CT, connective tissue
Cu, cupula
Ds, duct system (of membranous labyrinth)
Ep, epithelium
FN, facial nerve
HC, hair cell

M, modiolus
OL, oval ligament
S, stapes
SC, sustentacular celll
SG, spiral ganglia
V, vestibule
black arrow, Fig. 1, entry to cochlea
white arrow, Fig. 1, entry to semicircular canal

Fig. 1, guinea pig, × 20

Fig. 2, guinea pig, × 225

diolus (**M).** It contains the beginning of the cochlear nerve (**CN)** and the spiral ganglia (**SG).** Because of the plane of section and the spiral arrangement of the cochlear tunnel, the tunnel is cut crosswise in seven places (note, three and one-half turns). A more detailed examination of the cochlea and the organ of Corti is provided in Plate 130.

One of the semicircular canals and the crista ampullaris (**CA)** within the canal is seen in the lower right of **Figure 1.** A higher magnification of this area is provided in **Figure 2.** The receptor for movement, the crista ampullaris, (note its relationships in **Fig. 1)** is present in each of the semicircular canals. The epithelial (**Ep)** surface of the crista consists of two cell types, sustentacular (supporting) cells and hair (receptor) cells. (Two types of hair cells are distinguished with the electron microscope.) It is difficult to identify these cells on the basis of specific characteristics; however, they can be distinguished on the basis of location (see **inset),** the hair cells (**HC)** being situated in a more superficial location than the sustentacular cells (**SC).** A gelatinous mass, the cupula (**Cu),** surmounts the epithelium of the crista ampullaris. Each receptor cell sends a hair-like projection deep into the substance of the cupula.

The epithelium rests on a loose, cellular, connective tissue (**CT)** that also contains the nerve fibers associated with the receptor cells. The nerve fibers are difficult to identify because they are not organized as a discrete bundle.

PLATE 129

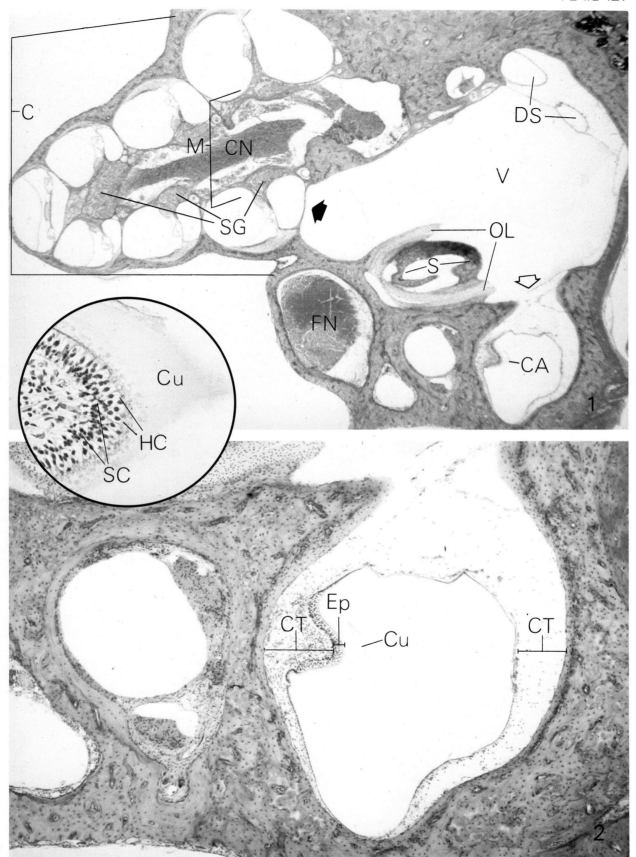

PLATE 130. Organ of Corti

A section through one of the turns of the cochlea is shown in **Figure 1.** The most important functional component of the cochlea is the organ of Corti. This region of the cochlear duct is enclosed by the **rectangle** and is shown at higher magnification in **Figure 2.** Other structures included in **Figure 1** are as follows. The spiral ligament **(SL)** is a thickening of the periosteum on the outer part of the tunnel. Two membranes, the basilar membrane **(BM)** and the vestibular membrane **(VM),** join with the spiral ligament and divide the cochlear tunnel into three parallel canals, namely the scala vestibuli **(SV),** the scala tympani **(ST),** and the cochlear duct **(CD).** Both the scala vestibuli and scala tympani are perilymphatic spaces; these communicate at the apex of the cochlea. The cochlear duct, on the other hand, is the space of the membranous labyrinth and is filled with endolymph. It is thought that the endolymph is formed by the portion of the spiral ligament that faces the cochlear duct, the stria vascularis **(StV).** This is highly vascularized and contains specialized cells considered to perform the above-mentioned function.

A shelf of bone, the osseous spiral lamina **(OSL),** extends from the modiolus to the basilar membrane. Branches of the cochlear nerve **(CN)** travel along the spiral lamina to the modiolus where the main trunk of the nerve is formed. [The components of the cochlear nerve are bipolar neurons whose cell bodies constitute the spiral ganglia **(SG).** The cell bodies are shown at higher magnification in the **inset,** upper right.] The spiral lamina supports an elevation of cells, the limbus spiralis **(LS).** The surface of the limbus is comprised of columnar cells.

The components of the organ of Corti are as follows **(Fig. 2),** beginning at the limbus spiralis **(LS):** inner border cells **(IBC);** inner phalangeal and hair cells **(IP and HC);** inner pillar cells **(IPC);** (the sequence continues, repeating itself in reverse) outer pillar cells **(OPC);** outer phalangeal and hair cells **(OP and HC);** and outer border cells **(CH),** cells of Hensen. Hair cells are receptor cells; the other cells are collectively referred to as supporting cells. The outer hair and phalangeal cells can be distinguished in **Figure 2** by their location (also see lower left **inset**) and because their nuclei

KEY	
BM, basilar membrane	OPC, outer pillar cells
CB, cells of Boettcher	OSL, osseous spiral
CC, cells of Claudius	lamina
CD, cochlea duct	OT, outer tunnel
CH, cells of Hensen	RM, reticular membrane
CN, cochlear nerve	SG, spiral ganglia
IBC, inner border cells	SL, spiral ligament
IP and HC, inner	ST, scala tympani
phalangeal and hair	StV, stria vascularis
cells	SV, scala vestibuli
IPC, inner pillar cells	TM, tectorial membrane
IST, internal spiral tunnel	VM, vestibular
IT, inner tunnel	membrane
LS, limbus spiralis	
OP and HC, outer	
phalangeal and hair	
cells	

Fig. 1, guinea pig, × 65	**Fig. 2,** guinea pig, × 180 (insets, × 380)

are well aligned. Because the hair cells rest on the phalangeal cells, it can be concluded that the upper three nuclei belong to outer hair cells, the lower three to outer phalangeal cells.

The supporting cells extend from the basilar membrane (this is not evident in **Figure 2** but can be seen in the **inset**) to the surface of the organ of Corti where they form a reticular membrane **(RM).** The free surface of the receptor cells fits into openings in the reticular membrane and the "hairs" of these cells project toward, and make contact with, the tectorial membrane **(TM).** The latter is a cuticular extension from the columnar cells of the limbus spiralis. In ideal preparations, nerve fibers can be traced from the hair cells to the cochlear nerve.

In their course from the basilar membrane to the reticular membrane, groups of supporting cells are separated from other groups by spaces that form spiral tunnels. These tunnels are named the inner tunnel **(IT),** the outer tunnel **(OT),** and the internal spiral tunnel **(IST).** Beyond the supporting cells are two additional groups of cells, the cells of Claudius **(CC)** and the cells of Boettcher **(CB).**

PLATE 130

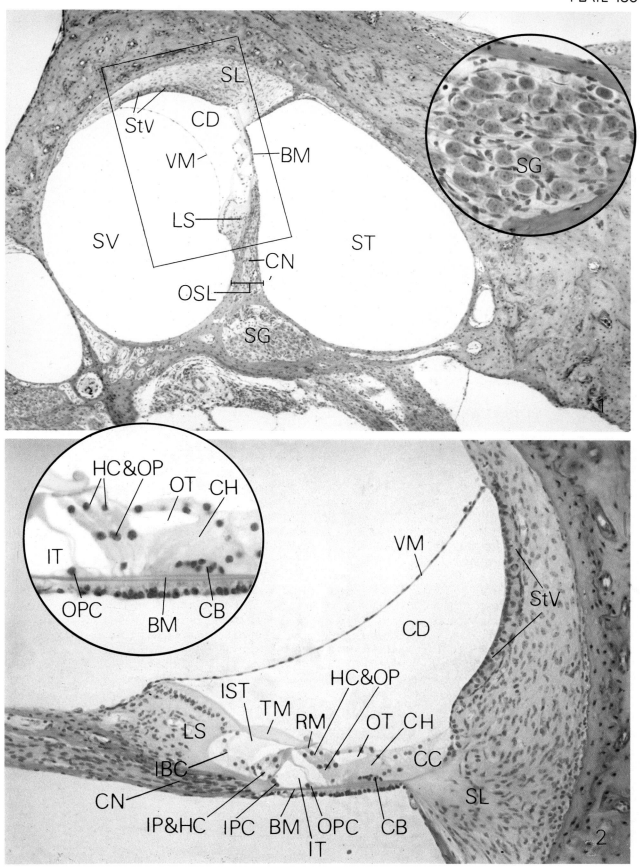

Index

Page numbers followed by "*t*" denote tables.